# Trauma
# Anesthesia

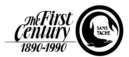

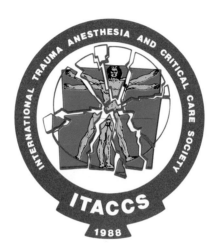

*The editors and contributors have arranged that all royalties and honoraria derived from participation in this book project be donated to the International Trauma Anesthesia and Critical Care Society (ITACCS).*

For more information on the Society, contact:
ITACCS
P.O. Box 4826
Baltimore, Maryland 21211, USA

# Trauma Anesthesia

*Edited by*

## John K. Stene, M.D., Ph.D.

President, ITACCS
Assistant Professor of Anesthesiology
Director of Perioperative Anesthesia Trauma Service
Department of Anesthesiology
The Pennsylvania State University College of Medicine
The Milton S. Hershey Medical Center
Hershey, Pennsylvania

## Christopher M. Grande, M.D.

Executive Director, ITACCS
Special Consultant and
Chief, Special Projects Branch
Department of Anesthesiology
The Shock Trauma Center
Maryland Institute for Emergency Medical Services Systems
University of Maryland at Baltimore
Baltimore, Maryland

*With 21 Contributors*

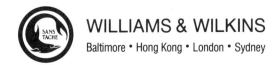

WILLIAMS & WILKINS
Baltimore • Hong Kong • London • Sydney

*Editor:* Timothy H. Grayson
*Associate Editor:* Carol Eckhart
*Copy Editor:* Linda Forlifer
*Designer:* Wilma Rosenberger
*Illustration Planner:* Ray Lowman
*Production Coordinator:* Charles E. Zeller

*The Publishers have made every effort to trace the copyright holders for borrowed material. If they have inadvertently overlooked any, they will be pleased to make the necessary arrangements at the first opportunity.*

*Accurate indications, adverse reactions, and dosage schedules for drugs are provided in this book, but it is possible that they may change. The reader is urged to review the package information data of the manufacturers of the medications mentioned.*

*Printed in the United States of America*

Library of Congress Cataloging in Publication Data

Trauma anesthesia / edited by John K. Stene, Christopher M. Grande; with 21 contributors.
     p.    cm.
   Includes bibliographical references.
   ISBN 0-683-07929-8
   1. Anesthesia.    2. Traumatology.    I. Stene, John K. II. Grande, Christopher M.
   [DNLM: 1. Anesthesia. 2. Critical Care. 3. Emergencies.
  4. Wounds & Injuries.    WO 200 T777]
  RD82.T73    1991
  617.9'6--dc20
  DNLM/DLC
  for Library of Congress                      90-12151
                                                               CIP

                                          90   91   92   93   94
                  1  2  3  4  5  6  7  8  9  10

*This book is dedicated to the improved care of trauma patients and to the further improvement of the profession of anesthesiology through the development of the subspecialty of "trauma anesthesia."*

# Foreword

Drs. J. K. Stene and C. M. Grande, authors-editors of this book, *Trauma Anesthesia*, are to be applauded for their efforts to revive the commitment of anesthesiologists to traumatology. The "complete anesthesiologist" is an essential member of the trauma management team, who may function with the assistance of nurse anesthetists under the doctor's direction. The anesthesiologist who has acquired knowledge, skills, and judgment in the resuscitation, anesthesia, and perianesthesia management of severe polytrauma victims and who has special skills, interest, and experience in trauma management can help reduce mortality and morbidity of patients brought to trauma centers. Such trauma-oriented anesthesiologists also have an influence on prehospital resuscitation and analgesia worldwide, mostly through education, organization, and development of guidelines for prehospital emergency care personnel. I will comment on the anesthesiologist and cases of severe polytrauma, not on anesthesia for emergencies in general; the latter include semielective procedures for minor injuries, which every anesthesiologist should be able to manage safely (1).

Since antiquity, trauma patients, particularly victims of wars, have been of variable interest to physicians. Anesthesia in World War I provided pain relief but little if any resuscitation and life support. It probably often contributed to mortality. Anesthesia in World War II made major lifesaving contributions (2). Since the 1950s, trauma has been recognized as "the neglected disease of modern society" (3). In the 1950s and 1960s, when I served on the standard-setting National Research Council committees concerning resuscitation and emergency medical services led by the late Sam Seeley (3), I

strived to expand the scope of trauma care beyond surgery and hoped to help improve trauma care by encouraging anesthesiologists to become reanimatologists (4), intensivists (5, 6), and community-wide leaders of emergency medical services (EMS) (7, 8).

Over the past 30 years, many have contributed to the development of modern resuscitation medicine, which is concerned with the reversibility of terminal states (such as asphyxiation or shock) and clinical death (cardiac arrest) (4). Resuscitation medicine consists of reanimatology (the science) (9), the cardiopulmonary-cerebral resuscitation system (the methods) (4), and the emergency and critical care medicine continuum (the service) (7, 8). Anesthesiologists have contributed to all three components of resuscitation medicine (10).

The appraisal below reflects my personal experiences and biases. As a medical student, I was enticed into surgical training through involvement in trauma care during World War II. The embryonic surgeon became an anesthesiologist when he recognized that life support was the greatest need for advances in surgery. The anesthesiologist became a reanimatologist and intensivist when he recognized that the life support skills of anesthesia were needed outside the operating room, particularly in multidisciplinary traumatology. My focus on the management of the critically ill or injured reflects regeneralization and multidisciplinary integration, not subspecialization.

In the 1960s, John Bonica, then President of the American Society of Anesthesiologists (ASA), and I agreed to help foster the "complete anesthesiologist" through a new ASA committee on acute medicine. It developed the world's first guidelines for the organization of community-wide EMS systems (7) and encouraged activism by anesthesiologists in the new multidisciplinary Society of Critical Care Medicine (11, 12). Subsequently, the leadership of American anesthesiologists in emergency and critical care medicine (and its components of traumatology) declined. There were a few exceptions—including individuals who tried to modernize prehospital first aid and advanced life support by mobile ICU ambulance services (13, 14), the continuum of life support throughout the life support chain of the EMS systems (8), and anesthesia within the hospital for cases of polytrauma (15–18). In Europe many more anesthesiologists expanded their roles as reanimatologists, emergency physicians, intensivists, and traumatologists (19). In the United States in recent years, we have witnessed a possible return of interest—so that this book is timely. The trend is fostered by the current designation of trauma centers, 20 years after our first national guidelines urged their establishment (7), and by an appreciation of the lifesaving potential of modern resuscitation in disasters (20, 21).

Why should the anesthesiologist be involved in traumatology?

*First*, it is the anesthesiologist's *duty*. A variable proportion of trauma patients are taken to the operating rooms of most acute care general hospitals. There, not only in superspecialized trauma centers, anesthesiologists are obligated to provide anesthesia and life support. National guidelines for anesthesia services include the perioperative activities of preanesthesia resuscitation of trauma victims and the support of their recovery through continued participation in life support in the recovery room and in the ICU.

*Second*, the anesthesiologist has unique *clinical expertise* that is needed inside and outside the hospital. The anesthesiologist should be the most experienced specialist in airway control (including conventional and fiberoptic intubation), artificial ventilation, vascular access, resuscitation from traumatic-hypovolemic shock, and other measures. In other words, the anesthesiologist acquires

in routine anesthesia practice and on elective cases a special expertise in the needed *titration* of life support by physiologic and pharmacologic means. This "titrated care" is crucial for patients with acute life-threatening injuries and differs from care by "rounding and prescription," which is adequate for general medical practice. The elective operating room anesthesia schedule is ideal for learning titrated analgesia, anesthesia, and life support. Making the patient pain-free is easy; keeping the patient alive is difficult.

There are numerous examples of resuscitative anesthesia measures that could be lethal in the hands of inexperienced persons and lifesaving in the hands of the skilled anesthesiologist. For example, consider the polytrauma victim with head injury who is vomiting, bleeding, convulsing or restless; has trismus and cyanosis; and needs rapid tracheal intubation. Simultaneously reoxygenating, moderately hyperventilating, intubating, clearing the bronchial tree, and optimizing cardiovascular-pulmonary functions, without causing aspiration or coughing that would increase intracranial bleeding, is not an easy task. The required psychomotor skills can only be acquired during the repeated administration of elective anesthesia.

The special clinical expertise of anesthesiologists has been successfully applied even outside hospitals in European EMS systems, where anesthesiologists staff mobile ICU (trauma) teams (19). Anesthesia groups can maintain continuity throughout the life-support chain, from the scene via transportation and the operating room to the hospital ICU, a continuity other specialists may not be able to provide. In the emergency department, the contributions of anesthesiologists would include resuscitative anesthesia for resuscitative surgery, as is occasionally required in cases of intrathoracic or intraabdominal exsanguination or of an intracranial hematoma.

*Third*, the anesthesiologist can contribute as a *teacher*. Operating room experience guided by an anesthesiologist is ideal for training prehospital, emergency room, and ICU personnel in titrated life support. Training goes far beyond practice in tracheal intubation to include cardiovascular-pulmonary-cerebral pharmacologic and physical support measures in general. These measures could not be learned in a similarly realistic setting through laboratory practice on animals or training on manikins.

As teacher and consultant, anesthesiologists could and should set standards in their areas of expertise (such as analgesia and resuscitation) for physicians and nonphysician personnel working in the prehospital setting and the emergency department. To become a consultant for prehospital personnel, the anesthesiologist should get firsthand experience in the field (22)—of course, after having taken advanced cardiac life support (4, 23) and advanced trauma life support (ATLS) (4, 24) courses. Those responsible for ATLS courses should differentiate among those measures that paramedics are also allowed to perform, additional nonsurgical measures for which a trained physician must be present, and "resuscitative anesthesia and surgery." Ideally, all members of the team should take such courses jointly. For the optimization of standards of trauma care, we recommend a revival of obligatory rotations of residents in anesthesiology, emergency medicine, and surgery, each through all three disciplines, for guided practical experience relevant to traumatology and reanimatology.

*Fourth*, the anesthesiologist can contribute as an *investigator*. Anesthesiologists' involvement in trauma-related research can contribute in laboratory, clinical, and public health research. In the laboratory, the anesthesiologist's expertise is needed to develop clinically relevant animal models. For clinical traumatology research, anesthesiologists should be essential research team members. Important topics for multidisciplinary laboratory or clinical research in traumatology include an exploration of dying patterns during the first 1 to 2 hours after injury; time limits for the treatment of intracranial hemorrhage; effects of extrace-

rebral organ failure on head trauma; optimal timing and type of fluid therapy for treatment of continued internal hemorrhage; resuscitation potentials of exsanguination cardiac arrest; analgesia in the field; acute therapeutic hypothermia for suspended animation to facilitate resuscitative surgery (25, 26); and "disaster reanimatology" (20, 21). The latter is the life-saving potential of life-supporting first aid, ATLS, and resuscitative surgery during the first few minutes and hours after a mass disaster, such as a major earthquake.

Research in general, and trauma research in particular, has traditionally been without specialty boundaries. Ideally, research programs in traumatology are needed at multiple levels: molecule, cell, organ, organism, and community. Research can become a force to help integrate the fragmented disciplines of acute medicine into the trauma system that the founders envisioned 30 years ago.

Should "trauma anesthesia" become another subspecialty of anesthesiology? There are arguments in favor of such a development. Subspecialization tends to enhance the sophistication and skills of a few leaders. Trauma centers might keep such subspecialists busy primarily but not exclusively with work on trauma cases. Surgical critical care medicine (CCM), with or without trauma surgery or other special areas of interest, has recently received subspeciality board status in the American Board of Surgery. Certification of trauma centers requires evidence of ongoing postgraduate education of specialists. The latter, of course, could be possible without a new subspeciality.

There are also arguments against a formal subspeciality. Subspecialization might further fragment anesthesiology and its service departments, with the expense of 24-hour coverage in most trauma centers, which must provide care primarily for nontrauma cases. It could create a small, elitist group of traumatologic anesthesiologists to the exclusion of others, instead of encouraging most anesthesiologists to become experienced in trauma care. The American Board of Surgery is opposed to a subspecialty of trauma surgery. Many trauma patients are treated in general hospitals not designated as trauma centers. There could be potential burnout of trauma anesthesiologists and a need for lateral mobility. The knowledge, skills, and judgment required for trauma cases and elective cases in neurosurgery, cardiothoracic surgery, pediatric surgery, and others are overlapping. There is a need for special anesthesia expertise in resuscitative trauma surgery, but the need is less in definitive or reconstructive surgery. A wide spectrum of needs exists for trauma cases, ranging from treatment of exsanguination to the setting of minor fractures and elective plastic surgery. Management of critical trauma cases requires a multidisciplinary core team, with subspecialists called in as needed.

The above arguments lead to the conclusion that cutting the pie of health care delivery into neat, increasingly small pieces is undesirable and perhaps impossible. There can and should, however, be an opportunity for interested anesthesiologists to receive fellowship experience in traumatology at trauma centers. Multidisciplinary fellowship training in traumatology, with experiences in trauma anesthesia, surgery, CCM, and research, would make more sense than unidisciplinary subspecialties of trauma anesthesia, trauma surgery, and so on.

Is a trauma anesthesia society needed? Such a society has already been shown to be attractive and viable (18). A society to stimulate anesthesiologists in general to pay more attention to trauma care can only be good, particularly if it opens its arms to include trauma surgeons and other trauma team members among its ranks. It should foster exchange of experiences and knowledge. This would greatly enhance the desirable team function throughout the life-support chain.

In the operating room we like to illustrate team function by using the analogy of a chamber music group. Its members require no conductor. Friends who are accustomed to playing together do the best job in support of the "opus," the patient. On the other hand, advanced emergency resuscitation of trauma victims depends on a team leader or coordinator. This person—who should be predesignated to avoid "fragmenting the case"—is usually a general surgeon committed to traumatology; however, this role may also be filled by a qualified trauma anesthesiologist as is the case in many parts of the world. This team leader must appreciate the analogy of the chamber music group—once the case has gone beyond emergency resuscitation—and the fact that modern care for victims of severe trauma requires more than surgical expertise in the operating room. The prehospital and intrahospital trauma resuscitation teams should include at least an anesthesiologist-intensivist with training in traumatology, a trauma-committed general surgeon, and nonphysician helpers. The nurse anesthetist, where available, should also be a member of the team, working under the guidance of the anesthesiologist. Other physician specialists should be drawn in as needed, as early as possible. The emergency physician should be able to stabilize the trauma victim in the prehospital arena and in the emergency department, particularly in nontrauma centers. In the United States, most anesthesiologists have withdrawn from these areas. The void has been filled by emergency physicians, who initiated emergency medicine as a new base specialty. Over the past 20 years they have developed attractive residency programs and a specialty board and are receiving increasing academic recognition. Emergency medicine residencies must and do provide experiences under the direction of anesthesiologists and intensivists. Emergency medicine specialists must also be allowed to train and to become certified in CCM, as do anesthesiologists, internists, pediatricians, and surgeons. Thus, anesthesiologists must understand their colleagues who staff emergency rooms and who have taken over the pioneering efforts in EMS that were initiated by anesthesiologists in the 1950s and 1960s.

At present, "turf problems" have evolved

in many hospitals because of overlapping areas of interest and expertise of anesthesiologists, nonanesthesia intensivists, surgeons, and emergency physicians. To avoid such turf problems, team leadership for resuscitation should be predesignated.

The new National Association for EMS Physicians, initiated by academic emergency physicians, is seeking as members anesthesiologists and other acute care specialists who would share leadership roles in community-wide EMS systems. Similarly, the new International Trauma Anesthesia and Critical Care Society, pioneered by the editors of this book and other prominent trauma anesthesiologists (18), offers membership to nonanesthesiologists. It would be desirable to have trauma surgeons and these two organizations conduct joint educational meetings.

Medical leadership of *EMS systems* by reanimatologists of any base specialty is crucial. Quality control of such systems should not be delegated to administrators or to physicians selected merely on the basis of political and organizational expertise. Such physician leaders should have some experience with medical care on the streets (22). Also, such physician leaders must coordinate numerous agencies into an EMS system. This requires activism and leadership of multiple role players (4, 7, 14). The base specialty is less important than leadership, competence, interest, and availability. EMS community leaders should defend the principle that the performance of advanced and prolonged life support is the practice of medicine; if carried out in the field by paramedics, it must be under the predirected and moment-to-moment radio-guided control of experienced physicians. Physician involvement is also required for research and the future introduction of novel methods into the prehospital arena. The Center for Emergency Medicine of Western Pennsylvania is an example of such an effort (27).

Trauma care of the individual patient is magnified in *disaster medicine*. In the past this has been primarily a concern of epide-miologists, public health specialists, and sociologists. Since the 1970s, with the creation of the Club of Mainz (World Association of Emergency and Disaster Medicine) (28), disaster medicine promoters have become more interested in reanimatology and traumatology. In 1981, we introduced "disaster reanimatology" as a new field of inquiry to explore for the enhancement of resuscitation potentials in mass disasters (20, 21). Disaster reanimatology represents a great challenge for anesthesiologists. Results of retrospective interview studies of recent earthquakes suggest that life-supporting first aid by uninjured bystanders, when combined with simple search and rescue and followed by advanced trauma life support at the scene and resuscitative surgery as early as possible, could save many lives (20, 21).

Anesthesiologists can contribute to disaster medicine not only with resuscitation but also with novel methods of analgesia and anesthesia. The latter, in disasters, may be needed in the field. In a mass disaster, anesthesia with minimal equipment must be provided in the field, during transportation, and in many more locations in the hospital than are usually staffed and equipped for elective surgery. Such field anesthesia techniques (29–32) should be taught in every anesthesia residency during elective surgical cases. Simple devices and techniques in themselves are not less safe than the expensive, complicated anesthesia and monitoring devices now in use in hospital operating rooms in rich countries. Mishaps are not caused by equipment but by those who use it. Electronic alarms cannot replace vigilance and in certain instances can distract attention away from the patient.

Preparedness for mass disasters includes the anesthesiologist as a member of the trauma-resuscitation team. Many such teams are recommended for trauma hospitals, for call-up in disasters, and to provide a tiered response within local, regional, and national disaster medical systems. These teams should function in major trauma hospitals and be available for rapid transport to the scenes of mass disasters. Professionals who are used to working together form the most effective teams. Experience should also be provided for military surgeons and anesthesiologists, who in peacetime should gain trauma experience in civilian trauma centers.

To conclude, we hope that this book, *Trauma Anesthesia*, will fulfill its laudable objectives. Medicine in general and resuscitation medicine (including traumatology) in particular are creations of humanism. Anesthesiologists are decisive factors in traumatology (the science) and in trauma care (the service). Medicine's common goal is to help an increasing proportion of human beings live full lives with healthy minds in healthy bodies. At present, probably one-fourth of all deaths worldwide occur before old age, without incurable illness and without irreparable injuries. The challenges are great. Man's potential biologic life span is more than 100 years. The promise of reanimatology including traumatology is the gift of added meaningful years. Its implementation needs scientists and physicians of many disciplines. Those who are logical promoters of increasingly effective trauma care because of their special expertise, interest, and availability—including anesthesiologists—should jointly pursue this common goal.

Peter Safar, M.D.
*Distinguished Service Professor of Resuscitation Medicine*
*Past Chairman of Anesthesiology and Critical Care Medicine*
*Director, International Resuscitation Research Center*
*University of Pittsburgh*

## References

1. Dripps RD, Eckenhoff JE, Vandam LR. Introduction to Anesthesia. Philadelphia, WB Saunders, 1988.
2. Beecher HK. Resuscitation and Anesthesia for Wounded Men. The Management of Traumatic Shock. Springfield, IL, Charles C Thomas, 1949.
3. Seeley S. Accidental Death and Disability: The Neglected Disease of Modern Society. Washington, DC, Committee on Trauma and Committee on Shock, Division of Medical Sciences, National Academy of Sciences, National Research Council, 1966.
4. Safar P, Bircher NG. Cardiopulmonary Cerebral Resuscitation: An Introduction to Resuscitation Medicine. London, WB Saunders, 1988.
5. Safar P, DeKornfeld TJ, Pearson JW, et al. Intensive care unit. Anaesthesia 1961;16:275.
6. Safar P. The anesthesiologist as "intensivist." In Eckenhoff JE (ed): Science and Practice in Anesthesia. Philadelphia, JB Lippincott, 1965.
7. American Society of Anesthesiologists, Committee on Acute Medicine (Safar P, Chairman): Community-wide emergency medical services. JAMA 1968;204:595.
8. Safar P. The critical care medicine continuum from scene to outcome. In Parrillo JE, Ayres SR (eds): Major Issues in Critical Care Medicine. Baltimore, Williams & Wilkins, 1984, pp 71–84.
9. Negovsky VA. Reanimatology—the science of resuscitation. In Stephenson H (ed): Cardiac Arrest and Resuscitation. St Louis, CV Mosby, 1974.
10. Safar P. History of cardiopulmonary-cerebral resuscitation. In Kaye W, Bircher N (eds): Cardiopulmonary Resuscitation. New York, Churchill Livingstone, 1989, pp 1–49.
11. Society of Critical Care Medicine (SCCM) (USA). Guidelines for organization of critical care units. JAMA 1972;222:1532.
12. Society of Critical Care Medicine (SCCM) (USA). Guidelines for training of physicians in critical care medicine. Crit Care Med 1973;1:39.
13. Nagel EL, Hirschman JC, Nussenfeld SR, et al. Telemetry-medical command in coronary and other mobile emergency care systems. JAMA 1970;214:332.
14. Safar P, Benson DM, Esposito G, Grenvik A, Sands PA. Emergency and critical care medicine: local implementation of national recommendations. In Safar P (ed): Public Health Aspects of Critical Care Medicine and Anesthesiology. Philadelphia, FA Davis, 1974, pp 66–125.
15. Giesecke AH (ed). Anesthesia for the Surgery of Trauma. Philadelphia, FA Davis, 1976.
16. Greene NM (ed). Anesthesia for Emergency Surgery. Philadelphia, FA Davis, 1963.
17. Katz RL (ed). Emergency and Trauma I and II, Seminars in Anesthesia Vol 8, No 3 and 4. Philadelphia, WB Saunders, 1989.
18. Grande CM, Stene JK, Barton CR. The trauma anesthesiologist. MD Med J 1988;37:531.
19. Frey R, Nagel E, Safar P (eds). Mobile intensive care units: advanced emergency care delivery systems (symposium, Mainz, 1973). Anesthesiology Resuscitation 1976;95.
20. Safar P. Resuscitation potentials in mass disasters. Prehosp Disaster Med 1986;2:34–47.
21. Klain M, Ricci E, Safar P, Semenov V, Pretto E, Tisherman S, Abrams J, Comfort L, and other

members of the Disaster Reanimatology Study Group. Disaster reanimatology potentials: a structured interview study in Armenia. I: Methodology and preliminary results. Prehosp Disaster Med 1989;4:135–154.

22. Caroline NL. Medical care in the streets. JAMA 1977;237:43.

23. American Heart Association (AHA) 1985 National Conference (Montgomery WH, Chairman; Donegan J; McIntyre KM; Albarran-Sotelo R; Jaffe AS; Ornato JP; Paraskos JA; et al): Standards and guidelines for cardiopulmonary resuscitation (CPR) and emergency cardiac care (ECC). JAMA 1986;255 (suppl):2841.

24. American College of Surgeons Committee on Trauma. Hospital and prehospital resources for optimal care of the injured patient. ACS Bull 1983;68:11–21.

25. Safar P, Grenvik A, Abramson NS, Bircher N (eds). Reversibility of clinical death: symposium on resuscitation research. Crit Care Med 1988; 16:919.

26. Tisherman SA, Safar P, Radovsky A, Peitzman A, Sterz F, Kuboyama K. Therapeutic deep hypothermic circulatory arrest in dogs: a resuscitation modality for hemorrhagic shock with "irreparable" injury. J Trauma 1990;30:836–847.

27. Stewart RB, Paris P, Heller MB. Design of a resident-in-field experience for an emergency medicine residency curriculum. Ann Emerg Med 1987;16:175.

28. Frey R. The Club of Mainz for improved worldwide emergency and critical care medicine systems and disaster preparedness. Crit Care Med 1978;6:389.

29. Macintosh RR. A plea for simplicity. Br Med J 1955;2:1054.

30. Pearson J, Safar P. General anesthesia with minimal equipment. Anesth Analg 1961;40:644.

31. Safar P, Gedang I. Inexpensive system for the administration of ether. Anesthesiology 1961; 22:323.

32. Jowitt MD. Resuscitation and anesthesia in a battle situation: the Falkland Islands campaign. J World Assoc Emerg Disaster Med 1985;1:43.

# Preface

Members of the anesthesiology profession have shown a resurgence of interest in the perioperative management of trauma patients over the past several years. Along with this renewed interest has come the realization that the magnitude of the problem has remained virtually unchanged over the past 20 years (1). Trauma is the primary cause of death among pediatric patients and young adults in the United States and the third leading cause of death (following cardiovascular disease and cancer) overall. Other far-reaching implications of trauma are revealed in the numbers of working hours lost by the country's labor force, the number of productive years of life lost, and the high cost of long-term rehabilitation (2).

From the standpoint of anesthesiology, very little progress has been made in improving the care of the injured. In conjunction with the resurgence of interest, the anesthesia literature has grown to encompass the introduction of new pharmacologic agents or equipment, but otherwise it represents a "rehash" of statements previously put forth. With few exceptions, the much-needed investigational work has been neglected.

The level of involvement of anesthesia specialists in the clinical and research arenas of trauma care is far below what it should be (3). If current trends are to be reversed, the subspecialty of *trauma anesthesia* must be recognized and fostered.

It is our intention that this book serve as an update/review of known information, as an introduction to areas not previously covered as part of trauma anesthesia, as a primer for individuals in training or working to expand their horizons, and as a "jumping-off" point for the critical investigational work that is needed. The book focuses on "major trauma," which is usually seen at a level I or II trauma center, and which normally, by virtue of the magnitude of the destructive forces involved, refers to the presence of injuries of multiple organ systems (e.g., orthopaedic, cardiac, and neurologic) within the same patient, colloquially termed "multitrauma." The book also stresses a high degree of involvement of the anesthesiologist in the primary management of the trauma patient from the time of injury until the patient leaves the critical care areas of the facility. Perhaps the most important contribution of the book is its title, *Trauma Anesthesia*. Although the point is subtle, this phrase stresses the significant difference between "trauma anesthesia" and the more commonly used phrases "anesthesia for trauma" and "emergency anesthesia." "Trauma anesthesia" implies a greater sense of commitment to dedicated trauma care by the anesthesia specialist. The reader is reminded that not all trauma is an emergency and not all emergencies are related to injury (3). The two entities can be, and often are, mutually exclusive.

It is our opinion that a book of this size could never be a truly definitive work on the subject (to that end, another project is under way). Instead, we hope to address the most basic and practical topics. Therefore, for educational and historical interest, the reader is referred to other complete works that have preceded this one (4–20). Following our own advice, we have tried to refrain, as much as possible, from "issuing any general 'blanket' statements as far as they regard management of trauma patients" (21). Rather than present a "cookbook" approach, we have tried to present the available information and the benefit of our experience and let the readers draw their own conclusions.

This volume covers topics that anesthesiologists must comprehend to care for trauma patients. Chapter 1 provides the framework for the functions of the "trauma anesthesiologist/critical care specialist" from the perspectives of the past, present, and future. Mechanisms of injury are covered in Chapter 2, especially the differences between blunt and penetrating trauma. Such knowledge aids the anesthesiologist in anticipating possible injuries as well as developing appropriate resuscitation and anesthesia protocols. Chapter 3 covers airway management in the trauma patient and discusses the balance among priorities of oxygenation, the "full stomach," and cervical spine stabilization. Shock resuscitation is covered in Chapter 4 and focuses on the pathophysiology of shock and initial fluid management. Transfusion therapy is specifically addressed in Chapter 5, which gives a rationale for the use of blood products and discusses the treatment of complications arising from transfusion.

The perioperative anesthetic management of the trauma patient (covered in Chapter 6) includes emergency room anesthetic management, preoperative preparation, monitoring devices, pharmacology, and postoperative recovery, as well as concerns particular to thoracoabdominal and orthopaedic injuries. Topics in anesthesia for special trauma patient populations are covered in Chapter 10 (the pregnant trauma patient) and Chapter 11 (the pediatric trauma patient).

Neurologic, maxillofacial (and ocular), and thermal trauma are covered in separate chapters (Chapters 7, 8, and 9). Chapter 13 focuses on the complications of temperature regulation and discusses the treatment and prevention of hypothermia and malignant hyperthermia. Other topics of interest include the transportation of critically ill patients (Chapter 15), hyperbaric oxygen therapy (Chapter 14), pain management (Chapter 12), medical legal issues (Chapter 18), information management systems (Chapter 17), and occupational hazards for trauma health care workers (Chapter 16).

The editors of this book sincerely hope that the information conveyed here will help anesthesiologists improve their care of the acutely injured patient. Having spent the majority of our professional lives exclusively dedicated to the perioperative management of trauma patients and to the development of "trauma anesthesia," we have derived a great sense of satisfaction. Of course, we can't "promise a rose garden" but we wholeheartedly encourage anyone interested in performing a vital function in an exciting environment to explore "trauma anesthesia."

*Go for it*!
J.K.S.
Hershey 1990
*Driving on*!
C.M.G.
Baltimore 1990

## References

1. McFee AS, Franklin ME. Evaluation of the patient with multiple injuries. In Zauder HL (ed): Anesthesia for Orthopedic Surgery. Philadelphia, FA Davis, 1980, pp 9–19.
2. Trunkey DD. Presidential address: on the nature of things that go bang in the night. Surgery 1982;92:123–132.
3. Grande CM, Stene JK, Barton CR. The trauma anesthesiologist. Md Med J 1988;37:531–536.
4. Beecher HK. Resuscitation and Anesthesia for Wounded Men. Springfield, IL, Charles C Thomas, 1949.
5. Wolfson LS. Anaesthesia for the Injured. Oxford, England, Blackwell Scientific Publications, 1962.
6. Greene NM (ed). Anesthesia for Emergency Surgery. Philadelphia, FA Davis, 1963.
7. Martin SJ (ed). Anesthesia for Trauma. Int Anesth Clin 1968;6(4).
8. Breechner VL (ed). Anesthesia in Emergency Surgery. Int Anesth Clin 1971;9(1).
9. Giesecke AH (ed). Anesthesia for the Surgery of Trauma. Philadelphia, FA Davis, 1976.
10. Sutcliffe AJ. Handbook of Emergency Anaesthesia, London, Butterworth, 1983.
11. Stoddart JC (ed). Trauma and the Anaesthetist. London, Ballière-Tindall, 1984.

12. Katz RL (ed). Anesthesia for Trauma and Emergencies. Semin Anesth 1985;4(2).

13. Adams AP, Hewitt PB, Rogers MC (eds). Emergency Anaesthesia. London, Edward Arnold, 1986.

14. Meyer AA (ed). Critical Care Management of the Trauma Patient. Crit Care Clin 1986;2(4).

15. Donegan JH (ed). Manual of Anesthesia for Emergency Surgery. New York, Churchill-Livingstone, 1987.

16. Kirby RR, Brown DL (eds). Anesthesia for Trauma. Int Anesthesiol Clin 1987.

17. Katz RL (ed). Emergency and Trauma I. Semin Anesth 1989;8(3).

18. Katz RL (ed): Emergency and Trauma II. Semin Anesth 1989;8(4).

19. Vanstrum GS (ed). Anesthesia in Emergency Medicine. Boston, Little, Brown & Co, 1989.

20. Grande CM, Stene JK, Bernhard WN (eds). Overview of Trauma Anesthesia and Critical Care. Crit Care Clin 1990;6(1).

21. Grande CM, Barton CR, Stene JK. Emergency airway management in trauma patients with a suspected cervical spine injury: in response. Anesth Analg 1989;68:416–418.

# Acknowledgments

ITACCS and the editors wish to express our gratitude to Dr. William N. Bernhard and the staff of the Department of Anesthesiology at the Maryland Institute for Emergency Medical Services Systems for their unswerving support of us, this project, and the development of "trauma anesthesia."

We also wish to thank Leanne Allgaier for her outstanding secretarial assistance and Linda Kesselring for invaluable technical editorial support. in preparing this book.

Dr. Stene wishes to express appreciation and gratitude to his wife, Joanne, who supported and encouraged the completion of the project while rearing 3 children born as the book was being written.

Dr. Grande recognizes and expresses gratitude and appreciation to the family members, true friends and close colleagues brethren in uniform who made completion of this book possible.

Thank you!

# Contributors

C. Russell Baker, C.R.N.A.
Associate Director, Nurse Anesthesia
The Shock Trauma Center
Maryland Institute for Emergency Medical
  Services Systems
Baltimore, Maryland

Charles R. Barton, C.R.N.A., B.A.
Chief Nurse Anesthetist
Union Hospital of Cecil County
Elkton, Maryland
Former Chief Nurse Anesthetist
Department of Anesthesia
Shock Trauma Center
Maryland Institute for Emergency Medical
  Services Systems
Baltimore, Maryland

William N. Bernhard, M.D.
Associate Professor of Anesthesiology
University of Maryland Medical School
Director, MIEMSS Anesthesiology
R Adams Cowley, M.D., Shock Trauma
  Center, MIEMSS
University of Maryland Medical System
Baltimore, Maryland
General Member of the Board of Directors,
  ITACCS

Barry Burns, Ph.D.
Graduate Faculty
University of Maryland at Baltimore
Former Director of Anesthesia Research
Department of Anesthesia
Maryland Institute for Emergency Medical
  Services Systems
Baltimore, Maryland

Bruce F. Cullen, M.D.
Professor of Anesthesiology
University of Washington School of Medi-
  cine

Anesthesiologist-in-Chief
Harborview Medical Center–Trauma
  Center
Seattle, Washington
Special Ad Hoc Advisor, ITACCS

Bennett Edelman, M.D.
Associate Professor
Pathology Department
University of Maryland School of Medicine
Baltimore, Maryland

Elizabeth A. M. Frost, M.D.
Professor of Anesthesiology
Albert Einstein College of Medicine
Montefiore Medical Center
Bronx, New York

William R. Furman, M.D.
Interim Director
Department of Anesthesiology
Francis Scott Key Medical Center and Balti-
  more Burn Center
Assistant Professor
Department of Anesthesiology & Critical
  Care Medicine
The Johns Hopkins University School of
  Medicine
Baltimore, Maryland

Adolph H. Giesecke, M.D.
Jenkins Professor and Chairman
Department of Anesthesiology
University of Texas
Southwestern Medical School
Dallas, Texas
Vice President, ITACCS

Christopher M. Grande, M.D.
Special Consultant and Chief, Special Proj-
  ects Branch
Department of Anesthesiology

Shock Trauma Center
Maryland Institute for Emergency Medical
  Services Systems
University of Maryland at Baltimore
Executive Director, ITACCS
Captain, Medical Corps, USAR
Flight Surgeon and Diving Medical Officer
11th Special Forces Group (Airborne)
1st U.S. Army Special Forces

Jonathan Greenberg, M.D., J.D.
Chief, Neurotrauma Services
Jackson Memorial Hospital
Miami, Florida
Former Attending Neurosurgeon
Maryland Institute for Emergency Medical
  Services Systems
Baltimore, Maryland

Andrew P. Harris, M.D.
Chief, Obstetrics/Gynecology Anesthesia
The Johns Hopkins Hospital
Assistant Professor
Department of Anesthesiology/Critical Care
  Medicine and Gynecology/Obstetrics
Baltimore, Maryland

Meyer R. Hayman, M.D.
Associate Professor of Medicine and Oncol-
  ogy
Division of Hematology, Department of
  Medicine, and the University of Maryland
  Cancer Center
University of Maryland School of Medicine
Baltimore, Maryland

Murray A. Kalish, M.D.
Assistant Professor of Anesthesiology
University of Maryland School of Medicine
Senior Attending Anesthesiologist
Shock Trauma Center
Maryland Institute for Emergency Medical
  Services Systems
Baltimore, Maryland

John I. Lauria, M.D.
Professor and Chairman
State University of New York at Buffalo
Department of Anesthesiology
School of Medicine and Biomedical Sciences
Buffalo, New York

Mark McCauley, M.S., R.R.T.
Director, Department of Respiratory Ther-
  apy
Shock Trauma Center
Maryland Institute for Emergency Medical
  Services Systems
Baltimore, Maryland

Roy A. M. Myers, M.D.
Director, Hyperbaric Medicine
Attending Traumatologist
Shock Trauma Center
Maryland Institute for Emergency Medical
  Services Systems
University of Maryland Medical System
Baltimore, Maryland

Henry E. Rice, M.D.
Resident
Department of Surgery
University of Washington
Seattle, Washington

John K. Stene, M.D., Ph.D.
Assistant Professor of Anesthesiology
Director of Perioperative Anesthesia Trauma
  Services
Department of Anesthesiology
The Pennsylvania State University College
  of Medicine
The Milton S. Hershey Medical Center
Hershey, Pennsylvania
President, ITACCS

Judith L. Stiff, M.D., M.P.H.
Attending Anesthesiologist
Francis Scott Key Medical Center and Balti-
  more Regional Burn Center
Associate Professor, Anesthesiology
The Johns Hopkins University School of
  Medicine
Baltimore, Maryland

Randall C. Wetzel, M.D.
Associate Professor
Departments of Anesthesiology/Critical Care
  Medicine and Pediatrics
Chief, Division of Pediatric Anesthesia
The Johns Hopkins Hospital
Baltimore, Maryland

Deborah Williams, B.A., C.R.T.T.
Respiratory Therapist
Homedco/Home Medical Equipment
Formerly Department of Respiratory Therapy
Shock Trauma Center
Maryland Institute for Emergency Medical Services Systems
Baltimore, Maryland

Chet I. Wyman, M.D.
Fellow in Trauma Anesthesia & Critical Care
Shock Trauma Center
Maryland Institute for Emergency Medical Services Systems
University of Maryland Medical System
Baltimore, Maryland

# Contents

# Trauma Anesthesia: Past, Present, and Future

*John K. Stene and Christopher M. Grande*

## INTRODUCTION TO TRAUMATIC DISEASE AND TRAUMA ANESTHESIA

Trauma accounts for more deaths in the United States during the first four decades of life than any other disease and ranks behind cardiovascular disease, cancer, and strokes as the fourth leading cause of death among the entire United States population. Because the incidence of infectious disease and heart disease has decreased in response to public health control measures, trauma has assumed a larger share of our national mortality rate. In recent years the mortality for trauma has remained under 100,000, but the overall incidence of serious injury has been increasing (1). The development of organized prehospital care systems for trauma care and of trauma centers has helped to reduce the mortality rate from acute injury. A well-trained cadre of trauma anesthesiologists will help further to control needless deaths secondary to acute injury.

Knowledge of the demographics of trauma will help physicians prepare for the type of care that will be required from them. Each geographic area has its own profile for the types of injury that occur; thus, what is appropriate for a trauma center in one area may not be appropriate in another. However, motor vehicle accidents account for the greatest number of serious injuries and traumatic deaths throughout the United States. Young males (15–25 years of age) suffer the highest mortality rate from trauma, but those victims over 70 years of age have an extremely high mortality per injury suffered.

Although homicides and suicides by gunshot wounds receive much press coverage, the overall effect of firearms is very small compared to vehicular trauma. However, many large city trauma centers (e.g., in Los Angeles) are receiving increasing numbers of patients with penetrating trauma secondary to drug trafficking and the increasingly sophisticated weaponry available to this criminal element. Injuries suffered in falls are frequent causes of trauma to the elderly and to those impaired by alcohol abuse (1).

The demographics of trauma deaths suggest prevention measures as well as providing information to prepare clinicians for the management of injured patients. Unfortunately, traumatic illness is sometimes a result of ingrained behavior patterns that are very difficult to change. Massive campaigns to reduce drinking and driving and to promote seat belt use have had short-term success but have been disappointing in terms of sustained behavior change. Data on alcohol abuse and driving demonstrate this point. A Vermont study of the blood alcohol concentration (BAC) of 1100 case control selected drivers revealed a distinct bimodal distribution (2). The majority of the drivers had BACs < 0.04% while a few had BACs > 0.15% and none had a level of 0.10%. The drivers with the high BAC had extensive histories of driving infractions and previous citations for driving while intoxicated. Therefore, a small number of drivers appear to be incorrigible in regard to modifying their drinking and driving behavior and thus continue to be involved in many accidents. Problem drinkers suffer traumatic injury so frequently that a pattern of repeat emergency room visits for injuries is one of the diagnostic criteria for alcoholism. Other types of behavior that lead to trauma are just as difficult to change as is alcohol abuse.

## Trauma Systems

Effective trauma care requires a community-wide, systematic approach to the care of trauma victims. Trauma systems have evolved to coordinate initial care of the injured in a uniform manner and to designate certain hospitals as trauma centers to maximize the use of scarce resources. High-quality trauma care to prevent unnecessary deaths is intensive in terms of personnel and equipment. However, the cost per patient saved can be reduced in a few sophisticated trauma centers where special equipment is used by highly trained personnel to treat many patients. Thus, other institutions that would admit very few trauma patients are spared the investment in expensive equipment that would remain idle much of the time. Obviously, such cost-sharing techniques require a system to triage patients rapidly to the appropriate facilities.

The validation of the concept of a trauma system was accomplished through a series of studies, the most notable of which were performed in California (3, 4). In the first study, the mortality rate in a group of more seriously injured trauma patients was lower in one county with a trauma system than the rate in less seriously injured patients in a second county without a trauma system (3). In a follow-up study, the mortality rate in this second county dropped once a trauma system was implemented (4).

Trauma systems are designed to place severely injured patients in the appropriate facility at the appropriate time. The state of Maryland has adopted a statewide system to coordinate both emergency medical services (EMS) and trauma care. Notably, Maryland is one of only two states actually to have implemented this type of recommended system, the other being Virginia (5). Within the Maryland Institute for Emergency Medical Services Systems (MIEMSS), a statewide medical director works with five regional medical directors to coordinate EMS policies and procedures so that patients in all 24 political subdivisions (23 counties and Baltimore City) are treated according to the same standards (6). The five regional medical directors oversee the function of the county-wide EMS programs in their regions. Each county system has an EMS medical director (sometimes designated as a fire surgeon), who is responsible to the State Board of Phy-

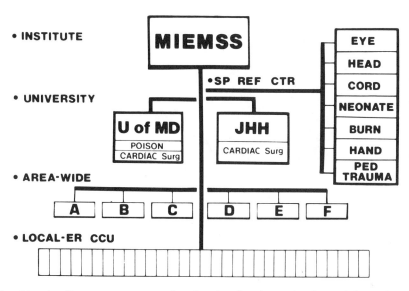

**Figure 1.1. Maryland's trauma system showing levels of care and specialty referral centers.** MIEMSS, Maryland Institute for Emergency Medical Services Systems; U of MD, University of Maryland Hospital; SP REF CTR, Specialty Referral Center; JHH, Johns Hopkins Hospital. (From Cowley RA. Systems of organization. In Cowley RA, Conn A, Dunham CM (eds). Trauma Care: Surgical Management. Philadelphia, JB Lippincott, 1987, vol 1, pp 1–40.)

sician Quality Assurance for the activities of the emergency medical technicians (EMTs) and paramedics (EMT-Ps) who work in the given county. As well as supervising EMS activity, MIEMSS is also responsible for designating hospitals as trauma centers. Triage criteria for field referral to a trauma center are designated to capture patients with expected serious and life-threatening injuries. Emergency rooms in non-trauma-center hospitals can be utilized for acute stabilization before transport to trauma centers following the Advanced Trauma Life Support (ATLS) protocols of the American College of Surgeons. The trauma centers are designated on an "echelons of care" scheme (Fig. 1.1) that requires multiple regional trauma centers geographically distributed around the state and specialized centers of particular excellence (e.g., ophthalmologic trauma) in a central location. Such centers include the University of Maryland Shock Trauma Unit, which is the MIEMSS headquarters as well as the specialized center for unstable multiple trauma patients, those with spinal cord injuries, and head-injured patients. Other special centers

include burn centers in Baltimore and Washington, DC; pediatric trauma centers at Johns Hopkins Hospital and Children's Hospital National Medical Center; the Curtis Hand Center at Union Memorial Hospital in Baltimore; and the Wilmer Eye Institute at Johns Hopkins Hospital (Fig. 1.1).

Review of ambulance runsheets by county and regional medical directors provides constant feedback to local EMTs and EMT-Ps about the appropriateness of their triage decisions. A further control on the flow of patients to appropriate facilities is the liaison between MIEMSS and the Maryland State Police Aviation Division. EMS helicopter transports in Maryland are provided by the state police, not by hospital-based helicopters (7). The police helicopters are dispatched by request of the ambulance-borne first responders (EMTs) at the scene of the accident. This system achieves some measure of cost control by combining EMS transport and police function in the same aircraft. However, EMS transport requests must have absolute priority for aircraft use if a creditable trauma system is to be retained.

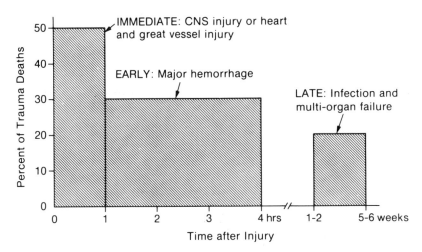

**Figure 1.2.   The trimodal distribution of traumatic disease.** (From Brown DL. Trauma management: the anesthesiologist's role. Int Anesthesiol Clin 1987;25:1–18.)

## Trauma Centers

Trauma centers were developed to provide state-of-the-art care in a timely manner to seriously injured patients in an effort to reduce the appalling mortality of injured patients who were still alive at the time they entered the medical care system (8). Trauma deaths occur in a trimodal distribution (9), with the immediate deaths due to brain or heart laceration not being amenable to medical therapy (Fig. 1.2). However, the second peak of trauma deaths (patients who hemorrhage to death from visceral injuries or fractures within 1 to 2 hours of their injury) can be prevented by the application of appropriate care by highly trained personnel in a trauma center. As EMS systems have become more sophisticated in the initial care of the trauma patient and as trauma center personnel have increased the sophistication of their resuscitative skills, the third peak (late trauma deaths) has assumed more importance. These late deaths (secondary to sepsis, multiorgan failure, and devastating brain injuries) peak about 2 weeks after injury. Much effort is being focused on improved early resuscitation to prevent these delayed lethal complications of trauma.

Trauma centers adhere to standards published by the American College of Surgeons (ACS) (10) that delineate personnel organization and function (Table 1.1). In most instances 85% of all trauma patients can be managed at a local level (either a conventional emergency room or a level III trauma center). Ten per cent will require the additional care provided at a level II center, and the 5% most seriously injured must be treated in a level I facility (Fig. 1.3). These guidelines are broad enough that hospitals can organize their trauma centers to meet special needs. Accrediting bodies such as MIEMSS or the Pennsylvania Trauma Systems Foundation periodically review trauma centers' level of adherence to the ACS guidelines. Among the essential personnel needed to respond to the emergency room in level I, II, and III trauma centers is an anesthesiologist or certified registered nurse anesthetist (CRNA) (Fig. 1.4).

As trauma centers have been developed in the United States, anesthesiologists have been slow to become professionally involved in their development. The ACS has developed standards for trauma centers because trauma is a "surgical disease." The ACS standards do recognize that an anesthesiologist is an essential medical specialist for the trauma center, although most anesthesiologists view their role as a consulting one. The situation is quite different in Europe (especially France, Belgium, Germany, and the U.S.S.R.), where anesthesiologists are

**Table 1.1.    Trauma Center Organization**

| | Level I | Level II | Level III |
|---|---|---|---|
| Philosophy | Identical community/hospital commitment to excellent care of severe and urgent injuries<br>Trauma quality assurance process<br>Trauma training programs<br>Trauma public education<br><br>Teaching program<br>Research<br><br>600–1000 cases/yr | 300–600 cases/yr | Best community commitment to stabilization and transport of severe and urgent injuries |
| Facilities | Lighted heliport | Lighted heliport | |
|   Emergency room | 24 hr/day with trauma-experienced M.D. staffing | 24 hr/day with trauma-experienced M.D. staffing | 24 hr/day with trauma-experienced M.D. staffing |
|   Operating room | Staffed and available for trauma 24 hr/day | Staffed and available for trauma 24 hr/day | Desirable to be staffed and available 24 hr/day |
| Anesthesia personnel | Anesthesiologist with trauma experience 24 hr/day | CRNA or anesthesiologist with trauma experience 24 hr/day | In-house anesthesia coverage (M.D. or CRNA) 24 hr/day |
| Surgery personnel | 24-hr/day general surgeon and neurosurgeon experienced in trauma; consultants rapidly available | 24-hr/day general surgeon and neurosurgeon experienced in trauma; consultants rapidly available | Promptly available general surgeon; 24-hr/day neurosurgeon availability highly desirable |
| Surgery case load | At least 50 severely and urgently injured patients per trauma general surgeon per year | At least 50 severely and urgently injured patients per trauma general surgeon per year | |
| | | Commitment to trauma training and research | |

## EMS PATIENT DISTRIBUTION — LEVELS OF CARE

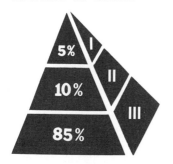

**Figure 1.3.    Typical distribution of trauma cases to levels I, II, and III trauma centers.** (From Cowley RA. Systems of organization. In Cowley RA, Conn A, Dunham CM (eds): Trauma Care: Surgical Management, Philadelphia, JB Lippincott, 1987, vol 1, pp 1–40.)

heavily involved as first responders to trauma patients. They direct emergency medical services as well as prehospital operations, emergency departments, operating rooms, and the intensive care of trauma victims (11–15).

Trauma patients require emergency surgery very frequently in the United States; however, many American anesthesiologists approach the trauma patient with ambivalence. Despite the fact that many anesthesiologists find trauma patients to be difficult and burdensome to anesthetize, anesthesiologists' training prepares them well to care for critically ill trauma patients. Successful treatment of patients with life-threatening injuries requires the application of critical care principles to all phases of acute resuscitation and treatment. Anesthesiologists are trained to provide critical care in the operating room and the intensive care unit and can easily adapt these principles to emergency rooms or the trauma admitting area. Anesthesia training also develops a mind-set that is useful in prehospital care (e.g., acute and

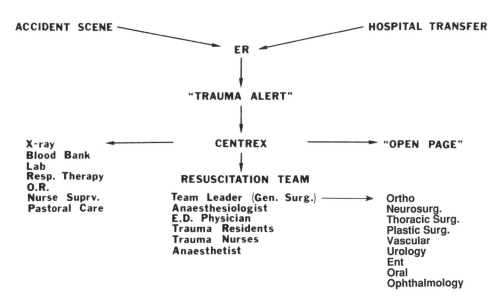

**Figure 1.4.  The trauma alert system.** The various components and individuals necessary for sophisticated trauma care. (From Rhodes M, Gillot AR. Operating room resuscitation of the severely injured trauma patient: direct transport to the operating room. In Maull KD (ed): Advances in Trauma, Chicago, Year Book, 1987, vol 2, pp 87–104.)

rapid intervention to prevent escalation of medical problems). The anesthesiologist is also trained to monitor patients closely, to care for acute perioperative medical problems, and to administer cardiopulmonary-cerebral resuscitative care.

In this introductory chapter, we focus on the history, status, and future of the specialty of trauma anesthesia itself. As editors of this book and as trauma anesthesiologists, we place great emphasis upon the involvement of anesthesiologists in the perioperative management of the trauma patient. In our minds, the acute perioperative period extends from the field environment, where the patient is first injured, to the time when the trauma patient is released from the critical care area of the hospital. The trauma patient will often undergo follow-up procedures during the critical care phase. The *elective* perioperative period focuses on the convalescing trauma patient, who will often return to the hospital for elective reconstructive procedures, and includes the preoperative interview, often conducted in the outpatient clinic, the day of the operation, and the recovery period.

## ECHOES FROM THE PAST

In 1988, we introduced the concept of the trauma anesthesia/critical care specialist (TA/CCS), but the concept that anesthesiologists should have a high degree of involvement in trauma care has been suggested many times in the past. In *Nei Ching*, the ancient book that summarizes Chinese medical knowledge circa 2600 BC, what may be the first battlefield anesthesia is described; distraction and hypnosis were used (16). Ironically, the newest subspecialty of anesthesiology, trauma anesthesia, is perhaps its oldest practice; some of the earliest historical records indicate that pharmacologic anesthesia was first used to manage battle casualties, one of the first inductions being performed by Dioscorides, a Greek physician in the Roman army in the first century AD. As martial action and trauma care have a round-robin relationship, various methods of inducing surgical anesthesia for victims of battlefield injuries were tried as the centuries passed. These included the use of herbs and plants (containing hyoscyamus and mandragora, opiates administered via various routes, or various concoctions with an ethanol base [e.g., mead, wine, whiskey]). After public demonstration of the clinical use of ether in a hospital setting by Morton in 1846, this agent was soon being used on battlefields around the world (e.g., the Mexican-American War of 1847, the Danish-German War of 1847, and the American Civil War in 1861). Chloroform was also available (after approximately 1847) and was used for military trauma anesthesia (17). From that time until the present, the civilian and military spheres have reciprocated in times of war and peace: developments made during peacetime are used (after some "latent period") on the "next" battlefield, where new observations are made and treatments are modified or new techniques evolve. When that war ends, these advances are then used in the civilian world.

This book is by no means the first time the value of the anesthesiologist in the perioperative care of the trauma patient has been discussed (see also the preface). To orient those unfamiliar with the concepts embodied in the field of trauma anesthesia, we present the following quotations as "echoes from the past," which extol the virtues of the trauma anesthesiologist. Paraphrasing would risk losing the original meaning, whereas quotation permits us to "give credit where credit is due."

## Anesthesia Is Necessary for Trauma Patients

First, some general comments on the importance of the role of the anesthesiologist in trauma care, beginning with one by Dr. W. T. G. Morton:

On previous occasions it had been my privilege to visit battlefields, and there to administer the pain-destroying agent which it pleased God to make me the human agent to introduce for the benefit of suffering humanity. How little did I think, however, when originally experimenting with the properties of sulfuric ether on my own person, that I should ever successfully administer it to hundreds in one day, and thus prevent an amount of agony fearful to contemplate (18).

Next are comments on Dr. Morton himself by Dr. John H. Brinton, who was present at the Battle of the Wilderness (May 1864) during the American Civil War:

Let me, from personal reminiscence, relate an anecdote in point: In the early summer of 1864, during the fierce contest in the Virginia Wilderness, I was present officially at the headquarters of Lieutenant-General Grant . . . an aide approached and said to him that a stranger, a civilian physician, wished to see him for the purpose of obtaining an ambulance for his personal use in visiting the field hospitals. The answer of the General was prompt and decided: "The ambulances are intended only for the sick and wounded, and under no circumstances can be taken for private use." This response was carried as given to the waiting applicant, a travel-stained man in brownish clothes, whom at the distance I thought I recognized. I went to him and found that he was Dr. W. T. G. Morton. I asked him to wait a minute, and returned to the General. On repeating this request I received the same answer. "But General," I ventured to say, "If you knew who that man is I think you would give what he asks for." "No, I will not," he replied. "I will not divert an ambulance to-day for any one; they are all required elsewhere." "General," I replied, "I am sure you will give him the wagon; he has done so much for mankind, so much for the soldier; more than any soldier or civilian has ever done before, and you will say so when you know his name." The General . . . asked: "Who is he?" "He is Dr. Morton, the discoverer of ether," I answered. The General paused a moment, then said: "You are right, Doctor, he has done more for the soldier than any one else, soldier or civilian, for he has taught you all to banish pain. Let him have the ambulance and anything else he wants." Not only this, but I have learned from a printed letter of Dr. Morton, recently sent me by his family, that the hospitalities of the headquarters—ambulances, tent, mess and servant—were afterward tendered him during his stay, by order of the general commanding (18).

More recent comments on the anesthesiologist's role in trauma care:

The anesthesiologist, with his or her background in acute perioperative medicine, offers key skills and familiarity with the many presentations of shock as a result of various disease processes or as a result of surgical trauma. He or she must deal with management dilemmas such as critical intracranial hypertension, coronary artery disease and myocardial dysfunction, the difficult airway, the open eye injury, the full stomach, and fractures in an emergency setting on a daily basis . . . The anesthesiologist, as part of the trauma team, must be involved in the patient's care early because of the immediate need for ongoing airway management and surgical intervention . . . If surgery is required, the anesthesiologist's initial role as a resuscitation team member is expanded to include comprehensive patient management in the operating room (19).

and

One of the emerging concepts of sophisticated trauma care is that of an anesthesiologist with supplemental knowledge and skills in traumatology, emergency medicine, and critical care who becomes the trauma anesthesia/critical care specialist (TA/CCS). At a trauma center, the TA/CCS performs unique functions compared to other medical specialists and anesthesia subspecialists. Analysis of the trauma patient population and other groups of patients will show significant differences that indicate the need for a dedicated anesthesia care provider specializing in traumatic disease to be a member of the trauma team. Although in the past anesthesiologists to manage trauma patients were recruited as needed from the ranks of practicing clinicians (even within the military itself in times of war), with today's high-quality trauma care systems the TA/CCS will find themselves with a full-time occupation as a professional consultant . . . Indeed, the recent past has witnessed a redefinition of the term *traumatologist*. Presently, traumatologists include not only trauma surgeons and emergency medicine physicians, but other physicians and nonphysician trauma care specialists, as well as nonclinical personnel (e.g., epidemiologists). The TA/CCS is anesthesiology's contribution to this collection of subspecialists (20).

and

It is contended that the anesthetist can usefully become a fully integrated member of the team treating injured patients, not only in the operating theatres, but in the management of respiratory and circulatory problems; resuscitation; in the relief of pain; and in a number of diagnostic and therapeutic procedures in which the techniques of anesthesia can be helpful (21).

## Skilled and Experienced Anesthesiologists Are Required for Trauma Care

A disparity exists between the level of training of the anesthesiologist who usually cares for the injured and the complexity of the trauma patients:

In view of possible underlying medical diseases, the absence of a history and the various choices available and the need to make quick decisions these patients should be anesthetized by experienced consultants and not by junior doctors. This is true for all the other people involved in treating multiply injured patients (22).

and

Reasonable accuracy of prediction is only likely with clinicians of considerable experience in dealing with major injuries, as unfortunately no formula has yet been evolved to take the place of experience of similar injuries previously treated and the judgement required to evaluate the clinical response to injury (23).

and

It is a paradox . . . that the responsibility for injured patients is often delegated to less skilled staff. When anesthetizing casualties with multiple injuries, a skilled assistant is essential (24).

## The Anesthesiologist's Contribution to Resuscitation

The anesthesiologist's contribution to resuscitation protocols includes:

Resuscitation techniques for patients with major multiple injuries have been developed in hospitals, largely by anesthetists, and, in the majority of centers, have become an extremely efficient routine. Patients who reach hospital alive and without irreversible damage to a vital organ can usually be well cared for (25).

and

The anaesthetist's aim is to provide anaesthesia for surgery with as little risk to the patient as possible. In order to do this he should be seen by his surgical colleagues as part of a team rather than someone who is called in at the last moment to give the gas. As with elective anaesthesia, the emergency anaesthetic starts long before the induction of anaesthesia. As a counsel of perfection, all patients should be seen preoperatively by the anaesthetist in person so that a full assessment of their physical and mental states can be made and any problems identified. This avoids "surprises" in the anaesthetic room because of incorrect or absent information. It also allows the anaesthetist to plan ahead and obtain any necessary equipment from other parts of the hospital . . . The distinguishing feature of an emergency anaesthetic is that it cannot be delayed if the life or quality of life of the patient is to be preserved . . . Anaesthesia should rarely be refused on the grounds of high risk (26).

and

Following admission of the patient to the emergency casualty department, the main lines of management are instituted immediately and in many instances overlap; resuscitation, overall assessment, diagnosis and specific treatment. This necessitates skilled team-work by many individuals but in particular the anaesthetist and the accident surgeon . . . While the accent must always be on securing of an impeccable airway and vigorous cardiopulmonary resuscitation, the anesthetist must also be familiar with the protean signs and symptoms of life-threatening primary damage to the brain, lungs, heart and intra-abdominal organs, and conscious of the need to avoid further secondary damage which, if it does not immediately result in death, may certainly determine the ultimate quality of survival. From the technical point of view, the anaesthetist is especially well suited to supervise the overall monitoring of vital functions necessary from the time of the patient's admission to ultimate recovery from the critical period of injury (27).

and

In individual, as well as macro- and maxi-emergencies, anesthetists-resuscitation specialists' training qualifies them for immediate action . . . These medical specialists' [anesthesiologists] work is of unique practical value, since their daily activities are specifically concerned with emergencies, either the usual emergencies which occur during surgical operations or the totally unpredictable, multidimensional emergencies, which occur during first-aid situations and in resuscitation or intensive care units . . . Only those specialists who remain in constant practice can perform resuscitation techniques accurately at

the right moment and under any, even the most precarious, environmental situations (28).

## The Anesthesiologist's Role in the Trauma Team

The anesthesiologist's participation in the trauma care team is essential:

The management of the severely injured patient requires a team approach. These critically ill patients are best treated in trauma centers that are equipped and staffed twenty-four hours a day to manage these complex problems. An experienced, efficient emergency-room staff of physicians and nurses is mandatory. One physician, usually a general surgeon or an anesthesiologist with expertise in multiple trauma, must coordinate the trauma team, which consists of general, vascular, orthopedic, thoracic, urological, and neurological surgeons. Only in this setting can correct decisions on resuscitation and surgical priorities be made expeditiously (29).

and

The goals of administration of anesthetic drugs are the same for trauma victims as for "normal" patients awaiting surgery: amnesia, analgesia, muscle relaxation, and control of cardiovascular and pulmonary responses. Traumatic injury may alter priorities with regard to the type or dosage of drugs administered . . . It should be evident that intraoperative care of the trauma patient involves far more than administering anesthetic agents. Resuscitation, assessment, and care begun in the field and the emergency room must continue through the operating room phase. The anesthesiologist must therefore be familiar with the natural history of the multisystem "disease" of trauma and with the many complications that can result (30).

and

In general, the anesthesiologist must be an active member of the trauma team. To provide maximal service and function most efficiently his or her involvement must begin at the earliest stage and continue through the immediate postoperative period. The ability to contribute, however, may be overshadowed by the ability to worsen the overall circumstance. This is certainly possible if he or she is not aware of the extent or magnitude of injury, results of the initial diagnostic evaluation, objectives for resuscitation, and ultimate intraoperative and postoperative stabilization. It is imperative that the overall anesthetic management and in particular his or her anesthetic plan is entirely consistent and in accord with these therapeutic objectives (31).

and

As surgical specialization in trauma care has improved patient outcome, so does anesthesia specialization in trauma care improve patient outcome; this specialization requires the anesthesiologist to participate in the initial resuscitation and diagnosis as well as the intraoperative anesthetic care . . . Many anesthesiologists equate trauma anesthesia with routine general anesthesia; however, trauma is a disease with unique features that affect anesthetic management. The victim of multiple blunt injuries suffered in a high-speed automobile accident has absorbed many thousands of foot-pounds of energy. Such a patient will have extensive cellular injury in many organ systems as well as several lesions requiring surgical correction for optimal healing. Thus, the trauma anesthesiologist will be required to provide anesthesia for many procedures and participate in prolonged critical care of this patient to provide the opportunity for a good recovery. The anesthesiologist inexperienced with trauma care will tend to underestimate the severity of the blunt trauma patient's illness on admission and be more concerned with a hypothetical full stomach than with the patient's total care (32).

and

Anesthetic management of the trauma victim should not be an isolated event but a significant component of the continuum of care if one is to provide the best chance of successful recovery for the victim. Its primary objective is to salvage a live individual with intact renal function. This is accomplished by preoperative, intraoperative, and postoperative management directed toward the establishment and maintenance of a normal physiological state. The pathway to this stabilization is multifaceted and encumbered with controversy . . . the approach must be systematic and preplanned but flexible. Constant awareness of potential catastrophes and attention to detail are mandatory. One should be thoroughly familiar with invasive monitoring techniques and their interpretation. Only then can the necessary therapy be instituted appropriately and without undue delay . . . In cases of trauma all too often the medical team is impressed by the grossly evident lesion and forgets to check for the more subtle, often more serious, injuries. Preoperative anesthetic management needs to be thorough

but expeditious. For this reason, a systematic evaluation is required . . . Knowledge of the medical history of the patient and the cause of trauma is imperative. Special efforts should be made to detect preexisting coronary artery disease, treated hypertension, diabetes mellitus, asthma, cirrhosis, renal and neurological diseases, and endocrine dysfunction. The patient should be questioned about allergies and chronic drug therapies. The ingestion of alcohol and/or psychotropic drugs not only may have precipitated the original accident but also may make an otherwise safe anesthetic a catastrophe . . . Knowledge of the cause of the trauma—a high-speed automobile accident, a 10-foot fall, or a lawn mower accident, for example—is very helpful in evaluating the physical state of the patient (33).

and

Trauma anesthesia, to paraphrase a military surgical expression, is "meatball anesthesia," i.e., dive-in-the-mess/save-the-life/make-it-pretty-later . . . interventions are always some combination of two related processes: resuscitation and repair. The faster the intervention, the more resuscitation will be involved, and the less the preoperative assessment and preparation and vice versa . . . First let's recognize that there is no such person as "THE trauma patient." . . . That's why only general guidelines can be offered (broad brush strokes to a canvas) . . .

What special knowledge is needed by the anesthesiologist who is not a seasoned trauma expert? First, one general body of knowledge unstressed in the anesthesia literature is the Advanced Trauma Life Support course sponsored by the American College of Surgeons and given in various areas of the country. This course stresses the initial interventions in the first, or "golden" hour, after the patient arrives in the emergency room. In many places, the anesthesiologist is not involved at this level. Nevertheless, this course is superb training, both for the initial interventions and for the carry-through into the OR, because it allows coupling of efficient trauma evaluations, procedures, and a way of thinking to one's existing anesthesia skills . . .

Second, we don't usually think of speed and organization as "special skills"; yet for the "rolling thunder" type of case, the need is supreme. The ability to keep a perspective, to plan, to change, and to replan second-by-second as the conditions change, without getting rattled, has to be there.

Third, the ability to quickly place intravenous lines in many sites by cutdown and percutaneous cannulation is necessary. Placing arterial lines is

handy . . . Last to be mentioned, but most important, are airway intubation skills. That means
oral and nasal intubation and cricothyroidotomy.
The latter is included to underscore its importance in the earliest thoughts of the anesthesiologist.

Fourth, it is essential to have help immediately
available. Good help, indeed, is always hard to
find. Sometimes any help is hard to find. Good
help need not be skilled help, necessarily. The
anesthesiologist in a major trauma case is busier
than a one-legged man in a rump-kicking contest. Minimally he needs a good "gofer," i.e.,
someone who knows where things are kept and
above all, can follow instructions. Such resource
people rarely get mentioned, but they are invaluable. To keep a pool of helpers may require some
on-going training, but the time spent will be well
rewarded. Who these helpers may be is irrelevant—from "sanitary engineer" to hospital administrator—provided they can follow directions. The concept of the "Iron Anesthesiologist"
who fights "The Force" alone needs to dissolve
into history alongside the "Iron Surgeon" (34).

## The Trauma Anesthesiologist Must
## Understand Mechanisms of Injury

On the trauma anesthesiologist's need for
a conceptual understanding of the mechanisms of injury:

In the emergency management of the trauma
patient, the dimension of time appears to
change. When faced with the trauma patient
with multiple injuries, time shrinks to a vanishing
point. Medically correct decisions must be made
based on the sum total of one's pertinent knowledge, experience, and skill. Deliberation and
equivocation are often out of the question.
Moreover, decisions made intuitively at this critical stage of the patient's care may have serious
legal implications. It is important, therefore, to
know the common combinations of injuries occurring in the trauma patient. We must recognize
that all associated injuries may not be diagnosed
at the time of anesthesia induction, and that associated injury may be a greater threat to life than
the primary target of the surgical procedure.
Above all, we must maintain that degree of suspicion that will lead us to search for occult explanations for serious alterations in vital signs.
The average anesthesiologist has the ability,
knowledge, and tools at hand to diagnose, for
example, a pneumothorax, pericardial tamponade, or intra-abdominal hemorrhage. In addition, however, one must train oneself to suspect
these commonly associated injuries in the patient with maxillofacial or extremity trauma. One

must further refrain from empirical treatment of
the observed hypotension with a vasopressor,
feeling secure that one has done what one can
(35).

and

Professional anesthesia care is an indispensable part of the care of the trauma patient.
Modern surgical care of the trauma patient requires rapid diagnosis concurrently with resuscitation and operation. Highly skilled anesthesia
practice is required to provide intraoperative
critical care for these patients to ensure prompt
definitive surgical treatment. The anesthesiologist needs to be aware of the types of injury the
patient may have in order to prepare properly for
intraoperative management . . . Appropriate anticipation of the expected injuries that occur with
different types of trauma will direct the anesthesiologist's attention toward appropriate care for
these patients. For example, a patient with a
gunshot wound to the chest might reasonably be
expected to require a chest tube to drain the
intrapleural hemorrhage and no further surgical
care. By contrast, a person involved in a high-
speed automobile accident with blunt chest
trauma, secondary to hitting the steering wheel,
could have several serious injuries, including pulmonary or myocardial contusions, a possible
ruptured aorta or bronchus, as well as multiple
broken ribs with a flail chest. The anesthesiologist should anticipate the need for early
intubation and mechanical ventilation in such a
patient . . . Mechanical ventilation stabilizes
broken ribs, maintains contused lung at optimum
volume for healing, and prevents splinting from
pleuritic pain. Also, anesthesiologists must be
aware of certain types of organ damage that
cluster together from certain injuries. Such
knowledge will help direct the appropriate critical care to the anesthetized patient . . . In summary, the anesthesiologist must be aware of patterns of trauma in the community in order to
anticipate the types of patients who will require
anesthesia management for surgical treatment of
their injuries. Since emergency surgical treatment of trauma rarely allows the anesthesiologist
time for extensive preoperative evaluation of the
patient, a knowledge of diseases to expect in the
patient's age group, of predisposing factors that
could lead to trauma, and of how the mechanisms of injury can lead to multiple organ systems
involvement is important. The anesthesiologist
armed with this kind of knowledge can make
appropriate preoperative judgments to provide
the best possible anesthesia management, and
anticipate possible complications that may arise.
Such high-quality anesthesia care will reduce

postoperative morbidity and mortality in trauma patients (36).

and

The injured patient often presents an unstable, rapidly changing, unpredictable situation. Anesthetists spend most of their time creating or adjusting unstable physiologic systems and can be most useful in a major emergency . . . For the severely injured patient, perhaps unconscious or with a crushed chest or in shock, the assistance of an anesthetist should be requested early . . . In the care of the severely traumatized patient, conditions often are unstable and unpredictable . . . The incidence of operative and postoperative anesthetic complications is high. To give us the best chance of providing safe and effective anesthesia at minimal risk, the anesthetist must be involved in the care of the patient at the earliest possible opportunity—in the emergency ward (37).

and

The aim of the anesthetist is to allow the necessary surgery to be performed properly, safely and quickly. Injured patients present a considerable number of problems superimposed on those of elective anaesthesia. Often tissue oxygenation is maintained only by homeostatic mechanisms which may be compromised by anaesthesia. A poor anaesthetic technique may cause further problems such as increasing intracranial pressure in patients with head injuries which may then prove fatal . . . Trauma may not be confined to a single part of the body and the full extent of the damage may only become apparent after some time (30).

and

The concepts of regional burn centers and of various levels of trauma centers equipped to deal quickly and efficiently with the acutely injured patient have not only improved care and outcome for these patients, but have heightened awareness among physicians, surgeons and the lay public of the problems entailed in transporting and treating victims of this "disease." Very frequently, initial trauma management includes surgery, which may be of an emergent and hurried nature. Since anesthesiologists will be intimately involved during this critical part of the patient's course, it is vital that they understand both the effects of trauma and the effects of anesthetics on the function of various organ systems . . . As in all phases of anesthesia, perhaps the most important aspect of administering an-

esthetics is to understand the natural history of the disease of the patient. It is only with the understanding of the underlying physiology and medical aspects of the patient's disease that we can monitor the appropriate functions and safely administer drugs and medical care to the victim. This applies as much to the traumatized patient as to the obstetric patient or the patient undergoing cardiac surgery (38).

and

Trauma is the leading cause of death for persons aged 1 to 38 years. Successful management is facilitated by prehospital endotracheal intubation, transport to regional trauma centers, rapid resuscitation by an on-site team of trained physicians, timely operative intervention, and provision of care by well-prepared anesthesiologists familiar with the potential complications typical of traumatized patients. No particular anesthetic agent or technique is ideal . . . The anesthesiologist should play an active role in all phases of trauma management, including provision of postoperative intensive care and pain relief . . . The availability and level of involvement of anesthesiologists within the emergency room of individual hospitals may vary greatly. However, even if the anesthesiologist does no more than intubate the trachea of a patient, a detailed knowledge of the pathophysiology of trauma is needed . . . The operating room should be in a constant state of preparedness for trauma. Many level I trauma centers hold one operating room open as a "crash" room . . . Similarly, the anesthesia team should be in a constant state of readiness with a general plan of attack set forth before the patient arrives in the operating room . . . The anesthesiologist's skills in pain control management are seldom needed to a greater extent than in the postoperative care of the injured patient . . . Finally, anesthesiologists must be willing to work at night, to care for patients who may lack funding, and to administer anesthetics under difficult circumstances. In addition, the anesthesiologists must heed the Boy Scouts' motto to "Be Prepared" (39).

and

If the massive investment in research in heart disease, cancer, and stroke results in a reduction in the mortality of these illnesses, we may see trauma emerging as the leading cause of death in all age groups except the very old. Under these circumstances, a large proportion of the anesthesiologist's time will be consumed in caring for the primary or secondary problems of the traumatized patient. A knowledge of this care will serve us well in the future (40).

and

The anesthetist's view of the traumatized patient differs from the medical-surgical view (41).

and

The recent trend to designate certain hospitals as trauma centers will profoundly affect the practice patterns of many anesthesiologists . . . High-energy blunt trauma such as that in an automobile accident usually causes multiple injuries. Experience has taught us that patients with multiple injuries have less postoperative morbidity if all of their injuries can be treated in one procedure. This philosophy will lead to patients being in the operating room for extended periods, especially if they have multiple fractures. Therefore, it will become imperative for the anesthesiologist to turn the operating room into an intensive care unit to keep the patients as fit as possible during prolonged surgery . . . Careful attention to appropriate preoperative and intraoperative anesthesia management will improve the survival rate of patients with serious life-threatening trauma who are admitted to a trauma center. This level of excellence in anesthesia care must be achieved if all unnecessary trauma deaths are to be prevented (42).

and

The need for improved care of trauma victims has been repeatedly demonstrated. As many as 40 per cent of victims of major trauma could be saved by appropriate, expeditious care at a trauma center (43).

and

There is no room for "turf wars": the TA/CCS is a member of the trauma team and, as such, works beside the trauma surgeon for the patient's ultimate benefit. Like the trauma surgeon, the TA/CCS must be familiar with the pathophysiology and subsequent management of a large range of traumatically induced diseases: penetrating and blunt trauma, burns and inhalation injuries; hypothermia due to exposure and drowning; and the fat embolism syndrome . . . Because of the time constraints involved with treating trauma patients, it is probably more important for the TA/CCS to have a thorough knowledge of traumatic disease than for other anesthesia subspecialists to understand their re-

spective diseases; with trauma patients, there is little time for verbalizing—communication between the TA/CCS and other team members must be almost "telepathic" (44).

and

The impact of trauma on the present and future practice of anesthesiology is clear . . . Indeed trauma may emerge as the leading overall cause of death. Already trauma is the leading cause of death during the first three decades of life. Many traumatic injuries require painful surgical intervention—sometimes electively, sometimes urgently, sometimes immediately, frequently at night, and weekends and holidays. If the mortality and morbidity of traumatic injuries are to be minimized, we must understand the special anesthetic problems presented by the traumatized patient . . . Anesthetic management of the patient will be influenced by the extent of injuries, the extent of hemorrhage and replacement, and adequacy of pulmonary ventilation, the preinjury state of health, previous drug therapy, the presence of acute intoxication, and the condition of the stomach (45).

and

Trauma tends to cut across the profile of society, involving all its members and nearly all medical and surgical specialties. Improvements in rescue, transport, and resuscitation of accident victims have given anesthesiologists the opportunity to see increasing numbers of traumatized patients in operating rooms for primary and secondary surgical correction of their injuries (46).

and

The natural reaction of most doctors, when confronted by a patient with multiple major injuries at the roadside or on the factory floor, is a feeling of inadequacy in the face of the enormous problems. Only training and practice can overcome this reaction and replace it with the calmness and confidence of knowing what to do urgently and being able to do it . . . Thanks largely to the teaching and skills of anaesthetists, it is now clear that the first priority in the management of any patient with major injuries is to assess and, if necessary, treat the respiratory and cardiovascular function. This may appear to us to be stating the obvious, but there are numerous instances in apparently excellent centres, where vital priorities have been overlooked in the face of other, perhaps traumatic, but nevertheless non-urgent, injuries . . . We must ask ourselves 3 questions: 1) What can I do to preserve this patient's life? 2) What can I do to reduce the complications arising from these injuries? 3) What can I do to relieve this patient's pain? (25).

## The Role of Anesthesiologists in the Care of Central Nervous System and Chest Injuries

On the contribution of the anesthesiologist to the care of trauma of specific systems such as the central nervous system and chest injury:

Anaesthetists are best suited of all specialists to manage patients in the acute state with spinal cord injury and associated multiple injuries. The anaesthetist has to start respiratory and circulatory resuscitation immediately to improve the general condition of the patient and to avoid or reduce post-traumatic damage to the spinal cord. Otherwise an injury at level C3–C5 or any post-traumatic complication of this segment of the spinal cord may result in death from respiratory insufficiency because all respiratory muscles, including the diaphragm, are paralysed (47).

and

Head injuries continue to be a major medical and social problem, accounting for over one-third of admissions to accident units . . . Many of these accidents take place some distance from a neurosurgical unit, and anaesthetists are becoming increasingly involved in the problem of immediate and intensive care, as well as the anaesthetic management. They should therefore understand the physiological and pathological changes that can take place following head injury . . . Anaesthetists, with their particular interest in intensive care and the respiratory and cardiovascular systems, can contribute a great deal as members of a team concerned with the management of a severe head injury (48).

and

The anaesthetist's contribution to the management of head-injured patients has expanded considerably in the past few years, reflecting change in the total management of these patients. The anaesthetist now has vital responsibilities in the immediate care of the patient in the emergency room, the radiology department, during surgical interventions, and in the critical care unit . . . If the patient reaches hospital alive then theoretically, treatment of prevention of the secondary injury should prevent death . . . Pivotal to the management of the secondary injury

is the management of the airway, breathing and circulation, all areas of expertise for the anaesthetist (49).

and

The majority of traumatic spinal injuries are not admitted directly to a spinal injury unit, but present initially at the accident and emergency unit. It is at this stage that the anaesthetist may become involved in resuscitation together with the management of the spinal and associated injuries. Whilst managing the airway and ventilation in injured patients he must be suspicious of the presence of spinal instability or cord damage and aware of the possible physiological disturbances. His role may be critical in limiting nerve damage, by avoiding hypoxia and hypotension, and preventing further trauma to the cord (50).

and

When confronted with a patient suffering from severe chest injury, the task of the anaesthetist may be 3-fold: therapeutic, organizational and pedagogic . . . His therapeutic role consists in resuscitation of the patient, evaluating his vital functions and supporting, or eventually supplementing, these functions should they fail . . . If the anaesthetist is not capable or willing to perform these supplementary tasks of organization and teaching, he will still be confronted with these patients but he will be without these facilities. Nevertheless, as the specialist most proficient in resuscitation, the anaesthetist still has the clinical responsibility of the care for the patient with crushed chest. The anaesthetists in our hospital have tried to organize this 3-fold task. In the first place, the co-author of this report is responsible for an ambulance system supplying the necessary medical care at the place of the accident . . . The good results obtained and the experience gained at our hospital in caring for patients with severe chest injury confirm our opinion that the anaesthetist is, generally speaking, the person "par excellence" to take up that 3-fold therapeutic, organizational and pedagogic task. His good example, his proficiency and the necessary propaganda, together with the help of the board of directors of the hospital, should make it possible to have the necessary facilities and personnel fulfil them (51).

## The Preoperative and Intraoperative Duties of a Trauma Anesthesiologist

The specific actions to be performed by the anesthesiologist when caring for a trauma patient whether preoperatively or intraoperatively include:

Except for the most desperate emergencies, a history of preexisting disease and previous drug therapy should be obtained prior to induction of anesthesia. Special efforts should be made to detect preexisting diabetes mellitus, asthma, coronary artery disease, hypertension, cirrhosis, renal disease, and neurologic disease. The patient should be questioned about allergies and chronic drug therapy with antihypertensives, diuretics, tranquilizers, steroids, and antiarrhythmics . . . The patients are usually semiconscious and may become comatose. Immediate surgery is a necessity. Anesthesiologists must accept the responsibility for the care of these patients even though preoperative data may not exist. They usually need no anesthetics. Even small doses of potent inhaled or intravenous anesthetics may precipitate complete and irreversible cardiovascular collapse. Pain appreciation is usually abolished in this state, and patients offer little resistance to endotracheal intubation, controlled ventilation, and, for that matter, the surgical procedure. Oxygen only should be given or, at the most, very small doses of anesthetic (i.e., 0.25 MAC isoflurane) (45).

and

The mortality of anesthesia and surgery in the traumatized patient is related to the preinjury state of health. Emergency surgery in a traumatized patient is associated with a mortality two to three times the mortality of a similar procedure under elective circumstances. For example, patients with diabetes mellitus are expected to have a mortality of 4.3 percent following elective surgical procedures. This is increased to 12.7 percent following emergency surgical procedures (40).

and

When considering the choice of anaesthetic technique for any surgical emergency, it is a sound rule for the anaesthetist to adhere to those methods with which he has become familiar, making such minor modifications as the particular circumstances demand. New techniques and drugs should be reserved for "cold" cases and only added to the emergency armamentarium after practice has brought familiarity and confidence. Sound clinical judgement and thecapacity to recognize and anticipate dangeroussituations are in the long run the most valuable assets of the emergency anaesthetist . . . Time, in planned surgery, is on the side of the anaesthetist. With increasing urgency of the surgical condition this valuable asset diminishes, and the anaesthetist may be faced with the task of compressing into the space of an hour or less, preparations for which a day might not seem excessive in planned surgery. In such circumstances, a compromise has to be reached between the ideal approach and that in which optimal anaesthetic conditions are subordinated to the urgency of the surgical intervention . . . It should not need saying that matters of simple convenience should never be allowed to influence judgement when assessing the urgency of a particular case; but how many of us have not, at some time, acquiesced in some minor in-fringement of this rule? . . . It is, of course, not always the major surgical emergency that presents the greatest anesthetic problem. A "whiff of gas" or a "shot of pentothal" [is] frequently requested for the incision of an abscess, but should this happen to be sited in the pharynx such simple methods of anaesthesia can be hazardous, and safety will demand a meticulous and expert technique. A minor surgical emergency may carry a major anaesthetic risk that need not be immediately apparent; there are, for instance, an increasing number of new drugs (and some older ones, such as cortisone) that are given to patients without any warning of their potential danger in anaesthesia. It is unfortunately in trivial cases that the anaesthetist is likely to be taken unawares, and a careful preliminary interrogation and examination of the patient is as important in minor as in major surgical emergencies (52).

and

Advances in anesthesia for trauma have often paralleled major military conflict. Both general and regional anesthesia has been used at times with equally beneficial and devastating effects. Present civilian practice tends toward the use of balanced general anesthesia. Regional techniques are useful for isolated limb injuries and injuries in which significant hypovolemia is not suspected, but techniques associated with major sympathetic blockade are relatively contraindicated in the face of hypovolemia (39).

and

Optimal surgical treatment of the multisystem blunt trauma patient often requires the operative correction of many injured systems at the initial setting. The operations are organized so that the most life-threatening problem is corrected first, followed by procedures that correct less life-threatening conditions. This may require the patient to be in the operating room for prolonged periods, occasionally longer than 24 hours. Such lengthy operations require the anesthesia team to provide an intensive care environment in the operating room. The benefits of such surgery (e.g., less postoperative morbidity) outweigh the disadvantages of prolonged procedures. Additional advantages include decreased blood loss from fractures that are surgically reduced and stabilized with internal fixation (compared with the loss from fractures that are stabilized with splints or casts) and greater pulmonary toilet with fewer pulmonary complications . . . a patient whose musculoskeletal system is repaired during the first operation is often able to get out of bed within 2 or 3 days postinjury. Such early mobilization allows rehabilitative physical therapy to start early in the hospital course, with improved results (32).

and

Patients requiring surgery for trauma are a varied group, ranging from the healthy individual whose injuries have not altered his normal physiology, to the individual with serious preexisting medical problems whose injury has caused further deterioration of his general medical condition. This latter type of patient may also be taking a number of different medications, some or all of which may interact with anesthetic agents. While the patient population varies a great deal, a number of problems are commonly encountered in patients with traumatic injuries. These may include: 1) inadequate time to perform a thorough preanesthetic workup; 2) those patients who are alert are very apprehensive; 3) full stomach; 4) intoxication; 5) hemodynamic instability and 6) multiple injuries, sometimes unrecognized. Thus, at no time is the skill and adaptability of the anesthesiologist more severely tested. The range of problems cannot always be anticipated since the full extent of the injuries may not be known preoperatively, past history may be sparse or nonexistent, and complicated medical problems may not be adequately controlled prior to surgery. This latter factor is often cited as the major reason for the higher mortality rate associated with emergency than with elective surgery . . . The anesthesiologist must have a systematic way of approaching the perioperative management of trauma victims and yet be able to rapidly diagnose and alter this management in response to changes in the patient's status (53).

and

In providing anesthesia for the multiply in-

jured patient the anaesthetist may find that he is faced with a variety of choices . . . After discussing some of the features of multiply injured patients, it can be concluded that anaesthesia in these victims is full of pitfalls. Because anaesthetic management of these patients must take into account many factors, including preexisting disease and medication, concomitant injuries outside the range of planned operations, the condition at the time of operation, the lesions found and the facilities available as well as the foreseen postoperative complications, no single method of anaesthesia can be described. The choice of anaesthesia in emergency accident surgery is seldom easy or straightforward and the way in which each individual patient should be treated can only be determined by the skilful experienced anesthetist . . . Quite often pre-existing conditions are unrecognized and then the choice of methods must rest on the nature of the injuries and the experience and skill of the anaesthetist (52).

and

As soon as possible after being summoned to prepare for a trauma case in the operating room, the anesthesiologist should conduct his own evaluation of the patient's condition. This involves a personal visit to the emergency room or to the bedside for a preanesthetic interview (54).

and

Frequently the anesthesiologist is summoned to aid in treating a severely injured patient in the emergency room. His primary responsibility should be to evaluate the patency of the airway and the adequacy of ventilation and circulation . . . The choice of anesthesia varies from the use of oxygen alone for the patient who is unconscious from shock, central nervous system trauma, or alcohol intoxication, to the full range of anesthetic agents for the patient in whom circulatory stability has been established (55).

and

The importance of trauma as a cause of death and disability in our society is increasing daily. The trauma patient presents challenges in establishment of adequate ventilation, resuscitation of shock, diagnosis of associated injuries and evaluation of preexisting medical conditions. The patient's prognosis depends on how well these challenges can be met in the time available prior to surgical correction (56).

## The Critical Care Role of the Trauma Anesthesiologist

On the role of the anesthesiologist in critical care areas and on providing critical care for trauma patients in the operating room:

Clinical anaesthesia is a form of intensive patient care in which the anaesthetist not only provides surgical anaesthesia for his patient, but also controls the supportive procedures. The anaesthetist has become experienced in the maintenance of artificial ventilation of the lungs, the prevention and treatment of shock, the art of resuscitation and the use of monitoring equipment. He is thus ideally suited to extend his knowledge into the postoperative period and the intensive care situation. In many hospitals, the anaesthetist has taken a lead in the planning and operation of intensive care units. This is in part due to accidental circumstances, and the need for an anaesthetist in other than a subsidiary role has been questioned . . . In summary, it may be said that the anaesthetist has a large part to play in intensive patient care. He is, however, only one member of the therapeutic team which must work together for the benefit of the patient. For efficient team work the anaesthetist must be prepared to learn from the disciplines of his colleagues and to teach in the areas where he can contribute from his special knowledge. Intensive care is no more than the intensive practice of good medicine in a favorable environment (57).

and

Since the advent of intensive care units in the 1960s anaesthetists have played a major part in their organization and development. Although these units, especially in district hospitals, are usually multidisciplinary, they all cater for critically ill patients, most of whom need some form of life support, either respiratory, cardiac, or renal. Anaesthetists, by virtue of their training in the use of mechanical ventilation, patient monitoring, applied pharmacology, and the management of fluid balance, are particularly suited to this type of work, both from the clinical and administrative points of view (58).

## The Prehospital Role of the Trauma Anesthesiologist

On the role of and deployment of anesthesiologists to the prehospital arena to provide sophisticated on-site trauma care:

A significant improvement in the morbidity and mortality figures is now likely to depend on the application of these resuscitative skills and techniques at the accident site and during transportation . . . The title of this symposium is "The role of anesthesiologists in the treatment of multiple injuries." . . . I would put it to you that our role is not only to practice in hospital the skills and techniques and therapy that we hear about at this symposium. We must also take an active part in resuscitation rescue schemes at the accident site in mobile resuscitation units, where we can practice our skills at the earliest possible moment and, therefore, to the best advantage of our patients. We can then see what the problems are of conducting resuscitation in the far from ideal conditions of the roadside, factory floor or inside an ambulance, and amend our techniques to suit these situations. Finally, it is also our place to provide training in resuscitation and care of the severely injured to general practitioners, the ambulance and emergency services and the members of the general public (25).

and

Most anesthesiologists' involvement in the transport and field phase of trauma care has been minimal. Since the management of this controversial phase of trauma care affects each anesthesiologist providing care to the injured, a review of the issue is warranted (59).

and

In the severely injured the greater number of hospital deaths occur within the first few hours following admission, at least one-third within 6 h and more than one-half within 24 h . . . Appropriate intensive management of this time is of vital importance and will largely depend on the immediate availability of adequate numbers of staff skilled in the techniques of resuscitation and experienced in the difficult matter of diagnosis in cases of multiple injuries, and recognition of priorities in emergency treatment. There is good evidence also that a proportion of these early hospital deaths [is] preventable if the fundamental principles of maintenance of a patent airway and adequate alveolar ventilation, along with control and adequate replacement of blood loss, are adhered to rigorously. Apart from the question of immediate survival, the quality of ultimate recovery may well depend on effective early management of the severely injured. Nowhere is this more obvious than in the treatment of head injuries . . . Depending on circumstances, the patient may be admitted to hospital having benefited from continuous resuscitation from the scene of the accident. The arguments in favor of mobile resuscitation teams attached to District General Hospitals are well known and the value of such an arrangement is clearly demonstrated where the number of accident victims justifies the organizational difficulties and expense involved . . . Nowhere has the anaesthetist a more critical or fundamental role than as part of the hospital accident team dealing with the immediate care of critically injured patients (27).

and

In France, the medical organization for the treatment of casualties is operated by anesthesiologists who are qualified to perform ALS, preanesthetic evaluation en route, anesthesia for the multitrauma patient, and postanesthetic resuscitation in a continuum from the accident scene to the ICU (11).

and

The TA/CCS also usually provides mobile coverage for the patient during intrahospital transfers, for example, to the computed tomography suite; he/she must anticipate and guard against any monitoring or stability problems that may be inherent with moving a critically ill patient (ventilatory and hemodynamic support) . . . In extreme cases when the unstable trauma patient absolutely cannot be moved, the TA/CCS may have to provide anesthetic coverage within the intensive care unit. In some locales in the United States, the TA/CCS is also being used to transport the seriously ill from the field to the trauma center or from one center to another aboard specially equipped aircraft (20).

and

Care of the critically ill or injured patient during transport—whether from the field, between care facilities, or intrahospital—plays an important role in ultimate patient outcome. Whatever the transport situation, it can engender various physiologic changes, depending on factors such as patient profile and logistics (for example, space, electrical power, available equipment). The individual in charge of patient care, therefore, must be able to ensure proper maintenance of the critical care equipment, monitor the patient's physiologic data, and render appropriate clinical intervention as necessary; that is, he or she must ensure that the level of care during transport equals that in a fixed intensive care unit (60).

and

In the Federal Republic of Germany an increasing number of emergency medical services are being organized. Adequately qualified physicians, often anaesthetists, are sent with well-trained emergency medical technicians in specially equipped vehicles or helicopters to the person requiring help . . . The chances of survival for multiple injury patients are significantly improved by exact medical care and monitoring, at the scene, during transport, and by cooperation between the emergency service and the clinic. In addition practice as an emergency physician offers excellent possibilities for training and proficiency of anaesthetists (61).

and

The basic alphabet of resuscitation (Airway, Breathing, Circulation) is familiar to most anaesthetists and is as applicable to the uncontrolled trauma of injuries as to the controlled events of active surgery. Anaesthetists, therefore, have something to offer in both the practice of and training for immediate care of the injured (62).

and

Experienced anesthesiologists who have become sophisticated life supporters for the most critically ill patients in the operating room have much more to offer outside the operating room. Their expertise should be applied to the care of patients in the emergency room and even the prehospital arena (63).

and

Paramedics should be taught the most effective means of airway control. One significant development in the care of the traumatized patient has been the emergency ambulance system and the emergency medical technicians . . . They are taught a variety of techniques of establishing an airway. Of these, oral endotracheal intubation leads to a high incidence of survivors of cardiac and respiratory arrest. Paramedics, properly trained, have a high incidence of successful intubation and a low incidence of serious complications . . . The OR experience is obviously a valuable addition to the paramedics' training and to the victim of a critical illness or injury who requires intubation in the field. The OR experience, which was originally offered by many community hospitals, has become less and less available. Progressively, the anesthesiology staffs have withdrawn from the training of paramedics. The reason given is fear of medico-legal difficulties and fear of an unacceptable complication rate. Many anesthesiologists engaged in this training can recount anecdotes of minor complications and potentially major problems, which are troublesome to the patient, unsettling to the anesthesiologist, and absolutely terrifying to the malpractice carrier. If anesthesiologists are unwilling to participate in the training of paramedics in this technique, where are they to receive the experience? (40).

## Battlefield Trauma Anesthesia

Some comments on military/battlefield anesthesia, which may be considered a specialization within trauma anesthesia:

Military (trauma) anaesthesia resembles anaesthesia in civil practice with the following exceptions—the patient is not prepared for operation; induction must be rapid and recovery must follow quickly; a large number of cases require treatment at one time, and, finally, the anaesthetic is often administered under trying conditions with improvised apparatus. If these difficulties are recognized and met, the well-trained anaesthetist in civil life will not fail to render his country a great service when called to the battle line (or a civilian disaster) (64).

and

In military practice many unprepared patients must be anesthetized speedily, frequently with improvised apparatus and in such a manner that their recovery is complete and rapid. Service patients usually are healthy, but frequently they are suffering from hemorrhage and shock, which, in addition to excitement, may cause them to vomit food eaten ten to twenty-four hours previously (65).

and

Had we discussed anesthesia for the surgery of trauma five years ago, we would have considered the increasing number of traffic, industrial and home accidents. Today, however, we must in addition to these, concern ourselves with the casualties associated with the world wide conflict in which our country is now involved. In this regard, we find our problem quite different from those of the first world war in that civilians as well as our armed forces are subject to attack . . . We are confronted with a problem quite different from the last war, namely, that of civilian casualties, besides the wounded soldiers. Developments in anesthesia during the past ten years have contributed much to the improved care of

civilian casualties in peace time. First the physician anesthetist has trained himself, not only in the improved anesthesia technic, but in the evaluation and treatment of the patient's general condition and in this way is able to relieve the surgeon of much responsibility (66).

and

An anaesthetist preparing equipment for such a mission should anticipate the type of service he will have to provide. Transport of drugs, fluids, and anaesthetic gases may be curtailed at any time and he should have the means to be completely self-sufficient for an indefinite period. The use of ketamine and local analgesic techniques is extremely valuable but a basic apparatus for general anesthesia and IPPV is also essential. Most disposable pieces of equipment can, in fact, be resterilized a limited number of times, but a supply of nondisposables is also recommended (67).

and

What are the basic requirements for the selection of an anesthesiologist who is to be stationed at the front line and who may suddenly find himself immersed in battle? The magic word is "experience." It may in part be gained by an anesthesiologist who regularly works in a situation very similar to the combat zone, e.g. in a sophisticated civilian trauma center that admits patients after high-speed vehicular accidents or casualties from a high-crime-rate neighborhood, where penetrating injuries are common . . . The battlefield anesthesiologist must also be experienced in intensive care doctrine and techniques. The role of the anesthetist in the battlefield situation is not restricted to the OR. A major part of his/her workload is in the admitting area with involvement in triage, immediate resuscitation, airway maintenance, and monitoring for the severely injured patient. For this purpose, experience in the prehospital emergency care of trauma is absolutely necessary . . . Working in these programs requires that the anesthesiologist be extremely competent with management of both elective and emergency cases, that he/she possesses the ability to quickly adapt to an adverse and often rapidly changing environment and to be familiar with a wide range of specialized equipment adapted for field use (68).

and

In the long past anesthesia has been looked upon as an operating room service solely. The term "anesthesiology" has been utilized in recent years to designate a larger service. It includes skill in the use of the various technical maneuvers and drug administration found useful in putting patients "at ease" during surgery, but it goes much further than that. The supervision of physiologic processes, especially the function of respiration, during depression following head and chest injuries; after drug administration for pain relief; after gas poisoning, in shock and in pneumonia, involves the use of methods familiar to the anesthetist. The insertion of artificial airways in the presence of blood and mutilation of the respiratory tract, the administration of artificial atmospheres, the cleansing of the tracheobronchial tree when contaminated, artificial respiration, the injection of locally acting anesthetic drugs to relieve the pain of fractured ribs and other bones, all these are technical procedures familiar to the well-trained anesthetist and useful for the safety and comfort of the injured. In military practice such service ought often to be rendered under field conditions. The need for medical officers especially trained along these lines is obvious . . . In the rush of plans to transpose surgery from a peacetime to a wartime basis, a certain element of hysteria is likely to creep in. We are apt to lose sight of details of prime importance. The matter of anesthesia is one such detail. In civil practice every surgeon has provided himself with what he believes to be a satisfactory solution of the anesthesia problem. Transferred to military duty, he can scarcely hope to take with him an intact surgical team as he has organized it at home. Even if this were possible, anesthesia for mutilated fighters and their victims is a more complicated problem than civilian practice of the relief of pain. The care of respiratory embarrassment in a patient in a civilian hospital is difficult. When the face is shot away or the pleural cavity laid open, maintenance of the respiratory function taxes the skill of the most adept . . . It is highly desirable that those who are formulating plans for medical military preparedness may include the assignment of at least one well-trained physician as anesthetist to each hospital unit. Arrangements ought also to be made for the training of an adequate number of medical officers in anesthesiology so that surgeons may be left free of the worry of providing such service for themselves. It is to be hoped that the present mobilization may include provision for such special training and assignment of medical officers from the beginning, without waiting for the demonstration of such need after field operations have begun (69).

and

The modern civilian anaesthetist employs his special skills for many purposes besides the ac-

tual administration of anaesthetics and, in the same way, the military anaesthetist has assumed responsibility for the resuscitation of battle casualties and has contributed to the management of Intensive Care Units (ICU) in field hospitals . . . The anaesthetist working in a service hospital treating battle casualties now assumes responsibilities relating to resuscitation of the injured, the administration of anaesthetics and postoperative intensive care (70).

## Research Agenda for Trauma Anesthesia

On future inroads in research that must be made to scientifically advance the field of trauma anesthesia:

Multiple trauma victims also require operative intervention frequently, and the potential impact of the anesthetic on the multiple trauma victim is considerable. This is an especially important problem when closed head trauma is present, because the various anesthetics have major effects on cerebral blood flow, cerebral oxygen consumption, and intracranial pressure. Patients with extensive burns often require multiple anesthetics during their treatment; these individuals may be especially fragile from an anesthetic viewpoint. This is especially evident in those with fluid and electrolyte imbalance, sepsis, and intraoperative blood loss associated with debridement and grafting of the burn. Patients with septic shock often require anesthesia for operations as well. Typical examples include abdominal surgery for resection of gangrenous bowel or drainage of abscesses in those with septicemia . . . In the laboratory, the influences of anesthetic agents on experimental results are perhaps not given adequate consideration. Without exception, the anesthetics have major influences on cardiac performance, peripheral circulatory control, regional blood flows, pulmonary function, respiration, metabolism, and oxygen consumption. Since changes in these may influence the outcome following shock, it is essential that the effects of the anesthetics be clearly understood by the laboratory investigator who is studying any of the various forms of shock . . . There is a need for further evaluation of the effects of anesthetics in both laboratory animals and in humans during the various shock states (71).

## Trauma Prevention

On the role of anesthesiologists in trauma prevention:

Trauma challenges the anesthesiologist with additional responsibilities and reminds us of our fullest duties as physicians. We need to prevent trauma. We need to spend more time preventing fights with handguns, to do more work educating the public about the risks of not using seat belts when driving, and to expend more energy to reduce the amount of alcohol being consumed before and while driving (45).

## Harsh Realities of Current Trauma Anesthesia Practice

And, finally, some comments on the harsh realities of today:

In many areas of the country, anesthesia is not readily available for emergency department interventions, and thus trauma anesthesia is delegated to the emergency department physician (72).

and

. . . a quick review of the research literature dealing with trauma reveals an appalling paucity of material when compared with the amounts generated about other diseases. And much of the trauma research that does exist has been developed by surgeons and paraprofessionals (e.g., paramedics); anesthesiologists must become more active in the researching and reporting of their role in trauma management as required by the ACS for Level I trauma centers . . . TA/CCSs, and anesthesiologists in general, need to improve their teaching performance. More need to become ATLS certified and progress to the instructor level (20).

and

The health care industry has recently joined many other major US industries that must survive in a fiercely competitive arena. In response, hospitals are managed like businesses, receiving advice from consultants and treating illnesses and patients as "product lines." It is essential to ensure excellent clinical care for severely injured patients during this period of transition (73).

To forge ahead against the opposition of a reluctant and even outraged medical profession as in the great tradition of the advocates of accident hospitals throughout their history . . . General surgeons, traditionally captains of the trauma-center team, are learning that as the complexity of injuries increases that they are called upon to provide more and more critical care and perform less and less surgery (74).

and

There is much for anesthesiologists to learn from emergency physicians, and the need for knowledge transfer in the opposite direction is just as apparent. For example, trauma patients may present to the operating room volume replenished, but with hypothermic solutions. Patients with elevated intracranial pressure may be intubated in the emergency department without pharmacologic attempt to ameliorate the resulting pressure increase. Muscle relaxants may or may not be optimally utilized. On the other hand, many anesthesiologists are unfamiliar with important advances in the pharmacology and treatment of cardiac arrest. Others may benefit from emergency physicians' expertise in many aspects of trauma management. Finally, there are areas in which the specialties need to combine forces, as in the use of inhalational agents for status asthmaticus and status epilepticus, or in disaster planning and management . . . Sixty seven per cent of the anesthesiologists assist in trauma resuscitation efforts in the ED, on either an on-call or in-house basis . . . The close association of emergency medicine with this field reinforces the need for cross-over of information between the two fields (75).

and

In trauma resuscitation, emergency physicians and anesthesiologists have an opportunity to utilize fully their many diagnostic and procedural skills. There is a sense of pride in working in a hospital that can effectively handle major trauma . . . On a specialist level, trauma center designation may mean changes in roles. The presence of an in-house trauma surgeon who assumes command of the resuscitation effort does leave the emergency physician with an uncertain role at times. Except in teaching hospitals, it is unusual for trauma anesthesiologists to be in-house, and thus emergency physicians, who routinely handle cardiac arrests, often become the local in-house airway expert. Of course, in a multiply injured patient, all three physicians can and do optimally work as a team simultaneously, with, for example, one intubating, one starting and maintaining lines, and one placing chest tubes (76).

and

In the presenting changing climate of health care provisions, there may be a decreasing willingness on the part of the hospital administrators to admit patients with severe multisystem injuries to their institutions for financial reasons despite the surgeon's wishes. This could have a devastating impact on the care of these patients (73).

and

Physicians face familiar economic challenges. In addition to the indigent and DRG problems, the trauma victim often requires a greater time commitment than do elective cases with similar rates of reimbursement. The trauma victim frequently arrives at inconvenient hours, is often unappreciative of the care given, and is perceived to pose an increased medicolegal risk. To surmount these problems, a select few physicians with a strong commitment to high-quality trauma care and willing to accept the fundamental limitations should constitute the nucleus of the trauma treatment team. If there is insufficient commitment by local physicians, out-of-region physicians should be recruited (5).

and

Unfortunately, while many hospitals have eagerly sought trauma center designation, hoping to gain favorable publicity and prestige, they often realize later the great expense involved in treatment of the many indigent patients who so often seem to get into traumatic situations (76).

and

Major trauma centers will continue to go by the wayside and the major burden of trauma care will fall on those few institutions that truly put "patients before pride" with the understanding that trauma care, although a socially rewarding experience, is not a financially rewarding experience (77).

## PRESENT STATE OF AFFAIRS

### "Trauma Anesthesia" versus "Anesthesia for Trauma"

Why should anesthesiologists be involved to such an extent with trauma care? After all, in the American system there are surgeons and emergency medicine specialists to do this. The answer is complex. First are all of the reasons cited above. Second, the anesthesiologist is the only individual who both is properly trained to render the necessary critical care (e.g., airway management, shock resuscitation including the use and interpre-

tation of invasive devices) and can perform these functions as a continuum from the moment transport to the trauma center begins through recovery in the intensive care units, both in and out of the operating rooms. Neither the surgeon nor the emergency medicine physician can do this. Anesthesiology is basically the perioperative medical management of the surgical patient. As many as 90% of trauma patients do not initially require a surgeon. The anesthesiologist who has received specialized training in intensive care medicine, trauma management, and field medicine is the ideal "life support physician" (20, 78, 79).

Third, our experience serving as evaluators for the designation and recertification of facilities as trauma centers has shown that those centers that do not utilize anesthesiologists as "frontline" care providers for trauma patients have a definite reduction in quality of care, which becomes obvious through such means as chart review. In these instances we have seen various examples of inappropriate and/or untimely application of critical techniques (e.g., lack of the use of appropriate pharmacologic adjuncts to airway management, delayed institution of invasive monitoring, grossly inadequate resuscitation), all of which basically stem from the absence of the "thinking processes" of an anesthesiologist serving as part of the trauma team. This is despite the fact that, in the early days of trauma system design, the presence of an anesthesiologist on the trauma team was strongly suggested (10).

Considering this same issue from the anesthesiologist's standpoint, we have already shown that the anesthesiologist performs a number of important duties when responding to a trauma patient in the emergency room (or sooner, in the field), such as airway control, pain management, and fluid resuscitation. Further, smooth and safe transfer to the operating room is enhanced by early involvement of the anesthesiologist in the trauma case. Anesthesiologists who opt to wait in the operating room for the trauma patient to surprise them will have to anesthetize a patient whom they know nothing about, will have to accept whatever monitoring and resuscitation lines are available, and will have to be prepared to accept chastisement from irate surgeons to "hurry up." On the other hand, involvement in the management of the trauma patient from the beginning will establish the anesthesiologist as a partner on the trauma team, allow the generation of a meaningful preanesthetic record, and allow the timely positioning of appropriate fluid administration and monitoring lines. The ACS standards (10) for trauma center organization require an anesthesiologist to respond to a trauma admission because the superiority of this scenario is well recognized.

Fourth, in many parts of the world outside the United States, anesthesiologists do in fact serve as the frontline trauma care providers, almost to the exclusion of surgeons and other specialists (except as specifically needed), and they do the job well (11–15, 80).

Fifth, these developments are only logical. As in other medical fields, various anesthesia subspecialties already exist (e.g., cardiac anesthesiology) to manage the pathophysiologic and epidemiologic peculiarities of different patient populations and to immerse practitioners completely in their condition-specific body of knowledge, equipment, and techniques. Cardiac patients are treated by a group of medical specialists who devote most of their time to the management of cardiac diseases: cardiologists, cardiac surgeons, and cardiac anesthesiologists. Similarly, there are neuroanesthesiologists, pediatric anesthesiologists, obstetric anesthesiologists, and anesthesiologists who devote most of their time to critical care medicine. From this perspective there is more than adequate reason to justify the development of trauma anesthesia (Tables 1.2 and 1.3).

Last, nurturing the development of "trauma anesthesia" will provide for the desirable third and fourth standard deviations of the Gaussian distribution representing current practice, thus "pushing back the envelope" with respect to creative innovations and contributions to the field. However, de-

**Table 1.2.   Characteristics of the Trauma Patient Population and Its Perioperative Management[a]**

Peak incidence: summer (July), weekend (Saturday), night
Often presents with a disease constellation (e.g., unconsciousness, increased intracranial pressure, hypoxia, and hypercarbia)
Patient identification/history often unknown
"Full stomach" airway considerations
Lengthy OR[b] procedures: multiple/serial/simultaneous, diagnostic/therapeutic
Frequent development of iatrogenic side effects (e.g., complications of massive transfusion)
Intraoperative anesthetic management often only "supportive" (i.e., administration of oxygen and muscle relaxant)
Wide range of advanced intraoperative management techniques often necessary (e.g., independent lung ventilation)
"Critical care" performed in the OR
High level of medicolegal problems

[a] From Grande CM, Stene JK, Barton CR. The trauma anesthesiologist. Md Med J 1988;37:531–536.
[b] OR, operating room.

spite any other "pro" or "con" arguments, this is an *ethical* issue. Knowing that so many people are injured appeals to our duty and responsibility as physicians to address the problem and provide the best solutions.

Although American surgeons have recognized the need for surgical specialists in trauma care for several years, for the most part American anesthesiologists have not recognized trauma anesthesia as a subspecialty of anesthesia. In many cases, anesthesiologists who function as TA/CCSs have have achieved better rapport with trauma surgeons and emergency medicine physicians than with other anesthesiologists. This is exemplified by common references by anesthesiologists to "anesthesia for trauma," which, although the difference is subtle, is distinct from "trauma anesthesia," which implies a true commitment to comprehensive trauma care. The development of better techniques for anesthetizing and providing critical care for trauma patients will require improved communication among TA/CCSs, other traumatologists, and other anesthesia specialists.

Some might argue that development of

**Table 1.3. Areas of Interest in the Subspecialty of Trauma Anesthesia and Critical Care**

Introduction to trauma and trauma care systems
  Trauma statistics and demographics
  Trauma centers, trauma programs, trauma
    systems
  Concepts of trauma care (e.g., "golden hour")
  Role of the trauma anesthesia/critical care
    specialist
  Economics of trauma
Prehospital phase
  Field stabilization (e.g., airway management/
    resuscitation)
  Anesthesia/analgesia in the field (e.g., equipment,
    pharmacologic agents, techniques)
  Emergency medical services systems
    administration/management
  Critical care transport (e.g., scene evacuation)
Intrahospital phase
  Preinduction/induction
  Mechanisms of injury
  Airway management (emergent and elective)
  Resuscitation
  Analgesia and sedation (e.g., pain control that
    does not interfere with serial neurologic
    evaluation yet permits completion of diagnostic
    studies such as computed tomography)
Intraoperative/anesthetic maintenance
  Perioperative anesthetic management of the
     trauma patient
    Inhalation agents
    Noninhalation agents
    Adjunctive agents
    Muscle relaxants
    Regional anesthesia
    Blood, blood component, and fluid therapy
     (e.g., various solutions, blood substitutes,
     effects of massive transfusion and their
     prevention, transfusion equipment)
  Perioperative anesthetic management of trauma
    of various organ systems
    Multisystem/multitrauma (e.g., priorities)
    Neurologic
    Maxillofacial/ophthalmologic
    Musculoskeletal (orthopedic)
    Thoracoabdominal
  Perioperative anesthetic management of special
    subpopulations of trauma patients
    Burns/inhalation injury
    Geriatric
    Pediatric
    Obstetric

Perioperative anesthetic management of trauma
    patients with common preexisting diseases
  Cardiovascular disease (e.g., hypertension,
    coronary artery disease)
  Diabetes
  Obesity
  Pulmonary disease (e.g., asthma, emphysema)
  Seizure disorder
  Sickle cell disease/trait
  Chronic renal failure
  Cirrhosis (ethanol abuse)
  Substance abuse
Immediate postoperative critical care/postanesthesia
  recovery
  Acute medical problems in the postoperative
    trauma patient
    Cardiovascular
    Respiratory
    Fluid/electrolyte/metabolic
    Bleeding and thrombosis
Extended postoperative critical care/recuperative
  phase
  Influence of anesthesia on the development of
    shock/multisystem failure
  Common critical care problems in the trauma
    patient
    Adult respiratory distress syndrome
    Acute renal failure
    Sepsis
    Postneurologic injury (e.g., persistent
     intracranial hypertension)
    Gastrointestinal complications
    Nutritional support
    Pain management
    Reoperation/follow-up surgery
Special considerations
  Critical care transport (i.e., long-range, extrahos-
    pital, interhospital, and intrahospital)
  Hyperbaric medicine
  Wilderness/environmental medicine (e.g.,
    hypothermia, frostbite)
  Quality assessment and assurance
  Ergonomics of trauma anesthesia
  Organ salvage and transplantation
  Anesthesia in difficult situations
    Military/battlefield anesthesia
    Natural/man-made disasters
    Civilian mass casualty
    "Third world" situations
    Environmental extremes (e.g., high altitude,
     post-nuclear event)

---

this newest subspecialty (which, in fact, may be the oldest) will cause further "fracturing" of the profession and that, with respect to anesthesia care providers, "everyone does trauma" (81). While these points may be true, the facts and present state of affairs speak for themselves.

For example, at a recent annual national meeting of anesthesiologists in the United States, a total of *2 hours* of a week-long meeting was devoted to the care of trauma patients (82). In past meetings, the subject of trauma has been neglected altogether. This is despite the fact that, depending upon locality, certifying agencies for trauma centers mandate that a specific number of continuing medical education (CME) credits in *specifically* trauma-related courses be obtained annually (e.g., 20 CME credits) by anesthesiologists responsible for the care of trauma patients (83).

Further, one of the main reasons for mismanagement of trauma patients is faulty judgment, possibly stemming from limited experience (84). Thus, perhaps not everyone should "do trauma," as "cardiac anesthesia" is practiced by a limited number of subspecialists. (As an analogy, consider that not all aircraft pilots are jet fighter pilots, experimental pilots, or astronauts.) Today, an increasing array of specialized equipment and management techniques (e.g., high-volume rapid fluid infusion/warming devices) requires the attention of a devoted individual. Also, it has been stated that, for clinical staff members to maintain proficiency, a minimum of 350 to 1000 patients should be admitted annually to the trauma center where they practice (depending upon the purported sophistication of care, i.e., level I versus level II). Many facilities that are currently designated as trauma centers certainly do not handle this volume of trauma cases (85).

There are many reasons for the secondary role of trauma anesthesiologists in American trauma centers. There has been a shortage of anesthesiologists during the critical period of trauma center development. Also, reimbursement patterns for anesthesiologists have rewarded them for staying in the operating room. Surgeons frequently are given monetary support to staff trauma centers; however, anesthesiologists are rarely given adequate renumeration for maintaining "standby" availability at trauma centers. Anesthesiologists receive very little cooperation from third-party payers for reimbursement of physicians' services in the emergency room or in prehospital care. The economic incentives for anesthesiologists are heavily weighted toward remaining solely in the operating room despite the professional incentives to improve patient care by preoperative and postoperative involvement.

Many anesthesiologists fear a higher risk of medical-legal complications. The possible association of undue medical-legal risks with trauma patients has not been borne out in fact (86). Critically injured patients with urgent treatment priorities are dying from their injuries; appropriate medical care may improve their outcome but only rarely make it worse. Long-term disability in trauma patients is usually a result of disease, not iatrogenic complications. Trauma care specialists frequently must testify in legal cases involving a suit over the cause of the injury, not medical malpractice. Furthermore, traumatic injuries are much more frequent in people from lower socioeconomic classes, who tend to sue less frequently than those in higher socioeconomic classes (86). Therefore, fear of malpractice lawsuits should not prevent anesthesiologists from involvement in trauma care.

Many anesthesiologists are unfamiliar with the pathophysiology of traumatic illness. Comprehension of the theories and realities of trauma care should help anesthesiologists understand that trauma anesthesia can be a rewarding and interesting specialty, but many are unwilling to spend the time and effort to gain this understanding.

Many anesthesiologists feel unwelcome in the unfamiliar settings of the emergency room, the ambulance, or the helicopter. Prehospital paramedical specialists have become very "turf-oriented," but this defensive attitude frequently can be overcome by an anesthesiologist who actively participates in paramedic training. Paramedics ideally should begin their airway management and intravenous access training in the operating room under the tutelage of anesthesiologists (40). Unfortunately, many anesthesiologists discourage the training of paramedics in airway management and endotracheal intubation within the operating room and actually may be forced to do so by hospital bylaws or insurance carriers. Forcing para-

**Table 1.4.   Most Frequent Errors in Anesthetic Management of Critically Injured Patients** [a]

1. Failing to take time and effort to evaluate the patient's vital status effectively
2. Delaying surgery for diagnostic studies on parameters either not vital for immediate surgicoanesthetic management or impossible to change in the time available
3. Allowing oneself to be rushed into a method of anesthetic management that, on reflection, one would not ordinarily choose
4. Proceeding without adequate blood products or substitutes or proceeding without adequate routes for administration of fluids (colloid and noncolloid) and electrolytes
5. Giving too much medication to patients scheduled for imminent operation, particularly during the induction phase of anesthetic management
6. Failing to have an emergency drug and equipment setup ready on a 24-hour basis
7. Failing to communicate with others involved in management of the patient
8. Failing to anesthetize the patient adequately before endotracheal intubation is begun
9. Failing to anticipate and be prepared for the possibility of regurgitation and resultant aspiration
10. Failing (on the part of the entire team) to maintain vigilance and direct personal attention during the period immediately after operation and after transfer to the recovery room or other special-care facility

[a] From Norton ML. Anesthesia for the trauma patient. In Walt AJ, Wilson RF (eds): Management of Trauma: Pitfalls and Practice. Philadelphia, Lea & Febiger, 1975, pp 163–181.

medics to learn endotracheal intubation outside the operating room may promote mutual antagonism between anesthesiologists and paramedics.

Finally, some anesthesiologists have "tunnel vision" that makes it difficult for them to participate in trauma care. For example, a patient with a blunt abdominal injury requiring urgent surgery may have recently received a large intragastric infusion of contrast medium to enhance the diagnostic utility of an abdominal computed tomographic (CT) scan, provoking a naive anesthesiologist to cancel the operation. Prejudices cause the anesthesiologist to place the highest priority on waiting many hours for the stomach to empty to prevent possible regurgitation and aspiration pneumonia, despite the fact that the theoretical risk of aspiration is actually 4.7 per 10,000 anesthetic inductions, with a mortality rate of 0.2 deaths per 10,000 anesthetic cases. This mortality rate is less than 5% for patients who actually aspirate (87). The anesthesiologist's attitude will conflict with that of the trauma surgeon, who feels that the patient will slowly bleed to death unless operated on and that there will also be an increased risk of peritonitis if operation is delayed. Anesthesiologists and surgeons who work together frequently in trauma care will both understand that the highest priority for such a patient is ensuring adequate pulmonary

gas exchange and tissue oxygenation. They will agree that this patient needs early intubation and anesthesia before a CT scan is obtained and will opt for the earliest possible transfer to the operating room. Other common errors in the trauma patient's anesthesia management, which were summarized in 1975, are probably still common today, mostly because of the lack of dedicated professionals who understand trauma anesthesia (Table 1.4) (88).

Other reasons opposing the commitment to "trauma anesthesia" include the incorrect perceptions that trauma patients are just injured people with "full stomachs"; that they are recipients of a "just punishment" (e.g., the injured drunk) or an "act of God"; that trauma patients often display pathologic behavior (e.g., belligerence, combativeness, or abusiveness, which may be the "cause" or the "effect" of their injury); that they are often substance abusers and carry a higher-than-normal incidence of transmittable disease (e.g., AIDS, hepatitis); that financial reimbursement can be poor; and that there is an increased likelihood of litigious episodes because trauma patients are part of the generalized emergency population (77, 89). Further, the hours are often long and late and the emotional expenditure is high (and many "burnouts" do occur).

Another common misconception is that trauma management is and should be the domain of surgeons (the "captain of the ship" concept) (90). This point of view is most often championed by surgeons themselves. An example can be found in the following quotation from a prominent trauma surgeon reporting on his findings in the trauma systems of the United Kingdom:

> In the accident and emergency department general surgeons were not present until called by the casualty surgeon . . . Critical care was a particularly vexing issue, as in many instances trauma was not managed by a surgeon but by a physician or anesthetist . . . I do not believe, however, that the casualty surgeons should be the central focus of trauma care. This belongs *rightfully* to the general surgeon, who should be available in designated trauma centres to coordinate resuscitation, operative care, and all postoperative care, including critical care (91).

This last statement is not true. As many as 90% of trauma patients initially do not require a surgeon. From another standpoint, in a 1980 survey, 46% of surgical program directors reported that more than 10% of all cases at their centers were due to trauma. In the same year, however, 95% of surgical residents reported that less than 5% of their experience was in trauma cases. Furthermore, 47% stated that they had managed fewer than 20 trauma cases during their residencies, and 18% had handled fewer than 10 cases (92). In the majority of medical facilities, when a major trauma victim arrives an experienced trauma surgeon will usually not be present; even if this were not the case, many experienced general surgeons must often call for the expertise of another surgical subspecialist (e.g., cardiothoracic, orthopedic, and neurosurgeons) (93, 94). These points imply that traumatology is a multidisciplinary specialty. While the Committee on Trauma of the ACS does serve as the major proponent for trauma care in the United States (perhaps because when this committee formed no other agency had already assumed this role), the fact that one is a surgeon does not automatically make one a specialist in trauma. Similar statements can be made regarding the conventional anesthesiologist.

Another entity to come on the scene in the recent past is the emergency medical physician. While these individuals must be recognized as highly trained professionals, their background in the majority of cases (we recognize that there are exceptions) leaves them unprepared to manage major trauma victims. Presently, they receive only rudimentary training in sophisticated airway management techniques (e.g., correct use of pharmacologic adjuncts) and they have minimal experience in intraoperative management and extended postoperative critical care—obvious necessities for optimal trauma management.

A third misconception relates to trauma management during war, mass casualties, or disaster situations. The civilian community seems to believe that these problems will "magically" be addressed by the military. On the other hand, to a large extent, the military regards the civilian medical community as the repository of knowledge and experience to be depended upon in the "next war." In our experience most anesthesia departments are completely unaware of what their role will be in these instances and thus can be only minimally prepared. Although it is unfortunate, we cannot conceive that the phenomena of war and other disasters will be eradicated in the near future. Therefore, it behooves us to prepare adequately for the medical fallout of these eventualities.

Generally reflecting our national ambivalence toward trauma care, public support for trauma centers is marginal. Society's attitude is then reflected in government and insurance support for trauma care which are again less than enthusiastic. One example of this is the exceedingly poor support for training in and research into traumatic illness. Americans seem to believe that trauma is a random event that occurs in an uncontrollable manner and is not preventable. Furthermore, many people feel that trauma affects the "other guy" and that they won't be injured because they have good luck and live right. In fact, injuries usually result from trauma-prone behavior and poor system design. Many injuries are preventable with behavior modification and improved system design. Witness the steady decrease in automobile fatalities that has resulted from driver education about alcohol abuse and seat belt use as well as improved crashworthiness of automobiles and roads (1).

## Formalized Training Programs for Trauma Anesthesia

Although early TA/CCSs "learned by doing," a few select centers now offer specialized fellowships in trauma anesthesiology and critical care, among them the R Adams Cowley Shock Trauma Center of MIEMSS (20). These fellowships require the same basic background as those for other physician anesthesia practitioners: a clinical base year (internal medicine, surgery, pediatrics, obstetrics/gynecology, or flexible internship); 2 to 3 years of clinical anesthesia training with a variety of techniques and patients, including neurologic, cardiothoracic, pediatric, and general surgical populations; exposure to the trauma patients admitted to the particular teaching hospital; and significant experience in intensive care settings (e.g., coronary care, medical, surgical, neurosurgical, cardiothoracic, pediatric, and neonatal), concentrating on the various aspects of critical care medicine. At the conclusion of this basic training, the candidate interested in pursuing a career as a TA/CCS should be proficient in giving a general or regional anesthetic, comfortable with various invasive techniques of airway management, and familiar with the principles of cardiopulmonary-cerebral physiology.

The next step is to seek a fellowship in trauma anesthesia and critical care at a major trauma center, as it is the only facility that can provide the TA/CCS trainee with the experience required to develop expertise. The candidate should consider the following factors when selecting a trauma center: (a) the political climate (e.g., relations with surgeons), (b) the functions and responsibilities that the TA/CCS will assume, and (c) the quality and sophistication of the trauma cen-

ter's EMS system and its internal facilities (admitting area, operating suites, and critical care areas). During the fellowship, the novice TA/CCS will develop expertise in advanced resuscitation/stabilization techniques, airway management, and critical care of the trauma patient. Important therapeutic skills include the use of vasoactive infusions, invasive cardiac monitoring, state-of-the-art respiratory therapy (e.g., high frequency and independent lung ventilation), and nutritional support.

In addition to these clinical skills, the fellow must gain conceptual knowledge of traumatology and emergency medicine, including certification in ATLS by the ACS, Committee on Trauma, and involvement with the EMS or field programs. Additional training might include elective time spent in hyperbaric medicine, infectious disease consultation, or research. Table 1.5 displays the "ideal" training schedule for a TA/CCS fellow at the R Adams Cowley Shock Trauma Center.

The functions the TA/CCS should be able to perform at the conclusion of the fellowship are listed in Table 1.6. At this point, the TA/CCS trainee is well equipped to either practice in an academic, sophisticated trauma center or serve as a consultant to a less developed trauma center and assist in its progress.

## Economic Dilemmas in Trauma Anesthesia

Today one of the most pressing issues facing trauma care systems is adverse economics (95). The problem is multifactorial and includes the following:

1. Many designated trauma centers were either unaware of the financial and logistical burden that such an operation entails or thought that these costs could be offset by revenues generated by other services offered at the center which would receive more utilization secondary to the publicity and prestige gained by being a trauma center (the "halo effect") (76). (This concept was later shown not to be supported [96]). These de-

**Table 1.5.    The Trauma Anesthesia and Critical Care Fellowship (TACCF) of the Maryland Institute for Emergency Medical Services Systems (MIEMSS)**[a]

The MIEMSS TACCF is designed to provide an anesthesiologist still in training (who has completed a minimum of 2 clinical years in an anesthesiology residency program) with a comprehensive, in-depth exposure to the entire spectrum of care through which a seriously injured patient should pass. This will include preoperative, intraoperative, and postoperative experience. The prospective fellow must be Advanced Cardiac Life Support (ACLS) and ATLS certified prior to the starting date of the fellowship.

*Fellowship Matrix/Model*

Month 1:          The fellow is assigned to a *Trauma Team* to learn general trauma management protocols, principles, and skills.
Months 2–4:       The fellow is assigned to the *Anesthesiology Department* to learn preoperative and intraoperative anesthesia management. During September and October, the fellow will be encouraged to attend:
                  1)  ATLS instructor course (2 days)
                  2)  ACLS instructor course (2 days)
                  3)  MIEMSS hyperbaric medicine course (4 days)
Month 5:          The fellow is assigned to *Hyperbaric Medicine Department* to learn clinical applications for hyperbaric oxygenation.
Months 6–7:       The fellow is assigned to the *Neurotrauma Intensive Care Unit (ICU)* to learn critical care doctrine and protocols as applied to this special patient population.
Months 8–9:       The fellow is assigned to the *Critical Care Respiratory Unit (CCRU)* to learn critical care doctrine as applied to patients with multiple injuries and associated medical problems.
Months 10–12:     The fellow is assigned to the *Elective* phase.
                  Electives include:
                  1)  Further training in:
                      a)  Anesthesia
                      b)  Critical care
                      c)  Hyperbaric medicine
                      d)  Trauma team
                  2)  Research
                  3)  Field EMS program
                  4)  Pediatric critical care
                  5)  Burn anesthesia and critical care
                  6)  Rehabilitation
                  7)  Infectious disease
                  8)  *Special visiting fellowship* at selected trauma centers

[a] Developed by C. Grande and W. N. Bernhard, October 1988. From Grande CM, Stene JK, Bernhard WN, Barton CR. Trauma anesthesia and critical care: the concept and rationale for a new subspecialty. In Grande CM, Stene JK, Bernhard WN (eds): Overview of trauma anesthesia and critical care. Crit Care Clin 1990;6(1):1–11.

cisions were initially made jointly, for the most part, by the hospital administration and medical staff. Once a trauma system was implemented at a given center, to a large extent administrators began focusing on cost-cutting measures, thus leaving health care providers and trauma patients in a difficult position. As the financial picture became clearer, support on the part of the administrators continued to be withdrawn until either a voluntary decision was made to no longer function as a trauma center or the center was stripped of its designation by cer-

tifying agencies because of suboptimal trauma care.

2. Trauma patients present with varying demographics, and reimbursement patterns reflect those characteristics. For instance, a trauma center whose geographic location predisposes it to admit largely victims of motor vehicle accidents may actually have a profitable operation (it should at least break even). This is because the majority of motorists are insured. In spite of various compulsory laws regarding motor vehicle insurance, however, a significant number of people continue to drive uninsured. These individ-

**Table 1.6.   Characteristics of the Trauma Anesthesia/Critical Care Specialist[a]**

*Mandatory*

1. Experienced with a large repertoire of general and regional anesthesia techniques for emergency and elective trauma cases
2. Expert in all forms of airway management, especially in emergency situations
3. Expert in resuscitation procedures (peripheral and central venous line placement, fluid management)
4. Able to perform functions under adverse conditions and in diverse locations (e.g., in transport vehicles)
5. Expert in diagnosis of crucial traumatic conditions (e.g., cervical spine fractures, pneumothorax)
6. Able to perform simple surgical procedures (e.g., cricothyroidotomy, intercostal thoracostomy)
7. Familiar with a wide range of specialized trauma care equipment (e.g., rapid infusion system)
8. Comfortable with the range of critical care medicine doctrine and management
9. Involved in providing postoperative analgesia (e.g., continuous epidural catheters) in various hospital environments (e.g., intensive care unit)
10. Background in the theory of traumatology and emergency medicine (e.g., Glasgow Coma Scale, Trauma Score)

*Desirable*

1. Able to perform more advanced surgical procedures (e.g., diagnostic peritoneal lavage, emergency thoracotomy)
2. Experienced in hyperbaric oxygen therapy
3. Involved directly with emergency medical services
4. Active in trauma prevention programs

[a] From Grande CM, Stene JK, Barton CR. The trauma anesthesiologist. Md Med J 1988;37:531–536.

uals, if injured, pose a financial burden (77, 97). If a trauma center admits primarily victims of "inner-city" penetrating trauma, the reimbursement patterns are extremely poor (77).

3. Federal regulations for hospital reimbursement—most importantly, the Diagnostic Related Groups (DRGs)—do not address the expensive extended care that many victims of major trauma require. Almost uniformly, DRGs underestimate the severity of patients' illnesses and just reimbursement (73, 98, 99).

4. Optimal staffing patterns for many trauma centers may be unrealistic in regard to affordability and true need, which, of course, also leads to financial waste (100).

The initial expansion of trauma systems included a good number of blatantly unqualified hospitals vying for trauma center designation. More recently, for essentially financial reasons, the systems have contracted, with many centers closing or being no longer willing to participate in trauma care (101). Only two states (Maryland and Virginia), however, have met the standards for regional trauma systems delineated al-

most 20 years ago (5). Therefore, unless the attitude of modern society toward health care in general changes, it will be a long time before trauma systems begin to receive the attention they deserve. Already a number of legislative remedies have been proposed to provide substantial monetary support for trauma systems as a temporizing maneuver (77, 97). Long-term changes from within the trauma systems themselves, including the medical and administration communities, must also be forthcoming.

We believe that the ongoing contraction of the systems will continue in certain areas until a critical point is reached where stability is achieved. This is appropriate and will improve the system because many hospitals currently designated as trauma centers should not justifiably hold the title. Once a facility receives its trauma center designation, it is "open for business." Remember that a basic tenet of dedicated trauma care is that patients should not be taken to the *nearest* center in terms of proximity but to the nearest *appropriate* center. Future revisions in trauma systems should correct these types of problems. Already these changes are being seen, for example, in the Houston area, where a single "all-trauma center" is proposed (102).

The following suggestions are made with these future improvements in mind:

1. Do not succumb to initial fiscal pressures to dilute the quality of a trauma system to obtain a trauma center designation (5).
2. Recruit a "select few" physicians who are firmly dedicated to high-quality trauma care, even if this means looking outside the immediate vicinity (5).
3. Institute continued and intensified public-awareness campaigns that underline the consequences of not having a regional trauma system (5).
4. Improve reimbursement by increasing the ratio of blunt to penetrating trauma and assembling a team of experts who are knowledgeable in renumeration schemes as they apply to trauma, such as making the appropriate applications to "crime subsidy" programs (77).
5. Reevaluate the DRG program as it applies to trauma centers and either revise the DRGs or adopt alternative programs (73).
6. Before making the commitment to organize a new trauma center, carefully scrutinize the true need for it by such means as evaluating the motor vehicle accident (MVA) rate in the surrounding area. From these figures estimations can be made as to the potential utilization of a trauma center (approximately 5% of all MVAs will cause someone to require care at a specialized trauma center) (100).

From a realistic point of view, recognizing that not all facilities are able to generate the ways, means, and need to operate an "optimal" *trauma center*, the concept of the *trauma program* has been proposed (100). The trauma program concept, generally applicable to community hospitals versus large university hospitals, downgrades previously proposed staffing patterns and focuses on cost containment while simultaneously providing a respectable level of care. The "backbone" of the trauma program still is 24-hour in-house coverage by a general surgeon, an *anesthesiologist*, and an emergency medicine physician, as this was thought to be "the minimum number of physicians neces-

sary to resuscitate and secure temporary operative control of hemorrhage in the critical trauma patient" (100).

Further, converse to the "trauma program" concept and consistent with the "all-trauma center" concept is the "accident hospital" concept, which actually precedes that of the trauma center, having been in existence since the late 1800s. An accident hospital is one that is freestanding and treats trauma patients exclusively, as opposed to most trauma centers, which are generally on the premises of a large general medical center that treats other types of patients (74). The accident hospital is "built around" the trauma patient and has all of the necessary equipment and facilities (e.g., radiology suites, operating rooms, intensive care units, outpatient clinic). There are other differences between a "trauma center" and an "accident hospital":

1. An accident hospital precludes the "echelons of care" schemata of level I, II, and III trauma centers. *All* trauma patients (both major and minor injuries) are treated within the accident hospital, and they are triaged at the facility.
2. The physicians working in an accident hospital are "traumatologists" in the true sense of the word, as they direct all of their professional efforts to the care of trauma patients only and some even subspecialize within the field. The MIEMSS Shock Trauma Center, in reality, more closely fits the description of an accident hospital. Other prominent accident hospitals include the Birmingham Accident Hospital in Birmingham, England, and the extensive accident hospital system in Austria operated by the General Accident Insurance Company (74).

There are advantages of an accident hospital compared to a trauma center:

1. In some locations the surplus of "trauma centers" both prevents any one center from receiving the number of trauma patients necessary to maintain its level of skills and permits the admission of seriously injured patients to inappropriate facilities.
2. Those individuals who abhor working in a trauma center, yet who must do so simply because their facility has been designated as such by its administrators, have more freedom of choice. Conversely, accident hospitals would attract truly dedicated professionals.

3. From an economic standpoint, there would be at least two advantages. First, special reimbursement policies (e.g., DRGs) for accident hospitals would be more easy to justify. Second, as the various industrial and governmental complexes are assuming a continually more prominent role in health care policy making (e.g., employment insurance), it would be feasible to present to them a proposal whereby a system of accident hospitals would function in a fashion similar to the Austrian experience (where industry and insurance companies have borne the financial burden). The attraction here is improved dividends to these entities as most trauma victims are young, with most of their lives and earning potential ahead of them. The accident hospital concept is aimed at maximizing trauma care, which includes rehabilitation and, ultimately, return to the workplace.

## New Horizons: The Future of Trauma Anesthesia

The TA/CCS now plays a prominent role in day-to-day trauma patient care, and the area of responsibility of a TA/CCS continues to expand. First and foremost, the TA/CCS functions in the clinical sphere as an important member of the trauma team. As surgical care expands to encompass more complex and challenging procedures, the TA/CCS must also grow to cope with the inherent new demands, not only in the operating room but also in the perioperative arena.

Second, as the role of the TA/CCS expands within the hospital, it also starts to encompass areas outside the facility environs, for example, the development and management of EMS systems (103). The role of the TA/CCS in the United States needs to mirror more closely that of its European counterpart, where the anesthesiologist is commonly found in the field. Although the TA/CCS has much to offer the trauma patient who has not yet reached the trauma center, a recent study showed a shamefully low representation of anesthesiologists in EMS in this country (104). These services (e.g., analgesia in the field via nitrous oxide/oxygen mixtures, such as Nitronox

[Entonox], or mixed narcotic agonist/antagonists, such as nalbuphine) can be administered either personally or through agents in this area ("physician extenders" such as paramedics).

In 1988 the International Trauma Anesthesia and Critical Care Society (ITACCS) was formed as a professional society to further the development of anesthesiologists as traumatologists; to be a forum for anesthesiologists to share ideas and techniques for managing trauma patients; to address issues such as those raised above that relate to subspecialists who dedicate a significant portion of their professional effort to the anesthesia and critical care of trauma patients; and to provide an educational framework to train TA/CCSs. Increased involvement of anesthesiologists in trauma care and in ITACCS will lead to the development of protocols for trauma anesthesia and other improvements in trauma management.

Examples of the efforts of ITACCS include the production of the *Annual Trauma Anesthesia and Critical Care Symposium Series* (with three successful symposia completed as of June 1990); the work that has been done in conjunction with the National Study Center for Trauma and Emergency Medical Systems to develop a dedicated training program, the "International Trauma Anesthesia and Critical Care Fellowship" (to be conducted at sites such as the MIEMSS Shock Trauma Center, the Birmingham Accident Center, and other renowned trauma centers around the world); and sponsorship of the publication of this book. Research in trauma anesthesia has thus far been deficient; another function of ITACCS is to reverse this trend.

With the proper support and a receptive atmosphere, the future of trauma anesthesia is bright. Undoubtedly, anesthesia practitioners have much to offer to the field of trauma management. Improvements must occur in the next few years for better utilization of the first ("golden") and second hours following injury (105). As the sophistication of intrahospital trauma care begins to peak, advancement in maximally utilizing the golden hour will involve improving the quality of care in the field. Examples include miniaturization of monitoring equipment so that critical care may begin at the scene. One of the key areas in which these developments will occur is in the military, where the ways, means, and current need exist. Other issues relating to the golden hour that must be addressed include further sophistication in airway management (e.g., evaluation of the pharyngeotracheal lumen airway), resuscitation (e.g., blood substitutes), analgesia (e.g., refinement of regional techniques for field use), and, in general, improved utilization of time such that definitive care is provided at the earliest possible moment (e.g., proper investigation of the effect of deployment of *properly trained* physicians to the field). During the second hour, when most conventional anesthetic management will begin, suboptimal but not necessarily substandard care will detract from the maximal outcome and will contribute to the "late phase manifestations" seen in the critical care areas (e.g., sepsis, renal failure, ARDS), which usually become evident during the first 2 weeks after injury. No longer will achieving the endpoint of a "good anesthetic" (i.e., sedation and analgesia) be acceptable. Other parameters that have been closely tied to morbidity and mortality (e.g., oxygen consumption index) will have to be addressed from the outset. This will occur through improved intraoperative management as applied to improved monitoring techniques (e.g., more aggressive, earlier invasive monitoring), investigation into the relative merits and detriments of agents and techniques (through properly conducted studies), and improved training and inclusion of anesthesia care providers as members of the "trauma team" (e.g., through the development, review, and certification of proper training programs such as the one mentioned above).

## SUMMARY

In this chapter we reviewed the basics of trauma as a specific disease entity, its demographics, and systems of trauma care. The role of the anesthesiologist was then focused upon, first reviewing, in the form of quotations, statements made by numerous individuals over the past 150 years. The present status of trauma anesthesiology throughout the world was presented, with notation of deficiencies in the performance and participation of the American anesthesiologist in comprehensive trauma care, despite an aptitude for such. Reasons for this problem were reviewed and include political, legal, economical, and logistical restraints. Recognition of this problem is an important first step in providing solutions. Besides the fact that the majority of anesthesiologists are depriving themselves of a unique, exciting, and rewarding professional experience, trauma patients are suffering as anesthesiologists "hide behind their masks" in the operating room instead of actively demonstrating their expertise in emergency rooms, on ambulance squads, and in critical care units. Such demonstrated expertise would make lobbying for support much more effective.

Regarding the future, we have concluded that, unless the ideology of the modern world drastically changes regarding the provision of health care to trauma patients, the trauma care system will initially contract to those tertiary care centers truly capable of providing the type of sophisticated care that is necessary (i.e., in accordance with the accident hospital philosophy).

The finding that dedicated trauma care lowers the morbidity and mortality due to injury has been well established (1). The need for high-quality trauma care is projected to increase as the modern life-style seems to promote violence and injury. Surely, because of the increase in civil violence related to terrorist acts, the increased number of handguns, and higher speed limits, the incidence of trauma will continue to mount. In view of these projections, the TA/CCS will be needed more and more. There will be a continually expanding spectrum of areas into which the TA/CCS can diversify. Although the number of these subspecialists is small at present, it is hoped that special training programs will enlarge their ranks.

The concept of the TA/CCS illustrates the common interest of anesthesiologists and emergency medicine physicians. Closer cooperation, especially in training, between these medical specialties will strengthen both fields. Anesthesiologists well trained as TA/CCSs can help to alleviate the presently unmet need for board-certified emergency medicine physicians in trauma centers. Thus, trauma anesthesia and critical care provide ideal opportunities for physicians who are interested in the nonsurgical care of the trauma patient. Under the auspices of ITACCS, the burgeoning field of trauma anesthesiology should continue to mature and flourish. To the profession of anesthesiology we now "throw down a gauntlet" to contribute to the improvement of trauma care!

# References

1. Accident Facts 1987. Chicago, National Safety Council, 1987.
2. Perrine MW. Alcohol involvement in highway crashes. Clin Plast Surg 1975;2:11–34.
3. West JG, Trunkey DD, Lim RC. Systems of trauma care: study of two counties. Arch Surg 1979;114:455–460.
4. West JG, Cales RH, Gazzaniga AB. Impact of regionalization: the Orange County experience. Arch Surg 1983;118:740–744.
5. West JG, Williams MJ, Trunkey DD, Wolferth CC. Trauma systems: current status—future challenges. JAMA 1988;259(24):3597–3600.
6. Ramzy AI. The Maryland Emergency Medical Services System: an update. Md Med J 1988; 37:517–520.
7. Cowley RA, Gretes AJ, Soderstrom CA. Providing safe Medevac helicopter transport: Maryland's 18 year experience. Md Med J 1988; 37:521–524.
8. Committee on Trauma and Committee on Shock. Accidental Death and Disability: The Neglected Disease of Modern Society. Rockville, MD, US Department of Health, Education, and Welfare, 1966.
9. Trunkey DD. Trauma. Sci Am 1983;249(2): 28–35.
10. Committee on Trauma. Hospital and prehospital resources for optimal care of the injured patient. Am Coll Surg Bull 1986;71:4–12.
11. Barrier G. Emergency medical services for treat-
12. Carn W, et al. The S.A.M.U. system of France. Disaster Med 1983;1.1.140.
13. Lust P. Resuscitation in the prehospital phase. Disaster Med 1983;1.1.127.
14. Damir E. Prehospital emergency medicine and intensive therapy in the USSR. Disaster Med 1983;1.1.157.
15. Commission on the Provision of Surgical Services. Report of the Working Party on the Management of Patients with Major Injuries. Royal College of Surgeons, November 1988.
16. Lyons AS, Petrucelli RJ. Medicine, an Illustrated History. New York, Harry N Abrams, Inc, Publishers, 1978.
17. Davis DA. Anesthesia in the World Wars. In Davis DA (ed): Clinical Anesthesia, Volume 2, Historical Vignettes of Modern Anesthesia. Philadelphia, FA Davis, 1968, pp 19–29.
18. Morton WTG. The first use of ether as an anesthetic at the Battle of the Wilderness in the Civil War. JAMA 1904;42:1068–1073.
19. Watson CB, Norfleet EA. Anesthesia for trauma. Crit Care Clin 1986;2:717–746.
20. Grande CM, Stene JK, Bernhard WN, Barton CR. Trauma anesthesia and critical care: the concept and rationale for a new subspecialty. Crit Care Clin 1989;6(1):1–11.
21. Wolfson LJ. Preface. In Wolfson LJ (ed): Anaesthesia for the Injured. Oxford, England, Blackwell Scientific Publications, 1962.
22. Booij LHDJ. Pitfalls in anaesthesia for multiply injured patients. Injury 1982;14:81–88.
23. Wolfson LJ. The anesthetist's management of the injured patient. Br J Anaesth 1966;38: 274–287.
24. Walters FJM, Nott MR. The hazards of anaesthesia in the injured patient. Br J Anaesth 1977; 49:707–720.
25. Baskett PJF. Priorities in the immediate management of major injuries. In Arias A, Llaurado R, Nalda MA, Lunn JN (eds): Recent Progress in Anaesthesiology and Resuscitation. Amsterdam, Excerpta Medica, 1975, pp 463–466.
26. Wandless JG. Emergency anaesthesia. Br J Hosp Med 1978;19:437–443.
27. Campell D. Immediate hospital care of the injured. Br J Anaesth 1977;49:673–679.
28. DeMedici M. Secondary prevention from individual to maxi emergencies: the role of the anesthetist—resuscitation specialist. Oplitai 1989;2:71–72.
29. Bone L, Bucholy R. The management of fractures in the patient with multiple trauma. J Bone Joint Surg [Am] 1986;68A:945–949.
30. Pavlin EG. Anesthesia. In Moore EE (ed): Early Care of the Injured Patient, ed 4. Toronto, BC Decker, 1990, pp 91–99.
31. Wilson RS. Anesthesia and the trauma patient. In

Burke JF, Boyd RJ, McCabe CJ (eds): Trauma Management: Early Management of Visceral, Nervous System and Musculoskeletal Injuries. Chicago, Year Book, 1988, pp 93–102.

32. Stene JK. Anesthetic management of the shock trauma patient. In Cowley RA, Dunham CM (eds): Trauma Care, Volume I, Surgical Management. Philadelphia, JB Lippincott, 1987, pp 204–211.

33. Horsewell JL, Cobb ML, Owens WD. Anesthetic management of the trauma victim. In Zuidema GD, Rutherford RB, Ballinger WF (eds): The Management of Trauma, ed 4. Philadelphia, WB Saunders, 1985, pp 127–138.

34. Courington FW. Anesthesia guidelines for the trauma patient. Semin Anesth 1985;4:92–101.

35. Trowbridge AM, Giesecke AH. Multiple injuries. Clin Anesth 1976;11:79–84.

36. Stene JK. Anesthesia for the critically ill trauma patient. In Siegel JH (ed): Trauma: Emergency Surgery and Critical Care. New York, Churchill Livingstone, 1987, pp 843–862.

37. Egbert LD. Trauma and the anesthetist. In Cave EF, Burke JF, Boyd RJ (eds): Trauma Management. Chicago, Year Book, 1974, pp 235–242.

38. Pavlin EG. Anaesthesia for the traumatized patient. Can Anaesth Soc J 1983;3:527–523.

39. Nicholls BJ, Cullen BF. Anesthesia for trauma. J Clin Anesth 1988;1:115–129.

40. Giesecke AH. The anesthesiologist and the traumatized patient. Semin Anesth 1985; 4:89–90.

41. Berry M. Anesthetist's view of the traumatized patient. Can Nurse 1968;64:38–41.

42. Stene JK. The anesthesiologists' role in trauma management. Pract Management Anesthesiol July 1989, 1–4.

43. Weiskopf RB. Anesthesia for major trauma. In 1987 Review Course Lectures Cleveland, International Anesthesia Research Society, 1987, pp 73–79.

44. Grande CM, Stene JK, Barton CR. The trauma anesthesiologist. Md Med J 1988;37:531–536.

45. Giesecke AH, Egbert LD. Anesthesia for trauma surgery. In Miller RD (ed): Anesthesia, ed 2. New York, Churchill Livingstone, 1986, pp 1819–1835.

46. Donnan GB, Giesecke AH. Anesthesia considerations. In Shires GT (ed): Principles of Trauma Care, ed 3. New York, McGraw-Hill, 1985, pp 62–84.

47. Morpurgo CV. The treatment of patients with multiple injuries associated with damage to the spinal cord. In Arias A, Leaurato R, Nalda MA, Lunn JN (eds): Recent Progress in Anaesthesiology and Resuscitation. Amsterdam, Excerpta Medica, 1975, pp 471–475.

48. Horton JM. The anesthetist's contribution to the care of head injuries. Br J Anaesth 1976; 48:767–770.

49. Gelb AW, Manninen PH, Mezon BJ, Durward QJ. The anesthetist and the head-injured patient. Can Anaesth Soc J 1984;31:98–108.

50. Fraser A, Edmonds-Seal J. Spinal cord injuries: review of the problems facing the anesthetist. Anaesthesia 1982;37:1084–1098.

51. Van de Walle J, Delooz H. The role of the anesthetist in the care of the patient with crushed chest. In Arias A, Llaurado R, Nalda MA, Lunn JN (eds): Recent Progress in Anaesthesiology and Resuscitation. Amsterdam, Excerpta Medica, 1975, pp 481–484.

52. Thorton HL, Knight PF. Introduction: the problems of emergency anaesthesia. In Thornton HL, Knight PF (eds): Emergency Anaesthesia. Baltimore, Williams & Wilkins, 1965.

53. Donegan JH. Anesthesia for the trauma victim. In 1985 Review Course Lectures, IARS 59th Congress. Cleveland, International Anesthesia Research Society, 1985, pp 68–72.

54. Rembert FC. Preanesthetic care: state of health at the time of injury. Clin Anesth 1976;11:17–24.

55. Giesecke AH, Hodgson RMH, Raj RP. Anesthesia for severely injured patients. Orthop Clin North Am 1970;1:21–48.

56. Giesecke AH, Lee JF. Anesthetic management of the severely trauma patient. Oklahoma State Med Assoc J 1969;62:464–470.

57. Atkinson RS. Place of the anesthetist in the intensive care unit. Int Anesthesiol Clin 1973; 11:271–288.

58. Telfer AB. Use of anesthesia: intensive care. Br Med J 1980;280:1593–1595.

59. Brown DL. Trauma management: the anesthesiologist's role. Int Anesthesiol Clin 1987;25:1–18.

60. Grande CM. Critical care transport: a trauma perspective. Crit Care Clin 1989;6(1):165–183.

61. Gorgass B, Ahnefeld FW, Dick W, Dolp R. The anesthetist as an emergency physician: his tasks in the treatment of multiple injuries at the scene of the accident and during transportation. In Arias A, Llaurado R, Nalda MA, Lunn JN (eds): Recent Progress in Anesthesiology and Resuscitation. Amsterdam, Excerpta Medica, 1975, pp 481–484.

62. Norman J, Moles M. Trauma and immediate care. Br J Anaesth 1977;49:641–642.

63. Safar P. Foreword. In Vanstrum GS (ed): Anesthesiology in Emergency Medicine. Boston, Little, Brown & Co, 1990.

64. Flagg PJ. The Art of Anesthesia, ed 2. Philadelphia, JB Lippincott, 1919.

65. Render JW, Lundy JS. Anesthesia in war surgery. War Med 1942;2:193–212.

66. Wiggin SC. Anesthesia for the surgery of trauma. Am J Surg 1943;59:363–369.

67. Carmichel MR. Anesthesia under civil war conditions. Anaesthesia 1981;36:1077–1088.

68. Donchin Y, Wiener M, Grande CM, Cotev S. Military medicine: trauma anesthesia and critical

care on the battlefield. Crit Care Clin 1989; 6(1):185–202.

69. Waters RM. Anesthesia in medical preparedness program. Surgery 1942;9:229–230.

70. Cole WHJ. The anesthetist in modern warfare: experience in the first Australian field hospital in South Vietnam. Anaesthesia 1973;28:113–117.

71. Longnecker DE. Anesthesia. In Altura BM, Lefer AM, Shumer W (eds): Handbook of Shock and Trauma, Volume I, Basic Science. New York, Raven Press, 1983, pp 449–459.

72. Bjornson K. Anesthesia in the trauma patient. Top Emerg Med 1987;43–51.

73. Jacobs LM, Schwartz RJ. The impact of prospective reimbursement on trauma centers. Arch Surg 1986;121:479–483.

74. Freeark RJ. Scudder Oration on Trauma: the accident hospital. ACS Bull October 1986; 24–30.

75. Vanstrum GS. Preface. In Vanstrum GS (ed): Anesthesia in Emergency Medicine. Boston, Little, Brown & Co, 1989, pp xvii–xix.

76. Vanstrum GS. Trauma management. In Vanstrum GS (ed): Anesthesia in Emergency Medicine. Boston, Little, Brown & Co, 1989, pp 303–339.

77. Shapiro MJ, Keegan M, Copeland J. The misconception of trauma reimbursement. Arch Surg 1989;124:1238–1241.

78. Lewis FR. Thoracic trauma. Surg Clin North Am 1982;62:97–192.

79. Mulder DS, Shennib H, Angood P. Thoracic injuries. In Maull KI, Cleveland HC, Strauch GO, Wolferth CC (eds): Advances in Trauma. Chicago, Year Book, 1986, pp 193–216.

80. Stoddart JC. Preface. In Stoddart JC (ed): Trauma and the Anaesthetist. London, Ballière-Tindall, 1984.

81. Heckel CG. Trauma—another subspecialty in anesthesiology? Md Med J 1988;37:715–716.

82. Committee on Refresher Courses. 40th Annual Refresher Course Lectures and Clinical Update Program. Park Ridge, IL, American Society of Anesthesiologists, 1989.

83. Emergency Medical Services, Orange County Health Care Agency, Santa Ana, California.

84. Committee on Trauma, Airway Management. Advanced Trauma Life Support Course: Instructor Manual, ed 3. Chicago, American College of Surgeons, 1989, pp 31–53.

85. Teufel WL, Trunkey DD. Trauma centers: a pragmatic approach to need, cost and staffing patterns. JACEP 1977;6:546–550.

86. McNulty M. Are poor patients likely to sue for malpractice? JAMA 1989;262:1391–1392.

87. Olsson GL, Hallen B, Hambraeus-Jonzon K. Aspiration during anaesthesia: a computer-aided study of 185,358 anaesthetics. Acta Anaesthesiol Scand 1986;30:84–92.

88. Norton ML. Anesthesia for the trauma patient. In Walt AJ, Wilson RF (eds): Management of Trauma: Pitfalls and Practice. Philadelphia, Lea & Febiger, 1975, pp 163–181.

89. Kolber JL. Malpractice law and emergency department medicine. Emerg Med Clin North Am 1985;3:625.

90. Maier RV. Evaluation and resuscitation. In Moore EE (ed): Early Care of the Injured Patient, ed 4. Toronto, BC Decker, 1990, pp 56–73.

91. Trunkey DD. Report to the Council of the Association of Surgeons of Great Britain and Ireland. Br Med J 1989;299:31–33.

92. McSwain NE, Kerstein MD. Preface. In McSwain NE, Kerstein MD (eds): Evaluation and Management of Trauma. East Norwalk, CT, Appleton-Century-Crofts, 1987, pp xv–xvi.

93. Lindsey D. Teaching the initial management of major multiple system trauma. J Trauma 1980; 20:160–162.

94. Hiatt JR, Tompkins RK. The importance of nonoperative trauma management in postgraduate surgical education. J Trauma 1987;22:769.

95. Munoz E. Economic costs of trauma, United States, 1982. J Trauma 1984;24:237–244.

96. Cales RH, Anderson PG, Heilig RW. Utilization of medical care in Orange County: the effect of implementation of a regional trauma system. Ann Emerg Med 1985;14:331–334.

97. Oakes DD, Holcomb SF, Sherck JP. Patterns of trauma care and reimbursements: the burden of uninsured motorists. J Trauma 1985; 25: 740–745.

98. Pories SE, Camelli RL, Vaeck P, Harris F, Lea D. Predicting hospital charges for trauma care. Arch Surg 1988;123:579–582.

99. Dimick AR, Potts LA, Clarles ED, Wayne J, Reed IM. The cost of burn care and implications for the future on quality of care. J Trauma 1986; 26:260–265.

100. Tuefel WL, Trunkey DD. Trauma centers: a pragmatic approach to need, cost, and staffing patterns. JACEP 1977;6:546–551.

101. Tokarski C. Worried Congress looks for ways to help the nation's troubled trauma-care system. Modern Healthcare, August 12, 1988, p 26.

102. Pinkney DS. Emergency crisis spurs call for Houston all-trauma center. American Medical News, November 3, 1989, pp 1, 32.

103. White RD. The role of the anesthesiologist in emergency medical services. Semin Anesth 1985;4:102–113.

104. Poulton TJ, Kisicki PA. Medical directors of critical care air transport services. Crit Care Med 1987;15:784–785.

105. Stene JK. Anesthesia for trauma. In Miller RD (ed): Anesthesia, ed 3. New York, Churchill Livingstone, 1990 (in press).

# 2

# Mechanisms of Injury: Etiologies of Trauma

*Christopher M. Grande and John K. Stene*

## WHY A KNOWLEDGE OF MECHANISMS AND PATTERNS OF INJURY IS CRITICAL TO TRAUMA MANAGEMENT

There is a shameful paucity of nonoperating traumatologists such as the trauma anesthesia/critical care specialist (TA/CCS) who truly have an interest in or appreciation of the various mechanisms and patterns of injury seen in traumatic disease. Many ask, "Why should I know this? Will it affect the way in which I treat the patient?" Most physicians do not permit this elective ignorance to extend to the etiologies of other diseases they may treat. For instance, the gastroenterologist does show an interest in why gallstones evolve, and the cardiologist is interested in the causative factors of coronary artery disease. Therefore, the epidemiology and etiology of trauma should demand the attention of the traumatologist (1).

To anticipate "pitfalls" and facilitate the diagnosis and treatment of traumatic injury, any anesthesiologist handling trauma patients on a repetitive basis should have at least a basic understanding of the various mechanisms of injury (1, 2). This understanding will impart the ability to evaluate a problem more thoroughly and to render more comprehensive therapy. Such knowledge will also aid in identifying occult problems and avoiding iatrogenic complications of the existing condition (3). Knowledge of the wounding mechanism may provide information as to the nature and the extent of the wound, which may be valuable in ongoing care. Knowledge of the mechanisms of injury is valuable for the anesthesiologist treating trauma patients to anticipate operative and critical care requirements. Treating trauma patients without an understanding of the mechanisms of injury is like walking in at the middle of a movie and never knowing how it began or like reading a novel in reverse (4). Frankly stated, to be involved in the management of a trauma patient and not have an appreciation for the mechanisms of injury and the pathology they cause is suboptimal practice (5).

The facts concerning the traumatic event and the wounding instrument should be sought actively when the trauma patient's history and other pertinent features of the recent sequence of events are being obtained. Similarly, to communicate in a common language with other traumatologists, the TA/CCS should be familiar with various trauma classification systems such as the Injury Severity Score and the Trauma Score and how to apply them.

## MECHANISMS OF INJURY

A person may be exposed to injury in many ways during the course of normal daily life. Trauma can occur when a person simply walks across the street and is hit by a motor vehicle or when a person climbs stairs and trips. Other accidental injuries may occur during engagement in sports or other recreational activities or occupationally in the workplace. Nonaccidental injuries may occur as a result of contemplated or premeditated intrapersonal violence. Intrapersonal violence can also occur as a result of "socially acceptable" or "noncriminal" military actions. In all cases, the final product, the injury, is reached by a common pathway.

There are limited subclassifications of

traumatic disease (Table 2.1). These include the major subclassifications most commonly seen in sophisticated trauma centers, such as blunt injury, penetrating injury, and thermal injury. Other categories such as environmental injury (e.g., snakebite) are more likely to be seen in local emergency departments and usually do not require the full-scale capabilities of the modern trauma team. Although each of these types of injury may have devastating results, they are considered "minor" trauma and will not be discussed in this chapter. Most common injuries are related to motion: rapid horizontal deceleration (e.g., motor vehicle accidents), rapid vertical deceleration (e.g., falls from great heights), and projectile penetration (e.g., gunshot wounds) (5). These are the types of injuries that will be discussed.

In each section of this chapter are described the mechanisms by which the injury occurs and the response induced in the host (victim), which subsequently will produce a constellation of signs and symptoms that can be appreciated as a discrete syndrome (6). Each of these mechanisms of injury can be viewed as a disease etiology for which the TA/CCS is a specialist in acute management.

### Obtaining the Medical History and Reconstructing the Sequence of Events

At some point in the management of the trauma patient, whether during the hectic moments of the primary assessment or resuscitation phase or later, during the secondary assessment, someone skilled in systematically elucidating pertinent informa-

**Table 2.1.   Various Forms of Trauma[a]**

Blunt (high velocity)
Penetrating (e.g., stab wounds, gunshot wounds)
Mixed blunt/penetrating (e.g., impalement)
Falls from great heights (vertical high-velocity blunt)
Burns (including thermal, electrical, chemical)
Chemical
Biologic
Nuclear
Environmental (e.g., snakebite)

[a] From Grande CM. Mechanisms and patterns of injury: the key to anticipation in trauma management. Crit Care Clin 6:25–35, 1990.

tion (e.g., TA/CCS, trauma nurse) must reconstruct the recent sequence of events, as well as obtain significant parts of the trauma patient's medical and surgical history, prior problems with anesthetics or blood transfusions, present medical regimens and allergies, and alcohol or "recreational drug" use (7).

Facts concerning the evolution of the current problem may have direct bearing on the ongoing management. These may be elucidated by questions such as the following: At what speed was the vehicle traveling at the time of impact? How long were the skid marks? Was there damage to the passenger compartment? Were seat belts used and properly worn? What was the height of the fall? What was the caliber of the firearm used? What was the distance between the assailant and the victim? What was the size of the knife?

More general questions include: Is a reliable estimate of blood loss available? How much time has elapsed since the injury? Was there loss of consciousness? Did the incident take place in a bar or "shooting gallery" (a secret location where illicit drugs are used and intravenous injection equipment is available for use at a cost), lending credence to drug involvement?

In the case of a trauma patient with a burn injury, one should seek evidence of smoke inhalation (such as the presence of acrid fumes), the location and type of materials undergoing incineration, or evidence of blunt or penetrating injury sustained from the blast effect associated with explosions occurring at the scene of a fire (8).

Sources of information are the emergency medical services paramedics and police officers who were at the scene and accompanied the trauma patient to the trauma center (as well as the reports they collected from bystanders and the forms such personnel are required to complete). Family and friends should also be questioned, including those who sustained concurrent injury and who are conscious and in a condition to participate in such questioning. If the primary physician of the trauma patient is known, he or she should also be contacted. It is also possible that the trauma patient has a medical record on file in the receiving hospital.

## Penetrating Trauma

Penetrating trauma can be thought of as a spectrum of disease that extends from a minor pinprick, which is frequently ignored, to the more devastating results caused by a high-powered firearm (9). Basically, the microscopic tissue pathology is the same, with the exception that, as the explosive characteristics of high-powered/highvelocity projectiles are considered, a new component of explosive or blast energy is introduced. Ultimately, the extent of damage caused will be governed by an interaction of three factors: (a) the character of the wounding instrument (e.g., knife, bomb fragment), (b) its velocity at the time of impact, and (c) the characteristics of the tissue through which it passes (9, 10).

### STAB WOUNDS

A crushing force is one that disrupts tissues. In a simplistic form of stab wound, caused by a narrow, pointed instrument (e.g., an icepick), the crush injury will be microscopic and confined to the path of the instrument's apex (9). If the instrument were tapered and flat (e.g., a dagger), there would also be fraying and crushing of the tissues as they stretched to accommodate the wide edge of the blade close to the shaft. If a blunter wounding instrument (e.g., an axe) is used, there will be a greater area of crushed tissue, and the force applied to achieve the same degree of penetration will introduce a component of "blunt" injury.

Historically, it has been difficult to categorize the various types of stab wounds and the morbidity and mortality they imply. These wounds must be examined individually and treated appropriately. In one study performed using a prison population, overall mortality was low (3%). Most fatalities were related to thoracic wounds (11).

## BALLISTICS

### Definitions

Ballistics is the branch of science that studies the motion of projectiles. It is divided into three main areas: interior ballistics, exterior ballistics, and terminal ballistics. *Interior ballistics* involves the behavior of projectiles while they are still within the barrel of the weapon from which they are fired. *Exterior ballistics* is the study of flight characteristics of these missiles as they travel through the air. *Terminal ballistics* is concerned with the behavior of the projectile once it has penetrated a medium more solid than air and with the interaction between that medium and the projectile. *Wound ballistics* is the subdivision of terminal ballistics dealing with the terminal ballistics of projectiles in animals.

Studies of wound ballistics are usually performed on animals that are alive and anesthetized or on artificial models. Such models usually consist of blocks of "ordnance gelatin," a medium found to simulate muscle tissue very well and in part developed by the Letterman Army Institute of Research (9). The behavior of missiles as they pass through the gelatin is recorded by high-speed cinematography, including the use of two-dimensional x-rays. These films are then used to construct a "wound profile" for a given projectile.

Ballistics are important for the TA/CCS confronted by a trauma patient with a gunshot wound. Knowledge of the type of firearm and ammunition used will allow the TA/CCS to predict the wound characteristics. The important factors are (*a*) velocity of impact-kinetic energy transfer, (*b*) shape of the projectile presented to the tissues (a tumbling, yawing bullet will produce a larger cavity than a sphere), (*c*) the trajectory within the body, (*d*) the degree of fragmentation, and (*e*) the body region that was hit (9, 10).

### Exterior Ballistics

The effects produced by a missile on gelatin, or on a human body, depend on several projectile characteristics: muzzle velocity, size (caliber), composition, flight characteristics (exterior ballistics), and the distance to the target. Muzzle velocity is that speed at which the bullet is traveling as it leaves the end of the barrel (muzzle) or the speed at which a fragment is launched from an exploding bomb. Under normal conditions, projectiles can only lose velocity from this point; therefore, the *residual velocity* of the projectile as it strikes is inversely proportional to the distance from the source to the target. Thus, a missile will have both an *effective range* (that distance within which the projectile can effect damage) and an *extreme range* (that distance at which a missile is still traveling but does not possess enough velocity or energy to be dangerous). In most cases of civilian trauma resulting from gunshot wounds, impact velocity closely approximates muzzle velocity because interpersonal distances are small (12).

A missile that impacts the target while within its extreme range will probably cause a "nonpenetrating" wound (a contusion or abrasion). Such a wound will occur when the impact velocity is less than 75 m/sec—at least 50 m/sec is necessary to penetrate the skin, and a somewhat higher velocity is required to go through clothing. The term "V-50" refers to the impact velocity at which 50% of a particular type of missile will penetrate a given material and is used to evaluate protective garments ("flak" jackets, ballistic armor).

A missile entering a body within its effective range will produce either a *penetrating* or a *perforating* wound. A penetrating wound occurs when the missile remains in the body and thus *only* an *entrance* wound can be found. A perforating wound occurs when the missile passes out of the body, thus creating both *entrance and exit* wounds. The size of the entrance wound will vary directly with the size (caliber) of the missile. The size and shape of the wound are also subject to the missile's flight pattern at the time of impact (yaw, nutation, precession, etc.) (Fig. 2.1) and the shape of the projectile (whether is it a smooth bullet or a jagged shell fragment)

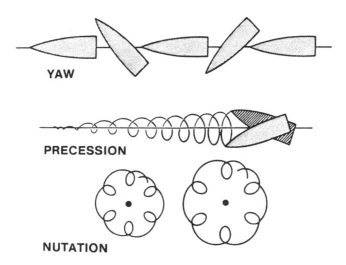

**Figure 2.1.    Variations from linear flight.** (From Ordog GJ. Wound ballistics. In Ordog GJ (ed): Management of Gunshot Wounds. New York, Elsevier, 1988, pp 25–60.)

(13). Once the missile is inside the body, the degree of damage is a result of the interaction of the body itself and the projectile and is dependent upon the consistency of the tissues being traversed by the missile and the characteristics of the weapon that launched it. The various types of weapons with which the TA/CCS should be familiar will be discussed separately.

Since approximately the turn of the century, there has been a move toward the creation of bullets that weigh less, yet have higher muzzle velocities and thus a much more devastating wounding capacity (10, 14). Originally, the reasons for this increased potential for wounding by small, high-velocity projectiles was not truly understood, yet developers tended in that direction on an empirical basis. Over the past 70 or 80 years, however, the reasons have become clearer.

First, one must consider the following formula:

$$\text{Kinetic energy} = \tfrac{1}{2}MV^2$$

where $M$ is mass and $V$ is velocity. Currently, most experts subscribe to the "kinetic energy theory" (13). Inspection of the kinetic energy equation reveals that doubling the velocity of a projectile will quadruple its energy, whereas doubling its mass will only double its energy.

*Velocity.* Wounding characteristics of projectiles, to a very large extent, are a reflection of their impact velocity. Three categories are used to classify projectiles based on their initial velocities: low velocity, high velocity, and very high velocity. Low-velocity missiles (LVMs) have speeds below 750 m/sec (2500 feet/sec) and usually are fired from side arms (pistols) or submachine guns (14). High-velocity missiles (HVMs) move in excess of 750 m/sec and up to 1200 m/sec (> 2500 feet/sec) and generally originate from modern rifles (Table 2.2) (14). Very-high-velocity missiles (VHMs) have speeds greater than 1200 m/sec and range up to 3000 m/sec (13, 14). Such projectiles usually originate from fragmentation munitions, but new small arms systems have also been designed to achieve these velocities.

The degree of wounding is directly related to the amount of kinetic energy transferred to the tissue medium being traversed. In the case of a perforating injury, the amount of energy deposited in the tissues will be equal to the difference between the amount of energy that a missile had before it entered the body (related to the impact velocity) and the energy it retains as it leaves the body (related to the residual velocity). In the case of a penetrating injury, *all* of the energy that the

**Table 2.2.    The Muzzle Velocity and Energy of Bullets Fired from Small Arms Weapons**

| Weapon | Bullet Weight | Muzzle Velocity | Muzzle Energy |
|---|---|---|---|
| | *grains* | *ft/sec* | *ft/lb* |
| Rifles | | | |
| Remington 22 | 49 | 1180 | 124 |
| M16 | 55 | 3200 | 1248 |
| M14 | 180 | 2610 | 2720 |
| M1 | 172 | 2700 | 2785 |
| Russian AK-47 | 150 | 2810 | 2635 |
| Russian AK-74 | 55 | 2970 | 1024 |
| 30-30 Winchester | 170 | 2200 | 1830 |
| Handguns | | | |
| 32 automatic | 71 | 863 | 91 |
| 45 automatic | 230 | 850 | 370 |
| 45 Colt | 250 | 860 | 410 |
| 38 Special Hi-Speed | 158 | 1090 | 425 |
| 38 Regular | 158 | 870 | 263 |
| 25 | 50 | 820 | 74 |
| 357 Magnum | 158 | 1415 | 695 |

missile possesses at the time of impact is transferred to the body (10).

Bullets launched from weapons with "rifled" barrels also have an angular velocity due to their spin (which increases their stability in flight). Thus, an additional amount of kinetic energy is present and is described by the formula:

$$KE = IW^2$$

where $I$ is the amount of inertia and $W$ is the angular velocity. Because of this angular velocity, when a projectile fragments within the body, particles are flung out at directions tangential to the line of flight (14).

*Air Resistance: Drag and Retardation.* While velocity may be thought of as a "positive force" propelling the missile forward, air resistance is a "negative force" retarding its forward motion. The amount of drag a missile will encounter is mainly dependent on its shape. The ideal shape of a projectile to minimize retardation is that of an arrow with its "area of presentation" minimized (13). Increases in the weight of the projectile minimize the effect of drag; thus, the heavier the bullet the better. For those ranges at which small arms may be fired accurately, however, the effective drag is minimal in *air*. Once this projectile enters a medium heavier than air, such as the tissues of the human body, its velocity will diminish more quickly and the

amount of kinetic energy transferred will be greater. This is the rationale behind the design of bullets that deform upon impact (see next section).

*Shape, Composition, and Design of the Missile.* Essentially, all war injuries are caused by one of four types of missiles: bullets and spheres (fired from small arms such as rifles and shotguns) and fragments and fléchettes (discharged by explosive devices known as fragmentation munitions). Bullets, spheres, and fléchettes have definite shapes and, thus, their ballistic behavior may be predicted, unlike that of fragments. A fifth type of projectile is a "secondary missile" (e.g., bone fragments) that has been accelerated by a "primary missile."

Bullets may be classified in various ways. The first system describes the composition of the bullet, of which four types exist: homogeneous, coated, jacketed, and semijacketed. Homogeneous bullets are made of a single substance such as lead. Coated bullets usually have a lead core but are coated with a thin layer of another metal, perhaps steel (13). Jacketed bullets also have a heavy metal core of lead or steel (steel is used when a high muzzle velocity is anticipated, as lead has a tendency to melt while the bullet is still in the barrel because of the heat produced by high velocities) but have a thick covering of "gilding metal"—usually copper, copper alloy, or steel. The construction of semi-jacketed bullets is essentially the same but, as opposed to a "full metal jacket" (full patch), a portion of the bullet's core is exposed, usually the nose. These missiles are designed so that the jacket will strip off, fragment within the target, and cause more serious damage. Semijacketed bullets are designed primarily for sporting use (game hunting) and are expressly forbidden for military use by a number of conventions (namely, the Hague Convention of 1899, the Geneva Convention of 1949, and a special meeting of the International Committee of the Red Cross in 1974) (9, 13). Fully jacketed bullets must be used by military forces for "humane" reasons.

Bullets may also be classified on the basis of their shape. Usually the bullet will receive its name based upon the shape of its nose: pointed noses, round noses, hollow-pointed noses, and flat noses (9, 13).

Certain types of round-nose bullets, called "soft points," are designed and constructed so that, upon impact, the bullet will flatten and "mushroom" back on itself, thereby increasing the degree of damage (see below) (9, 13). Hollow-point bullets are manufactured with a depression at the tip of their noses and are also designed to deform upon impact; whether they actually increase the amount of damage caused is not clear (15). "Dum-dum" bullets, a type of flat-nosed bullet, were developed by the British in 1897 at their garrison in Dum Dum, India (14). Such bullets will also flatten and deform. Dum-dum bullets were outlawed for military use by the Hague Convention.

Other special types of bullets (e.g., those that are hourglass-shaped) are designed to increase the amount of damage they cause by tumbling (see "Exterior Ballistics"). Another special type of bullet is the "exploding" bullet. The noses of these bullets are filled with explosive substances such as black powder (Pyrolex) or a synthetic powder, lead azide (Devastator) (14, 16). These devices increase destruction by generating a secondary explosion within the tissues (controversial) (17). In fact, this type of bullet was used in the attempted assassination of United States President Ronald Reagan by John Hinckley; however, the explosive bullet reportedly failed to detonate (16).

This raises a very important point concerning the health professionals who may be working with a trauma patient who has sustained a gunshot wound due to exploding ammunition. The device may not have been detonated and may do so when manipulated by the physician (18, 19). Serious hand or eye injuries may result. Thus, protective equipment such as goggles should be worn during the removal of explosive bullets and long-handled instruments should be used. These bullets may be identified by their pointed tips or by x-ray (cavities may be seen within the nose) (18, 19).

Another special type of bullet is filled with liquid mercury fulminate. It is used for precision sniping (deliberate assassination). When this bullet decelerates upon impact with the target, the mercury is ejected in a forward direction out from the nose and dispersed in many directions. Additional internal fragmentation damage will occur. If the victim survives, mercury poisoning will ensue. This type of bullet was used by "Jackal" in his attempt to assassinate French President General Charles de Gaulle. Injury may also occur during the construction of these exploding and mercury-filled bullets, as they are usually handmade.

Glaser Safety Slugs are a specialty bullet, favored by many law enforcement officers in the United States. They are actually hollow-point bullets that have their noses filled with #12 shot and are capped with a fiberglass-Teflon plug. The practical advantage is that very few of these bullets will result in penetrating wounds, and thus innocent bystanders are spared injury. However, this is one of the most lethal bullets in use today and its results are devastating (20) because the degree of energy transference is maximized.

*Variations from Linear Flight.* The caliber of the bullet directly affects the size of the entrance wound. A larger caliber bullet produces a larger wound. The size of the wound is also affected by *yaw*. Yaw is a characteristic of the missile's flight pattern, the degree of rotation around its center of gravity. Yaw may range from 0 to 90°. Therefore, a small caliber bullet can produce an inordinately large entrance wound if it possesses a large degree of yaw as it makes contact with the skin. Significant yaw *before* tissue penetration is a characteristic of LVMs, with a muzzle velocity of less than 900 feet/sec, which are usually fired from handguns (14). However, certain rounds fired from handguns are designed with supplemental power (such as the .357 Magnum or the .44 Magnum) and assume the wounding characteristic of HVMs, usually fired from rifles. HVMs usually impact with less than 4% yaw (14). Table 2.2 shows the characteristics of bullets fired from common small arms.

### Terminal Ballistics

Once the bullet strikes the tissue, a new set of events may occur. Usually a LVM cuts and crushes tissue in its path to form a "drill hole" wound if bone is not encountered. Thus, a "simple" tract, the *permanent cavity*, of approximately the same diameter as the bullet is created (Fig. 2.2). If a LVM produces a *temporary cavity*, it is usually small. The LVM is typified by the United States Army Colt .45 caliber automatic pistol (model 1911).

A HVM wound will be associated with two pressure-related phenomena in addition to the force that forms the permanent cavity (9, 13). The first precedes the path of the HVM and is termed the *shock wave* (Fig. 2.3). The shock wave may produce pressures of 60 atm or 1000 pounds per square inch (9). Whether this shock wave is responsible for any tissue damage is questionable. In the wake of the HVM, a *temporary cavity* forms, several milliseconds later, which may be 10 to 15 times (and up to 40 times) the size of the permanent cavity (Fig. 2.4) (10, 14). This "cavitation effect" consists of a series of rapid expansions of the space followed by collapse, oscillating in a pulsatile fashion. By this mechanism, tissues undergoing these changes, which may be as far as 10 cm from the permanent cavity, are stretched and torn. Thus, nerves and blood vessels may be stretched temporarily or ruptured permanently. During the collapse of the temporary cavity, a vacuum is created and a variety of debris may be sucked into the wound, causing further contamination. The formation of the temporary cavity may be viewed as a "miniature internal explosion."

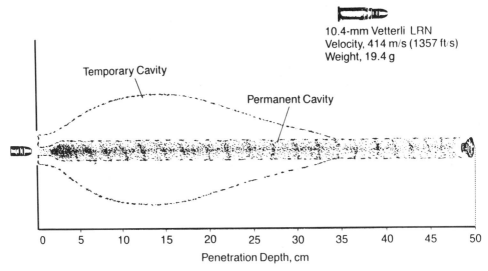

Figure 2.2.   **Typical wounding profile of a low velocity missile.** Note temporary and permanent cavities and the deformation of the bullet to a "mushroom" shape. (From Fackler ML. Wound ballistics: a review of common misconceptions. JAMA 259:2730–2736, 1988.)

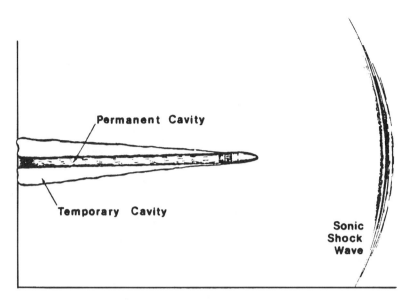

**Figure 2.3.    Passage of a high-velocity bullet through tissue.** Note temporary cavity, permanent cavity, and sonic shock wave. (Courtesy of Medical Audio Visual Services, Letterman Army Institute of Research, Presidio of San Francisco, California, file #179-84-8.)

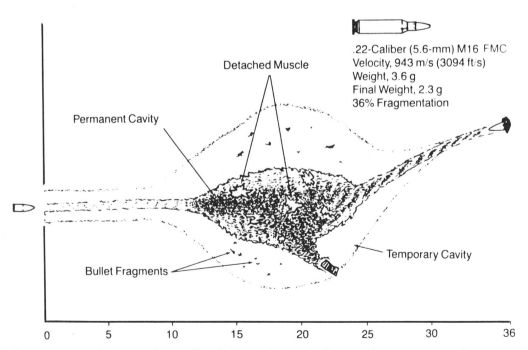

**Figure 2.4.    Typical wounding profile of a high velocity missile.** Note the permanent and temporary cavities; bullet fragments displaced radially, including the metal jacket; and the deformed bullet now traveling with its base forward. (From Fackler ML. Wound ballistics. In Ordog GJ (ed): Management of Gunshot Wounds. New York, Elsevier, 1988, pp 25–60.)

The HVM usually begins to yaw appreciably 12 to 15 cm after penetration, with the yaw varying up to 90° and sometimes beyond 180° (termed "tumbling"), so that the base of the bullet is then facing in the forward direction (14). Yawing enlarges the size of both the permanent and the temporary cavity. Specially designed hourglass bullets actually tumble end over end. Wounds resulting from LVMs and HVMs are compared in Figure 2.5.

Depending upon the composition of the bullet, it may become deformed or it may fragment. As fragments break off, the centripetal force of the rotating bullet disperses them in a radial distribution, each creating its own pathway through the tissue (21). Fragmentation is usually well defined on roentgenograms, which indicate areas of potential damage.

Another concept that is important in determining the development of the temporary cavity is the *rate* of energy transfer from the projectile to the tissue, which is independent of velocity (22). The rate at which

energy is transferred (and absorbed by the tissue) increases as the angle of yaw increases and is maximal at 90°.

Many other types of "specialty" ammunition, such as Teflon-coated armor-piercing rounds, the subsonic ammunition used by Air Marshals against hijackers (which are also amenable to use in silenced weapons), and the rubber bullets used by riot control squads, are available and may have their own particular wounding characteristics (13).

Recently, the relative importance of items such as the effect of velocity on the magnitude of wounding and temporary cavity formation and on the maximal size of the temporary cavity itself has been reexamined (23). These issues are now controversial, and more research is required to clarify them.

### TYPES OF WOUNDING INSTRUMENTS

#### Small Arms: Low- and High-Velocity Weapons

Small arms by definition have barrel bore diameters of less than 0.6 inch. This cate-

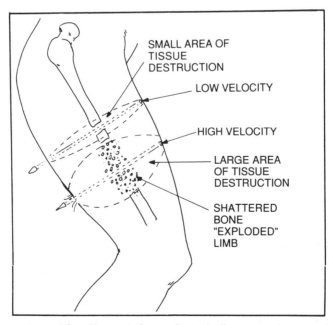

**Figure 2.5.    Comparison of the effects of a low-velocity bullet versus those of a high-velocity bullet on the lower extremity.** (From Creel JH. Mechanisms of injuries due to motion. In Campbell JE (ed): Basic Trauma Life Support: Advanced Prehospital Care. Englewood Cliffs, NJ, Prentice-Hall, 1988, pp 1–20.)

gory includes handguns, shotguns, and rifles. The term *caliber* defines bore diameter in hundredths of an inch. Thus, the ".45 caliber pistol" has a 0.45-inch barrel bore. Also, the bore diameter may be designated in millimeters (e.g., 9.0 mm). Small arms may be further classified as "high velocity" or "low velocity." The two groups are separated by a muzzle velocity of 2500 feet/sec.

### Shotguns

The barrel diameter of the shotgun is described in terms of "gauge" (Fig. 2.6). Gauge is defined as the number of lead balls, each just fitting within the internal diameter of the barrel, which are required to weigh 1 pound. Smaller bores require a smaller ball and thus a larger number of balls to equal a pound. This gives rise to a higher gauge representing a smaller barrel diameter. The number and size of pellets per ounce packed in a shotgun cartridge are represented by the cartridge number (i.e., 00, 0, 1, 2, 3, 4). The choke control on the shotgun regulates the degree of pellet dispersion, acting like a nozzle on a hose. Maximal dispersion is caused by opening the choke all the way (13).

A shotgun may also be loaded with rifled deer slugs ("pumpkin balls"), single, high-caliber rounds. Rifled slugs are designated by gauge and varying weight (1/5 to 1¾ ounces).

## SHOT

| NUMBER | DIAM. IN INCHES | APPROX. PELLETS IN 1 OZ. |
|---|---|---|
| 12 | .05 | 2385 |
| 9 | .08 | 585 |
| 8 | .09 | 410 |
| 7½ | .09½ | 350 |
| 6 | .11 | 225 |
| 5 | .12 | 170 |
| 4 | .13 | 135 |
| 2 | .15 | 90 |
| BB | .18 | 50 |

## BUCKSHOT

| NUMBER | DIAM. IN INCHES | APPROX. PELLETS IN 1 LB. |
|---|---|---|
| 4 | .24 | 340 |
| 3 | .25 | 300 |
| 1 | .30 | 175 |
| 0 | .32 | 145 |
| 00 | .33 | 130 |

**Figure 2.6.** Correlation of number, size (actual) and diameter of shot, and approximate number of pellets in 1 pound. (From Ordog GJ. Wound ballistics. In Ordog GJ (ed): Management of Gunshot Wounds. New York, Elsevier, 1988, pp 25–60.)

Projectiles fired from a shotgun will have a muzzle velocity of approximately 1200 feet/sec (14). When the weapon is fired at ranges below 10 yards, its load will simulate the effect of HVMs. Below 20 yards the pellets behave like LVMs. At extremely short ranges, below 10 feet, or at "point blank range" (1 foot), an additional "blast effect" is present. Here entire areas of the target are "punched out" and debris (e.g., clothing, cardboard, wadding) may be driven into the wound. One can clearly understand why many combat veterans claim that a "sawed-off" (barrel length reduced to a minimum, thus making the weapon more wieldy) 12 gauge shotgun is the most effective close-quarter weapon available. It also explains the extremely low salvage rates in cases of short-range shotgun wounds in the civilian setting (13, 14) (Table 2.3). Additionally, there is a wide range of special ammunition being manufactured for the shotgun today. Included are hollow-point rifled slugs, sabot slugs, fléchettes, gas projectiles, and rubber bullets.

### Fragmentation Munitions

Missile injuries in military personnel (and more recently, in civilian terrorist incidents) may occur because of the disintegration/fragmentation of the metal casing of explosive devices or because of the specially designed shrapnel loads within other similar equipment. Sources include hand-, rifle-, and rocket-propelled grenades, land mines, aerial bombs, and artillery projectiles. As previously stated, the exterior ballistics of these fragments are difficult to predict because the fragments vary in number, size, and shape. However, it can be generally stated that the initial velocities are usually "very high" (> 1200 m/sec) (8).

As opposed to the aerodynamic shaping of bullets, fragments for the most part are irregularly shaped and, thus, the air resistance they face (the "drag") is considerable. Therefore, such projectiles usually have a much more limited effective range when compared to the projectiles fired from small arms (usually less than 15 m). The effective range can be increased by incorporating a fuse that will detonate the shell in the air before it hits the ground ("airburst").

In the case of special "antitank" munitions designed to penetrate the heavy armor of tracked vehicles, additional trauma to the crews may occur because of a delayed, second explosion of a charge within the shell (blast effect and fire) or because of secondary fragmentation of the tank armor itself.

### WOUND BALLISTICS

Now that the general ways in which projectiles cause damage have been discussed, their specific effects on the various regions of the body and its organs will be described. The way a particular organ will respond to a missile depends on the missile's properties and that tissue's density and elastic recoil potential (5, 10, 14, 24). HVMs usually pulp less-elastic organs such as the liver, spleen, kidney, brain, or heart because of the effect of the temporary cavity. The lung, bowel, skin, and muscle, which are more elastic, usually have limited injury unless fragmentation occurs (10, 14).

### Neck

There are many structures in the neck, such as large arteries and veins, nerve

**Table 2.3.   Classification of Shotgun Wounds[a]**

| Range[b] | Injury | Mortality |
|---|---|---|
| | | % |
| Type I: Long (>12 m) | Penetrates only subcutaneous tissue and deep fascia | 0–5 |
| Type II: Close (<12 m) | Penetrates beyond deep fascia | 15–20 |
| Type III: Point blank (<5 m) | Extensive tissue damage | 85–90 |

[a] From Ordog GJ. Wound ballistics. In Ordog CJ (ed): Management of Gunshot Wounds. New York, Elsevier, 1988, pp 25–60.
[b] Distance will vary with each type of shotgun and will be reduced significantly for sawed-off shotguns.

complexes, and the vertebral column. The airway may be damaged easily by direct impact or by the effects of cavitation because of the close proximity of structures. As a general rule, penetrating injuries of the neck require mandatory exploration, although there are some proponents of selective management (4).

### Central Nervous System

Cavitation that occurs within the brain from a HVM usually results in instant death. The effect of transmitted energy from a tangential shot may result in skull fractures or brain contusions or lacerations. Fragmentation of the bullet or skull will compound the damage. A LVM makes a permanent cavity as it traverses the cranial vault. The bullet may remain in the brain substance or in the contralateral skull, or it may exit the head. The sequelae of such passages are dependent upon which areas of the brain are involved.

Peripheral nerves may be stretched or torn or may hemorrhage because of the cavitation of a HVM, which will result in varying degrees of permanent dysfunction. LVMs usually just push nerves aside without much resultant injury, although direct hits may completely sever the nerves.

### Thorax

The heart is virtually shattered by HVMs; death is instantaneous. A LVM may cause a small hole that is amenable to repair, provided death from tamponade or exsanguination does not occur first. If a major vessel is hit, it will be transected and death usually ensues quickly, unless the bleeding is controlled by abutting structures. Tangential hits or cavitation effects may cause limited partial-thickness damage to the vessel walls so that only the media or intima is damaged. Pseudoaneurysms may then form. Such vessel damage may be repaired by surgical anastomosis. LVM damage is usually limited to simple perforation and is associated with a better prognosis.

If the lung alone is hit, it may be treated by simple tube thoracostomy if there is no significant bronchial airway or blood vessel

damage. Fragmentation may macerate the lung and necessitate lobectomy (25).

HVM passage in the lower chest may cause rupture of the diaphragm, with associated damage to the upper abdominal organs due to cavitation. In fact, these organs may be damaged by transference of energy even though the diaphragm is totally intact (14). Tangential gunshot wounds of the chest wall by HVMs have a large potential for causing the same type of energy transference; this may result in a pulmonary contusion or hemothorax if an intercostal or mammary vessel is injured even if the pleura is intact.

### Abdomen

The liver, spleen, and kidney are all pulped by the temporary cavity of the HVM. LVM wounds are usually limited to "drill holes" unless blood vessels within the organs are affected. The bowel will suffer perforation, contusion, or hemorrhage from high-velocity damage. Intramural hemorrhage in either colon or small bowel may proceed to delayed perforation after 2 to 7 days (26). Contused areas share this prognosis. Delayed perforation may then progress to acute peritonitis or intraabdominal abscess formation.

### Extremities

Consideration of the major structures found within a limb leads to a conceptual understanding of the extremity injuries that are possible. Applying one's knowledge of terminal ballistics to an anatomic area will yield a good idea of firearm effects. For example, if the area of the proximal humerus sustains a "hit" from a .357 Magnum, then traumatic amputation of the entire arm is possible. In this case exsanguination from the major arteries and veins becomes the major problem. Injuries caused by smaller caliber LVMs will usually cause drill-hole wounds through muscle, bone, and subcutaneous tissue. HVMs may cause bone fragmentation within a limb (Fig. 2.5). Adjacent arteries and veins may form fistulas, partly due to the searing heat of the bullet (10, 14). Remember that the presence or absence of distal pulses is not a reliable indicator of vascular integrity. Vigilance must be maintained for the development of compartment syndrome.

## Blunt Trauma

### FORCES: ΔV AND GRAVITY

Direct impact, deceleration, continuous pressure, shearing forces, and rotary forces all contribute to the end product of blunt trauma and are all associated with high-speed crashes and high-altitude falls (1). The majority of trauma related to motion can be explained by Newton's First Law, which states that an object in motion has a tendency to remain in motion until acted upon by an outside force. In motor vehicle accidents (MVAs), this force is destructive and acts to decelerate the object (i.e., the motor vehicle and its occupants). This force is a form of gravity, which can occur in any one of the axes of three-dimensional space: forward/rearward (x axis), sideways (y axis), or up/down (z axis) (Fig. 2.7). Therefore, during abrupt deceleration, negative gravitational forces are created (−G). In a head-on collision, negative gravitational forces in the x axis will be generated (−Gx). In a collision occurring with a sideways component, −Gy forces come into play. A person who jumps from a roof and lands upon his feet will be subjected to −Gz forces. As the human body decelerates, the organs continue forward at the original velocity. Under such conditions the body and its organs assume "apparent weights"

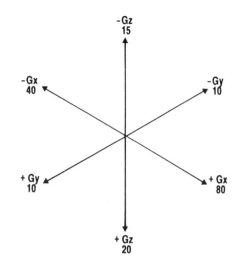

Figure 2.7.  Human tolerance to gravitational forces in three dimensions: Gx, Gy, Gz. (From Grande CM. Mechanisms and patterns of injury: the key to anticipation in trauma management. Crit Care Clin 6:25–35, 1990.)

that vary with velocity (Table 2.4) (21). As they move forward, the organs are torn from their attachments as rotary and shearing forces come into play (3, 5). Connective tissue, blood vessels, and nerves are disrupted. Table 2.5 shows the effects of various Gx forces as correlated with specific injuries.

The severity of injuries may also be correlated with the ΔV, which is defined as the change in velocity when a moving object makes abrupt contact with an object (21). ΔV values of less than 12 miles per hour (mph) are rarely associated with significant injuries. ΔV values of greater than 20 mph

**Table 2.4.    Apparent Weights of the Organs of the Human Body during Violent Impacts at Various Velocities[a]**

| Organ (Actual Weight in kg) | Apparent Weight[b] (kg) | | |
|---|---|---|---|
| | 36 km/hr | 72 km/hr | 108 km/hr |
| Spleen (0.25) | 2.5 | 10 | 22.5 |
| Heart (0.35) | 3.5 | 14 | 31.5 |
| Encephalon (1.5) | 15 | 60 | 135 |
| Liver (1.8) | 18 | 72 | 162 |
| Blood (5.0) | 50 | 200 | 450 |
| Whole body (70) | 700 | 2800 | 6300 |

[a] From Besson A, Saegesser F. Color Atlas of Chest Trauma and Associated Injuries. Oradell, NJ, Medical Economics Books, 1983.
[b] At 36 km/hr the inertial weight of the body and its parts is increased 10-fold over resting weight; at 72 km/hr the increase is 90-fold.

**Table 2.5.   Scale of Typical Injuries Produced by Various G Forces[a]**

| Injury | G Force |
|---|---|
| Compression fractures of vertebral column | 20–30 |
| Atlantoocciptal disruption | 20–40 |
| Transection of vertebra | 200–300 |
| Intimal tear of aorta | 50 |
| Transection of aorta | 80–100 |
| Fractured pelvis | 100–200 |

[a] From Grande CM. Mechanisms and patterns of injury: the key to anticipation in trauma management. Crit Care Clin 6:25–35, 1990.

usually cause severe injuries, depending upon the circumstances. When the $\Delta V$ exceeds 30 mph, the trauma patient is likely to have severe injury. It may be difficult to evaluate the $\Delta V$ at the scene of an accident, but helpful clues may be present (Table 2.6).

Studies have shown that the human body is able to cope with G forces generated in one plane better than with those generated in another. It can sustain more Gx than Gz and more Gz than Gy. This is probably because of the internal arrangement of organs and their attachments. The magnitude of G forces generated by a particular MVA can be calculated using the following formula:

**Table 2.6.   Indications of Major Blunt Trauma and of High-Impact $\Delta V$**

Two or more long bone fractures
Unstable pelvis
Flail chest
Sternal, scapular, clavicular, upper rib fractures
Falls of 15 feet or more (adult), 12 feet or more (child)
$\Delta V$:  20 mph without restraints
       25 mph with restraints
Rearward displacement of car by 20 feet
Rearward displacement of front axle
Engine intrusion into passenger compartment
Frame intrusion into passenger compartment:
   15 inches on patient side of car
   20 inches on opposite side of car
Ejection of passenger
Roll-over
Death of another passenger
Pedestrian struck at 20 mph or more
"Spiderweb" in windshield
Prolonged extrication

$$G \text{ force} = \frac{(\text{mph})^2}{30 \times \text{stopping distance (feet)}}$$

The number 30 serves as a conversion factor that converts feet/second to miles/hour and incorporates gravity (32 feet/sec$^2$). The tremendous G forces associated with even low-speed MVAs can be appreciated by a device called "The Convincer," which simulates the effect of a MVA occurring at a speed of 7 to 8 mph (Fig. 2.8).

The following five factors affect crash survival. The first five letters of each word form "CREEP" (thus, "creep concept"):
   C—containers
   R—restraint
   E—environment
   E—energy absorption
   P—postcrash factors

Points regarding the "container" include the protective steel/alloy "cage" that surrounds the passenger compartment and any padding. Restraints (e.g., seat belts) are discussed below. The "environment" relates to items such as obstacles (e.g., other cars, trees) in the impact area. Energy absorption will vary depending upon factors such as the rate of deceleration and the use of airbags. Postcrash factors include ejection, fires, explosions, and drowning.

## ETIOLOGIES

### Motor Vehicle Accidents

MVAs are usually classified into five types (3, 5):
   Head-on
   Rear impact
   Side impact
   Rotational impact
   Roll-over

Each type produces a distinct pattern of injury (6). A key concept is that, since the passengers of a motor vehicle are going in the same direction as the vehicle, they will have injuries in locations corresponding to damage points on the vehicle. However, there may also be "contre coup" injuries on the opposite side of the body. At times, depending upon the vector forces, the

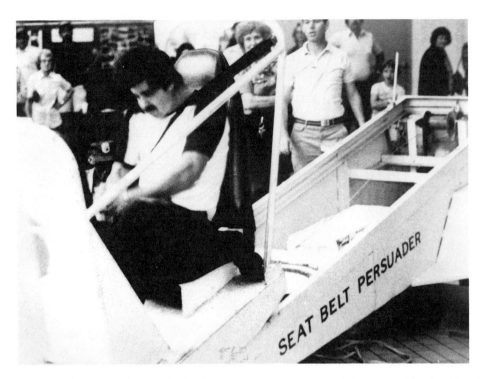

**Figure 2.8.   "The Persuader" crash simulator.** (Courtesy of Regional Programs, Maryland Institute for Emergency Medical Services Systems.)

different types of MVAs may be combined and the injury patterns will be superimposed on each other. For example, a car may have a side impact with another car and then may undergo rotational impact after colliding with a third car.

All of the following injury patterns will be assumed to occur in the unrestrained or improperly restrained passenger.

*Head-on.* If a motor vehicle suddenly impacts an object, its speed is essentially the same as it had been a moment earlier prior to impact. On the other hand, if the operator of the vehicle has time to anticipate the collision, the most common reaction (particularly by untrained operators) is to "lock" the brakes. When the brakes are locked, contact of the wheels with road is lost, and there is little frictional force and thus very little loss in velocity. Therefore impact velocity may still be close to what it had been originally.

In the case of a passenger in an automobile undergoing a head-on impact, one of four patterns will occur: (*a*) the down-and-under or (*b*) the up-and-over; (*c*) in the case of an improperly restrained passenger, one of the "seat belt syndromes." (*d*) The properly restrained passenger can be protected adequately by the passenger compartment and escape with minor injuries.

The *down-and-under pattern* (3, 5) begins with the passenger "slumping" into the seat with knees moving forward. The body's first point of contact is the knees. Force is then transmitted up through the femur to the hips. Possible injuries secondary to this phase of movement include fracture/dislocations of the knees, fractures of the femur, and fracture/dislocations of the acetabulum. If the feet are placed in the floor pan or on the brake pedal, fractures and dislocations of the tibia and fibula may occur, or the ankle may be sprained severely. The upper portion of the body will then also move forward, colliding with the dashboard, steering wheel, and/or windshield, producing injuries of the head, neck, thorax, abdomen, and upper extremities.

Evidence of the down-and-under pattern includes imprints of the knees in the dashboard, "starburst" (spiderweb, bull's eye) patterns in the windshield, and steering wheel imprints on the chest.

In the *up-and-over pattern* (3, 5), the body arcs forward so that the head is first to impact, usually with the windshield. The thorax impacts next, with a large amount of energy being absorbed by the neck (cervical spine) as well. Depending upon the position of the head in relation to the cervical spine at the moment of impact, vertebral fractures may be produced by hyperflexion, hyperextension, or a direct compression mechanism (Figs. 2.9 and 2.10). If the trachea is impacted directly, the "padded dash syndrome" (laryngeal fracture) may be seen (27).

*Rear Impact (3, 5).*    If an automobile is struck from behind while it is stopped or moving slower than the other vehicle, it will have a tendency to accelerate forward abruptly. Portions of the body normally in contact with the car (i.e., all parts except the head and neck) will accelerate also. The head will be "left behind" and then snapped

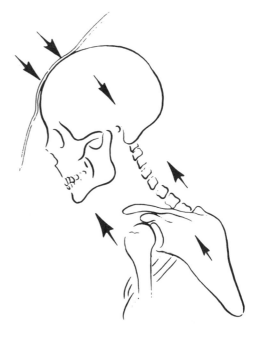

**Figure 2.9.    Forces acting upon the cervical spine when the head makes contact with the windshield during a MVA.** (From McSwain NE. Mechanisms of injuries in trauma. In McSwain NE, Kerstein MD (eds): The evaluation and management of trauma. East Norwalk, CT, Appleton-Century-Crofts, 1987, pp 1–24.)

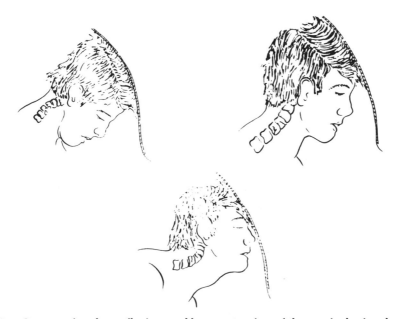

**Figure 2.10.    Compression, hyperflexion, and hyperextension of the cervical spine during impact of the head with the windshield during a MVA.** (From McSwain NE. Mechanisms of injuries in trauma. In McSwain NE, Kerstein MD (eds): The Evaluation and Management of Trauma. East Norwalk, CT, Appleton-Century-Crofts, 1987, pp 1–24.)

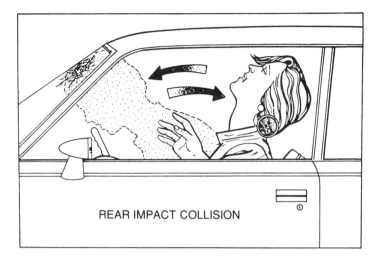

**Figure 2.11.   Mechanisms by which "whiplash" is produced during rear-impact collision.** (From Creel JH. Mechanisms of injuries due to motion. In Campbell JE (ed): Basic Trauma Life Support: Advanced Prehospital Care. Englewood Cliffs, NJ, Prentice-Hall, 1988, pp 1–20.)

along by the neck (Fig. 2.11). This action may produce the "whiplash" syndrome due to stretching, straining, and tearing of cervical muscles and ligaments. If severe enough, spinal fractures can occur. Whiplash can be prevented by correct use of the headrest (head restraint).

If the automobile impacts an object (e.g., another car) in front after having been struck from behind, conditions for a head-on pattern exist.

*Side Impact (3, 5).*   The side-impact MVA is typical of those seen in an intersection where one car runs a yellow or red light or on a side street when a car is pulling out of a driveway and is struck by oncoming traffic. In a manner similar to that described for whiplash injury, when an automobile undergoes side impact, the car is pushed out "from underneath" the passengers.

The occupant on the side closest to the impact may collide with the door or other parts of the frame. If the $\Delta V$ is large enough, the body of the car may actually intrude into the passenger compartment (Table 2.6). Any portions of the "exposed" side of the body may be injured: head, neck, thorax, abdomen, and upper and lower extremities. Because of the mechanics of the impact, the neck may be subject to a sideways version of whiplash injury (with spinal fractures being

more common here than in the rear-impact type) (3). The lateral organs of the abdomen may be punctured by the inwardly moving rib fragments. If the greater trochanter of the femur is struck, the femoral head may be driven through the acetabulum (Fig. 2.12). Also, the pelvis may be disrupted.

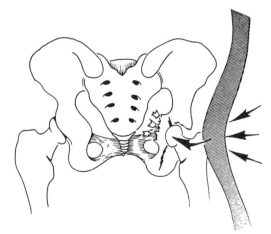

**Figure 2.12.   The head of the femur is driven into the acetabulum because of force on the greater trochanter secondary to side-impact collision.** (From McSwain NE. Mechanisms of injury in trauma. In McSwain NE, Kerstein MD (eds): The Evaluation and Management of Trauma, East Norwalk, CT, Appleton-Century-Crofts, 1987, pp 1–24.)

The passenger on the side opposite the impact will be moved toward the contralateral side of the car. Thus, there may be a collision of passengers who, because of gravitational effects, may have enormous "apparent" weights and thus crush each other.

*Rotational Impact (3).* Impacts occurring at a corner of the automobile will impart a rotational component of movement depending upon which part of the car is hit. If a secondary collision occurs (e.g., as the car then collides with a telephone pole), any combination of the three above MVA patterns may emerge.

*Roll-over (3, 5).* In a rollover MVA the passenger may be subject to any combination of the first three patterns of MVAs except that they may be applied to all three dimensions as opposed to only two. The occupant may be struck by unsecured objects moving in the passenger compartment as missiles. There is also a significant probability for ejection.

*Ejection (3).* Ejection from an automobile may be total or partial. In partial ejection a limb may be thrust out through a window and subsequently caught between the car and another object (e.g., another car, the road), undergoing crush, laceration, degloving, and almost any other type of trauma. If a passenger is completely ejected, there is a sixfold increased chance of injury or death.

### Seatbelts: Effect on Morbidity/Mortality and the "Seatbelt Syndrome"

Currently there are three passenger restraint devices available for use in automobiles: seatbelts, airbags, and the belt/knee bar combination (28). They may be used in combination. The most commonly available is the seatbelt. Although the "five-point" restraint configuration (two shoulder straps, waist/lap belt, and a crotch strap to prevent "submarining") does exist, the two most common are the lap belt and the lap belt/chest (diagonal) strap. Eighty-seven per cent of the population of the United States does not use any passenger restraint (3).

If worn properly, seatbelts drastically reduce the overall incidence of injury, especially head injury (29, 30). This has been demonstrated by the Australian experience since their regulations that mandate 100% compliance with seatbelt wearing took effect (31, 32). Similar experiences have been seen in other countries and in American states that enforce mandatory seatbelt use (33). If not properly worn, seatbelts themselves can induce morbidity and mortality (34).

A lap belt should be worn so that it crosses over the groin area between the femur and the anterior-superior ileac spine. If positioned above this area, strain will be placed on the lumbar spine and intraabdominal organs. The lumbar spine (and lower portions of the thoracic spine) will be prone to acute forward flexion and subsequent angulation around the seatbelt. Disruption of spinal ligaments and anterior compression fractures of the vertebral bodies may then occur (35, 36).

Use of a lap belt without a diagonal strap will still permit portions of the upper body to make contact with the windshield, dashboard, and steering wheel (3). Injuries to any of these areas may occur. Of course, this can be prevented by wearing the diagonal strap in conjunction with the lap belt (three-point restraint).

If the diagonal belt (shoulder belt) is worn without the lap belt or without a knee bar, the lower body will continue to move forward on impact. Most often the diagonal belt will then loop under the chin, causing neck injuries, strangulation, or decapitation (3). Alternatively, there may be angulation of the normally rigid thoracic spine around the belt, leading to problems in this anatomic region, as well as raising the possibility of contact of the head and neck with structures such as the windshield and steering wheel. In some instances, passengers choose to wear the diagonal belt in an underarm position to alleviate neck irritation and other discomforts. During an impact this places great strain on the lower thorax and upper abdomen, similar to that seen when the lap belt is worn too high. Injury to the lower thoracic/upper lumbar spine and intraabdominal organs may then occur (37). Other "unauthorized" variations of seatbelt use exist and result in a number of different patterns of injury (34).

Even if the three-point restraint system is used properly, characteristic injuries may occur. The most common are fractures of the ribs, clavicle, or sternum (38, 39). Several articles have reported injury to solid intrathoracic and intraabdominal organs in conjunction with the use of the restraints, but these appear to occur only in extreme cases (40). Clearly, in most instances the injuries caused by the proper use of seatbelts are less major than those that would occur had they not been worn.

### Motorcycle Accidents

When a passenger of a motorcycle (or for that matter any unenclosed vehicle) is involved in a collision, the situation is very much like that of a passenger ejected from an automobile in a MVA. The individual is subject to forces acting in any of the three dimensions, the only protection being articles such as a helmet, a face plate, leather clothing, or metal plating. In recent years, a number of states have repealed or changed laws regarding motorcycle helmet usage (41). The majority of this legislation has led to more situations that require minimal or no helmet wearing. The epidemiology of head injuries since these legislative changes occurred has been studied and shows an increase in volume and financial expenditures for long-term care (41).

In motorcycle accidents there are characteristic patterns similar to those for MVAs. Motorcycle accidents usually involve deceleration and impact in one of several directions: forward, sideways, or rearward (3). Usually these incidents will cause injuries (e.g., fractures) of the lower extremities as they collide with other objects. If the passenger is ejected from the motorcycle, injuries may involve the head, neck, and upper extremities. In one special type of motorcycle accident, known as "laying the bike down," the driver orients the vehicle perpendicular to the direction of travel, "lays" down the vehicle away from the direction of travel, and then "steps off," thereby separating himself from the motorcycle and reducing the chance of injury. Severe abrasions or "road rash" of areas of the body not adequately protected (e.g., by leather garments) will be seen.

### Degloving and Compartment Syndrome

Shearing forces are the major cause of degloving injuries. This type of trauma may be seen in a trauma patient who has been run over by a motor vehicle. As the vehicle passes over the body, the skin and subcutaneous tissues are "sheared" away from their blood vessels and the muscles below, causing extensive tissue loss.

Low-velocity trauma associated with sustained pressure can lead to development of the crush syndrome. In this case local compression of the muscle and blood vessels is followed by ischemia and stasis injury to the capillaries. Increased permeability of the minute blood vessels follows, with leakage of fluid into the interstitium. Fascial compartmental tamponade then occurs. Muscle necrosis, nerve damage, and paralysis ensue. If cell death is prominent, myoglobin and hemoglobin may be released and precipitate acute renal tubular necrosis. Early signs and symptoms of compartment syndrome should be recognized to avoid serious sequelae. Pain and tense swelling in the affected extremity signal compartment syndrome. If severe enough, third-space losses will result in hypovolemia, oliguria, and an increased hematocrit. Treatment by early fasciotomy and necrotic tissue excision is mandatory. Hyperbaric oxygenation may also be helpful (see Chapter 14).

### Falls From Great Heights (FGH)

FGH may be considered a form of blunt trauma in which injury may be caused by all of the decelerating forces discussed earlier in the chapter. Two differences are that movement is in the vertical plane and that, if

**Table 2.7.   Relation of Distance Fallen to Velocity at Impact[a]**

| Duration of Fall | Distance Fallen | Velocity at Impact | |
|---|---|---|---|
| | | ft/sec | mph |
| sec | ft | | |
| 1 | 16.1 | 32.2 | 21.9 |
| 2 | 64.4 | 64.4 | 43.9 |
| 3 | 144.9 | 96.9 | 65.8 |
| 4 | 257.6 | 128.8 | 87.8 |
| 5 | 402.5 | 161.0 | 109.8 |
| 6 | 579.6 | 193.2 | 131.7 |

[a] Modified from Besson A, Saegesser F. Color Atlas of Chest Trauma and Associated Injuries. Oradell, NJ, Medical Economics Books, 1983.

"terminal velocity" (approximately 120 mph) has not yet been reached, the body may still be accelerating (Table 2.7) (42). FGH may also be associated with combined forms of blunt and penetrating trauma, such as impalement. Consider the trauma patient who has fallen out of a fourth story window and landed on a picket fence (43).

FGH may be classified by various systems. One may be based on the position and alignment of the body structure at the time of impact. Another may be based on causative factors (44, 45).

With regard to the first system, the subject may impact in one of several standardized positions: (a) standing, (b) sitting, (c) supine, (d) prone, or (e) diving. Each can be correlated with a resultant injury constellation. For example, the trauma patient who is in the standing position at the time of impact will be expected to have compression/torsion injuries of the calcaneus, tibia, fibula, femur, pelvis, and spinal column (Fig. 2.13). Con-

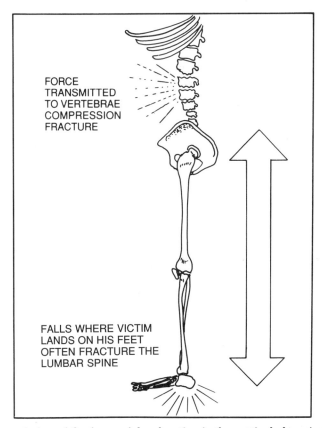

FORCE TRANSMITTED TO VERTEBRAE COMPRESSION FRACTURE

FALLS WHERE VICTIM LANDS ON HIS FEET OFTEN FRACTURE THE LUMBAR SPINE

**Figure 2.13.   Transmission of the force of deceleration in the vertical plane (−Gz) when the body impacts in the "standing" position after a fall from a great height.** (From Creel JH. Mechanisms of injuries due to motion. In Campbell JE (ed): Basic Trauma Life Support: Advanced Prehospital Care, Englewood Cliffs, NJ, Prentice-Hall, 1988, pp 1–20.)

ceptually, the decelerating forces (−Gz) are acting linearly through these aligned skeletal structures. The "diving" or "head-first" position (again −Gz) will be associated with injuries of the cranium or brain, the face, and/or the cervical spine, as well as possible injuries of the upper extremities, shoulder girdle, or lumbar spine if these portions of the body absorb much of the impact.

Survivability of a fall is based on at least three factors: (a) distance of fall (or velocity at impact), (b) anatomic areas that impact, and (c) characteristics of the surface struck. The most important surface characteristics include "surface density" (concrete versus sawdust) and irregularity (smooth floor versus stairway) (5).

In the alternative system, injuries correlate with the background reason for the fall; the "lover's leap," the "jumper" syndrome, the "Don Juan" syndrome, and the "paratrooper" syndrome are associated with discrete injury constellations (5, 45).

Regardless of the position at impact, various heights have been correlated with "estimated lethal doses" (ED). The ED in 50% (ED50) of the population is four stories (one story = 12 feet). The ED in 90% of the population (ED90) is seven stories (46).

## TRAUMA CLASSIFICATION SYSTEMS

In the early 1970s objective systems to characterize the trauma patient were first devised. The purposes of such schemes were (a) to provide a "common language" to equate injuries of varied anatomic locations in terms of severity, (b) to direct triage and subsequent care more objectively and consistently, (c) to evaluate methods of treatment, (d) to document progress, (e) to predict outcome in terms of morbidity and mortality with respect to certain injuries, (f) to identify problem areas in terms of trauma care delivery, and (g) to guide the allotment of resources (47).

With the recently introduced concept of Diagnostic Related Groups (DRGs), comparison of the data produced by such systems will allow more reasonable reimbursement

(see Chapter 1). For example, a center such as the Shock Trauma Center of the Maryland Institute for Emergency Medical Services Systems (MIEMSS), which handles a large percentage of more seriously ill trauma patients, cannot be categorized with less sophisticated trauma centers or with community hospitals. The fact that the MIEMSS Shock Trauma Center does deal with such a population of trauma patients will be revealed through the use of one of these systems.

Also, mistakes in field triage by paraprofessionals are thought to be a significant problem. In this capacity, an objective method of evaluation might optimally serve to identify those patients who are sick enough to be adversely affected by poor care but are not so sick as to die if appropriate care is provided (47).

Today, many such systems exist. The most popular and useful of these are the Injury Severity Score (ISS) and the Trauma Score (TS) (48, 49). The ISS is based on anatomic evaluation and quantitates the severity of physical injury, whereas the TS uses physiologic parameters like blood pressure and respiratory rate. Further modifications of these systems, such as the Trauma Chart, have followed (50).

### The Injury Severity Score (ISS)

The ISS (also known as the Maryland Scoring System) was developed in 1974 from the Abbreviated Injury Scale (AIS) in an effort to compare persons whose injuries, although not necessarily the same anatomically, were of similar severity (Table 2.8)

**TABLE 2.8.    Abbreviated Injury Scale (AIS)**

| AIS Score | Definition |
|---|---|
| 0 | No injury |
| 1 | Minimal injury |
| 2 | Moderate injury |
| 3 | Severe injury (non-life-threatening) |
| 4 | Severe injury (life-threatening) |
| 5 | Critical injury (low probability of survival) |
| 6 | Maximal injury (fatal/currently untreatable) |

(51). It was found that, if the three highest AIS scores were squared and then added together, the sum correlated very well with mortality and morbidity rates. Studies show that using a single AIS code, the square of a single AIS code, or the sums of the squares of two AIS codes does not correlate as well (49). Additionally, using a fourth AIS rating instead of three does not improve accuracy significantly (49).

The highest AIS score for a person with trauma to a single area is 25. This is based on the fact that the highest nonlethal AIS score that may be assigned to any nonlethal injury is 5 ($5^2 = 25$). A lethal injury such as decapitation receives an AIS score of 6 and automatically gives an ISS of 75. The highest score a person with three or more injuries can be assigned is 75 (three scores of 25 added together). The relationships of the ISS to mortality and to disability are shown in Tables 2.9 and 2.10. These correlations change with age. Intuitively, it would be reasonable to assume that an older person with a given ISS should have a worse prognosis than a younger person with the same score, a relationship that has been demonstrated to be true (52, 53). Death rates are higher among 50- to 69-year-olds than among younger patients and are much higher in the group over 70 years old. This age-associated differential is more exaggerated for less severe injuries; that is, the rate of death in persons over 70 years old relative

TABLE 2.10.   ISS for Different Degrees of Disability[a]

| Disability | ISS (mean ± S.E.) |
| --- | --- |
| Very severe | 32.4 ± 4.70 |
| Severe | 18.5 ± 1.61 |
| Moderate | 12.7 ± 0.62 |
| Slight | 10.1 ± 0.61 |
| Nil | 5.8 ± 0.12 |

[a] From Bull JP. Measures of severity of injury. Injury 9:184–187, 1978.

to persons under 50 increases as ISS decreases. Conversely, for the most severe trauma constituting an ISS score of greater than 50, this age differential is negligible. Incidentally, it appears that the elderly (65 years and older) are less likely to be injured than younger people but are more likely to die of those injuries that do occur.

The ISS becomes valuable when used as part of the initial triage decision process. Trauma patients with an ISS score greater than 15 should be transported directly to a trauma center (54). Those with an ISS score below 50 may have the greatest potential for improved survival if treated at a trauma center with minimal delays, as the majority of these trauma patients are still alive at the end of the "golden hour."

Criticism of the ISS stems mainly from the impression that it is useful only in cases of blunt trauma (although recent developments have widened its applicability somewhat) (47, 55). Another point is that the ISS is noncontinuous; that is, individual num-

TABLE 2.9.   Approximate Probability of Mortality for Different Combinations of ISS and Age[a]

| ISS | Mortality Probability at Age: | | | | | | |
| --- | --- | --- | --- | --- | --- | --- | --- |
| | 15–<25 | 25–<35 | 35–<45 | 45–<55 | 55–<65 | 65–<75 | 75–<85 |
| 55–<60 | 1.0 | 1.0 | 1.0 | 1.0 | 1.0 | 1.0 | 1.0 |
| 50–<55 | 0.9 | 0.9 | 1.0 | 1.0 | 1.0 | 1.0 | 1.0 |
| 45–<50 | 0.7 | 0.8 | 0.9 | 1.0 | 1.0 | 1.0 | 1.0 |
| 40–<45 | 0.6 | 0.7 | 0.8 | 0.9 | 1.0 | 1.0 | 1.0 |
| 35–<40 | 0.4 | 0.5 | 0.6 | 0.8 | 0.9 | 1.0 | 1.0 |
| 30–<35 | 0.3 | 0.3 | 0.5 | 0.6 | 0.8 | 0.9 | 1.0 |
| 25–<30 | 0.2 | 0.2 | 0.2 | 0.4 | 0.7 | 0.8 | 0.9 |
| 20–<25 | 0.1 | 0.1 | 0.1 | 0.2 | 0.3 | 0.5 | 0.8 |
| 15–<20 | 0 | 0 | 0 | 0.1 | 0.1 | 0.3 | 0.5 |
| 10–<15 | 0 | 0 | 0 | 0 | 0 | 0.1 | 0.3 |
| 5–<10 | 0 | 0 | 0 | 0 | 0 | 0 | 0.1 |
| 0–<5 | 0 | 0 | 0 | 0 | 0 | 0 | 0 |

[a] From Bull JP: Measures of severity of injury. Injury 9:184–187, 1987.

bers are skipped between 1 and 75 (55). The importance of this fact is questionable.

## The Trauma Score

The Trauma Score (TS) is a modification of the previously described Triage Score and is currently advocated for use by the American College of Surgeons, being taught as part of the Advanced Trauma Life Support curriculum (56). In calculating the TS, respiratory rate, respiratory effort, systolic blood pressure, capillary refill, and neurologic status (evaluated by the Glasgow Coma Scale) are considered. Table 2.11 demonstrates the way to arrive at the TS. Trauma patients most likely to receive the greatest benefit from rapid definitive care at a trauma center are those with a TS of 13 or less (54). Table 2.12 shows the correlation of probability of survival with TS values.

**Table 2.11.    Trauma Score[a]**

|  | Rate | Code | Score |
|---|---|---|---|
| A. *Respiratory rate* | 10–24 | 4 | |
| Number of respirations in 15 sec; multiply by | 25–35 | 3 | |
| 4 | ≥36 | 2 | |
| | 1–9 | 1 | |
| | 0 | 0 | A.____ |
| B. *Respiratory effort* | | | |
| *Retractive*—Use of accessory muscles or | Normal | 1 | |
| intercostal retraction | Retractive/none | 0 | B.____ |
| C. *Systolic blood pressure* | ≥90 | 4 | |
| *Systolic cuff pressure*—either arm auscultate or | 70–89 | 3 | |
| palpate | 50–69 | 2 | |
| | 0–49 | 1 | |
| No carotid pulse | 0 | 0 | C.____ |
| D. *Capillary refill* | | | |
| *Normal*—Forehead or lip mucosa color refill | Normal | 2 | |
| in 2 sec | | | |
| *Delayed*—More than 2 sec capillary refill | Delayed | 1 | |
| *None*—No capillary refill | None | 0 | D.____ |
| E. *Glasgow Coma Scale* | | | |
| 1. *Eye opening* | | *Total GCS Points* | *Score* |
| Spontaneous ____4 | | 14–15 | 5 |
| To voice ____3 | | 11–13 | 4 |
| To pain ____2 | | 8–10 | 3 |
| None ____1 | | 5–7 | 2 |
| | | 3–4 | 1    E.____ |
| 2. *Verbal response* | | | |
| Oriented ____5 | | | |
| Confused ____4 | | | |
| Inappropriate words ____3 | | | |
| Incomprehensible sounds ____2 | | | |
| None ____1 | | | |
| 3. *Motor response* | | | |
| Obeys commands ____6 | | | |
| Localizes pain ____5 | | | |
| Withdraw (pain) ____4 | | | |
| Flexion (pain) ____3 | | | |
| Extension (pain) ____2 | | | |
| None ____1 | | | |
| *Total GCS points* (1 + 2 + 3) ____ | (Total points A + B + C + D + E) *Trauma Score* ____ | | |

[a] From Champion HR, Sacco WL. Trauma scoring. In Mattox KL, Moore EE, Feliciano DV (eds): Trauma. Norwalk, CT, Appleton-Lange, 1988, pp 63–77. After Champion HR, Sacco WJ, Carnazzo AJ, et al. Trauma score. Crit Care Med 9:672, 1981.

**TABLE 2.12.   Probability of Survival (P_s) for Trauma Score Values[a]**

| Trauma Score on Admission | $P_s$ |
|---|---|
| | % |
| 1 | 2.3 |
| 2 | 6.1 |
| 3 | 6.2 |
| 4 | 14.3 |
| 5 | 21.6 |
| 6 | 31.7 |
| 7 | 38.3 |
| 8 | 52.2 |
| 9 | 61.7 |
| 10 | 66.7 |
| 11 | 75.2 |
| 12 | 80.4 |
| 13 | 90.7 |
| 14 | 95.0 |
| 15 | 97.6 |
| 16 | 99.1 |

[a] Data from 25,327 patients submitted by 51 institutions to the Major Trauma Outcome Study. From Champion HR, Sacco WL. Trauma scoring. In Mattox KL, Moore EE, Feliciano DV (eds): Trauma. Norwalk, CT, Appleton and Lange, 1988, pp. 63–67.

## TRISS

Correlations of the ISS and the TS and their ability to predict survival rates yield $R$ values between 0.7 and 0.9. Using a combination of both the ISS and the TS with the addition of age will produce $R$ values of at least 0.9. The combination of these three parameters is called the TRISS index (47).

## SUMMARY

In this chapter the reader has been presented with an introduction to the complex study of mechanisms of injury. As stated in the introduction, this knowledge will permit the TA/CCS to render better care to the trauma patients for whom he or she is responsible. Understanding the various common measurements of injury will assist the anesthesiologist by giving a "head start" in the hectic moments when the trauma patient is first received; will allow more realistic planning, preparation, and allocation of resources; and will help to avoid iatrogenic pitfalls. Ultimately this knowledge may have its greatest value when applied to the *prevention* of trauma. The trauma anesthesi-

ologist should also be an active participant in this phase of care.

Although this chapter basically focuses upon penetrating and blunt trauma, one should be aware of the many other forms of injury. It behooves the practicing trauma anesthesiologist to make a study of the demographics of trauma in his or her particular location and to become familiar with local "etiologies" (e.g., lower extremity fractures due to skiing accidents in a resort area) (57).

One should also be aware that, for the most part, the mechanisms of injury described here relate to trauma on an *organ* level. These mechanisms of injury and the trauma they produce lead to secondary mechanisms of injury at a *cellular* level (e.g., hypoxia). These cellular mechanisms of injury are described in Chapter 4.

## References

1. Odling-Smee W, Crockard A. The trauma problem. In Odling-Smee W, Crockard A (eds): Trauma Care. London, Academic Press, 1981, pp 3–18.
2. Trowbridge AM, Giesecke AH. Multiple injuries. Clin Anesth 1976;11:79–84.
3. McSwain NE. Mechanisms of injuries in blunt trauma. In McSwain NE, Kerstein MD (eds): Evaluation and Management of Trauma. East Norwalk, CT, Appleton-Century-Crofts, 1987, pp 1–24.
4. McSwain NE. Kinematics of penetrating injury. J Prehosp Care October/November 1986;10–13.
5. Creel JH. Mechanisms of injuries due to motion. In Campbell JE (ed): Basic Trauma Life Support: Advanced Prehospital Care. Englewood Cliffs, NJ, Prentice-Hall, 1988, pp 1–20.
6. Feliciano DV. Patterns of injury. In Mattox KL, Moore EE, Feliciano DV (eds): Trauma. Norwalk, CT, Appleton and Lange, 1988, pp 91–103.
7. Grande CM, Tissot M, Bhatt V, Patasky A, Rivlin M, Kurtti N. Pre-existing compromising conditions. In Capan LM, Miller S, Turndorf H (eds): Trauma: Anesthesia and Perioperative Care. Philadelphia, JB Lippincott (in press).
8. Wiener SL, Barrett J. Explosions and explosive device-related injuries. In Wiener SL, Barrett J (eds): Trauma Management for Civilian and Military Physicians. Philadelphia, WB Saunders, 1986, pp 13–26.
9. Fackler ML. Physics of missile injuries. In McSwain NE, Kersteon MD (eds): Evaluation and

Management of Trauma. East Norwalk, CT, Appleton-Century-Crofts, 1987, pp 25–41.

10. Owen-Smith MS. High velocity and military gunshot wounds. In Ordog GJ (ed): Management of Gunshot Wounds. New York, Elsevier, 1988, pp 61–94.

11. Walton CB, Blaisdell FN, Jordan RG, Bodai BI. The injury potential and lethality of stab wounds: Folsom Prison study. J Trauma 1989;29:99–101.

12. Barach E, Tomlanovich M, Nowak R. Ballistics: a pathophysiologic examination of mechanisms of firearms: part II. J Trauma 1986;26:374–383.

13. Ordog GJ. Wound ballistics. In Ordog GJ (ed): Management of Gunshot Wounds. New York, Elsevier, 1988, pp 25–60.

14. Wiener SL, Barrett J. Wound ballistics. In Weiner SL, Barrett J (eds): Trauma Management for Civilian and Military Physicians. Philadelphia, WB Saunders, 1986, pp 1–12.

15. Harrel JB. Hollowpoint ammunition injuries: experience in a police group. J Trauma 1979;19: 115–116.

16. Eckert WG. Exploding bullets: a hazard to the victim, physician, and investigator. Am J Forensic Med Pathol 1981;2:103–104.

17. Tate ZG, DiMaio VJM, Davis JH. Rebirth of exploding ammunition—a report of six human casualties J Forensic Sci 1981;26:636–644.

18. Abidin MR. Letter on exploding ammunition. J Trauma 1989;29:896.

19. Amatuzio JC, Coe JI. Homicide by exploded ammunition. Am J Forensic Med Pathol 1981;2: 111–113.

20. Menzies RC, Anderson LE. The Glaser safety slug and the Velex/Velet exploding bullet. J Forensic Sci 1980;25:44–52.

21. Trunkey DD. Wound ballistics. In Trunkey DD, Lewis FR (eds): Current Therapy of Trauma—2. Toronto, BC Decker, 1986, pp 94–104.

22. Rybeck B, Janzon B. Absorption of missile energy in soft tissue. Acta Chir Scand 1976;142:201–207.

23. Fackler ML. Wound ballistics: a review of common misconceptions. JAMA 1988;259:2730–2736.

24. Amato JT, Billy LJ, Lawson NS, Rich NM. High velocity missile injury: an experimental study of the retentive forces of tissue. Am J Surg 1974; 127:454–459.

25. DeMuth WE. High velocity bullet wounds of the thorax. Am J Surg 1968;115:616–625.

26. Johansson L, Holmstrom A, Norrby K, Nystrom PO, Lennquist S. Intramural hemorrhage of the intestine as an indirect effect of abdominal missile trauma—classification and prognosis. Acta Chir Scand [Suppl] 1982;508:175–177.

27. Butler RM, Moster FH. The padded dash syndrome and blunt trauma to the larynx and trachea. Laryngoscope 1968;78:1172–1182.

28. Herbert DC. Injury reduction by diagonal and other vehicle safety belts. Med J Aust 1964;1: 61–72.

29. Evans L. Fatality risk reduction from safety belt use. J Trauma 1987;27:746–749.

30. Huekle DF, Sherman HW. Seat belt effectiveness: case examples from real-world crash investigations. J Trauma 1987;27:750–753.

31. Henderson M, Wood R. Compulsory wearing of seat belts in New South Wales, Australia: an evaluation of its effects on vehicle occupant deaths in the first year. Med J Aust 1973; 2:797–801.

32. Marburger EA, Friedel B. Seat belt legislation and seat belt effectiveness in the Federal Republic of Germany. J Trauma 1987;27:703–705.

33. Petrucelli E. Seat belt laws: the New York experience—preliminary data and some observations. J Trauma 1987;27:706–710.

34. Sato TB. Effects of seat belt and injuries resulting from improper use. J Trauma 1987;27:754–758.

35. Smith WS, Kaufer H. Patterns and mechanisms of lumbar injuries associated with seat belts. J Bone Joint Surg [Am] 1969;51A:239–251.

36. Burke DC. Spinal cord injuries and seat belts. Med J Aust 1973;2:801–806.

37. States JD, Huelke DF, Dance MD, Green RN. Fatal injuries caused by underarm use of shoulder belts. J Trauma 1987;27:740–746.

38. Michelinakis E. Safety-belt syndrome. Practitioner 1977;207:77–80.

39. Williams JS, Kirkpatrick JR. The nature of seat belt injuries. J Trauma 1971;11:207–218.

40. Woelfel GF, Moore EE, Cogbill TH. Severe thoracic and abdominal injuries associated with lap-harness seatbelts. J Trauma 1984;24:166–167.

41. McSwain NE, Lumis M. The impact of the repeal of motorcycle helmet law. Surg Gynecol Obstet 1980;151:215–225.

42. Synder RG. Terminal velocity impacts into snow. Milit Med October 1966;1290–1298.

43. Horowitz MD, Dove DB, Eismont FJ, Green BA. Impalement injuries. J Trauma 1985;25:914–916.

44. Maull KI, Whitley RE, Cardea JA. Vertical deceleration injuries. Surg Gynecol Obstet 1981;153: 233–236.

45. Ciccone R, Richmar R. The mechanisms of injury and the distribution of three thousand fractures and dislocations caused by parachute jumping. J Bone Joint Surg [Am] 1948;30A:77–79.

46. Kazarian KK, Bole P, Ketchum SW, Mersheimer WL. High-flyer syndrome. NY State J Med 1976;76:982–985.

47. Champion HR, Sacco WL. Trauma scoring. In Mattox KL, Moore EE, Feliciano DV (eds): Trauma. Norwalk, CT, Appleton and Lange, 1988, pp 63–77.

48. Champion HR, Sacco WJ, Carnazzo AJ, Copes W, Fouty WJ. Trauma score. Crit Care Med 1981; 9:672–676.

49. Baker SP, O'Neill B, Haddon W Jr, Long WB. The injury severity score: a method for describing

patients with multiple injuries and evaluating emergency care. J Trauma 1974;14:187–196.

50. Greenspan L, McLellan BA, Greig H. Abbreviated injury scale and injury severity score: a scoring chart. J Trauma 1985;25:60–64.

51. Committee on Medical Aspects of Automotive Safety: Rating the severity of tissue damage. I. The abbreviated scale. JAMA 1971;215:277–280.

52. Oreskovich MR, Howard JD, Copass MK, et al. Geriatric trauma: injury patterns and outcome. J Trauma 1984;24:565–572.

53. Lauer AR. Age and sex in relation to accidents. Safety Res Rev 1959;3:21–25.

54. Champion HR, Sacco WJ. Triage of trauma victims. In Trunkey DD, Lewis FR (eds): Current Therapy of Trauma. Philadelphia, BC Decker, 1986, pp 5–13.

55. Bull JP. Injury severity scoring systems. Injury 1982;14:2–6.

56. Committee on Trauma. Advanced Trauma Life Support, ed 3. Chicago, American College of Surgeons, 1989.

57. Morpugo CV. L'anestesia per il servizio traumatologico invernale in montagne [anesthesia for a winter trauma service in the mountains]. Arch Ortop 1956;6:565–569.

# 3

# Airway Management for the Trauma Patient

*John K. Stene, Christopher M. Grande, and Charles R. Barton*

Unlike the general surgical patient, the trauma patient usually presents a complex scenario for airway management: the patient has suffered multiple life- and limb-threatening injuries, is unprepared for surgical interventions, and usually has a "full stomach." Although many anesthesiologists tend to focus their attention on this last condition (aspiration prophylaxis), it is only one of the many problems associated with posttraumatic airway management.

There are many reasons for the trauma patient to be in respiratory failure (Table 3.1). The anesthesiologist must first determine whether the patient requires artificial ventilation. Many patients who are breathing spontaneously when admitted to the hospital will have less morbidity if airway intervention and mechanical ventilation are instituted early in the admission process (1,

2). Patients who present with cardiac or respiratory arrest require immediate artificial ventilation. Comatose patients require tracheal intubation to protect their airways from aspiration and to facilitate ventilation, which will in turn reduce arterial carbon dioxide ($PaCO_2$) and intracranial pressure (ICP). Patients with long bone fractures resulting from high-energy impacts are less likely to develop the fat emboli syndrome if they receive an initial period of mechanical pulmonary ventilation (3). Patients in traumatic shock require comprehensive resuscitation, which includes mechanical ventilation as well as massive fluid replacement (2).

These considerations form part of the decision-making basis for the anesthesiologist. However, management decisions must also be based on a thorough understanding not only of airway anatomy but also of the

**Table 3.1.    Etiologies of Respiratory Failure in the Trauma Patient**

Aspiration
Foreign body obstruction
Soft tissue obstruction (e.g., tongue)
    Prolapse due to the relaxation of unconsciousness
    Prolapse due to mandibular fracture or maxillo-facial injury
    Edema/hematoma formation
Pulmonary injury
    Hemothorax
    Pneumothorax
    Hemopneumothorax
    Lung contusion
Mediastinal emphysema
Upper airway collapse due to cervical hematoma, etc.
Rib fractures
Flail chest
Largyngeal fracture
Laryngotracheal separation
Tracheobronchial laceration
Pulmonary edema (cardiac)
Adult respiratory distress syndrome (e.g., traumatic, neurologic etiologies)
Hypoventilation secondary to:
    Cervical trauma
    Cranial trauma
    Diaphragmatic hernia
    Thoracic wall injury
Central nervous system depression (e.g., secondary to drug overdose, hypoxia)
Electrocution
Inhalation injury
Cardiac injury
Preexisting medical condition

[a] From Grande CM, Stene JK, Bernhard WN. Airway management: considerations in the trauma patient. Crit Care Clin 1990;6:37–59.

physiology of trauma as a disease. The ability to create rapid solutions to airway obstruction ultimately may determine the patient's survival.

## ANATOMY AND PHYSIOLOGY

The anesthetist's ability to secure a patient's airway can be affected by direct injury to the airway or by the secondary systemic physiologic changes initiated by injury. Airway anatomy and physiology are described in depth in other sources (4–6); therefore, this chapter will concentrate on traumatic effects influencing airway management.

The upper airway (consisting of the nose; the mouth; the nasal, oral, and laryngeal portions of the pharynx; and the larynx) is particularly vulnerable to maxillofacial trauma (7, 8). Fractures of the nasal bones can obstruct the nasal airway. Midface fractures can permit posterior movement of the hard palate, creating airway obstruction. Mandibular fractures, especially bilateral fractures, can allow the tongue to obstruct the pharynx. Soft tissue injury accompanying these fractures can aggravate airway obstruction (9–11) (see Chapter 8).

Injury to the temporomandibular joint, which is both a gliding joint and a hinge joint, may impede adequate mouth opening. The mandible may need to be extended with a jaw thrust to "sublux" the temporomandibular joint and enhance mouth opening (12–14). The difficulties presented to laryngeal exposure by inadequate mouth opening relative to tongue size have been emphasized by several authors (15–17). The most reliable anatomic indicator of a difficult intubation is a tongue that obscures visualization of the posterior pharynx during the preinduction examination.

The lower airway, consisting of the conducting airways (trachea and bronchi) and the gas-exchanging parenchyma (alveoli, alveolar ducts, and terminal bronchioles), is particularly prone to injury during thoracic trauma. This trauma varies from lung contusions and lacerations to tracheobronchial tree rupture. The distal portion of the larynx is susceptible to injury and dysfunction after trauma to the neck. Penetrating trauma to the airway obviously requires emergency measures to control hemorrhage and airway obstruction.

Trauma to the lower airway varies from the Macklin phenomenon of hyperexpansion alveolar rupture to acute traumatic laceration of the tracheobronchial tree (18). Injury to the lower airway results in release of air or blood into the pleural space. Sudden hyperexpansion of the lung (such as gasping in pain) tends to rupture perivascular alveoli as negative pressure is created when the expanding lung pulls away from the nonexpanding blood vessels (18, 19).

The negative perivascular pressure creates an extremely large transmural pressure in these alveoli, causing rupture. The air released from these alveoli dissects along the vascular sheaths (interstitial emphysema) to the mediastinum to cause the Macklin effect—pneumomediastinum and/or subcutaneous emphysema (18). This effect is also seen with ventilator-induced barotrauma. Alternatively, air may dissect from the mediastinum into the pleural spaces, causing pneumothorax. Pneumothorax follows traumatic rupture of alveoli contiguous with the visceral pleura. However, rib fractures with lung laceration are the most common cause of pneumothorax. Tracheobronchial laceration is a rare cause of persistent air leak into the pleural and mediastinal spaces. Complete transection of the trachea will be rapidly fatal unless a continuous air column between mouth and lungs can be established and maintained. A continuous air leak into the pleural space without an escape route leads to tension pneumothorax. If this condition is not relieved rapidly, circulatory and ventilatory collapse and death will follow.

Laceration of the lung by ribs or penetrating trauma frequently causes hemorrhage into the pleural space, resulting in hemothorax as well as pneumothorax. Pulmonary laceration of both air spaces and pulmonary veins can allow air entry into the low-pressure venous drainage system, which will transport the air bubble to the left atrium (20). The resultant air bubbles are particularly dangerous because they gain direct arterial access from the left heart and can become emboli in coronary and cerebral vessels.

The muscles of the chest wall perform a vital function in providing the work of ventilation. Penetration of the chest wall, resulting in a sucking chest wound, will reduce pulmonary ventilation as chest wall motion preferentially moves air through the penetrating wound instead of the larynx. Contusions of the chest wall impair the ventilatory function of the respiratory muscles. Flail segments are caused by numerous rib fractures that impair the stability of the thoracic cage. High cervical spinal cord injury will paralyze the muscles of the chest wall, leading to ventilatory failure. Ventilatory failure secondary to chest wall injury is an indication for immediate intubation and mechanical ventilatory support (see Chapter 6).

## ASSESSMENT

Assessment of immediate airway problems in patients who are acutely traumatized is different from that in patients who are returning for follow-up surgical procedures. Patients with initial airway trauma who return to surgery for other procedures are usually stabilized sufficiently so that there is time to determine the best approach to subsequent airway management. Follow-up patients can also be prepared more ideally for various attempts at airway interventions, similar to elective surgical patients. Aspiration prophylaxis consists of a fasting state (nothing by mouth after midnight) (21) and may include using various pharmacologic agents to neutralize gastric acid (see "The 'Full Stomach'") (22, 23). Acute trauma patients, on the other hand, frequently require rapid assessment and intervention to prevent or relieve asphyxia or respiratory depression.

All trauma victims should be assessed for adequacy of ventilation immediately upon arrival at a treatment facility to determine the urgency of intervention. Patients who are obviously apneic or cyanotic require simultaneous assessment and intervention to establish a patent airway for effective ventilation. The patient's mouth should be inspected for dentures or foreign material, which should be removed if found. Blood and secretions should be suctioned to aid in visualization and to help clear obstructions of the airway. Consideration of possible spinal cord injuries or direct traumatic tracheal injuries should not prevent lifesaving attempts at translaryngeal intubation for such patients. If manual attempts to open the airway and provide mask ventilation are unsuccessful, immediate oral endotracheal intubation should be attempted (3, 24). Occasionally, even experienced anesthetists will be faced with patients who cannot be managed by direct oral intubation attempts, such as those presenting with severe blunt or penetrating injuries of the trachea or mouth that distort normal anatomic relationships. Provisions for an emergency cricothyroidotomy should always be available in such circumstances.

Arterial blood gas tensions should be measured in the trauma patient immediately after arrival in the hospital. These blood gases are just as important to management and diagnosis of the trauma patient as hematologic and chemistry laboratory results. The measured arterial oxygen tension ($PaO_2$) should be compared with the expected $PaO_2$, utilizing the ratio of $PaO_2$ to alveolar oxygen partial pressure ($PAO_2$). The normal $PaO_2/PAO_2$ ratio is $> 0.75$. Lower values suggest increased right-to-left pulmonary shunting of blood or venous admixture. Significant venous admixture is common after trauma and is best treated by intubation and mechanical ventilation (2). Several indices have been used to compare actual $PaO_2$ with expected $PaO_2$. The $PaO_2/FIO_2$ ratio is simple to calculate; a value of $< 200$ is consistent with an elevated pulmonary shunt. The alveolar-to-arterial difference of the partial pressure of oxygen ($A-aDO_2$) is increased with elevated venous admixture. However, the ratio of arterial to alveolar $PO_2$ ($PaO_2/PAO_2$) is a more sensitive indicator of pulmonary dysfunction and can be used to predict the $FIO_2$ needed to maintain a desired $PaO_2$ because it remains constant with different levels of $FIO_2$, unlike the $A-aDO_2$ and the $PaO_2/FIO_2$ (25). Values less than 0.75 suggest significant venous admixture. The requirement to calculate the $PAO_2$ is the major drawback to the use of this ratio, but bedside computers can simplify the process.

Chest x-ray films are another essential diagnostic tool for the trauma patient (24). Pneumothoraces are most accurately diagnosed radiographically. Persistent air leak despite adequate thoracostomy tube (chest tube) drainage suggests perforation of the tracheobronchial tree. Such perforations can occur anywhere from the intrathoracic trachea to the small bronchi in the pulmonary parenchyma. Air leaking from the lung parenchyma tends to increase during positive-pressure ventilation. Thus, even small pneumothoraces should be corrected by the placement of a chest tube, especially if the patient will be taken to the operating room, be covered with a sterile field, and subsequently be relatively inaccessible. Many penetrating chest wounds can be treated with thoracostomy tube drainage alone. Large-volume hemothoraces and tension pneumothoraces must be evacuated properly to allow normal ventilation.

When managing the airways of polytrauma patients, one should maintain a high index of suspicion for the possibility of both head and spinal cord injuries. Patients sustaining severe polytrauma are frequently confused and obtunded on admission. This may be caused by central nervous system injuries, hypoxia due to inadequate respiratory exchange, ingestion of drugs, or a combination of these factors. Early establishment of a secure airway in these patients is important to limit or prevent hypoxic insult and to minimize swelling of the brain. The adequacy of ventilation should be evaluated by arterial blood gas analysis. The relationship between increased ICP and accentuation of this pressure by hypercarbia is well known (26). Head injury produces loss of control of ventilation/perfusion ($\dot{V}/\dot{Q}$) ratios and leads to impaired gas exchange (27). Head-injured patients should be viewed as respiratory emergencies.

The Committee on Trauma Research has stated that "the most important topic to be addressed with regards to treatment of trauma patients is control of swelling of the brain; improvement could substantially reduce injury mortality" (1). Early intubation and hyperventilation are paramount intervention techniques to reduce cerebral swelling and prevent further brain injury. Widespread appreciation of the value of rapid airway control and hyperventilation to reduce intracranial swelling should have a positive effect on the mortality and morbidity associated with high-energy automobile collisions and other traumatic events.

Proper technique (circumstances permitting) for oral intubation should include the use of a hypnotic drug (if the patient is not significantly obtunded), administration of a neuromuscular blocking agent, application of cricoid pressure (cricoesophageal compression, Sellick's maneuver) (28–30), establishment of manual cervical spine stabilization (31), and readiness to perform a cricothyroidotomy. Proper use of this technique has never been associated with aspiration or increased neurologic deficit at the Shock Trauma Center of the Maryland Institute for Emergency Medical Services Systems (MIEMSS).

## TECHNIQUES

### Manual Techniques

As soon as the anesthesiologist decides that the patient needs airway support, the appropriate method must be determined. Many patients with single-system trauma, intact airway reflexes, and a brief period of hypoxia (low $PaO_2/PAO_2$) can be treated with an oxygen mask and close observation, including serial blood gas determinations. Patients who are unconscious or semiconscious are at high risk for tracheal aspiration of gastric contents (21, 22, 32). Apneic or obviously cyanotic patients need immediate intervention to restore airway patency and ventilation. Patients who have difficulty maintaining a patent airway or adequate ventilation will require endotracheal intubation. Both airway patency and mechanical ventilation can be provided through an endotracheal tube. Simple mechanical means of opening the airway and providing ventilation should not be overlooked in the rush to intubate. Whenever possible, inadequate ventilation should be corrected with a bag-valve-mask before intubation is attempted (3, 24). A surprising number of trauma patients will have marginally saturated oxyhemoglobin, if not frank desaturation.

Of the three generally accepted maneuvers to open a patient's airway, only two are generally applicable to the trauma patient (the "head tilt" maneuver should be avoided) (12). The "chin lift" maneuver is performed by placing the fingers of one hand under the anterior base of the mandible while *gently* lifting upward to move the chin forward. Using the thumb of the same hand, the lower lip is displaced downward to open the mouth. This maneuver should be used with caution to prevent any movement of the cervical spine from its neutral position. An alternative method to open the natural airway is the "jaw thrust." This involves securing the angles of the mandible bilaterally to displace it forward. If the lips tend to close, the lower lip can be displaced downward to open the mouth. If needed, an oropharyngeal or nasopharyngeal airway or another device (Table 3.2) can be used to improve ventilation. Placement of these devices can precipitate gagging and subsequent vomiting if the patient still has active airway reflexes (see "Trauma Patient 8").

It seems intuitively obvious that the chin lift and jaw thrust techniques of opening an obstructed airway for cardiopulmonary resuscitation will cause minimal motion of the cervical spine. However, an experimental study demonstrated that a surgically created unstable anterior cervical spine lesion moved less with the head tilt maneuver than with the jaw thrust or chin lift (33). In this study, head tilt was accompanied by a caudal axial push, which may have effectively pushed together the unstable anterior cervical spine elements. However, the chin lift and jaw thrust techniques have been demonstrated in anesthetized humans to be superior to the head tilt method for opening an obstructed airway (12).

The anesthesiologist who is faced with resuscitating a trauma patient must weigh the priorities of achieving an adequate airway and protecting the cervical spine.

**Table 3.2.    Summary of Airway Management Techniques**[a]

| Techniques | Modifications |
|---|---|
| *Nondefinitive Airway Adjuncts* | |
| 1. Noninvasive | |
| a. Mouth-to-mask | Oral airway |
| b. Bag-valve-mask | Nasal airway |
| | Binasal airway |
| 2. Invasive | |
| a. Oropharyngeal airway (oral airway) | |
| b. Nasopharyngeal airway (nasal airway) | |
| c. Esophageal obturator airway | |
| d. Esophageal gastric tube airway | Oxygen-powered breathing device |
| e. Pharyngeotracheal airway | |
| *Definitive Airway Adjuncts* | |
| Intubation | |
| 1. Nasal | |
| a. Direct visualization | |
| i.  Laryngoscope and Magill forceps | Jet insufflation via suction port of broncho-scope |
| ii. Fiberoptic | |
| b. Blind | |
| i.  Traditional | Trigger ETT[b] |
| ii. With audio-assist device[c] | |
| iii. Tactile (digital) | |
| 2. Oral | |
| a. Direct visualization | Laryngeal mask |
| i.  Direct laryngoscope | Variety of blades, ETTs |
| | Stylet |
| | Flexible stylet[d] |
| A. Awake | |
| B. Sedated | |
| C. Rapid sequence | |
| D. Traditional | |
| ii. Fiberoptic | Williams Airway Intubator |
| | Railroad stylet or Seldinger-TTX[e] |
| | Jet insufflation via suction port of bronchoscope |
| b. Blind | |
| i.  Completely blind | With transillumination (light wand)[f] |
| ii. Audio-assist device | |
| iii. Tactile (digital) | |
| iv. Retrograde | |
| Surgical (operative) airway | |
| 1. Transtracheal (percutaneous) needle | |
| 2. Cricothyroidotomy | Weiss airway, Nutrach with ETT or tracheal tube |
| 3. Tracheostomy | |

[a] From Grande CM. Airway management of the trauma patient in the resuscitation area of a trauma center. Trauma Q 1988;5:30–49.
[b] Endotrol (Mallinckrodt, Inc., St. Louis, MO).
[c] Ballistic Airway Airflow Monitor (Great Plains Ballistic Co., Lubbock, TX).
[d] Flexiguide.
[e] Tracheal Tube Exchanger (Sheridan Catheter Corp., Argyle, NY).
[f] Tube-STAT (Concept Corp., Clearwater, FL).

The Advanced Trauma Life Support (ATLS) protocols recognize this dilemma, and the "A" in the "A B C D E" acronym for initial assessment stands for "airway and cervical spine stabilization" (24). Adequate oxygenation of the trauma patient must have the highest priority, but the trauma anesthesia/critical care specialist (TA/CCS) must be aware of the potential for an unstable cervical spine fracture and must use techniques that minimize motion of the cervical spine (34).

Although penetrating trauma, especially of the neck, has a high incidence of airway injuries that need immediate attention, unstable cervical spine fractures are not commonly caused by penetrating trauma (10, 35). A retrospective review of battlefield injuries from the Viet Nam conflict demonstrated that, if medics took the time to immobilize the cervical spines of wounded soldiers, there was a 10% increase in fatal wounds from enemy fire, whereas only 1.4% of the wounded soldiers had injuries that would have benefited from such immobilization (35). A similar review of the MIEMSS trauma registry by this chapter's authors revealed a low percentage of cervical spine fractures in trauma patients (mostly blunt trauma) who arrived at the hospital with respiratory arrest requiring immediate intubation. The MIEMSS experience is supported by other reports that cervical spine stabilization during airway manipulation prevents further spinal cord injury (34).

Unstable cervical spine fractures occur when all supporting elements in either the anterior portion (vertebral bodies, intervertebral discs, anterior and posterior longitudinal ligaments) or the posterior portion (facet joints with capsules, interspinous and supraspinous ligaments) are disrupted along with one element of the other portion of the spine (34, 36). Movement of the neck causes dislocation at the site of an unstable cervical spine fracture with a decrease in area available for the spinal cord. This spinal dislocation may permanently damage the spinal cord. Flexion of the neck tends to accentuate instability through the posterior elements of the spinal cord, whereas extension accentuates instability in its anterior elements.

Immobilization of the cervical spine is best performed with a combination of sandbags taped on each side of the patient's head, a Philadelphia collar, and a spine board (Fig. 3.1) (37). Orotracheal intubation, nasotracheal intubation, and tracheostomy can all be performed successfully without spinal cord damage as long as the neck is immobilized adequately (34, 38). The fiberoptic bronchoscope is a very useful instru-

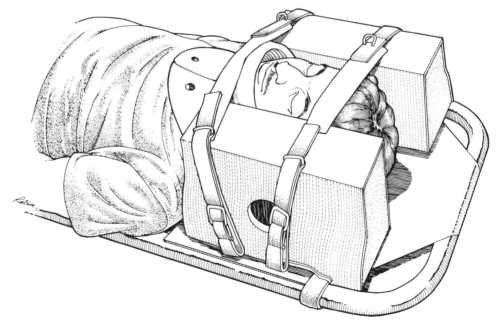

**Figure 3.1. Proper stabilization of suspected cervical spine injury.** The combination of a long spine board, a cervical collar, and bilateral padded immobilization devices is used.

ment for the TA/CCS to use for oral or nasal intubation of the patient requiring cervical spine immobilization (39, 40). However, the bronchoscope has limitations in use for the apneic patient or the patient with copious intraoral bleeding. Traditional blind nasal intubation has several drawbacks and should be used only in patients who can cooperate with deep breaths and who will not require prolonged nasotracheal intubation (38, 41, 42).

## Endotracheal Intubation

After determining that an artificial airway and assisted ventilation are indicated, the anesthesiologist must choose an appropriate airway control mechanism. A secure, cuffed intratracheal tube often offers the best method of airway control, providing a route for mechanical ventilation and pulmonary toilet as well as protection from aspiration (4). Exceptions to this rule are the mandatory use of uncuffed tubes in children less than 6 years of age and the short-term use of needle cricothyroidotomy with jet ventilation in patients with facial trauma (7, 8, 43, 44).

A cuffed intratracheal tube may be placed by one of three routes: nasally, orally, or through a tracheostomy. Each of these routes has advantages and disadvantages, and the appropriate choice should be used where indicated (Table 3.3).

Some anesthesiologists consider nasal intubation to be the ideal method for securing the airway in a trauma patient with cervical spine injury. However, for the acute trauma patient with obvious or presumed injuries of the craniocervicofacial complex, we tend to disagree. If time permits, all polytrauma patients should have radiographic evaluation of the cervical spine to rule out associated injuries before intubation (i.e., at least an acceptable cross-table lateral view).

Although many clinicians recommend the nasal route for intubation, the authors' experience with hundreds of patients with suspected cervical spinal cord injuries leads

**Table 3.3. Comparison of Routes of Intubation for Trauma Patients**

Oral
 Advantages—rapid, direct visualization of larynx; use of a larger tube possible; enhanced suctioning not dependent on patient's respiration
 Disadvantages—oral access needed, laryngoscopy, laryngeal trauma, esophageal intubation

Nasal
 Advantages—blind intubation techniques, surgical access to mouth
 Disadvantages—nasal trauma, laryngeal trauma, time required more than for oral, thorough suction difficult, sinusitis, nose bleeds

Tracheostomy (cricothyroidotomy)
 Advantages—direct route into the trachea; ability to bypass mouth and nose, requiring minimal neck motion; only route possible in patients with massive facial and/or cervical trauma
 Disadvantages—surgical errors, laryngeal damage with scarring, hemorrhage, high placement through hyo-thyroid membrane, esophageal intubation

us to avoid this approach. In general, we have recommended that the nasal route be avoided in the acute trauma patient with evidence of maxillofacial injury or whose mechanism of injury indicates that this type of associated trauma is a likelihood. Any patient with a suspected head injury could have a basilar skull fracture (Table 3.3). There are documented cases of nasogastric tubes being pushed through cribriform plate fractures into the brain substance of the cranial vault (45). It is conceivable that a nasal endotracheal tube could traverse a severe basilar skull fracture defect. A nasal endotracheal tube can also introduce bacteria through a basilar skull fracture or can produce sepsis postoperatively as the result of severe persistent sinusitis, which frequently develops in trauma patients because of their immunosuppressed status (46, 47).

Additionally, all forms of nasal intubation are associated with characteristic complications and limitations. (a) Nasal intubation may induce nosebleeds, which may be aggravated by dilutional coagulopathy in many trauma patients. (b) Nasal intubation is very difficult to perform in frightened, inebriated, obtunded, or combative patients, who may thrash about and cause further damage to a spinal cord injury. (c) Stimulation of airway reflexes in the pharynx during the multiple manipulations that may be necessary to place the endotracheal tube (ETT) in the trachea may induce retching and vomiting; these reactions may increase ICP or cause laryngospasm or bronchospasm. (d) Attempts at blind nasotracheal intubation often lead to greater cervical movement than does controlled oral intubation with proper technique. Blind nasotracheal intubation requires the endotracheal tube to emerge from the posterior nasopharynx in line with the glottic opening. If the tube does not line up with the glottis, the neck must be flexed and angulated toward the ipsilateral side of the endotracheal tube (5). A study performed by emergency medicine physicians comparing oral and nasal intubation in unconscious, drug-intoxicated patients emphasized the difference in efficacy between oral and nasal intubations in emergency situations (42). The authors concluded that oral intubation was preferable because it had a greater success rate (oral, 100%; nasal, 65%), was quicker, required fewer attempts (oral, 1.3 per patient; nasal, 3.7 per patient), and had drastically fewer complications (oral, 0%; nasal, 69%).

Blind nasotracheal intubation, for the most part, requires a breathing patient for a significant degree of success, although supplementary devices exist (e.g., Ballistic Airway Airflow Monitor; Great Plains Ballistic Company, Lubbock, TX) (Table 2). Blind passage of a nasal tube, even when aided by adequate breath sounds, has a significant failure rate. Additionally, a deviated nasal septum may guide the tube into the piriform sinus instead of the larynx. Either lateral flexion of the neck toward the side of the tube (contraindicated in patients with suspected cervical spine injury) or direct laryngoscopy to guide the tube with Magill forceps is required to bring the tube tip back to midline. Nasotracheal intubation is also fraught with more complications than is orotracheal intubation (41, 42, 46, 47).

Experience at the MIEMSS Shock Trauma Center with trauma patients who have a cervical cord injury and need intubation has supported the place of nasal intubation in the airway management repertoire. However, nasotracheal intubation has become inappropriately common in the care of patients with neck injury—partly because of "reflex action" based on rote association of the nasotracheal route of intubation with cervical spine trauma and partly from a lack of knowledge and facility with reliable alternatives. Oral intubation is a feasible alternative to intubation using the manual in-line axial traction (MIAT) technique, also referred to as manual C-spine immobilization or stabilization (31, 34). These three terms require clarification since "traction" and "immobilization" are sometimes incorrectly used interchangeably when referring to "stabilization" of suspected cervical spine injury (48). Ultimately, the goal of these manual maneuvers is to stabilize the spine and thus prevent further injury. Stabilization often may involve a dynamic interplay between traction and immobilization, i.e., an ideal amount of force is applied against the force generated by the intubator (49). (To our knowledge, there is no report documenting this ideal amount of force.) It is equally important that the force be applied in the correct plane relative to a particular injury. In any case, it is probably impossible to make a general statement of how much traction should be applied unless feedback information is available (e.g., from fluoroscopy). Ideally, a neurosurgeon should be present for immediate consultation and guidance. MIAT has been accepted by the American College of Surgeons as part of the ATLS protocol for emergency intubation (Fig. 3.2) (24).

Most trauma patients are now routinely transported from the field with some combination of cervical collar, spine board, and sandbags to stabilize the cervical spine. When oral intubation is attempted, obstructions to mouth opening and cricoid pressure (such as the anterior portion of the Philadelphia cervical collar) are usually removed

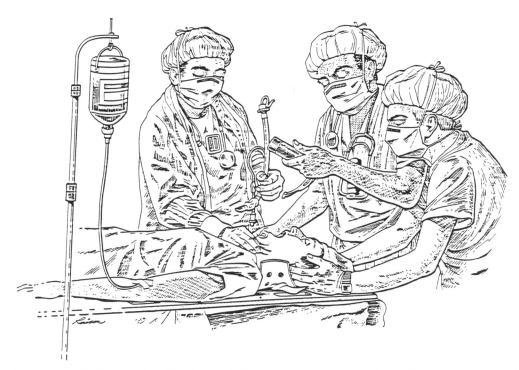

**Figure 3.2.    Technique of oral intubation in the emergency trauma patient using laryngoscopy and "manual in-line axial traction."**  The individual on the *left* is applying cricoid pressure while holding the endotracheal tube ready. The intubator (*center*) holds the laryngoscope in the left hand while opening the patient's mouth with his right hand. The assistant on the *right* is using both hands to maintain the patient's head and neck in a neutral position. The anterior portion of the cervical collar has been removed, and the patient is on a long spine board. (From Stene JK. Anesthesia for the critically ill trauma patient. In Siegel JH (ed). Trauma: Emergency Surgery and Critical Care. New York, Churchill Livingstone, 1987, pp 843–862.)

to facilitate movement of the mandible for laryngoscopy and application of cricoid pressure. Cricoid pressure is a technique in which the thumb and forefinger are pinched together and then applied in a downward fashion over the cricoid cartilage of the trachea (Fig. 3.3). This pressure closes the esophagus and significantly reduces the possibility of gastric regurgitation (28–30, 50–52). Analysis reveals that 44 newtons of force upon the cricoid cartilage impinges it upon the anterior body of C6; thus, the esophagus is effectively closed. Pressure must be applied to the cricoid cartilage only, as it alone is a contiguous cartilagenous ring and thereby permits the transmission of force necessary to seal the esophagus. Before intubation, the patient can be protected from regurgitation/vomiting by cricoid pressure (29). Use of the "cricoid yoke"

will provide consistently optimal cricoid pressure (50, 51). If establishment of a surgical airway becomes necessary, access to the anterior neck is ensured. An assistant can maintain the head in a neutral position with MIAT during intubation, and the appropriate instruments should be ready to perform a cricothyroidotomy if needed.

If there is a delay in establishing the airway, the patient may be ventilated by mask while cricoid pressure is maintained until the airway is secured. Conversely, cricoid pressure may also be used to prevent inflation of the stomach (a potential cause of regurgitation) resulting from positive-pressure ventilation applied through a face mask (29, 30, 52). The intubator can "time" the process by taking a deep breath before beginning an intubation sequence ("breath-hold" rule). If the patient is not intubated by

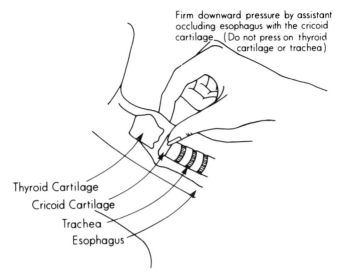

Firm downward pressure by assistant occluding esophagus with the cricoid cartilage. (Do not press on thyroid cartilage or trachea)

Thyroid Cartilage
Cricoid Cartilage
Trachea
Esophagus

**Figure 3.3.    The application of cricoid pressure (also known as cricoesophageal compression and Sellick's maneuver).** The thumb and forefinger are used to press the cartilaginous cricoid ring posteriorly toward the sixth cervical vertebra, thereby sealing the esophagus. (From Horswell JL, Cobb, ML, Owens MD. Anesthetic management of the trauma victim. In Zuidema GD, Rutherford RB, Ballinger WF (eds). The Management of Trauma, ed 4. Philadelphia, WB Saunders, 1985, pp 127–136.)

the time the intubator feels the need to breathe (as $CO_2$ levels rise and $O_2$ levels fall), that particular attempt should be aborted. Ventilation of the patient should then be continued through cricoid pressure until the next attempt. Such practice prohibits extraordinarily long intubation trials and prevents the patient from becoming markedly hypoxic or hypercarbic. Furthermore, monitoring the patient's arterial oxygen saturation ($SaO_2$) with a pulse oximeter will help the TA/CCS avoid hypoxia associated with long intubation attempts (53).

Thus, severely traumatized patients who are hypoxic on arrival at the MIEMSS Shock Trauma Center are ventilated by mask, with application of cricoid pressure, until intubation is completed (i.e., the "modified rapid sequence technique"). We submit that this procedure has prevented the additional hypoxic insults that can occur during intubation and has minimized the incidence of arrhythmias. Often there is not time for the luxury of adequate preoxygenation of an already compromised hypoxic patient with respiratory insufficiency. These patients should be ventilated continuously with

oxygen while cricoid pressure is used to prevent gastric inflation. We have used this technique for many years (on more than 3000 patients). Approximately 1% of these patients have been diagnosed subsequently to have fractures of the cervical spine. None of them developed any change in the level of spinal cord function during intubation.

Will the application of cricoid pressure itself affect an unstable cervical spine? To the best of our knowledge, this question has never been examined formally and thus no quantifiable answers exist. Intuitively, the possibility is present if efforts are overly vigorous (33).

Oral translaryngeal intubation has become the standard technique for intubating the trachea in trauma patients at the MIEMSS Shock Trauma Center. In less urgent cases, patients with *known* cervical spine trauma are intubated while awake with a fiberoptic bronchoscope passed orally through a Williams intubating airway as long as they can breathe spontaneously. Apneic patients and those with *suspected* cervical spine injury are intubated with direct laryngoscopy while the neck is maintained in neutral alignment with manual stabilization and other stabilizing devices such as a Vac Pak (Canadian Howmedica, Ltd.) or sandbags bilaterally and a long spine board (Fig. 3.1) (3, 38).

Cervical spine stability is ensured by instructing the patient and/or holding the patient's occiput and shoulders onto the spine board. The patient is given 100% oxygen by mask or is ventilated with a bag-valve-mask apparatus. Firm cricoid pressure, which effectively seals off the esophagus from the mouth (28–30, 50–52), is applied before the patient becomes unconscious. With the application of cricoid pressure, gentle mask ventilation rarely inflates the stomach. Experience with several thousand trauma patients at the MIEMSS Shock Trauma Center supports Sellick's (28) contention that a smooth induction with mask ventilation while cricoid pressure is maintained is possible while simultaneously protecting the airway and preventing regurgitation and aspiration. In most patients, muscle relaxants facilitate mouth opening and translaryngeal passage of the endotracheal tube (3, 42, 54, 55). The muscle relaxant is frequently preceded by a "sleep dose" of a hypnotic drug (e.g., thiopental, 25–100 mg i.v.). To avoid excessive doses, the drug is titrated to the patient's "sleep" response before administration of the muscle relaxant. The patient's airway is tested to be sure that ventilation can be established if the trachea cannot be intubated. The muscle relaxant is infused rapidly through the intravenous line if the patient has a patent airway. Gentle mask ventilation is continued until the time of intubation to enhance preoxygenation. As stated above, adequate oxygen saturation is often a problem in multitrauma patients who have sustained intrathoracic injuries (e.g., pulmonary contusions) or who have other reasons for $\dot{V}/\dot{Q}$ mismatching.

Laryngoscopy proceeds in a standard manner after the patient is relaxed. Firm cricoid pressure is maintained until the endotracheal tube is verified to be in the trachea and the cuff is inflated. Manual cervical stabilization is continued throughout the intubation sequence. Maintaining the neck in neutral alignment often reduces visibility during direct laryngoscopy. Frequently, the large Macintosh (MAC) blade provides better visualization than straight blades, but this will vary from case to case (56). A stylet can be bent appropriately (e.g., hockey-stick-shaped) to guide the tube between the arytenoids and the epiglottis if that is all that is visualized during laryngoscopy. Other devices, such as the Huffman prism, will also facilitate visualization of the glottic aperture while minimizing the amount of cervical movement necessary. Another device that may be of use in these situations is the Bullard fiberoptic laryngoscope (57, 58).

## Verification of Intubation

The endotracheal tube must be placed properly with its distal opening near the midpoint of the trachea (59). Since unrecognized esophageal intubations have devastating consequences, it is of the utmost importance to verify *intratracheal* placement of the endotracheal tube. The "gold standard" for verifying proper endotracheal tube placement is to observe the tube advancing through the vocal cords (60). However, in patients in whom neutral neck alignment is maintained, it may not be possible to observe the endotracheal tube passing through the vocal cords. Furthermore, it is possible for an endotracheal tube to become dislodged from the trachea and be repositioned into the esophagus when the laryngoscope is withdrawn.

Two other methods of verifying intratracheal position of the endotracheal tube are also considered reliable. The quickest means is to observe the end-tidal $CO_2$ waveform using capnography (60–62). The trachea is the only orifice in the body that systematically will produce a characteristic $CO_2$ waveform due to the tidal excretion of gaseous $CO_2$. As a second choice, direct observation of intratracheal mucosa (identified by observing tracheal rings) through a bronchoscope passed via the endotracheal tube is considered confirming evidence for intratracheal position of the endotracheal tube. All other signs of intratracheal tube placement, including chest x-ray films, have an appreciable incidence of false-positive findings (60, 63–69). Obviously, an endotracheal tube placed in the esophagus must be recognized and repositioned into the trachea immediately. If capnography is unavailable to confirm endotracheal tube position, one must look for as many positive signs of tracheal tube placement as possible (Table 3.4). Only a high index of suspicion and insistence on stringent verification of endotracheal tube placement will save the patient from a disastrous esophageal intubation. An apnea monitor that qualitatively detects the expired $CO_2$ waveform can be used as a portable device to verify endotracheal tube placement (70). There is also a chemical capnometer that changes color semiquantitatively with varying $CO_2$ concentrations (FEF end-tidal $CO_2$ detector; Fenem, Inc., New York, NY) (71).

## Failure to Intubate

Trauma patients present various difficulties that may prevent intubation by direct laryngoscopy. Causes of difficult intubation have been reviewed (15). These same difficulties are found in the trauma patient with the added aggravating factors of a potential cervical spine injury, acute traumatic anatomic distortion, and regurgitation or vomiting resulting from a full stomach (9, 72). A large tongue obstructing visualization of the larynx has been confirmed by others (16, 17) as significantly increasing the difficulty of intubation.

Alternatives to direct laryngoscopy and intubation include blind nasotracheal intubation, digitally guided oral or nasal intubation, retrograde stylet-guided intubation, and tracheostomy (73). Nasotracheal intubation has already been discussed.

Digital guidance of oral (and, more recently, nasal) endotracheal intubation has been promoted as a safe way to guide an endotracheal tube into the larynx of an apneic patient without moving the cervical spine (9). Variations on this theme for field

**Table 3.4.    Signs of Endotracheal Tube Placement**

| Sign | Tracheal Intubation | Esophageal Intubation |
| --- | --- | --- |
| Breath sounds (auscultation of chest) | Easily heard over trachea and at lung bases | Air entry in esophagus may mimic breath sounds at lung bases |
| Auscultation over epigastrium | No gastric air entry | Characteristic gurgling of gastric air entry |
| Chest wall movement | Good bilateral upper chest wall movement | Expansion and contraction of esophagus may cause chest wall movement |
| Exhaled vapor[a] | Easily seen in clear plastic tubes | Usually weakly present or absent |
| $SaO_2$ | Remains at baseline values to 100% | Decreases from baseline |
| $CO_2$ waveform[a] | Characteristic respiratory tidal waveform for $CO_2$ | Usually absent but may exhibit a rounded off waveform with low end-tidal value for a few breaths; rapidly disappears |
| Chest x-ray (portable anterior-posterior) | Endotracheal tube appears in tracheal air shadow | Endotracheal tube may overlie tracheal air shadow; lateral view is needed to verify placement |
| Colorimeter $CO_2$ indicator (FEF) | Characteristic purple to yellow color change with each breath indicating strong $CO_2$ signal | Brief, weak color change (purple to brown) to no color change (remains purple) |
| Bronchoscopic | Characteristic tracheal rings and mucosa | Esophageal mucosa and folds |

[a] Cardiopulmonary arrest alters the endotracheal excretion of water vapor and carbon dioxide. Direct visualization may be the only reliable indicator.

use include transilluminating the larynx with a high-intensity lighted stylet. Of course, the success of this technique, like any other, is highly dependent upon the facility of the performer, which is developed through practice. The emergent case is not the situation in which first to attempt such a technique. Nevertheless, this technique remains more popular in field situations in which a laryngoscope is unavailable. Field airways (see "Trauma Patient 8"), such as the esophageal obturator airway (74), the esophageal gastric tube airway, and the pharyngeotracheal lumen (PTL) airway (75, 76), probably have limited utility in the emergency room, as they are primarily field devices that should be converted as quickly as possible to a standard intrahospital airway device (i.e., endotracheal or tracheostomy tube).

Emergency surgical airway techniques in the trauma patient are usually performed via the cricothyroid membrane. Cricothyroidotomy is preferred over formal tracheostomy because it is easier and quicker to perform (i.e., fewer complications such as bleeding). This technique is well described in the ATLS manual (24). Cricothyroidotomy is contraindicated in children younger than 6 years. In these patients the cricoid ring is the narrowest portion of the airway. Edema or reactive granuloma formation as a result of cricothyroidotomy may drastically reduce the internal diameter of this area and thus cause serious airway obstruction. In the pediatric patient, either a formal tracheostomy or a percutaneous needle cricothyroidotomy is recommended. Every anesthesiologist who cares for trauma patients should be certified as an ATLS provider and be familiar with performing cricothyroidotomy. In addition, before beginning any form of intubation, the anesthesiologist should become familiar with the anatomy and landmarks of a given patient's anterior neck, locate the cricothyroid space, and have all necessary equipment to perform a cricothyroidotomy (also known as cricothyrotomy and coniotomy). Emergency support of oxygenation with limited $CO_2$ removal can

be performed with placement of a percutaneous needle through the cricothyroid membrane and jet ventilation (43, 44). Although a well-proven, reliable method, percutaneous cricothyrotomy probably does not play a large role in the admitting area of a sophisticated trauma center, where persons adept at performing more advanced surgical techniques (such as cricothyroidotomies) abound; therefore, it will not be discussed extensively here. This technique, although relatively safe, is associated with several potential complications (Table 3.5). Many surgeons believe that it is necessary to replace a cricothyroidotomy with a formal tracheostomy during the elective phase.

## The "Full Stomach"

A basic concept in perioperative airway management of the trauma patient is the "full stomach." This term cannot always be taken literally but implies that more and varied gastric contents would be present than in the fasting, elective surgical patient. The full stomach is a product of two factors: (a) injury is accidental and unplanned, and therefore the patient may have eaten or drunk immediately before the event; (b) trauma itself, as well as the anxiety and pain secondary to injury, and alcohol consumption all act to delay or arrest gastric emptying (77). Concerns regarding the full stomach stem from the risk of regurgitation of gastric contents, which rises as intragas-

**Table 3.5. Complications of Transtracheal Ventilation by Percutaneous Cricothyrotomy**

*Emergent*
  Asphyxia due to prolonged technique
  Aspiration
  Exsanguinating hemorrhage
  Inadequate ventilation leading to hypoxia and inadequate exhalation leading to $CO_2$ retention
  Barotrauma
*Urgent*
  Esophageal perforation
  Subcutaneous and/or mediastinal emphysema ± pneumothorax
  Thyroid perforation
*Delayed*
  Cellulitis
  Hematoma

tric volume is increased, and the severity of aspiration pneumonitis if these contents enter the lungs, which increases with factors such as increasing volume (>0.4 ml/kg body weight), increasing acidity (classically a pH of <2.5), and the presence of particulate matter (78). The full stomach can be created iatrogenically, for example, by performing contrast radiography of the abdomen after a barium swallow. Often the interval between the time of last intake and the time of injury is more important than the interval between intake and intubation (79, 80). Gastric filling and distension can increase intragastric pressure and overcome the lower esophageal sphincter sealing pressure, leading to gastroesophageal regurgitation. Patients with head injury and elevated ICP are prone to vomiting. An obtunded patient who vomits or an anesthetized patient who regurgitates is at increased risk of aspirating gastric contents into the lungs. Inhaled gastric contents can "drown" the patient if the volume is great enough or may induce aspiration pneumonitis if the volume and pH are beyond critical values (21, 22). The most dangerous complication of aspiration is obstruction of major portions of the lower airway by inhaled food particles.

Many suggestions have been made regarding the management of the full stomach. The most obvious is simply to wait and allow the stomach to empty itself. Various arbitrary waiting periods have been suggested (81). However, none of these waiting periods is always reliable, as the stomach may not be evacuated completely for 24 to 48 hours postinjury. With the severe multitrauma patient, waiting is often not an option. In this situation, the use of regional anesthesia has merit but is not always possible (23, 32).

Another approach focuses on actively evacuating the stomach. Two methods have been suggested. The first is to induce vomiting, for example, by the use of an apomorphine derivative or syrup of ipecac. The second is to place an orogastric or nasogastric tube. The first choice is often discounted on the basis that it is a "barbaric"

practice. All of these methods also are associated with retching and coughing, known contributors to the raising of ICP (a concern in any head-injured patient) and intraocular pressure (a concern in the patient with open globe injury [see Chapter 8]). Placing a tube carries the possibility of traversing a fractured cribriform plate if a nasal tube is used (45) or of intubating a false passage if either the nose or mouth is used. Additionally, the presence of a gastric tube may defeat the competence of the lower esophageal sphincter and serve as a "wick" around which gastric contents may regurgitate. This is controversial. Additionally, the presence of such a tube may render cricoid pressure ineffective (82). However, one study demonstrated that the nasogastric tube did not affect the utility of cricoid pressure (83). In any case, it is well known that complete evacuation of gastric contents cannot be ensured by using any of these techniques.

The third approach focuses on the use of pharmacologic agents to assist the stomach in emptying (metaclopromide), reduce the likelihood of vomiting (e.g., droperidol), or alter the pH of the stomach contents (antacids and $H_2$-blockers). Metoclopramide stimulates gastric emptying, reduces the tone of the pyloric sphincter, and stimulates anterograde movement of gastric contents. (This action can be inhibited by narcotics.) One investigator has even suggested a method in which metaclopromide, intragastric barium, and serial x-ray films can be used to evaluate the degree of gastric emptying objectively (81).

Cimetidine, ranitidene, and famotidine histamine, $H_2$-antagonists, will inhibit the secretion of gastric acid and thus, over time, will raise the mean pH of the intragastric contents. However, their action is not immediate and requires some time to be effective, as it has no influence on contents already in the stomach.

Antacids may also be given with the objective of raising mean intragastric pH. There are two general types: particulate and nonparticulate. Aspiration of a particulate antacid (e.g., milk of magnesia) carries a risk of inducing aspiration pneumonitis. This risk is reduced when a nonparticulate antacid such as sodium citrate is used.

The use of anticholinergic agents (e.g., atropine, glycopyrrolate) has also been suggested to reduce gastric acidity and volume; however, these compounds have the adverse effect of reducing the tone of the lower esophageal sphincter (84).

Another method that has been suggested is intentionally intubating the esophagus before proceeding with endotracheal cannulation (85). The motive here is to provide a predictable conduit for the expulsion of gastric contents. This technique may make endotracheal intubation more difficult, but it should be no more difficult than intubating around an esophageal obturator airway.

Another technique involves using gravity to protect the airway from aspiration (79). In the conscious patient before the administration of anesthetic agents, the right lateral/head-down position is utilized to permit vomitus to run out of the mouth. Once consciousness is lost, a 40° foot-down tilt is assumed, as active vomiting is not probable in the chemically paralyzed patient. However, this foot-down position may be associated with postural hypotension in the hypovolemic trauma patient.

However, the gold standard is the application of cricoid pressure, as discussed above. Many anesthesiologists have well-founded fears about trauma patients regurgitating or vomiting and then aspirating gastric contents during the induction of anesthesia. Although massive vomiting during anesthetic induction may result in the horror of acute asphyxiation (drowning) (21), the prevalent use of muscle relaxants during intubation in recent years has reduced the frequency of this problem (32). Additionally, review of large numbers of anesthetized patients demonstrates the low incidence of aspiration pneumonia when modern anesthetic techniques are used (22, 23, 32). The overall incidence is approximately 5 cases of aspiration per 10,000 anesthetics, but nighttime emergency cases,

especially patients with elevated ICP, those requiring emergency abdominal surgery, obstetric patients, and patients less than 9 years old, have an increased incidence—up to 8 per 10,000 anesthetics (32). The mortality rate from aspiration pneumonia is approximately 5%, for an overall mortality rate of 0.2 per 10,000 anesthetics (32).

Protection of the trauma patient's airway requires the placement of an endotracheal or tracheostomy tube with the cuff inflated sufficiently for a complete seal (in the adult). This protection can be afforded to children, in whom the cricoid ring fits more closely around the endotracheal tube than in adults, with an uncuffed tube utilizing positive-pressure ventilation.

If aspiration occurs, mechanical ventilation with positive end-expiratory pressure (PEEP) to reduce venous admixture and good tracheobroncheal toilet (including bronchoscopy) to remove airway obstruction are necessary to support the patient. If aspiration occurs, early intervention to support oxygenation and ventilation usually will improve results. Steroids probably have no beneficial effect in aspiration pneumonitis or in preventing adult respiratory distress syndrome (ARDS) after trauma (23, 86).

## Complications of Intubation

Intubation of the trachea in trauma patients shares complications with all endotracheal intubations but also has some idiosyncrasies. These complications (Table 3.6) include esophageal intubation, endobronchial intubation, damage to the endotracheal tube cuff, obstruction of the endotracheal tube by foreign materials, aspiration during intubation, and laceration of the airway or the esophageal mucosa (4, 5, 9, 13, 22, 60, 66, 72, 87–89).

Patients with upper and lower airway trauma can develop unique complications of intubation. Among these are conversion of a simple pneumothorax to a tension pneumothorax because of the institution of positive-pressure ventilation, loss of ventilation

**Table 3.6.   Complications of Intubations in Trauma Patients**

Oral Intubation
  Trauma from laryngoscopy
  Excessive cervical spine motion
  Esophageal intubation
  Pneumothorax
  Damage to endotracheal tube
  Vomiting/aspiration
  Broken teeth
  Inadvertent extubation
  Laryngeal trauma
  Right main bronchus intubation
  Mouth debris forced down trachea
  Esophageal perforation
  Laryngotracheal disruption
  Blood clots obstructing tube
Nasal Intubation
  All complications listed above plus:
  False passage in posterior pharynx
  Air entry from paranasal sinuses into subcutaneous tissues
  Nose bleed
  Prolonged intubation
    Sinusitis
    Necrosis of nose

through a large bronchopleural fistula, systemic air embolism, subcutaneous emphysema, pneumomediastinum, pneumopericardium, pneumoperitoneum, obstruction of the endotracheal tube by blood clots, intubation and/or creation of a false passage in the soft tissues, or intubation of cranial vault contents in the case of a cribriform plate fracture if a nasal route is chosen (24, 45). Direct injury to the larynx due to preadmission traumatic events will require special care in maintaining a secure airway (8, 90, 91).

Maxillofacial injuries may provide the anesthesiologist with a real airway challenge (7) (see Chapter 8). Loss of skeletal stability around the mouth, nose, and larynx often allows soft tissues to obstruct the airway during inspiration. Likewise, tissue, bone, and teeth fragments may be aspirated or may obstruct the upper airway. Before securing the airway, placing the patient in the lateral decubitus position may allow gravity to keep the airway free of tissues, blood, and debris. Practicing intubation of elective patients in the lateral position will

prepare the anesthesiologist for emergency situations.

Patients with facial injuries often require an "awake" technique of airway management, as anesthesia and muscle relaxants will obliterate any remaining airway patency and make mask ventilation impossible. These patients are often surprisingly easy to intubate orally as the laryngoscope blade will provide an excellent passage through the injured tissues. However, a surgical airway may be the only alternative in these patients if laryngoscopy fails to demonstrate the glottic aperture. Depending on the nature of the injury and the type of surgical intervention, a cricothyroidotomy or tracheostomy may be necessary. However, performing either of these is far easier to accomplish electively once an endotracheal tube has been placed.

If the trachea has been intubated successfully, one may appreciate precipitous evidence of the complications of positive-pressure ventilation in patients with thoracic trauma, which include progressive tension pneumothorax and intravascular air embolism. If the trauma patient has sustained rib fractures or other injuries that are predisposing him or her to a simple pneumothorax, the patient's condition will deteriorate as air is virtually pumped into the pleural space, giving rise to an eventual tension pneumothorax. The proper management for this problem would be to place an intercostal thoracostomy tube (chest tube) on the ipsilateral side (24). This is a relatively simple problem to solve if it is detected in a timely fashion. Detection depends, to a large degree, on the level of clinical suspicion and on the anticipatory potential of the person performing airway management.

On the other hand, systemic air embolism is a much more serious problem with more dire long-term implications (20). The trauma patient is predisposed to this condition if the vasculature of the lungs near the hili or more peripherally has been injured. Systemic air embolism, once thought to be rare, may actually occur in more than 10% of all major thoracic injuries. If air is entrained through a vein, it may affect right-heart performance. Air embolism may also traverse the pulmonary circulation, enter the arterial system, and then be transported to the periphery, where it may interfere with the coronary, cerebral, or peripheral circulation. Again, a high degree of clinical suspicion is necessary to make the diagnosis of systemic air embolism. Associated signs include hemoptysis, air visualized in the retinal veins during funduscopic examination, or froth obtained during aspiration of arterial blood for blood gas analysis. Treatment of a systemic air embolism involves emergency thoracotomy and, if possible, hyperbaric oxygen therapy. Prognosis is extremely poor.

## FOLLOW-UP CARE

Once a definitive airway has been achieved, it must be secured. In the case of an orotracheal or nasotracheal intubation, the endotracheal tube should be fastened firmly to the face with adhesive tape. Prior application of tincture of benzoin to the appropriate areas of the face will increase the effectiveness of the tape and protect the skin. Alternatively, one may use umbilical tape to tie the endotracheal tube in place. This is often a necessity in cases of facial burns, in which the use of adhesive tape is impossible.

For cricothyroidotomy or tracheostomy tubes, it is wise to place stay sutures on either side of the wound. Thus, if the tube is dislodged accidentally, it will be easier to realign the tissues and replace the tube. Also, the tube should be secured with the holder supplied as part of the kit and then tied around the neck.

Next, the intratracheal tube should be suctioned to remove secretions that may have collected and to evaluate the sample for consistency. Indication that the trauma patient has aspirated is important information from an infectious disease standpoint.

The TA/CCS is responsible for providing adequate levels of ventilation, inspired oxygen, and humidity to the intubated patient

because the patient's own physiologic mechanisms are bypassed. Trauma patients frequently require a minute ventilation ($V_E$) greater than normal to maintain appropriate $PaCO_2$ and pH levels. An increased pulmonary dead space ($V_D/V_T$) accompanies hemorrhagic shock and increases $V_E$ requirements. Head-injured patients require a low $PaCO_2$ (<30–35) to reduce cerebral blood volume and ICP (26). Ventilator settings can be adjusted according to frequently measured arterial blood gases. ICP should be monitored to be sure that ventilatory maneuvers are achieving the desired effect and are not complicating matters (i.e., inducing cerebral ischemia as a by-product of overzealous hyperventilation).

Oxygenation of arterial blood may also be monitored by frequent arterial blood gas determinations or by continuous pulse oximetry, which measures arterial oxyhemoglobin saturation ($SaO_2$) (53). One should usually initiate ventilation with 100% $O_2$ and then adjust the inspired oxygen concentration ($FIO_2$) by following the trend of the $PAO_2$. The probability of oxygen toxicity is minimized by keeping the $FIO_2 < 0.5$; therefore, the PEEP is adjusted to achieve an adequate $PaO_2$ and $SaO_2$ while using the minimal $FIO_2$. Trauma patients need the ability to elevate oxygen consumption to repay shock-induced oxygen debt (92). Therefore, the authors attempt to keep $PaO_2 > 120$ torr to ensure fully saturated arterial hemoglobin ($SaO_2 = 100\%$). During the acute phase of trauma care, it is usually possible to adjust the ventilator to provide a $PaO_2$ of 120 torr with an $FIO_2$ of 0.4. If the patient develops ARDS, increased levels of airway pressure are required to achieve adequate oxygenation.

Weaning the patient from mechanical ventilation occurs with fewer complications if the $FIO_2$ is first decreased to 0.35 or less. One may then decrease the frequency of mechanical breaths to spontaneous breathing supported by continuous positive airway pressure. Finally, the PEEP is reduced to 5 cm $H_2O$. Small airways with low ventilation to perfusion ($\dot{V}/\dot{Q}$) ratios will close due to adsorption atelectasis at elevated $FIO_2$ values (93). Therefore, we try to keep these small airways open by promoting an improved $\dot{V}/\dot{Q}$ with PEEP and mechanical breaths until oxygen exchange and the alveolar stability improve, with a lower alveolar $PAO_2$ and higher alveolar pressure of $N_2$ ($PAN_2$). Reducing PEEP will not collapse these small airways if they are stabilized with a low $PAO_2$ and a high $PAN_2$. An alternative to this standard method is using the newer mode of pressure support ventilation or a combination of pressure support and PEEP (94). Once the patient can be weaned from mechanical ventilatory support, extubation is considered. For extubation of trauma patients, one must meet the same criteria as for other anesthetized patients. Our criteria include adequate arterial oxygenation during support with $FIO_2$ of <0.4 and PEEP of <5 cm $H_2O$, adequate $CO_2$ excretion with spontaneous ventilation, the muscle strength to generate a negative inspiratory pressure of at least −25 cm $H_2O$, and a vital capacity of >15 ml/kg. Extubating the trauma patient provides more efficient natural humidification of the airway and more effective coughing to clear secretions than with an artificial airway. Patients who have had a translaryngeal tube in place for a prolonged time frequently have some laryngeal edema and vocal cord dysfunction after extubation. These patients often benefit from nebulized racemic epinephrine inhalation, incentive spirometry to keep the small airways open and stimulate coughing, and limitation of oral food intake until competent swallowing is demonstrated.

The late complications of intubation include vocal cord paralysis (arytenoid ankylosis) and tracheal stenosis. Both of these should be kept in mind when dealing with patients who are returning for reconstructive/follow-up surgery after variable amounts of time.

## CASE STUDIES: AIRWAY MANAGEMENT OF TRAUMA PATIENTS

To emphasize points that may not have been covered above and to reemphasize important points, several representative case studies will now be examined.

### Trauma Patient 1: Conscious Patient with Cervical Injury

The first patient, conscious and cooperative, has adequate spontaneous respirations, no facial trauma, and a presumed cervical spine injury. At admission, the clinician has time to consider carefully the presenting problems and the options that will constitute the plan of action for this patient, including "baseline" arterial blood gas analysis, supplemental oxygen supplied via face mask, a lateral cervical spine x-ray film to determine the extent of cervical spine instability, and placement of a gastric tube. In the absence of associated head or facial injury, the gastric tube may be passed through the nose. The slightest possibility of a basilar skull fracture (i.e., the presence of a LeFort II or III fracture [see Chapter 8]) mandates tube placement through the mouth. A nasogastric tube may disrupt the cribriform plate at the base of the nose in the presence of a basilar skull fracture, or it may traverse the fractured cribriform plate and impale the brain substance.

After the gastric tube is positioned, it is attached to suction and the contents of the stomach are evacuated to lessen the risk of aspiration. However, this does not *guarantee* that the stomach has been fully emptied (see "The 'Full Stomach' ").

At this point, the cervical spine x-ray film will usually have been developed and, for the sake of this discussion, shows pathologic findings. There are three route options: oral intubation, nasal intubation, or surgical airway. The "classic" choice for this type of patient is nasal intubation. For this method, one may anesthetize the mucosa of the nasal pharynx and apply a vasoconstrictor to minimize the possibility of epistaxis. The tube is then advanced blindly or with the aid of an appropriate device. Clinicians at the MIEMSS Shock Trauma Center believe that this technique may be contraindicated in the majority of traumatically injured patients for the reasons stated above (see Chapters 7 and 8) (38).

## Trauma Patient 2: Respiratory Distress with Cervical Injury

This patient initially presents essentially in the manner as trauma patient 1, except that inadequate spontaneous respirations are present, markedly diminishing the amount of preparatory time. The value of keeping all necessary equipment in readiness is quite apparent with such a patient (Table 3.7).

Basically, the choices for handling the airway management of this trauma patient are the same as for trauma patient 1: nasotracheal intubation versus orotracheal intubation (using MIAT) versus a surgical airway. One of the first two choices should probably be exercised before resorting to the last but, again, the choice depends on the individual practitioner's preference and the particulars of a given case.

With nasal intubation, there will be limited time to prepare the nasal mucosa adequately; if at all possible, a lubricant should be used on the endotracheal tube. Any one of the modifications of nasotracheal intubation that will permit rapid placement of the endotracheal tube may be used (Table 3.2). If several attempts at this route are unsuccessful, it is prudent to try another technique—probably MIAT.

On the other hand, MIAT may be the primary choice, as is often the case at the

**Table 3.7. Necessary Equipment for Emergency Airway Management[a]**

Laryngoscope with blades of various sizes and shapes
Endotracheal tubes (various sizes)
Endotracheal tube stylet
Oral or nasal airways
Face mask (various sizes)
Tonsil-tipped suction handle or suction source
Ambu bag (attached to oxygen source)
Pharmacologic adjuncts (drugs drawn up in syringes)

[a] From Grande CM. Airway management of the trauma patient in the resuscitation area of a trauma center. Trauma Q 1988;5:30–49.

MIEMSS Shock Trauma Center. Variables for this technique include the choice of laryngoscope blade and medications. The choice of medication and the way in which it is used will be governed primarily by the trauma patient's hemodynamic presentation. Unlike elective oral intubations in uncomplicated patients, failure to orally intubate a trauma patient with suspected cervical spine injury via MIAT usually requires the establishment of an emergency surgical airway.

For all trauma patients, especially those with suspected cervical spine injury, the airway "manager" should not hesitate to perform a cricothyroidotomy (preferable) or a tracheostomy because of problems (such as oxygen desaturation) during prolonged attempts at intubation airway management. Often the patient cannot afford repetitive attempts to intubate the trachea via the translaryngeal route and the care provider should quickly proceed to a surgical airway. Cost/benefit analysis of the morbidity and mortality considerations relative to all of the options supports this decision. The transtracheal (percutaneous) needle airway may also be used in the emergent situation.

## Trauma Patient 3: Comatose Patient with Head and Facial Trauma

This trauma patient presents at the trauma center with an altered mental status: stuporous, obtunded, or comatose. Other evidence of head injury includes lacerations of the scalp or forehead, pupillary changes, "raccoon eyes" or "Battle's sign," and hemotympanum (evidence of basilar skull fracture).

Airway management should proceed with an immediate evaluation of the urgency of intubation. Because head injury with altered levels of consciousness is the leading cause of respiratory compromise in trauma patients, any patient with head injury and presumed elevation of ICP is regarded as an acute respiratory emergency (26, 27). Signs of partial airway obstruction such as stridor and stertorous breathing are often present; associated problems include altered servoregulation of blood gas tensions and diminished or absent protective airway reflexes. If not rapidly reversed, resultant hypercarbia and hypoxemia greatly affect the prognosis of head injury (see Chapter 7). Therefore, the clinician must act immediately to obtain definitive airway control.

The care giver should remember that the traumatic event responsible for the head injury will also frequently produce cervical pathology, most significantly to the cervical spine, the upper airway, or the major vessels of the neck. Precautions should be taken and maintained to protect the cervical spine until the extent of injury can be evaluated definitively. Exterior physical examination of the neck should determine the absence or presence of tracheal deviation, the presence of fractures of the laryngeal or tracheal cartilage, and the status of the carotid pulses.

Because of routine concerns for the constellation of skull, facial, and cervical injury, cribriform plate fractures must be assumed. Thus, as stated above, nasal intubation is probably best avoided. Choices for these patients, therefore, are similar to those for trauma patients 1 and 2, including oral intubation with cervical spine stabilization (MIAT) and a surgical airway. The patient should be hyperventilated immediately by bag-valve-mask apparatus through constant cricoid pressure; this hyperventilation will lower $PaCO_2$ levels acutely and induce cerebral vasoconstriction.

Pharmacologic adjuncts to airway management become important for head-injured patients—especially with regard to alleviating elevated ICP (Fig. 3.4). In addition, several drugs (such as thiopental, etomidate, propofol, midazolam, lidocaine, and muscle relaxants) also attenuate the detrimental effect of increased ICP due to airway manipulations such as laryngoscopy, intubation, or tracheostomy. Thiopental, etomidate, propofol, and lidocaine directly induce vasoconstriction of the cerebral vasculature and reduce ICP and secondarily

provide various levels of anesthesia, which blunt the effect on ICP of adrenergic stimulation (increased heart rate and blood pressure) caused by sensory stimulation of the airway (95–97).

Therefore, drug choice becomes a matter of judgment on the part of the clinician, based on at least three important factors: (a) the patient's hemodynamic status, (b) the circumstances (e.g., time allowed for action), and (c) the clinician's experience. Thiopental and propofol, for example, have shown a tendency to reduce blood pressure—which not only reduces overall cerebral perfusion pressure but also may lead to cardiopulmonary arrest in the hypovolemic trauma patient. However, thiopental can be used safely in reduced, incremental doses. On the other hand, etomidate is reported to have minimal effects on hemodynamics and, in some cases, has elicited a direct adrenergic response that would have implications similar to the effects of airway manipulation (see below).

Although very popular in some locales, etomidate seems to have several liabilities as an induction agent in both the general surgical and the trauma populations (96). Etomidate frequently causes pain on injection, myoclonic movements that can be disconcerting in the head-injured patient, and postoperative nausea. Further, etomidate is contraindicated in the management of pregnant patients. It therefore should not be used in any female trauma patient in the childbearing age range if definitive pregnancy tests cannot be performed before the need for induction of anesthesia. Additionally, our clinical experience in the anesthetic management of trauma patients revealed that patients frequently showed signs of awakening before tracheal intubation could be completed following anesthetic induction with etomidate. Probably the most troublesome characteristic of this agent is that it is capable of inhibiting adrenal steroidogenesis, even at the recommended induction dose of 0.3 to 0.4 mg/kg (98). Another study indicated that use of etomidate for induction and maintenance of anesthesia was associ-

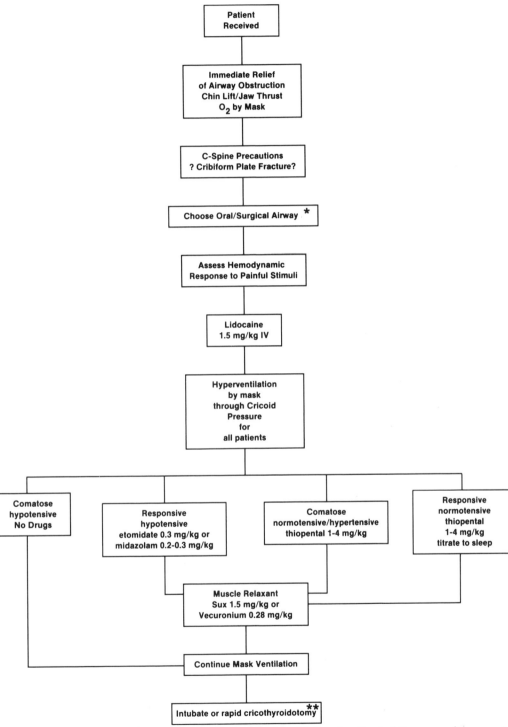

**Figure 3.4.   Emergency airway management of the head-injured patient.** * Because of the possibility of cribriform plate fractures in all head-injured patients, the nasal route of intubation should probably be avoided, unless this concern has been addressed definitively. ** In the case of failed intubation, hyperventilation should be maintained and whether to proceed with another intubation attempt or with a surgical airway must be decided quickly. This algorithm is presented as a learning tool; it is recognized that variations may exist.

ated with significantly depressed plasma cortisol concentrations during both anesthesia and the immediate postanesthesia period (99). Finally, other investigators described an increase in mortality rates due to infection in critically ill patients with multiple trauma after the administration of intravenous etomidate infusions over extended periods for sedation (100).

Propofol, an intravenous anesthetic agent, has recently been approved for use within the United States. Advantages of propofol are shorter recovery room time due to more rapid recovery of psychomotor activity and orientation and a low incidence of nausea and vomiting (101). These properties of propofol would appear to make it attractive for use in stable trauma patients who need to undergo several short surgical procedures during their hospitalization. The mild to moderate cardiovascular depressant effects of this drug need to be evaluated more extensively in the trauma population to determine its suitability for use in the acute trauma patient with an unstable hemodynamic profile. Experience with the use of propofol in a variety of trauma patients will ultimately help define its best utility in this population.

Intravenous lidocaine in standard dosages (1.5 mg/kg) is usually hemodynamically inert and should be given to all patients with head injury (unless there is documented allergy or history of malignant hyperthermia). If the patient is hemodynamically stable but comatose and seemingly unresponsive to painful stimuli, one may proceed with small intermittent boluses of thiopental. Conversely, if the patient is hypotensive but sensory pathways are still intact, etomidate would be a good choice.

Thus, evaluation must be made regarding the particular patient's overall hemodynamic condition. Objectively, this would include blood pressure, heart rate, strength and profile of pulses, estimation of blood loss, preexisting medical conditions (such as cardiovascular disease), and the patient's response to painful stimuli (such as the placement of intravascular catheters or an oral airway). Subjective evaluation includes the "gestalt" perceived by the trauma anesthesiologist regarding the particular patient's course, gained from previous clinical experience.

Muscle relaxants serve two purposes in this scenario. First, they facilitate laryngoscopy and thereby shorten the duration of sensory stimulation and exposure to the detriments of hypoxia (42, 102). Second, once the patient is intubated, they prevent "bucking" on the endotracheal tube, which is also correlated with "spikes" in ICP, much as during coughing.

Choice of an ideal muscle relaxant for use in acute trauma patients and in follow-up surgical care of these patients is a major consideration in formulating a safe plan for anesthetic management. Rapid tracheal intubation is often needed early in the resuscitation process as well as prior to surgical intervention. Because of its rapid onset, succinylcholine has for years been the drug of choice for tracheal intubation in emergency patients. Unfortunately, as a depolarizing muscle relaxant, succinylcholine has several undesirable side effects. Succinylcholine causes elevation of intragastric pressure, which may increase the risk of regurgitation and subsequent aspiration in the unprepared emergency trauma patient with a "full stomach." Additionally, it increases both the intraocular and the intracranial pressure under certain circumstances. Succinylcholine also causes exaggerated potassium release from skeletal muscle in patients who have sustained burns and spinal cord injuries (103).

More recently, the use of "high-dose" nondepolarizing agents has provided a viable alternative to the use of succinylcholine. The authors have demonstrated in a large group of trauma patients that the onset of good intubating conditions requires approximately the same amount of time for either succinylcholine (1.5 mg/kg) or vecuronium (0.28 mg/kg) (104). Both drugs produced greater than 90% neuromuscular block between 60 and 90 seconds after injection. The time from neuromuscular block produced by vecuronium (0.28 mg/kg) to 25% recovery of neuromuscular transmission was approximately 89 minutes. Other advantages over other nondepolarizing muscle relaxants are that vecuronium does not cause deleterious autonomic reflexes and does not promote histamine release (105). Nondepolarizing muscle relaxants such as pancuronium do not have the drawbacks associated with succinylcholine, but large "intubating doses" cause deleterious autonomic reflexes and prolonged paralysis (106).

Hyperventilation by mask should continue after muscle relaxant injection until intubation conditions are ideal (90 seconds). Once newer, nondepolarizing neuromuscular blocking drugs that have a profile of action similar to that of succinylcholine become available, they will probably replace this older depolarizing agent.

Some might argue that using a nondepolarizing muscle relaxant in a "high-dose" fashion will predispose the trauma patient, who "only needed an intubation," to an unnecessarily prolonged recovery period. In our experience, this factor would not usually be of major importance in the multitrauma patient, in whom perioperative management (e.g., diagnostic studies and surgery) is normally extensive.

After hemodynamic resuscitation is accomplished, constant levels of anesthesia and muscle relaxants should be maintained as appropriate. Thus, rebound of elevations in ICP will be avoided.

### Trauma Patient 4: Conscious Patient with Severe Facial Injuries

This conscious trauma patient presents with adequate spontaneous respirations but with severe facial injuries, including LeFort and mandibular fractures. Again, in such a patient, one must have a relatively high index of suspicion for *both* associated head injury and cervical spine trauma and act accordingly. In some cases, this should mean immediately proceeding to a surgical airway. However, the existing adequate respirations "buy some time" to evaluate the extent of injury by way of lateral cervical spine and skull roentgenograms, neurologic examination, and perhaps a computed tomographic (CT) scan or magnetic resonance image of the head. Nevertheless, all forms of nasal intubation would be at least relatively contraindicated, and possibly absolutely contraindicated, on the basis of occult cribriform plate fracture and the need to visualize the airway directly. To perform a blind technique in the face of soft-tissue trauma to the cervical area, which has not been fully disclosed (e.g., laceration of the mucosa of the hypopharynx), is to invite costly complications such as the creation of false passages by the endotracheal tube. Therefore, the only alternative (aside from a surgical airway) is oral intubation using MIAT. If the possibility of a spinal cord injury can be directly eliminated, then one may opt to use any of the other methods of oral intubation (Table 3.2).

Once again, use of pharmacologic adjuncts is governed by the hemodynamic situation. Commonly, trauma patients presenting in this condition have other associated injuries that cause them to be quite hypotensive, often requiring application/inflation of military/medical antishock trousers (MAST). If so, one approach would be to place the laryngoscope in the trauma patient's mouth and determine whether airway reflexes are indeed intact, judging by the degree of hemodynamic stress response (tachycardia, hypertension) (97). The stress response (increased ICP and decreased cerebral blood flow) elicited by stimulation of airway reflexes during laryngoscopy can be detrimental to head-injured patients. This reflex tachycardia and hypertension can be attenuated to a certain degree by the judicious use of lidocaine and thiopental (lidocaine is more hemodynamically inert) for their anesthetic and cerebral vasoconstrictor effects. Additionally, hyperventilation by face mask through cricoid pressure to reduce carbon dioxide levels acutely should also be performed to reduce the vasodilating effects of hypercarbia.

## Trauma Patient 5: Respiratory Distress with Severe Facial Injuries

This trauma patient is much the same as trauma patient 4 but either has inadequate spontaneous respirations or is apneic. Swift definitive action is obviously needed. In this case, head and facial injury present together with suspected cervical spine injury. For reasons cited above, nasal intubation is again not a choice, although MIAT may be attempted. Hemodynamics will dictate the use of pharmacologic adjuncts. For these patients, time and circumstances often do not permit the use of any drugs, and intubation is accomplished without pharmacologic assistance. Profound muscle relaxation is often a side effect of the hypoxia and hypercarbia seen in unconscious, apneic patients. After intubation is accomplished, 100% oxygen and a muscle relaxant should be administered (the so-called "oxygen-and-a-prayer" technique). The muscle relaxant will prevent coughing, bucking, and any involuntary movements made by the patient.

## Trauma Patient 6: Disoriented, Combative Patient

This patient does not have any of the "serious" problems of the preceding patients: no obvious head, cervical, or facial injury and adequate spontaneous respirations. However, this trauma patient is disoriented, combative, occasionally somnolent, and probably under the influence of ethanol or some other substance(s), as is frequently the case with trauma admissions. This patient needs various diagnostic/therapeutic procedures (e.g., head CT scanning, suturing of lacerations), which are made difficult or impossible by the patient's unstable neurologic condition.

In some instances, one might be inclined to administer a narcotic antagonist, like naloxone, to reverse the effects of the assumed etiologic factor. The drawbacks of this maneuver would be that (a) ICP would be raised acutely (while the possibility of occult head injury still exists); (b) vomiting might occur; or (c) the patient, who may be a chronic substance abuser, could be placed iatrogenically into a withdrawal state.

If the reversal agent does not have its desired effect or if the practitioner opts not to use such an agent, two choices are left: to sedate or to intubate the trauma patient. It is our opinion that gradual sedation with one or more of the appropriate drugs, alone or in combination (narcotic/benzodiazepine) initially may be a reasonable approach. In this case, respiratory function must be followed closely by conventional observation and/or the use of monitoring devices such as a pulse oximeter and capnograph in conjunction with a nasal catheter. However, relative oversedation of an unintubated trauma patient may be described as providing a general anesthetic without the benefit of an endotracheal tube. In other words, the trauma patient's airway will be completely unprotected (in conjunction with a full stomach) and respirations cannot be controlled properly.

The other choice would be to proceed directly with definitive airway management via endotracheal intubation. In this type of trauma patient, the extensive use of any intravenous pharmacologic agent can be avoided by providing local anesthesia to the nasal mucosa and performing blind nasal intubation by any number of methods, as time permits. Or, with the assistance of either topical preparation of the oropharynx with local anesthetics or intravenous adjuncts, oral intubation may be performed by an appropriate technique.

## Trauma Patient 7: Patient Injured by Explosion and Fire in a Closed Space

This patient was involved in an explosion and fire in a closed space and was brought to the trauma center with adequate spontaneous respirations. Since adequate ventilation is present initially, time is available to evaluate the circumstances. In this case, there are at least three concerns: (a) since the fire was in a closed space, the patient may have upper airway burns; (b) because the fire occurred in a closed area, there is a high probability that the patient inhaled fumes; and (c) because of the explosion, associated nonthermal trauma may be present (107, 108).

If the patient is conscious, questioning as to the particulars of the fire is possible. If the patient is unconscious, one will have to rely upon clinical deductive skills or question other witnesses (e.g., relatives or fire/police officials). Evidence of upper airway burns indicates that a degree of urgency must be exercised in assuming definitive airway control, even if respiration is normal at the time of examination. Burns to the face, carbonaceous material around the mouth or nares or in the pharynx, or singed facial or nasal hairs are all signs of close proximity to a fire. One may listen to the pattern of air exchange for stertorous sounds. Laryngoscopy may be performed to assess the degree of upper airway burns. The lower airway is generally spared from exposure to thermal injury because of the heat-absorptive properties of the upper airway. The exceptions to this rule are steam inhalation, chemical burns (e.g., phosgene gas), and inhalation of hot beverages (109).

Thermal injury induces the body's natural sequence of responses, which includes the development of edema in the affected area. Edema in the face/neck area may progress to an extent that airflow is compromised—especially in anatomic areas that are normally narrow, such as the larynx and its associated structures (e.g., epiglottis, cricoid ring). Edema of these structures may limit air exchange severely and may develop quite rapidly over the course of minutes. Therefore, after objective evaluation of the airway, one must act quickly. It is safer to assume a more conservative posture and to achieve definitive airway control than to opt for continued clinical observation in such cases. If any of the signs of impending obstruction are present, such as stridor, rapid airway control is even more essential.

Lower airway injury may be evaluated by direct visualization using a flexible fiberop-tic bronchoscope or by performing a xenon scan. Overall, airway function may be evaluated by airflow studies and other pulmonary function tests, as described in further detail in Chapter 9.

If the patient has adequate respirations at the time of evaluation, the clinician may choose one of several courses of action. If time permits, the standard protocols for trauma patients, such as obtaining a cervical x-ray film, should be followed. Depending upon the presence or absence of other injuries, one may intubate by either of the two transtracheal routes (oral or nasal); since some degree of subclinical laryngeal edema already may be present, laryngeal narrowing should be anticipated and a smaller endotracheal tube should be used. One may attempt to use an aerosolized form of racemic epinephrine for inhalation in an attempt to limit or reverse some degree of airway swelling, although this is not a reliably successful maneuver. If other associated facial, pharyngeal, laryngeal, or cervical trauma does not permit transtracheal intubation, one may quickly proceed to the creation of a surgical airway: cricothyroidotomy, tracheostomy, or percutaneous needle ventilation. One should be aware that, in patients with burns of the lower face, anterior neck, and upper thorax, creating one of these surgical airways may be more difficult than usual because of problems caused by soft tissue edema and contractures. During the recovery phase, the hypopharynx should be evaluated formally before extubation by either indirect or direct laryngoscopy.

Other points to be considered and investigated at this time are the possibility of carbon monoxide poisoning and the various sequelae of exposure to an explosion. Explosions in closed areas induce injuries by blunt, penetrating, and/or combination mechanisms (107, 108). As an example of blunt trauma, the patient may have been displaced physically by the blast effect of the explosion. When the person collides with a stationary object such as a wall or floor, additional blunt injury may be sustained, as well as indirect blunt trauma caused by secondary shock waves. This combination of blunt trauma mechanisms may induce injuries to the neck, face, chest (e.g., pneumothorax); abdomen (e.g., splenic rupture); or extremities (e.g., fractures). The initial explosion may accelerate other stationary objects, creating projectiles capable of causing penetrating injuries. Mixed mechanical (blunt/penetrating) trauma such as impalement may also occur. Thus, when dealing with the burn patient, one must have a high index of suspicion for various types of trauma, not just thermal injury (107, 108).

## Trauma Patient 8: Injured Patient with Previously Unsuccessful Airway Control

The trauma patient may have any combination of the first seven conditions profiled, but he or she has had previous airway manipulations, which may include any of the "noninvasive" airway management techniques listed in Table 3.2.

If the trauma patient has been receiving positive-pressure ventilation via mask without application of cricoid pressure (many care providers are unaware of this technique), there is a high probability that a significant amount of air has insufflated the stomach. This air increases the volume of the stomach along with the probability of regurgitation (and aspiration). If the trauma patient has regurgitated into the pharynx and mask ventilation continues without suctioning, the vomitus may be forced into the lungs.

The placement of oral and nasal airways may stimulate vomiting. Improperly placed oral airways may actually worsen airway mechanics by folding the tongue back on itself. Nasal airways, if not used correctly, may damage the nasal mucosa and cause epistaxis, with possible aspiration of blood and subsequent bronchospasm. However, in general, prior placement of oral or nasal airways should imply to the airway "manager" that the correct placement of those devices should be verified.

Placement of the more invasive airway adjuncts such as the esophageal obturator airway (EOA), esophageal gastric tube airway (EGTA), and the pharyngeotracheal lumen airway (PTL) requires more deft handling to avoid complications (74–76, 110–112). All of these devices are used in conjunction with either mouth-to-tube ventilation, a bag-valve-mask apparatus, or a pressure-driven oxygen inflator. These devices have all been developed with field care providers (e.g., paramedics) in mind. These individuals may be working in locations where endotracheal intubation by these persons is not permitted by state or municipal regulations. The EOA and EGTA may be considered as one category. Each has a low margin of safety for use and a low degree of efficacy. For this reason, many localities now permit intubation by field care providers because the risk of failed intubation by these individuals is considered to be less than the risk of using one of these devices. The basic device, the EOA, consists of a blunt tube, which is not patent and which has a distal cuff. It is meant to be inserted into the esophagus, thereby sealing off the gastric contents. At the EOA's proximal end is a universal connector (15 mm), which is attached to any of the above ventilation devices. A clear face mask provides the oronasal seal. Gas supplied to the EOA then exits via multiple fenestrations in the upper third of the tube, which, if the tube is positioned properly, will be in the vicinity of the larynx (Fig. 3.5). The face mask, by sealing the airway, permits ventilation of the lungs via mass action. The problem with the EOA is that, if it is placed inadvertently into the trachea, it will seal off the lungs and not permit ventilation. However, the authors have seen two patients with EOAs placed through the larynx receiving one-lung ventilation and oxygenation because the distal cuff on the EOA was advanced past the carina into one of the mainstem bronchi. The proximal ventilation holes in the EOA were in the trachea, thus ventilating the unobstructed lung.

The EGTA is a next-generation improve-

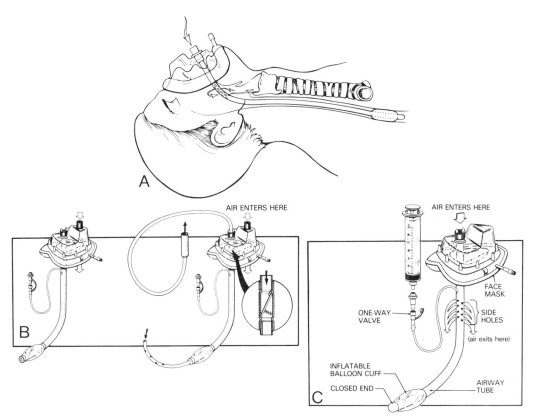

AIR ENTERS HERE

AIR ENTERS HERE

A

B

ONE-WAY VALVE

FACE MASK

SIDE HOLES
(air exits here)

INFLATABLE BALLOON CUFF

CLOSED END

AIRWAY TUBE

C

**Figure 3.5.    Esophageal obturator airway (A,** *top* **and C,** *right*) **and esophageal gastric tube airway (B,** *left*). (**A** from Clinton JE, Ruiz E. Emergency airway management. In Roberts JR, Hedge JR (eds): Clinical Procedures in Emergency Medicine. Philadelphia, WB Saunders, 1985, pp 2–29. **B** and **C** from Stewart RD. Field airway control for the trauma patient. In Campbell JE (ed): Basic Trauma Life Support: Advanced Prehospital Care, ed 2. Englewood Cliffs, NJ, Prentice Hall, 1988, pp 42–90.)

ment of the EOA. The difference is that the lumen of the EGTA is patent and will permit the passage of a narrow suction catheter into the stomach. As the incidence of regurgitation is high with either the EOA or the EGTA, this feature improves the situation. The first step when approaching the airway management of these patients is to auscultate breath sounds with a stethoscope. If breath sounds are poor or absent, the scenario becomes more emergent. For example, this may mean that the EOA or EGTA has been placed into the trachea itself. Advancing the EOA to its limit may place the cuff into a bronchus, improving breath sounds over one lung. An intratracheal EOA must be removed to allow endotracheal intubation.

The trachea should then be intubated via the appropriate route to maintain ventilation and to protect the patient from aspiration as the esophageal airway is removed. When using the left-handed laryngoscope, this entails moving the EOA/EGTA to the left side of the mouth, positioning the laryngoscope in the right side of the mouth, and intubating around the EOA/EGTA within the cramped confines of the mouth. This procedure may be made easier by using Magill forceps to assist in placing the endotracheal tube.

Assuming successful intubation, the EOA/EGTA should then be removed as follows (Table 3.8): in the case of an EOA, the esophagus is suctioned proximal to the EOA cuff; in the case of an EGTA, the stomach is suctioned via the gastric port and the esophagus is suctioned proximal to the

**Table 3.8.   Removal of Esophageal Obturator Airway and Esophageal Tube Airway**[a]

Patient unconscious
1. Ensure that EOA/EGTA balloon is inflated.
2. Suction stomach if possible (EGTA) and/or the esophagus proximal to balloon (EOA/EGTA) with NGT. Leave NGT in place.
3. Have adequate suction available with Yankauer tip attached.
4. Intubate trachea with appropriate technique chosen from Table 3.2.
5. Confirm placement of ETT.
6. Remove EOA/EGTA.
7. Observe closely for signs of complications developing due to intubation or the EOA/EGTA.

Patient conscious with adequate respirations
1. Ensure that airway reflexes are intact and that ventilation is adequate.
2. Follow steps 2 and 3 above.
3. Turn patient's head to side if appropriate (cervical spine injury precautions).
4. Remove EOA/EGTA.
5. Suction oropharynx, apply oxygen mask, and confirm that acceptable respirations are present.

[a] EOA, esophageal obturator airway; EGTA, esophageal gastric tube airway; NGT, nasogastric tube; ETT, endotracheal tube.

cuff. Next, the oropharynx and hypopharynx should be suctioned thoroughly. Finally, the EOA/EGTA cuff is deflated, and the device is removed. The trauma patient should be monitored for the development of any of the characteristic complications associated with the use of these devices (e.g., esophageal perforation).

The PTL, a fairly new type of "field" airway, is theoretically safe, easy to use, and effective (Fig. 3.6) but is still undergoing evaluation; preliminary results are not definitive (75, 76). The device (which exists in several variants and may thus be known by other names, e.g., "Combitube") is supposed to be "fail-safe" and "foolproof." It consists of two parallel tubes, one long and one short. Ideally, the long tube should cannulate the esophagus. Inflating the distal cuff of the long tube would effectively seal the esophagus, as well as provide a route for the egress of vomitus and for gastric suctioning. The distal lumen of the short tube will be in the hypopharynx, in the vicinity of the larynx. The large proximal cuff is then inflated, which can serve two purposes. The first would be to tamponade any bleeding in the oropharynx and hypopharynx. As this device functions basically as a mass-action ventilation system, the second purpose would be to reduce the amount of dead space in the pharynx. Conversely, if the long tube is placed into the trachea instead of the esophagus, the situation is essentially an endotracheal intu-

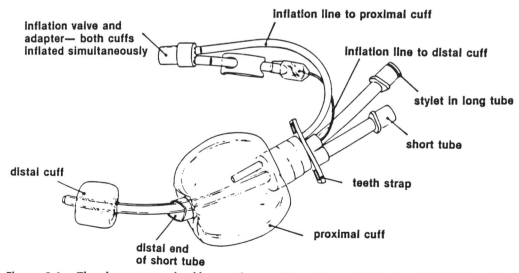

**Figure 3.6.   The pharyngeotracheal lumen airway.** (From Nieman JT, Rosborough JP, Myers R, et al: The pharyngeotracheal lumen airway: preliminary investigation of a new adjunct. Ann Emerg Med 1984;13:591–596).

bation. As a secondary benefit, one now also has a route for suctioning the stomach via the short tube.

Two important points must be realized about the PTL: (*a*) Its successful use is highly dependent upon recognizing the location of the long tube (i.e., in the trachea or the esophagus). An error here could easily spell disaster (i.e., an unrecognized esophageal intubation). In the field situation, the determination is made by listening to breath sounds, by observing movements of the chest wall and epigastric area, and possibly by evaluating suctioned contents from the various tubes. In the hospital setting, radiography can also be used. (*b*) The PTL is essentially a "blind" technique and may cause further damage to soft tissues or result in intubation of false passages.

The PTL probably will perform well in the field as an airway adjunct when tracheal intubation with an endotracheal tube and laryngoscope is not possible, for example, in cramped spaces (e.g., intubating a victim trapped beneath an automobile).

When a trauma patient with a PTL in place arrives in the admitting area, the first step is to check breath sounds. By doing so, one may determine whether the long tube is in the trachea or esophagus. A gastric tube should be passed through the appropriate lumen to decompress the stomach. Next, the large oral cuff should be deflated and excess air evacuated by using a syringe to collapse the cuff fully. A laryngoscope is then inserted into the oropharynx and the trachea is intubated. The PTL is then removed. (We are not aware of any literature describing nasal intubation for patients with PTLs, nor does the manufacturer mention it. The PTL is designed for oral use only.)

If one determines by auscultation of breath sounds that the long tube of the PTL is in the trachea, one has two options. First, a tube-changing stylet such as the tracheal tube exchanger (TTX; Sheridan Catheter Corp.) may be used. The stomach still may be suctioned if a gastric tube can be passed via the lumen of the short tube. Both cuffs of the PTL may be deflated and the PTL can be

removed cautiously while ensuring that the intratracheal stylet remains in place.

The second option is to suction the stomach as above, suction the oropharynx, remove the PTL, and intubate the trachea using a laryngoscope. This choice is probably less attractive than the first option because one is unnecessarily surrendering a certain degree of airway control already obtained by the long tube of the PTL.

## Trauma Patient 9: Injuries to the Upper Airway

This trauma patient is discussed to demonstrate airway management in cases of injuries of the larynx, trachea, and major airways. The true incidence of injuries to these areas is difficult to estimate because many of these patients die at the scene of the traumatic event. Of those patients who do survive transport to a trauma center (78% are dead on arrival), many will die upon arrival (21% of survivors expire in the first 120 minutes) (91, 113). Manifestations can be protean, and presentation may be delayed up to several days.

Textbook signs and symptoms include cyanosis, voice changes, dyspnea, hemoptysis, appreciable evidence of injury upon physical examination of the cervical region (including subcutaneous emphysema), and pneumothorax or pneumohemothorax (113, 114). In this situation the most important tool that the anesthesiologist possesses is a sound understanding of the concepts of mechanisms of injury and their application and association with the history of a given case (see Chapter 2).

Most of these cases will occur in conjunction with a history of either a penetrating wound of the neck (caused by either a bladed weapon or a gunshot) or some form of blunt trauma. The high degree of association of these types of injuries with the riding of open vehicles such as motorcycles, snowmobiles, minibikes, and all-terrain vehicles (ATVs) has led to the coining of terms such as "clothesline injury" and "snowmobile injury." In these instances, the neck of the unprotected passenger makes abrupt contact with a wire, a clothesline, or a tree branch (115). The passengers of these vehicles usually position their heads with a backward tilt orientation, thereby further exposing the neck, which is usually protected by the mandible.

In the case of automobile accidents, similar injuries may be seen in victims who are wearing only a lapbelt. Upon impact, the upper body, head, and neck continue in a forward motion, usually with the head striking first at the windshield. Thus, the head is again tilted rearward, exposing the neck. The neck makes contact with the sharp edge of the dashboard (the "padded dash" syndrome) (114). These injuries may also occur secondary to blows to the neck with a variety of instruments (e.g., club, hand).

The extent of injury is variable, ranging from isolated damage to the various cartilaginous structures, soft tissue, and dentition of the upper airway to complete crushing of the entire larynx and trachea or even laryngotracheal separation.

Injuries to lower airway structures such as the intrathoracic trachea or bronchi usually occur as a result of either abrupt deceleration of structures tethered by ligaments or barotrauma. In the latter scenario, "blow-out" injuries may occur, especially if the glottis is closed during impact, as the result of reflex gasping in anticipation of the crash (115).

Upon receipt of this type of trauma patient, an initial evaluation is performed, focusing on the patient's ability to exchange air. Blood gas analysis, which should be performed initially, may reveal hypoxia, which in a large number of cases is due to concomitant pulmonary contusion with secondary ventilation/perfusion ($\dot{V}/\dot{Q}$) mismatching (see Chapter 6).

If the situation allows, further diagnosis should be attempted before engaging in manipulation of the airway, while supplemental oxygen is supplied. The range of evaluation techniques includes direct and indirect laryngoscopy, bronchoscopy, radi-ography, CT scanning, and, most recently, magnetic resonance imaging (MRI).

As to specific choices of airway management techniques, the range is wide, including translaryngeal intubation (both antero-grade and retrograde), cricothyroidotomy, tracheostomy, and percutaneous needle ventilation. Whatever technique is used, it is important that precautions be taken to ensure that the method of choice does not complicate the situation. If possible, a backup procedure should be identified and available for immediate application.

If translaryngeal intubation is chosen, one should almost always proceed via the oral route. "Awake-sedated," "rapid-sequence," use of a bronchoscope as a stylet, and use of inhalation induction have all been suggested (91, 115). It is essential that the endotracheal tube itself does not cause further tissue damage or disruption of structure (thus the avoidance of the nasal route).

Translaryngeal intubation has been criticized from the standpoint of the possibility of the endotracheal tube entering false tissue passages and complicating management. Use of a flexible fiberoptic broncho-scope in conjunction with translaryngeal intubation for any cases of suspected sub-glottic injury has been advocated with the ability for constant visualization in mind (115). Cricothyroidotomy may be chosen if the injury is above the level of the cricothy-roid membrane. It may later be necessary to perform an elective tracheostomy if the cricothyroidotomy is interfering with recon-structive surgery of the larynx and upper trachea. The cricothyroidotomy itself may be absolutely contraindicated if complete laryngotracheal separation has occurred, although exceptions to the rule can be imagined.

Tracheostomy is the route that will most often be chosen, especially if the upper trachea is damaged. Theoretically, a trache-ostomy may be performed as low as the sixth tracheal ring, where the trachea enters the thorax.

For intrathoracic tracheal injuries one

may generally proceed in either one of two ways. The first would be to intubate the trachea via the larynx or by tracheostomy. In either case, the objective is to bypass the location of the injury and create a patent airway by inflation of the endotracheal tube cuff. In the case of an injury to the lower trachea or the right main bronchus, this may involve choosing a long single-lumen endotracheal tube and advancing it as necessary (i.e., a deliberate main bronchus intubation) or using a double-lumen endotracheal tube. In the case of a left main bronchus injury, it is probably best to use a double-lumen tube from the outset.

Alternatively, if the injury is too distal to be reached by an endotracheal tube, if the extrathoracic larynx is crushed to such an extent as to prohibit the passage of any tracheal tube, or if a foreign object is obstructing the intrathoracic airway, one may first attempt percutaneous needle jet ventilation. If this is unsuccessful, one must resort to ventilation without using the lungs (i.e., some form of extracorporeal oxygenation or partial cardiopulmonary bypass). In this regard, a simple-to-use and quick-to-employ device still cannot be found in the resuscitation area of a trauma center (116). Success in these types of cases without such a device is often a matter of good fortune.

A recent innovation in extrapulmonary gas exchange is the intravenous oxygenator (IVOX; Cardiopulmonics, Salt Lake City, UT). This device supplements the oxygenation of patients with severe lung disease by transferring the $O_2$ and $CO_2$ directly in the vena cava and right atrium (117). With further development this type of device (which is inserted percutaneously, much like an aortic balloon pump) may find its way into the emergency room to support gas exchange temporarily and expeditiously in patients with badly obstructed or damaged airways or severely traumatized lungs.

In all of the above cases, once the airway has been secured, the patient will undergo further evaluation to delineate the extent of the injury. This should include esophagoscopy to investigate the possibility of concomitant injury to the esophagus (10). Extensive reconstruction procedures also may be necessary.

## SUMMARY

In this chapter, perioperative airway management has been discussed comprehensively from a conceptual standpoint. Patients with cervical, cranial, and airway trauma and the intrahospital management of various field airway devices have been presented. Recommended techniques have also been presented, while reminding the reader that the proper approach to one patient may not be the best for another as far as trauma care especially airway management, is concerned. Thus, we stress that the individual practitioner's prior experience, preferences, and medical ideologies are very important in the decision-making process. At the same time, we also stress that each trauma patient must be approached individually and that "cookbook" methods should be avoided. Trauma mismanagement is often a result of improper judgment and limited experience (118).

## References

1. Committee on Trauma Research: Injury in America: A Continuing Public Health Problem. Washington, DC, National Academy Press, 1985.
2. Peters RM. Fluid resuscitation and oxygen exchange in hypovolemia. In Siegel JH (ed): Trauma: Emergency Surgery and Critical Care. New York, Churchill Livingstone, 1987, pp 157–179.
3. Stene JK. Anesthesia for the critically ill trauma patient. In Siegel JH (ed): Trauma: Emergency Surgery and Critical Care. New York, Churchill Livingstone, 1987, pp 843–862.
4. Stoelting RK. Endotracheal intubation. In Miller RD (ed): Anesthesia, ed 2. New York, Churchill Livingstone, 1986, pp 523–552.
5. Roberts JT: Fundamentals of Tracheal Intubation. New York, Grune & Stratton, 1983.
6. Grande CM, Ramanathan S, Turndorf H. Structural correlates of airway function. In Bishop MJ (ed): Problems in Anesthesia. Philadelphia, JB Lippincott, 1988, vol 2, pp 175–190.
7. Broadbent TR, Woolf RM. Gunshot wounds of

the face: initial care. J Trauma 1972;12:229–232.

8. Flood LM, Astley B. Anaesthetic management of acute laryngeal trauma. Br J Anaesth 1982;54:1339–1342.

9. Boegtz MS, Katz JA. Airway management of the trauma patient. Semin Anesth 1985;4:114–123.

10. Herrin TJ, Brzusfowics R, Hendrickson M. Anesthetic management of neck trauma. South Med J 1979;72:1102–1106.

11. Miller J, Iovino W, Fine J, Klain M. High-frequency jet ventilation in oral and maxillofacial surgery. J Oral Maxillofac Surg 1982;40:790–793.

12. Guildner CW. Resuscitation—opening the airway: a comparative study of techniques for opening an airway obstructed by the tongue. JACEP 1976;5:588–590.

13. Sosis M, Lazar S. Jaw dislocation during general anaesthesia. Can J Anaesth 1987;34:407–408.

14. Redick LF. The temporomandibular joint and tracheal intubation. Anesth Analg 1987;66:675–676.

15. McIntyre JWR. The difficult tracheal intubation. Can J Anaesth 1987;34:204–213.

16. Mallampati SR, Gratt SP, Gugino LD, Desai SP, Waraksa B, Freiberger D, Liu PL. A clinical sign to predict difficult tracheal intubation: a prospective study. Can Anaesth Soc J 1985;32:429–434.

17. Arora RD, Patterson L, Hagen JF, Pinchak AC. Prediction of difficult intubation. Anesthesiology 1987;67:A472.

18. Macklin MT, Macklin CC. Malignant interstitial emphysema of the lungs and mediastinum as an important occult complication in many respiratory diseases and other conditions: an interpretation of the clinical literature in the light of laboratory experiment. Medicine (Baltimore) 1944;23:281–358.

19. Howell JBL, Permutt S, Proctor DF, Riley RL. Effect of inflation of the lung on different parts of pulmonary vascular bed. J Appl Physiol 1961;16:71–76.

20. Graham JM, Beall AC Jr, Mattox KL, Vaughan GD. Systemic air embolism following penetrating trauma to the lung. Chest 1977;72:449–454.

21. Bannister WK, Sattilaro AJ: Vomiting and aspiration during anesthesia. Anesthesiology 1962;23:251–264.

22. Hardy JF. Large volume gastroesophageal reflux: a rationale for risk reduction in the perioperative period. Can J Anaesth 1988;35:162–173.

23. Gorback M. Pulmonary acid aspiration. I: pathophysiology, clinical settings, consequences, and role of proper anesthetic technique. J Drug Dev 1989;2(Suppl 3):4–17.

24. ACS Committee on Trauma: Airway management and ventilation. In Advanced Trauma Life Support Program, Instructor Manual. Chicago, American College of Surgeons, 1989, pp 31–56.

25. Gilbert R, Keighley JF. The arterial alveolar

26. Archer DP. Intracranial pressure and the anesthetist. Can J Anaesth 1987;34:S51–S54.

27. Schumacher PT, Rhodes GR, Newell JC, Dutton RE, Shah DM, Scovill WA, Powers SR. Ventilation perfusion imbalance after head trauma. Am Rev Respir Dis 1979;119:33–43.

28. Sellick BA. Cricoid pressure to control regurgitation of stomach contents during induction of anaesthesia. Lancet 1961;2:404–406.

29. Salem MR, Sellick BA, Elam JO. The historical background of cricoid pressure in anesthesia and resuscitation. Anesth Analg 1974;53:230–232.

30. Lawes EG, Campbell I, Mercer D. Inflation pressure, gastric insufflation and rapid sequence induction. Br J Anaesth 1987;59:315–318.

31. Olsson GL, Hallen B, Hambraeus-Jonzon K. Aspiration during anaesthesia: a computer-aided study of 185,358 anaesthetics. Acta Anaesthesiol Scand 1986;30:84–92.

32. Majernick TG, Bieniek R, Houston JB, Hughes HG. Cervical spine movement during orotracheal intubation. Ann Emerg Med 1986;15:417–420.

33. Aprahamian C, Thompson BM, Finger WA, Darin JC. Experimental cervical spine injury model: evaluation of airway management and splinting techniques. Ann Emerg Med 1984;13:584–587.

34. Crosby ET, Liu A. The adult cervical spine: implications for airway management. Can J Anaesth 1990;37:77–93.

35. Arishita GI, Vayer JS, Bellamy RF. Cervical spine immobilization of penetrating neck wounds in a hostile environment. J Trauma 1989;29:332–337.

36. Doolan LA, O'Brien JF. Safe intubation in cervical spine injury. Anaesth Intensive Care 1985;13:319–324.

37. Podolsky S, Baraff LJ, Simon RR, Hoffman JR, Larmon B, Ablon W. Efficacy of cervical spine immobilization methods. J Trauma 1983;23:461–465.

38. Grande CM, Barton CR, Stene JK. Appropriate techniques for airway management of emergency patients with suspected spinal cord injury. Anesth Analg 1988;67:714–715.

39. Wang JF, Reves JG, Gutierrez FA. Awake fiberoptic laryngoscopic tracheal intubation for anterior cervical spinal fusion in patients with cervical cord trauma. Int Surg 1979;64:69–72.

40. Messeter KH, Pettersson KI. Endotracheal intubation with the fibre-optic bronchoscope. Anaesthesia 1980;35:294–298.

41. Layman PR. An alternative to blind nasal intubation. Anaesthesia 1983;38:165.

42. Dronen SC, Merigian KS, Hedges JR, Hoekstra

JW, Borron SW. A comparison of blind naso-tracheal and succinylcholine-assisted intubation in the poisoned patient. Ann Emerg Med 1987;16:650–652.

43. Smith RB, Schaer WB, Pfaeffle H. Percutaneous transtracheal ventilation for anaesthesia and resuscitation: a review and report of complications. Can Anesth Soc J 1975;22:607–612.

44. Jacoby JJ, Hamelberg W, Ziegler CH, Flory FA, Jones JR. Transtracheal resuscitation. JAMA 1956;162:625–628.

45. Seebacher J, Nozik D, Mathieu A. Inadvertent intracranial introduction of a nasgastric tube, a complication of severe maxillofacial trauma. Anesthesiology 1975;42:100–102.

46. Boyle S, Ockerman R, Barton CR, McVey JR. Venous air embolism during anesthesia for maxillary sinus irrigation: a case study. J Assoc Nurse Anesth 1986;54:126–129.

47. Dinner M, Tjeuw M, Artusio JF. Bacteremia as a complication of nasotracheal intubation. Anesth Analg 1987;66:460–462.

48. Bivins HB, Ford S, Bezmalinovac Z, Price HM, Williams JL. The effect of axial traction during orotracheal intubation of the trauma victim with an unstable cervical spine. Ann Emerg Med 1988;17:25–29.

49. Grande CM, Barton CR, Stene JK. Emergency airway management in trauma patients with a suspected cervical spine injury: in response. Anesth Analg 1989;68:416–418.

50. Lawes EG, Duncan PW, Bland B, Gemmel L, Downing JW. The cricoid yoke: a device for providing consistent and reproducible cricoid pressure. Br J Anaesth 1986;58:925–931.

51. Lawes EG. Cricoid pressure with or without the "cricoid yoke." Br J Anaesth 1986; 58:1376–1379.

52. Admani M, Yeh TF, Jain R, Mora A, Pildes RS. Prevention of gastric inflation during mask ventilation in newborn infants. Crit Care Med 1985;13:592–593.

53. Yelderman M, New W Jr. Evaluation of pulse oximetry. Anesthesiology 1983;59:349–352.

54. Grande CM, Stene JK, Bernhard WN. Airway management: considerations in the trauma patient. Crit Care Clin 1990;6:37–59.

55. Cordell WH, Nugent SK, Ehrenwerth J. Neuromuscular blocking agents as an aid to tracheal intubation. Emerg Med Rept 1984;5(19): 141–148.

56. Stoddart JC. Trauma and the Anaesthetist. London, Baillière-Tindall, 1984.

57. Circon Acmi: Brochure. Circon Acmi, 300 Stillwater Avenue, PO Box 1971, Stanford, CT 06904.

58. Borland LM, Casselbrant M. The Bullard laryngoscope: a new indirect oral laryngoscope (pediatric version). Anesth Analg 1990; 70:105–108.

59. Spadafora MP, Roberts JR. Technique for determining proper depth of oral tracheal tube placement in the critically ill adult patient. Ann Emerg Med 1987;15:657.

60. Birmingham PK, Cheney FW, Ward RJ. Esophageal intubation: a review of detection techniques. Anesth Analg 1986;65:886–891.

61. Linko K, Paloheimo M, Tammisto T. Capnography for detection of accidental oesophageal intubation. Acta Anaesthesiol Scand 1983;27: 199–202.

62. Sum-Ping ST, Mehta MP, Anderton JM. A comparative study of methods of detection of esophageal intubation. Anesth Analg 1989;69: 627–632.

63. Huang KC, Kraman SS, Wright BD. Video stethoscope—a simple method for assuring continuous bilateral lung ventilation during anesthesia. Anesth Analg 1983;62:586–589.

64. Heiselman D, Polacek DJ, Snyder JV, Grenvik A. Detection of esophageal intubation in patients with intrathoracic stomach. Crit Care Med 1985;13:1069–1070.

65. Howells TH, Riethmuller RJ. Signs of endotracheal intubation. Anaesthesia 1980;35: 984–986.

66. Gatrell CB. Unrecognized esophageal intubation with both esophageal obturator airway and endotracheal tube. Ann Emerg Med 1984;13: 624–626.

67. Owen RL. Endotracheal vs. esophageal intubation. Crit Care Med 1986;14:754.

68. Pollard BJ, Junius F. Accidental intubation of the oesophagus. Anaesth Intensive Care 1980;8: 183–186.

69. Batra AK, Cohn MA. Uneventful prolonged misdiagnosis of esophageal intubation. Crit Care Med 1983;11:763–764.

70. Owen RL, Cheney FW Jr. Use of an apnea monitor to verify endotracheal intubation. Respiratory Care 1985;30:974–976.

71. Goldberg JS, Rawle PR, Zehnder JL, Sladen RA. Colorimetric end-tidal carbon dioxide monitoring for tracheal intubation. Anesth Analg 1990; 70:191–194.

72. Taryle DA, Chandler JE, Good JT, Potts DE, Sahn SA. Emergency room intubations—complications and survival. Chest 1979;75:541–543.

73. Stewart RD. Airway management. In Trunkey DD, Lewis FR (eds): Current Therapy of Trauma—2. Toronto, BC Decker, 1986, pp 30–44.

74. Johnson KR Jr, Genovesi MG, Lassar KH. Esophageal obturator airway: use and complications. JACEP 1976;5:36–39.

75. Nieman JT, Rosborough JP, Myers R, Scarberry EN. The pharyngeo-tracheal lumen airway: preliminary investigation of a new adjunct. Ann Emerg Med 1984;13:591–596.

76. Bartlett RL, Martin SD, Perina D, Raymond JI. The pharyngeo-tracheal lumen airway: an as-

sessment of airway control in the setting of upper airway hemorrhage. Ann Emerg Med 1987;16: 343–346.

77. Howard JM. Gastric and salivary secretion following injury: the systemic response to injury. Ann Surg 1955;141:342–346.

78. Bynum LJ, Pierce AK. Pulmonary aspiration of gastric contents. Am Rev Respir Dis 1976;114: 1129–1136.

79. Giesecke AH, Hodgson RMH, Phulchand PR. Anesthesia for severely injured patients. Orthop Clin North Am 1970;1:21–48.

80. Clarke RSJ. The unprepared patient. In Nunn JF, Utting JE, Brown BR (eds): General Anaesthesia, ed 5. London, Butterworths, 1989, pp 682–685.

81. Davies JAH, Howell TH. The management of anesthesia for the full stomach case in the casualty department. Postgrad Med J 1973; 49(suppl 4):58–63.

82. Satiani B, Bonner JT, Stone HH. Factors influencing intraoperative gastric regurgitation. Arch Surg 1978;113:721–723.

83. Salem MR, Joseph NJ, Heyman HJ, Belani B, Paulissian R, Ferrara TP. Cricoid compression is effective in obliterating the esophageal lumen in the presence of a nasogastric tube. Anesthesiology 1985;63:443–446.

84. Brock-Utne JG, Rubin J, Welman S, Dimopoulos GE, Moshal MG, Downing JW. The effect of glycopyrrolate (Robinul) on the lower oesophageal sphincter. Can Anaesth Soc J 1978;25: 144–146.

85. Cucchiara RF. A simple technic to minimize tracheal aspiration. Anesth Analg 1976;55: 816–817.

86. Bernard GR, Luce JM, Sprung CL, Rinaldo JE, Tate RM, Sibbald WJ, Kariman K, Higgins S, Bradley R, Metz CA, Harris TR, Brigham KL. High-dose corticosteroids in patients with the adult respiratory distress syndrome. N Engl J Med 1987;317:1565–1570.

87. Cooper JB, Newbower RS, Long CD, McPeek B. Preventable anesthesia mishaps. Anesthesiology 1978;49:399–406.

88. O'Neill JE, Giffin JP, Cottrell JE. Pharyngeal and esophageal perforation following endotracheal intubation. Anesthesiology 1984;60:487–488.

89. Johnson KG, Hood DD. Esophageal perforation associated with endotracheal intubation. Anesthesiology 1986;64:281–283.

90. Mathisen DJ, Grillo H. Laryngotracheal trauma (abstract). Ann Thorac Surg 1987;43:254–262.

91. Seed RF. Traumatic injury to the larynx and trachea. Anaesthesia 1971;26:55–65.

92. Shoemaker WC, Appel PL, Kram HB. Tissue oxygen debt as a determinant of lethal and nonlethal postoperative organ failure. Crit Care Med 1988;16:1117–1120.

93. Dantzker DR, Wagner PD, West JB. Instability of lung units with low $\dot{V}A/\dot{Q}$. ratios during $O_2$ breathing. J Appl Physiol 1975;38:886–895.

94. MacIntyre NR. Respiratory function during pressure support ventilation. Chest 1986;89: 677–683.

95. Fragen RJ, Avram MJ. Comparative pharmacology of drugs used in the induction of anesthesia. In Stoelting RK, Barash PG, Gallagher TJ (eds): Advances in Anesthesia. Chicago, Year Book, 1986, vol 3, pp 103–132.

96. Dundee JW, Wyant GM. Intravenous Anaesthesia, ed 2. Edinburgh, Churchill Livingstone, 1988.

97. Ng WS. Pathophysiological effects of tracheal intubation. In Latto IP, Rosen M (eds): Difficulties in Tracheal Intubation. London, Ballière-Tindall, 1984, pp 12–35.

98. Wagner RL, White PF. Etomidate inhibits adrenocortical function in surgical patients. Anesthesiology 1984;61:647–651.

99. Sear JW, Allen MC, Bales M, McQuay HJ, Kay NH, McKenzie PJ, Moore RA. Suppression by etomidate of normal cortisol response to anaesthesia and surgery. Lancet 1983;2:1028.

100. Ledingham IM, Watt I. Influence of sedation on mortality in critically ill multiple trauma patients. Lancet 1983;1:1270.

101. White PF. Propofol: pharmacokinetics and pharmacodynamics. Semin Anesth 1988;7(1)(Suppl 1):4–20.

102. DeGarmo BH, Dronen SC. Pharmacology and clinical uses of neuromuscular blocking agents. Ann Emerg Med 1983;12:48–55.

103. Gronert GA, Theye RA. Pathophysiology of hyperkalemia induced by succinylcholine. Anesthesiology 1975;43:89–99.

104. Stene JK, Barton CR, Grande CM, et al. Time course of relaxation from high dose (0.28 mg/kg) vecuronium (abst). In Proceedings of the 9th World Congress of Anaesthesiologists, Washington, DC, May 1988, vol II, A0540.

105. Basta SJ, Savarese JJ, Ali HH, Moss J, Gionfriddo M. Histamine releasing potencies of atracurium besylate (BW 33A), metocurine, and d-tubocurine. Anesthesiology 1982;57:A261.

106. Morris RB, Cahalan MK, Miller RD, Wilkinson PL, Quasha AL, Robinson SL. The cardiovascular effects of vecuronium (ORGNC45) and pancuronium in patients undergoing coronary artery bypass grafting. Anesthesiology 1983;58: 438–440.

107. Grande CM, Wong L, Bernhard WN, et al. Mechanisms of injury in the burn patient: thermal, nonthermal and mixed multiple trauma. Crit Care Rep (in press).

108. Wong L, Grande CM, Munster AM. Burns and associated nonthermal trauma: an analysis of management, outcome, and relation to the injury severity score. J Burn Rehabil Care 1989;10: 512–516.

109. Garland JS, Rice TB, Kelly KJ. Airway burns in an infant following aspiration of microwave-heated tea. Chest 1986;90:621–622.

110. Schofferman J, Oill P, Lewis AJ. The esophageal obturator airway: a clinical evaluation. Chest 1976;69:67–71.

111. Auerbach PS, Geehr EC. Inadequate oxygenation and ventilation using the esophageal gastric tube airway in the prehospital setting. JAMA 1983;250:3067–3071.

112. Kassels SJ, Robinson WA, O'Bara KJ. Esophageal perforation associated with the esophageal obturator airway. Crit Care Med 1980;8: 386–389.

113. Kelly JP, Webb WR, Moulder PV, Everson C, Burch BH, Lindsey ES. Management of airway trauma. I. Tracheobroncheal injuries. Ann Thorac Surg 1985;40:551–555.

114. Butler RM, Moser FH. The padded dash syndrome: blunt trauma to the larynx and trachea. Laryngoscope 1968;78:1172–1182.

115. Roberge RJ, Squyres NS, Demetropoulos S, McAuliffe M, Vukich D. Transtracheal transection following blunt trauma. Ann Emerg Med 1988;17:95–100.

116. Snider MT, Campbell DB, Kofke WA, High KM, Russell GB, Keamy MF, Williams DR. Venovenous perfusion of adults and children with severe acute respiratory distress syndrome: the Pennsylvania State University experience from 1982–1987. Trans Am Soc Artif Intern Organs 1988;34:1014–1020.

117. Mortensen JD. An intravenacaval blood gas exchange (IVEBGE). Trans Am Soc Artif Intern Organs 1987;33:570–573.

118. Grande CM. Airway management of the trauma patient in the resuscitation area of a trauma center. Trauma Q 1988;5:30–49.

# Shock Resuscitation

*John K. Stene, Christopher M. Grande, and Adolph Giesecke*

## PATHOPHYSIOLOGY OF TRAUMATIC SHOCK

Shock is commonly associated with serious trauma. This association is so strong that many trauma centers have been named "shock trauma units." Although not all trauma patients are in shock, acute hemorrhagic shock is the lethal factor in many traumatic deaths. The "golden hour" concept that popularized trauma centers incorporates the idea that effective traumatic shock resuscitation must be done without delay to promote a high trauma survival rate (Fig. 4.1).

The trimodal distribution of trauma deaths validates the concern with traumatic shock (1) (see Fig. 1.2). The first peak of trauma deaths occurs within a few minutes of the injury and is secondary to laceration of the heart or central nervous system. This group of patients who die "instantly" will receive little or no benefit from state-of-the-art trauma care. The second peak of deaths, occurring approximately 1 and a

half hours after injury, is caused by uncorrected hemorrhagic shock secondary to visceral injuries or extensive fractures. Prompt institution of shock resuscitation and Advanced Trauma Life Support (ATLS) principles should prevent many unnecessary deaths in this group of patients (2). Anesthesiologists caring for these patients must be familiar with principles of shock resuscitation to improve patient care in both the emergency department and the operating room. The third peak of trauma deaths occurs approximately 7 to 10 days after injury; these deaths are caused by severe head injury, sepsis, or multiorgan failure. Slow and inadequate shock resuscitation during the initial phase of trauma care in the emergency department and the operating room will set the stage for sepsis and multiorgan failure.

An understanding of the pathophysiology of shock is required to provide appropriate titrated treatment to the injured patient in shock. Failure to appreciate these pathophysiologic principles leads to empirical care, such as the inappropriate use of

# THE GOLDEN HOUR

## Probability of Survival

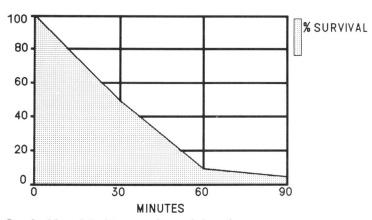

Survival is related to severity and duration.

**Figure 4.1.    The Golden Hour: the principles developed by R Adams Cowley, MD.** As more time elapses between the point at which an injured patient develops serious posttraumatic shock and the start of resuscitation, the percentage of surviving patients decreases. The survival rate after 1 hour of severe untreated shock is very low. The "golden hour" is the time in which resuscitation of severely injured patients must begin to achieve maximal survival.

vasopressors. The lethal factor in shock is irreversible anoxic cellular injury that kills a critical mass of cells (3, 4). Inadequate cellular oxygen delivery via the microcirculation leads to this irreversible cellular damage. Thus, successful resuscitation requires the restoration of cellular oxygen delivery via the microcirculation by increasing the flow of oxygenated blood through the capillaries (5).

Hemorrhagic (hypovolemic) shock is the most common form of shock to affect trauma patients. Inadequate blood flow and tissue oxygenation—the final common pathway of shock—have many etiologies including sepsis, spinal cord injury, and cardiac failure (Table 4.1). Septic shock usually occurs as a late complication of trauma-induced infection and prolonged hemorrhagic shock resuscitation; therefore, it rarely will be seen in the acute, recently injured trauma patient. Spinal shock secondary to spinal cord injury occurs frequently with cervical spine fractures that damage the spinal cord. This form of shock is frequently associated with cutaneous

vasodilation and prominent peripheral pulses despite a low blood pressure. Exogenous sympathomimetic catecholamines are needed to replace inadequate endogenous sympathetic nervous system activity. Cardiogenic shock caused by inadequate cardiac output occurs in the trauma patient secondary to pericardial tamponade, direct cardiac injury, or occasionally myocardial infarction. Most of the discussion in this chapter is concerned with the pathophysiology and treatment of hemorrhagic shock. The terms traumatic, hemorrhagic, and hypovolemic shock are used interchangeably here.

## Cardiovascular Response to Hemorrhage

Acute hemorrhagic loss of circulating blood volume decreases the vascular filling pressure (termed *mean systemic pressure* [MSP] [6]), which is determined by the ratio of intravascular blood volume to the vascular compliance. Venous return to the heart (VR) is determined by the difference between MSP and right atrial pressure (PRA) and determined inversely by the resistance

**Table 4.1.   Differential Diagnosis of Shock in the Trauma Patient**

| | |
|---|---|
| Hemorrhagic shock | Cardiogenic shock |
|   Caused by |   Caused by |
|     External blood loss |     Myocardial infarction |
|     Occult blood loss |     Myocardial contusion |
|     Inadequate resuscitation |     Coronary artery injury |
|     Massive tissue edema |     Valvular disruption |
|     Aortic/great vessel injury |   Diagnosed by signs of inadequate cardiac output |
|   Diagnosed by signs of hypovolemia |     Tachycardia or bradycardia |
|     Tachycardia |     Characteristic ECG[a] changes |
|     Hypotension |     Hypotension |
|     Cool, diaphoretic skin |     Cool, diaphoretic skin |
|     Decreased level of consciousness |     Increased venous pressure |
|     Low urine output |     Acute murmur heard with valvular injuries |
| Cardiac tamponade | Anaphylactic shock |
|   Caused by |   Caused by antigen-antibody reaction |
|     Hemopericardium |   Diagnosed by signs of vasodilation |
|     Pneumopericardium |     Tachycardia |
|   Diagnosed by signs of low cardiac output |     Hypotension |
|     Tachycardia |     Warm, erythematous skin |
|     Hypotension |     Bounding peripheral pulses |
|     Cool, diaphoretic skin |     Wheezing heard over the chest |
|     Decreased level of consciousness | Spinal shock |
|     Increased venous pressure |   Caused by transection of the spinal cord and anatomic sympathectomy |
|     Decreased heart sounds |   Diagnosed by signs of decreased sympathetic nervous system function |
| Increased intrathoracic pressure |     Bradycardia |
|   Caused by |     Hypotension |
|     Tension pneumothorax |     Warm skin |
|     Massive hemothorax |     Bounding peripheral pulses |
|     Massive hydrothorax |     Normal breath sounds and heart sounds |
|     Massive chylothorax |     Associated neurologic deficit |
|   Diagnosed by signs of inadequate cardiac output |     Normal level of consciousness |
|     Tachycardia | Vasovagal syndrome |
|     Hypotension |   Caused by reflex increase in vagal tone |
|     Cool, diaphoretic skin |   Diagnosed by signs of increased vagal tone |
|     Decreased breath sounds |     Bradycardia |
|     Increased venous pressure |     Hypotension |
| |     Cool skin |
| |     Weak peripheral pulses |

[a] ECG, electrocardiogram.

to venous return (6):

$$VR = MSP - PRA/\text{resistance to VR}$$

Therefore, hemorrhage will acutely decrease VR flow, which fills the right atrium. Cardiac preload or ventricular filling is decreased by the reduction in VR. Because the circulatory system is a closed loop, cardiac output (CO) from the left ventricle must equal VR into the right heart during the steady state. The pulmonary and cardiac (end-systolic) blood volume acts as a fluid capacitor to adjust for differences between VR and CO that occasionally occur within a

few heart beats. For example, if CO is greater than VR, pulmonary and residual cardiac blood volume will be decreased as blood is translocated to the systemic veins, raising MSP and VR. In this case, a new steady state is reached with an increased blood volume in the systemic veins (raising MSP and VR) and a decreased cardiopulmonary blood volume (reducing CO) (7). Central blood volume adjusts rapidly as VR and CO achieve equilibrium. However, massive hemorrhage may lead to such a large blood volume loss that translocation of central cardiopulmonary volume to the

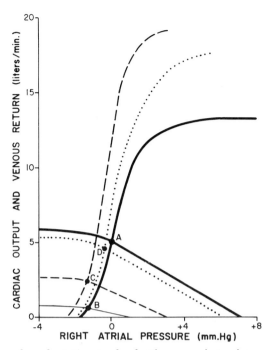

**Figure 4.2.   Cardiovascular adaptation to shock.** The normal circulatory system will regulate CO and PRA at *point A*. The cardiac function curve (Starling curve) ascends upward to the *right* because an increase in PRA will cause the heart to increase CO. The venous return curve decreases to the *right*. (Both normal curves are indicated as *heavy black lines*.) When PRA increases, venous return from the systemic circulation decreases linearly until it is reduced to zero at a PRA equal to MSP. At a very low PRA ($\leq-2$ mm Hg), venous return is constant because the great veins collapse, providing a constant back-pressure to venous return.

After major hemorrhage, MSP decreases from 7 to 1 mm Hg, which causes the circulation to regulate to *point B* with a CO of 1 liter/min and a PRA of $-2$ mm Hg. Reflex stimulation of the heart moves the cardiac function curve to the *left*, representing an increased inotropic state. Reflex stimulation of the circulatory system increases MSP and decreases resistance to venous return, which increases the slope of the venous return curve. The venous return curve now intersects the cardiac function curve at *point C* with a CO of 2.5 liters/min and a PRA of $-2$ mm Hg. Transcapillary refill and fluid therapy restore venous return to follow the *dotted curve* and reduce the stimulation of the heart to the *dotted cardiac function curve*. The circulation regulates at *point D* with a CO of 4.5 liters/min and a PRA of 1 mm Hg. (From Guyton AC, Jones CE, Coleman TG. Circulatory Physiology: Cardiac Output and Its Regulation. Philadelphia, WB Saunders, 1973, p 374.)

systemic veins cannot compensate for the loss. Thus, CO is reduced by hemorrhagic blood loss, which stimulates reflex cardiovascular compensation for hemorrhage.

Tachycardia and improved contractility, leading to an increased ejection fraction, are compensatory reflex changes that occur as the heart is stimulated both chronotropically and inotropically by the sympathetic nervous system (Fig. 4.2). This cardiac stimulation maximizes VR and CO by two additional mechanisms: (*a*) PRA is reduced to subatmospheric levels, maximizing the available VR (6, 8), and (*b*) a greater proportion of end-systolic blood volume is translocated from the heart and lungs to the peripheral blood vessels, which increases MSP and VR (7) (Fig. 4.2). Reflex constriction of peripheral vessels, a fourth compensatory mechanism, increases arterial pressure (BP) and MSP and decreases resistance to VR (9). Thus, the sympathetic nervous system compensates for hemorrhage by restoring CO and BP toward normal.

At the microcirculatory level, however, these compensatory changes mediated through the sympathetic nervous system may not be as felicitous as in the larger blood vessels. Arterial vasoconstriction maintains central aortic BP at the expense of reduced flow through several different capillary beds including the kidney, liver, and skeletal muscle. Reduced capillary blood flow allows white blood cell aggregation, platelet clumping, and obstruction of red blood cell flow. Local ischemia in obstructed capillary beds causes endothelial cell swelling, which further impedes capillary blood flow (5). Capillary obstruction is probably involved in the "no-reflow" phenomenon that is especially prominent in the brain (10). Reintroduction of oxygenated blood flow into ischemic capillary beds enhances the generation of free radicals of oxygen, which further damages endothelial cells and obstructs capillaries (3).

Arteriolar vasoconstriction relaxes during prolonged shock, but venular vasoconstriction is maintained much longer. This predominance of venular vasoconstriction causes intracapillary pressure to rise late in the shock state. Edema formation becomes prominent at this point as a result of this imbalanced vasoconstriction (11).

Plasma-volume refill, or posthemorrhagic hemodilution, is the fifth compensatory mechanism for replacement of hemorrhagic losses (12). After *moderate* hemorrhage, extravascular interstitial fluid replenishes the plasma volume through the capillaries or postcapillary venules in a volume almost exactly equal to the volume of shed blood. The rate of plasma volume refill is initially 90 to 120 ml/hr and then decreases with an upwardly convex slope until refill is complete after 30 to 40 hours (12). Intravenous balanced salt infusion will rapidly complete the plasma volume refill and replace deficits in the interstitial fluid compartment. Moore found that about twice as much balanced salt solution remained in the intravascular space after administration to subjects with mild hemorrhage than after administration to normal resting volunteers (12). The physiologic mechanisms to restore plasma volume are so well developed that enterally administered tap water can be used to replace experimental hemorrhage in human volunteers. These volunteers replaced their lost blood volume and maintained their blood volume regardless of the source of water replacement. When hypotonic fluids were used, blood volume was restored, but serum sodium concentration and osmolarity, as well as hematocrit, were diminished (12).

The combination of the compensatory mechanisms just described, reflex stimulation of the heart and blood vessels, and plasma-volume refill offsets the effects of hemorrhage (*compensated shock*) until a critical level of hypovolemia occurs. *Progressive shock* will develop after a critical degree of hemorrhage. The transition from compensated to progressive shock is associated with a decreasing CO and BP. Unless therapy is introduced rapidly to stop further blood loss and replace lost blood volume, the patient will develop *irreversible shock* as progressive shock continues to cause inadequate tissue perfusion. Irreversible shock is characterized by a progressive reduction in CO and BP until the patient dies despite therapy to replace blood loss. Once the patient develops progressive shock, improvements in CO and BP may occur with heroic resuscitation efforts, but the patient is still at elevated risk of ultimately succumbing to multiorgan failure (13, 14).

Although experimental animals differ greatly in the volume of hemorrhagic loss required to initiate progressive and irreversible shock, there is a marked uniformity, at least within species, in the magnitude of cumulative oxygen debt that is lethal (15). In dogs, the oxygen debt that was lethal for 50% of the animals (LD$_{50}$) was 120 ml of O$_2$ per kg body weight (Fig. 4.3). That this cumulative oxygen debt required both a reduced CO and a certain time to reach the lethal level is consistent with the clinical finding that, the more rapidly shock resuscitation is commenced, the greater the probability of a successful outcome. This concept is codified in the "golden hour" concept (Fig. 4.1).

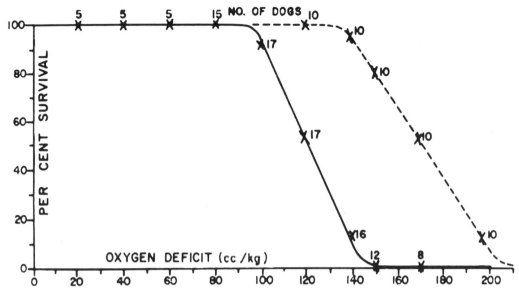

**Figure 4.3.    Dependence of irreversible shock on oxygen deficit.** Cumulative oxygen debt is measured by continuous oxygen consumption ($\dot{V}O_2$) during experimental shock in dogs. $\dot{V}O_2$ decreases during shock, so cumulative oxygen debt is measured by the area between the extrapolated baseline $\dot{V}O_2$ and the actual $\dot{V}O_2$ during shock. Reinfusion of shed blood was associated with restoration of $\dot{V}O_2$, repayment of oxygen debt, and survival until the cumulative oxygen debt reached 120 ml/kg, the $LD_{50}$ for oxygen debt. Treatment of the animals with a digitalis glycoside (*dashed line*) increased the tolerance for oxygen debt to an $LD_{50}$ of 170 ml/kg. (From Crowell JW, Smith EE: Oxygen deficit and irreversible hemorrhagic shock. Am J Physiol 1964;206:313–316.)

Progressive and irreversible heart failure is responsible for irreversible shock in both animals and humans (15–18). Dogs that received digitalis survived a more severe oxygen debt than control animals because their hearts tolerated a more severe oxygen debt (15). Despite the accumulation of a lethal oxygen debt, the effects of irreversible shock on the peripheral blood vessels can be easily reversed by blood transfusion. Thus, the MSP and venous return can be increased by blood transfusion until the heart stops pumping after the development of irreversible shock (16, 17). The goal of shock resuscitation is to restore oxygen consumption to levels needed to repay the shock-induced oxygen debt before the heart suffers an irreversible injury (Fig. 4.4).

Although terminal heart failure causes the lethal outcome in irreversible shock, clinical experience with trauma patients suggests that multiorgan failure also follows high oxygen debts and progressive shock

(13, 14, 19, 20). The overall effect of multiple ischemic organ failure is frequently delayed and manifests as "late death" in the intensive care unit.

The cardiovascular system's response to increasing hemorrhage produces characteristic clinical signs that can be used to classify the approximate quantity of blood loss (2). Table 4.2 outlines the classification of hemorrhage described below.

*Class I hemorrhage* is defined as the loss of as much as 15% of blood volume. It is associated with minimal physiologic changes.

*Class II hemorrhage* is defined as a 15 to 30% loss of blood volume. Class II hemorrhages are associated with modest elevations in heart rate and decreases in pulse pressure as diastolic pressures rise with smaller stroke volumes. Systolic pressures tend to be maintained, but digital, capillary refill is slightly retarded. Urinary output is only mildly depressed. Postural hypoten-

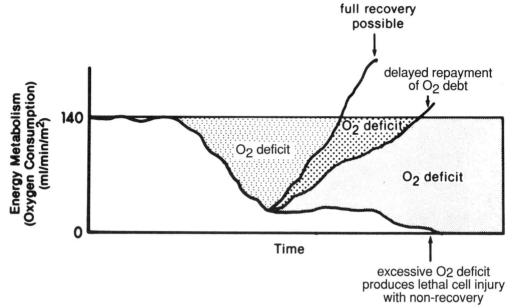

**Figure 4.4.** **Oxygen consumption (V̇O₂) in shock,** which decreases below the baseline level—140 ml/min/mm² in this illustration. This decreased V̇O₂ creates an oxygen debt measured as the area between the normal V̇O₂ level and the shock-induced V̇O₂ level. (From Siegel JH, Linberg SE, Wiles CE III: Therapy of low-flow shock states. In Siegel JH (ed): Trauma: Emergency Surgery and Critical Care. New York, Churchill Livingstone, 1987, pp 201–284.)

sion may be associated with class II hemorrhage, as may subtle central nervous system changes such as fright and hostility.

*Class III hemorrhage* is defined as loss of 30 to 40% of blood volume. Patients with class III hemorrhage present with tachycardia, systolic and diastolic hypotension, delayed capillary refill (>2 seconds), reduced urinary output, and an apprehensive, slightly clouded sensorium.

*Class IV hemorrhage* is defined as a loss of 40% or more of blood volume and causes frank shock with cool, diaphoretic, ashen skin, tachycardia, hypotension or unobtainable blood pressure, anuria, and a reduced level of consciousness.

Patients with class III and IV hemorrhages require immediate intravenous fluid administration to survive. Patients with class IV hemorrhage will require blood transfusion for recovery, but class III hemorrhage patients may tolerate postresuscitation anemia if further hemorrhage is controlled immediately after fluid resuscitation is started. Recent clinical experience with a wide variety of surgical patients suggests

that hematocrits as low as 20 to 25% may be well tolerated if total blood volume is adequate.

Other causes of fluid loss such as massive tissue edema as an aftereffect of blunt trauma will cause more profound shock with lesser amounts of hemorrhagic blood loss. The inflammatory response to shed blood in body cavities or soft tissues will promote an extensive "third space" loss of extracellular fluid (21). The use of clinical signs to estimate traumatic blood loss is very important because soft tissues and body cavities frequently can hold large quantities of blood with minimal external body changes (see Chapter 6) (21).

## Respiratory Effects of Hemorrhagic Shock

Hypovolemic shock reduces blood flow to skeletal muscles, including the respiratory muscles. Experimental animals in shock have an increased mortality when allowed to breathe spontaneously (22). Minute ventilatory requirements are increased during shock as reduced pulmonary blood flow

**Table 4.2.    Classification of Hemorrhage**

Class I hemorrhage
  Up to 15% of blood volume lost
  Vital signs unchanged, may exhibit transient postural hypotension
  Rx—rapidly infuse 1–2 liters of balanced salt solution; then infuse maintenance fluids
Class II hemorrhage
  15–30% of blood volume lost
  Vital signs—mild tachycardia, normal systolic BP, elevated diastolic BP, decreased pulse pressure, postural
    hypotension, mild tachypnea
  Rx—rapidly infuse 2 liters of balanced salt solution; reevaluate continued replacement as needed
Class III hemorrhage
  30–40% of blood volume lost
  Vital signs (minimal hemorrhage that will consistently decrease systolic BP)—tachycardia (>120 beats/
    min), decreased systolic BP and pulse pressure, tachypnea, delayed capillary refill, decreased urine
    output
  Rx—rapidly infuse 2 liters of balanced salt solution; reevaluate; replace blood losses with three volumes
    of balanced salt solution or blood (packed cells and colloid or whole blood); maintain urine output at
    >0.5 ml/kg/hr; restore oxygen consumption to >100 ml/min/m$^2$
Class IV hemorrhage
  ≥40% blood volume
  Vital signs—"shady," cool, ashen skin; decreased level of consciousness; tachycardia; profound hypo-
    tension; delayed capillary refill; anuria
  Rx—rapidly infuse 2 liters of balanced salt solution; reevaluate; replace blood losses with three volumes
    of balanced salt solution or blood (packed cells and colloid or whole blood); maintain urine output at
    >0.5 ml/kg/hr; restore oxygen consumption to >100 ml/min/m$^2$

increases the fraction of dead space ventilation ($V_D/V_T$). Therefore, the muscular work of breathing must increase to maintain adequate alveolar ventilation. However, shock reduces the blood flow to the respiratory musculature, which causes these muscles to fail in supporting needed ventilation.

Initially, arterial blood gas levels characteristically demonstrate hypoxia, hypocarbia, and metabolic acidosis (23, 24). The acidosis may be reflected only by a negative base excess as respiratory alkalosis keeps the pH near normal. However, extreme hypovolemia will decrease CO to levels at which $CO_2$ excretion is impaired; thus, profound metabolic and respiratory acidosis can occur in patients with a class IV hemorrhage.

### Renal Effects of Hemorrhagic Shock

Hemorrhagic shock is one of the few causes of acute anuria, which occurs when renal blood flow is reduced to preserve central perfusion (25, 26). The kidney is able to compensate for a significant reduction in arterial BP and CO by vasodilation of the glomerular afferent arterioles mediated by prostacycline, which is released in response to reduced blood pressure. While prostacycline dilates the afferent arterioles to reduce the total renal blood flow resistance, angiotension II, which is already circulating in increased amounts in response to renin release from the macula densa, constricts the glomerular efferent arterioles. This combination of afferent arteriolar dilation and efferent arteriolar constriction maintains both the glomerular filtration pressure and the rate of filtration. The limits of renal blood flow autoregulation are reached and eventually surpassed as shock becomes progressive. Catecholamine and vasopressin secretion are markedly elevated during shock and tend to reduce renal blood flow and glomerular filtration rate. Maximal conservation of water and salt occurs with the reduced level of glomerular filtration, which further decreases urinary output. As the glomerular filtrate entering the renal tubules is reduced, toxic pigments such as free hemoglobin can then crystallize, leading to tubular cell damage and acute tubular necrosis. Prolonged renal ischemia during shock will eventually cause a lethal hypoxic injury to renal cells. This ischemia-induced necrosis of renal cells then causes a prolonged oliguric renal failure in survivors of progressive hemorrhagic shock.

## Cellular Response to Hemorrhagic Shock

The cellular response to hemorrhagic shock is a result of ischemia-induced, anoxic/hypoxic cellular injury. This injury can be sublethal and reversible or can be lethal, leading to cell necrosis, depending upon the magnitude of the insult (3) (Fig. 4.5). Cellular hypoxia associated with shock-induced hypoperfusion causes mitochondria to reduce adenosine triphosphate (ATP) production, which reduces the activity of the Na/K-ATPase. Decreased activity of the Na/K-ATPase causes intracellular [Na$^+$] to rise and intracellular [K$^+$] to fall, which changes cell membrane potential ($-90$ to $-60$ mV) during hemorrhagic shock (3, 27). These electrolyte shifts accompany a transfer of water from the extravascular, extracellular space to the intracellular space (28, 29).

Microscopically, cells collected from patients dying from traumatic shock exhibit characteristic changes in response to the hypoxic injury (4) (Fig. 4.5). Early changes in cell morphology include loss of granules in mitochondria, dilation of the endoplasmic reticulum, and slight clumping of nuclear chromatin. With prolonged ischemia, the cells swell as a result of water accumulation as Na/K-ATPase is inhibited by the reduced availability of ATP. Intracellular [Ca$^{++}$] increases at this point, aggravates the cellu-

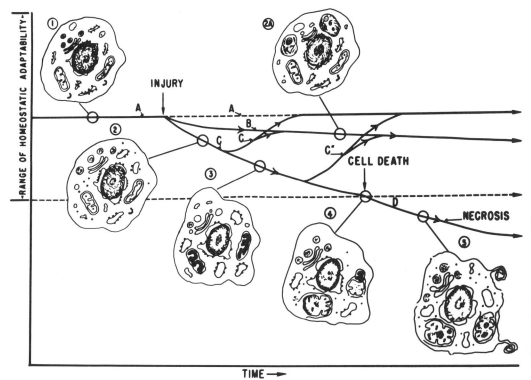

**Figure 4.5. Cellular response to shock:** the change in transmission electron microscopy ultrastructure of human cells subjected to anoxia from shock. As the degree of anoxic injury increases, the cells exhibit characteristic changes. These changes include alterations in mitochondria (first contraction, then dilation), dilation of endoplasmic reticulum, cytoplasmic swelling, and lysosomal rupture. If oxygen is restored at any point before cell death, the cell either will completely recover or will be restored to a level of function less than normal if it suffered a chronic sublethal injury. (From Trump BF, Vilzgorsky JM, Dees JH, et al: Cellular changes in human disease: a new method of pathological analysis. Hum Pathol 1973;4:89–109.)

lar swelling, and changes membrane fluidity. Mitochondria first condense and then markedly swell, with dilation of the cristae and occasional membrane disruption. As the cell passes from the reversible to the irreversible necrotic phase, flocculent densities appear in the mitochondria, lysosomes become leaky and rupture to begin the process of autolysis, and marked cell swelling is noted as the cell membrane loses its integrity.

These changes in cellular morphology vary under different conditions. For example, the cellular responses to anoxic injury during shock-induced ischemia occur at different rates in different organs (e.g., the kidney develops irreversible changes faster than does the bronchial epithelium) (3, 30). Hypothermia increases cellular tolerance for hypoxia and prolongs the time to irreversible injury. Acidosis—an increase in both intracellular and extracellular [H$^+$]—retards the transition into the necrotic, irreversible phase of cell injury response. If blood flow and oxygenation are restored during the sublethal, reversible phase of injury, cells and organs will probably heal.

The final pathway leading to death from shock is the cumulative effect of enough cells reaching the irreversible necrotic phase of anoxic injury so that the trauma patient dies (Fig. 4.6).

### Metabolic Response To Trauma

Serious injury triggers a characteristic neuroendocrine response (Fig. 4.7) that tends to compensate acutely for the effects of hemorrhagic hypotension (31). Over the longer term, the effects of the neuroendocrine response to trauma lead to metabolic effects (e.g., hyperglycemia) that complicate pharmacologic treatment of shock during the postoperative critical care of the trauma patient. The acute response becomes amplified as patients develop sepsis followed by multiorgan failure (13, 14). Laboratory studies performed on blood samples obtained during shock resuscitation and operation will reflect many metabolic changes.

As described above, an acute reduction in circulatory blood volume stimulates the sympathetic nervous system to constrict both arteries and veins and thus maintain systolic arterial pressure. The heart is stimulated by the sympathetic nervous system to maintain CO by reducing PRA (Fig. 4.2). This usually results in a rapid heart rate with smaller stroke volumes. The level of circulating plasma epinephrine is also increased as the adrenal medulla increases its secretion of epinephrine. The circulating epinephrine reduces perfusion to the splanchnic, renal, and cutaneous circulation, which tends to increase venous return (9).

Adrenocorticotropic hormone released from the pituitary stimulates the release of cortisol from the adrenal cortex (31). Growth hormone is likewise secreted in increased amounts from the pituitary. Glucagon secretion from the pancreas increases while insulin secretion decreases. In response to the catecholamines, glucocorticoids, growth hormone, and glucagon, hepatic glucose output is increased by both glycogenolysis and gluconeogenesis. Therefore, the blood sugar is elevated in the so-called "diabetes of trauma" (Fig. 4.8) (32). Pancreatic insulin secretion, which is initially depressed, slowly rebounds (32). However, it takes hours to days for insulin secretion to surpass glucagon secretion (Fig. 4.7) and reduce blood sugar. Much of the neuroendocrine response to trauma can be blocked with epidural anesthesia, indicating that the response is associated with nerve impulses from the peripheral site of injury and is not just an effect of hypovolemic shock (33).

Other metabolic effects of traumatic injury include β-adrenergic-stimulated hypokalemia and lipolysis with the release of free fatty acids (34–37). Synthesis of acute phase proteins such as fibrinogen, haptoglobin, complement components, and C-reactive protein is stimulated by the stress response to trauma (38). Rapid correction of traumatic shock, in conjunction with necessary surgical repair to injuries with subsequent hemostasis, will allow the metabolic

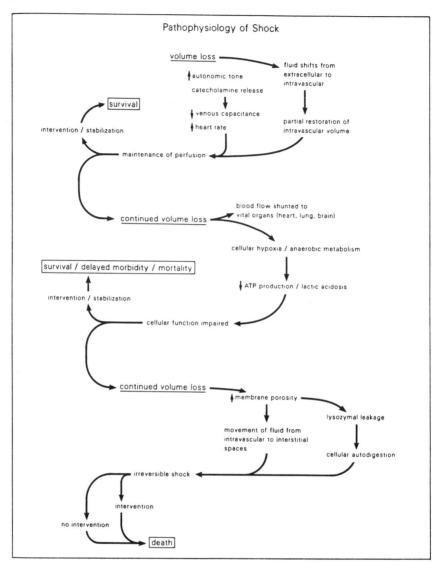

**Figure 4.6.  Flow diagram of pathophysiologic changes with traumatic shock.** (From Guss DA: Hemorrhagic shock. In Baxt WG (ed): Trauma—the First Hour. East Norwalk, CT, Appleton-Century-Crofts, 1985, p 5.)

responses to traumatic stress to initiate the healing process and gradually change into a recuperative metabolic profile (39).

## CLINICAL APPROACH TO THE PATIENT IN TRAUMATIC SHOCK

The initial approach to treating the patient with traumatic shock is to assess the degree of blood volume loss. During the primary survey (ATLS) (2), a quick exami-

nation of the patient for vital signs, capillary refill, and urinary output can be used to estimate the degree of blood loss by classifying hemorrhage as described above (i.e., class I versus class II) (2, 40). As soon as volume loss has been estimated, the anesthesiologist must develop a plan for the replacement of hemorrhagic losses. The ATLS course teaches that the diagnosis of acute hemorrhagic loss and the replacement of these losses should be almost simultaneous.

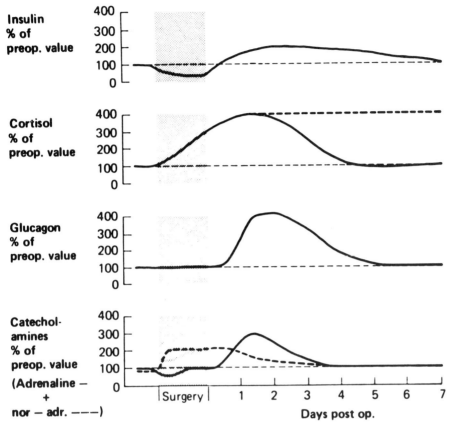

**Figure 4.7. Neuroendocrine effects of shock. A,** Changes in insulin, cortisol, glucagon, and catecholamines after surgically induced trauma and hemorrhage. **B,** Changes in adrenocorticotropic hormone (*ACTH*), growth hormone, vasopressin, thyroid-stimulating hormone (*TSH*), and catecholamines after surgical trauma and hemorrhage. (From Elliot MJ, Alberti KGMM: Carbohydrate metabolism—effects of preoperative starvation and trauma. Clin Anesthesiol 1983;1:527–550.)

## Intravascular Line Placement for Volume Resuscitation

Members of the "trauma team," which includes anesthesiologists, must insert intravenous catheters for the replacement of hemorrhagic blood loss. Blood should be drawn from the first intravenous catheter inserted for the required laboratory studies such as hemoglobin and hematocrit, platelet count, coagulation profile, type and cross-match for transfusion, electrolytes, creatinine, blood urea nitrogen, glucose, and toxicology screen. Peripheral veins should be the first choice because cannulation of peripheral veins can be performed faster than central venous cannulation or surgical cutdown. However, if peripheral venous cannulation fails, percutaneous subclavian vein catheterization is faster than surgical cutdown and has a similar complication rate (41). Figure 4.9 illustrates the physical layout of a trauma resuscitation room that allows simultaneous diagnosis and treatment of shock.

Many devices for vein catheterization are available. These vary from the standard "catheter-over-needle" to pediatric feeding tubes or urologic irrigation tubes placed through surgical cutdowns. Introducer sheaths (7F–8.5F) designed to facilitate pulmonary artery catheterization may be placed percutaneously into a large central vein. The subclavian, internal jugular, or

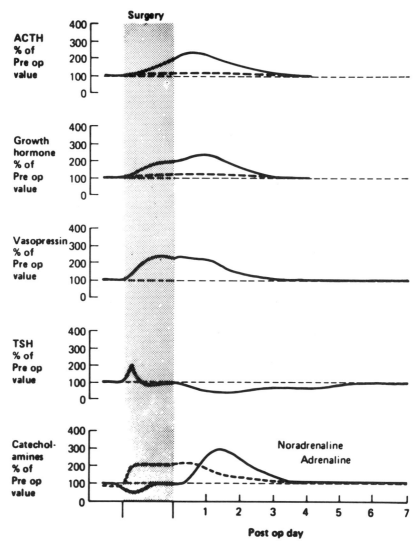

**Figure 4.7.   B.**

femoral vein will provide large-bore vascular access similar to a surgical cutdown.

If a vein cannot be cannulated percutaneously, open surgical cannulation should be performed without hesitation. The best site for surgical cutdown is controversial: some experts advocate the saphenous vein at the ankle or saphenous opening on the thigh, whereas others advocate the antecubital venous system—the basilic or cephalic vein. The objections to using the lower extremity veins include the probability that the veins are smaller and may be occluded from chronic venous stasis and that military/medical antishock trousers (MAST)

may interfere with venous drainage. Objections to using the subclavian or internal jugular vein are the possibility of complications such as pneumothorax and interference with the surgical field around the patient's head and neck. However, it is advantageous to have at least one intravenous site below the diaphragm and one above the diaphragm, especially if the patient's trunk has been injured. If venous return through either the inferior or the superior vena cava has been disrupted, fluid infused through that venous system will be ineffective in filling the heart. Therefore, a catheter placed to infuse fluids through the

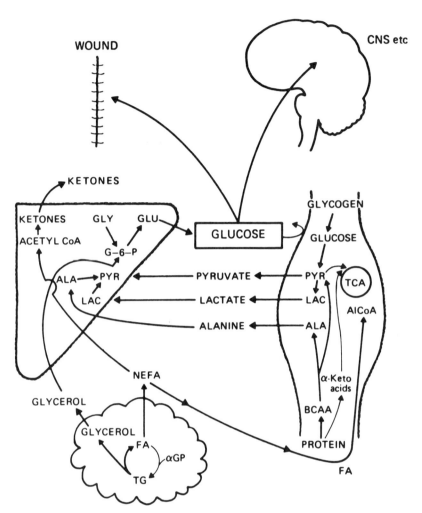

**Figure 4.8.** *"Diabetes of trauma."* Metabolic pathways during injury and shock reflect increased production of glucose and decreased utilization of glucose in the skeletal muscles. *Outlines* represent the liver, skeletal muscle, and the adipose tissue, as well as brain. (From Elliot MJ, Alberti KGMM: Carbohydrate metabolism—effects of preoperative starvation and trauma. Clin Anesthesiol 1983;1:527–550.)

other vena cava will be useful to maintain venous return.

Large-bore intravenous catheters permit much higher flow rates than small-bore catheters (Fig. 4.10). The rate of intravenous fluid administration can also be increased by using large-bore intravenous tubing with an internal diameter that is at least as large as the intravenous catheter. Several infusion sets marketed as "trauma sets" have large internal diameters (even at typical areas of constriction such as injection ports and connectors). Fluid flow increases by the fourth power of the cross-sectional radius for laminar flow or the second power for turbulent flow. Moreover, turbulent flow is less likely in large-bore tubing than small-bore tubing. Therefore, intravenous infusion sets and intravenous catheters with large internal diameters will facilitate rapid fluid replacement for the trauma patient (Fig. 4.11). The anesthesiologist must be sure that the patient receives at least two large-bore intravenous catheters and that the intravenous infusion sets have minimal resistance to fluid flow.

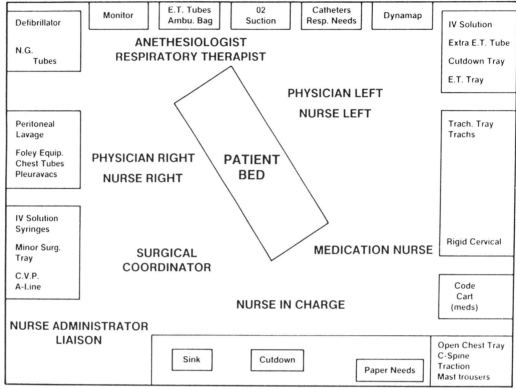

**Figure 4.9.    Floor plan for a trauma admitting area** (resuscitation bay). (From Eichelberger MR, Zwick HA, Pratsch GL, McGinley TP, Mangubat EA: Pediatric trauma protocol: a team approach. In Eichelberger MR, Pratsch Gl (eds): Pediatric Trauma Care. Rockville, MD, Aspen Systems, 1988, pp 11–13.)

### Adjuncts to Venous Catheterization

Profound shock after trauma and extensive hemorrhage causes collapse of the peripheral veins. It is very tedious to cannulate collapsed veins of a patient in profound shock, either through a cutdown or percutaneously. Therefore, alternative techniques of initiating fluid therapy are occasionally required. Emergency fluid resuscitation can be initiated through the bone marrow of the tibia in children or the marrow of the anterior superior iliac spine or the sternum in adults. The vascular spaces in the bone marrow connect with the venous drainage from the bone, providing a direct route for intravenous fluid to enter the circulation. Impressive flow rates have been reported for intraosseous infusions, but the reported infusion rates vary widely (42). Bone marrow fluid infusion is an emergency temporizing procedure; an intravenous catheter should be placed as soon as possible either via cutdown or percutaneously to replace the bone marrow needle (42). The goal is to replace enough hemorrhagic loss to dilate veins enough to be directly cannulated or at least to "buy some time" while searching for a vein to cannulate. The complications from intraosseous fluid administration include osteomyelitis, pneumothorax from sternal puncture, arterial thrombosis, and subcutaneous abscess.

### Military Antishock Trousers (MAST)

Another temporizing maneuver to improve cardiac and venous filling to enhance the ability to cannulate a vein is the pneumatic antishock garment, formerly known as military antishock trousers (MAST) (43) (Table 4.3). MAST evolved from the compression G-suit used by pilots to prevent gravity-induced redistribution of

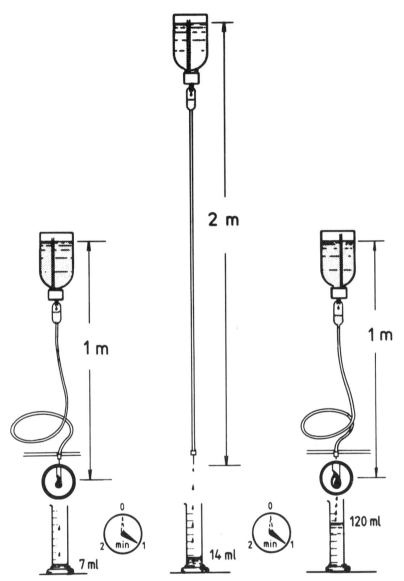

**Figure 4.10.    Effects of gravity and catheter size on intravenous flow rate.** *Left*, an intravenous bottle is draining through a catheter with a 0.36-mm internal diameter with a pressure head of 1 meter. *Middle*, increasing the pressure to 2 meters doubles the fluid flow rate. *Right*, increasing the internal diameter of the catheter to 0.93 mm increases the flow rate 17 times at a pressure of 1 meter. (From Mushin WW, Jones PL: Macintosh, Mushin, and Epstein Physics for the Anaesthetist, ed 4. Oxford, England, Blackwell Scientific Publications, 1987, p 261.)

peripheral blood flow. Inflated MAST will externally compress the arterial inflow to the legs and effectively raise both the arterial resistance and BP in the arms. It also allegedly translocates blood from the lower extremity veins to the upper body and the central circulation. The transfer of blood volume from lower extremities to upper extremities has never been demonstrated experimentally in patients in shock. The effect of MAST is seen in the improved ability to gain intravenous access in the severely hypovolemic patient as arterial and venous pressure is "boosted" in the upper extremities due to temporary obstruction to blood flow in the aorta.

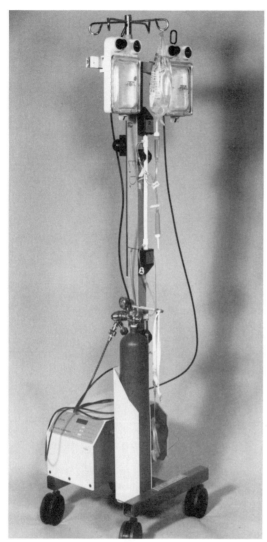
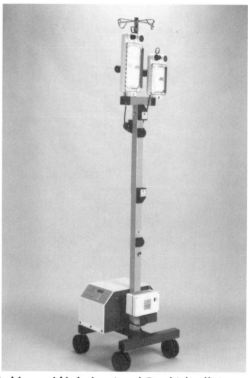

**Figure 4.11.    High-efficiency fluid warmer modified for rapid infusion.** Level One high-efficiency fluid warmer designed to warm 500 ml/min modified with rapid pressure infusion devices (Alton Dean Company, Salt Lake City, UT). **A**, An E cylinder of oxygen provides gas pressure to infuse fluids rapidly. **B**, An air compressor mounted at the bottom of the pole provides pressure to infuse fluids rapidly. (Figure 4.9**B** courtesy of Level One Company, Braintree, MA.)

Recently, MAST have been determined to be most useful to stabilize fractures of the lower extremities and pelvis (44). Use of MAST has become controversial because of associated complications (43). Prolonged inflation produces ischemia of the skin and superficial tissues under the suit. Acidosis and hyperkalemia have been associated with MAST-induced tissue ischemia. Other complications from MAST include ventilatory embarrassment from tightly binding the abdomen, cardiac rate and rhythm disturbances, muscle damage, increased capillary permeability, coagulopathy, and elevated levels of thrombolytic products (43).

Concerns over the tissue ischemia and serious questions about the efficacy of MAST in recent years have discouraged traumatologists from recommending routine, unqualified use of MAST. Recent recommendations from the American Col-

Table 4.3.    MAST: Potential Advantages and Disadvantages

| Advantages | Disadvantages |
|---|---|
| Raise/maintain perfusion pressure when IV[a] cannot be started or when volume replacement is inadequate | Are time-consuming: delay evacuation, obstruct physical examination of lower body |
| | Raise intracranial pressure |
| Tamponade hemorrhage | Cause respiratory embarrassment secondary to intraabdominal pressure |
| Stabilize pelvic/lower extremity fractures | Delay vascular access to lower extremities |
| | Cause ischemia/compartment syndrome to develop beneath suit |
| | Augment bleeding above level of suit |
| | Decrease splanchnic perfusion |
| | Elevate risk of deep vein thrombosis |
| | Elevate risk of vomiting/aspiration secondary to raised intraabdominal pressure |
| | Cause skin necrosis beneath suit |
| | Cause profound hypotension when rapidly deflated |

*Contraindications*: Cardiogenic shock, pregnancy, pulmonary edema, impaled object in abdomen, evisceration, esophageal varices, traumatic quadriplegia, head injury, ruptured diaphragm

[a] IV, intravenous access.

lege of Surgeons discourage the use of MAST in trauma centers; therefore, prehospital care providers will be the major users of this device in the future (45) (see also Chapter 15 for transportation uses). MAST is no substitute for the rapid infusion of intravenous fluid to replace hemorrhagic losses. However, as stated above, pelvic and lower extremity fractures may be splinted effectively by utilizing MAST if inflation pressure is carefully controlled to prevent tissue ischemia.

The greatest danger to a patient who requires MAST in the field is sudden and inappropriate deflation by inexperienced personnel (43). Intravenous fluid infusion must be started before the deflation procedure is initiated (2). The arterial BP is monitored while the abdominal compartment is first deflated gradually. If the systolic blood pressure decreases more than 10 mm Hg, deflation is stopped and the intravenous fluid infusion rate is increased. Ultimately, the leg compartments are deflated slowly—one leg at a time—while the BP is monitored.

### Trendelenburg Position

The Trendelenburg position was originally developed to facilitate surgery on the genitourinary system. It was popularized for

the treatment of hemorrhagic shock in World War I (46). Direct measurement of BP and CO in patients has failed to demonstrate that this position increases either BP or CO consistently (46–48). Many complications are associated with the Trendelenburg position, including increased intracranial pressure, increased intraocular pressure, displacement of endotracheal tubes, and elevation of the diaphragm, which compromises ventilation (46–48). Because of the number of complications associated with this position and the absence of demonstrated efficacy, it probably should be avoided. However, elevating a supine patient's legs is recommended if the trauma anesthesiologist wishes to augment VR and CO with postural changes (49).

### Fluid Administration: Crystalloid versus Colloid

Volume replacement for hemorrhagic shock starts with either a crystalloid or a colloid intravenous fluid (Table 4.4). The traditional crystalloid fluids used for volume replacement are 0.9% NaCl solution, lactated Ringer's solution, and Plasmalyte (40). Hemorrhagic shock leads to water shifts that cause interstitial space dehydration associated with electrolyte shifts from the extravascular, extracellular space to the intracel-

**Table 4.4.   Common Resuscitation Fluids**

Crystalloid
  Ringer's lactate
  Normal saline (0.9% NaCl)
  Normasol
  Plasmalyte
Colloid
  Albumin (5%, 25%)
  Hydroxyethyl starch (hetastarch [4,500,000 $M_r$/
    0.7 MS], pentastarch [264,000 $M_r$/0.48 MS])[a]
  Dextran 40
  Dextran 70
Blood components
  Fresh whole blood
    Fully cross-matched
    Type-specific
    Autotransfused
  Packed red blood cells
    Fully cross-matched
    Type-specific
    Type O, Rh neg; type O, Rh pos
  Fresh frozen plasma
    Platelets
    Cryoprecipitate
    Factor concentrate
Experimental (to be used only under specific protocol)
  Hypertonic crystalloid (7.5% NaCl)
  Fluorocarbon solution (Fluosol-DA 20%)
  Pyridoxilated stroma-free hemoglobin solution

[a] $M_r$, molecular weight; MS, molecular substitution—the number of ethylated OH groups on the hydroxyethyl starch.

lular compartment (29). Balanced salt solutions (e.g., lactated Ringer's) will restore hemorrhagic losses of water, especially water and salt lost from the interstitial space. Because intravenously administered water and electrolytes distribute throughout all water compartments in the body, large volumes of balanced salt solution must be administered to replace hemorrhagic losses. A study that utilized physiologic endpoints of resuscitation demonstrated the need to administer twice as much crystalloid as colloid solution (50). This is consistent with the previously mentioned finding that subjects in whom mild hemorrhage had been induced retained almost twice as much balanced salt solution in the intravascular space than did nonhemorrhagic controls (12). However, initial resuscitation theoretically may require three or more volumes of crystalloid per volume of shed blood (2). An initial rapid infusion of lactated Ringer's

solution (1 to 2 liters for adults and 20 ml/kg for children) is recommended by the ATLS protocols for the acute trauma patient (2). Many authors would continue to administer lactated Ringer's solution and use whole blood to replace lost hemoglobin (29, 51–54). Other authors suggest that a colloidal intravenous fluid be used to supplement crystalloid and packed red blood cell administration (55–60).

The rationale for administering colloidal solutions for hemorrhagic shock resuscitation traditionally has been to maintain colloid oncotic pressure of the plasma and reduce the amount of water administered to the patient to save the patient from "shock lung." Results of large patient series, as well as randomized trials of surgical fluid replacement, have demonstrated that using large-volume crystalloid shock resuscitation does not predispose the patient to the development of the adult respiratory distress syndrome (ARDS) or shock lung (52). Permeability changes to the pulmonary endothelium, as from endotoxic shock or sepsis, are required to initiate ARDS after trauma resuscitation (61–63).

Studies of fluid resuscitation in sheep with chronic pulmonary lymph fistulas demonstrated that hypoproteinemic crystalloid fluid resuscitation for hemorrhagic shock caused parallel changes in colloid oncotic pressure in both the intravascular and the pulmonary extravascular compartments during shock resuscitation. The colloid oncotic pressure in these two compartments changed in the same direction as the plasma protein concentration (64). Thus, the rate of water filtration from the blood vessels to the perivascular space and to the lymphatic system remains dependent only on the hydrostatic pressure in the pulmonary capillaries. In the sheep model, an increase in microvascular permeability induced with endotoxin caused a high rate of fluid flow from intravascular to extravascular compartments and into the lymphatics. In the septic sheep model, the high rate of water transfer to the interstitium was not dependent on intravascular hydrostatic pressure or protein concentration but was dependent on increased vascular permeability. Thus, there is probably little rationale either clinically or experimentally for the use of colloid instead of crystalloid solely on the basis of preventing ARDS.

Conversely, from another standpoint, several recent studies from Europe in both injured humans and experimental animals have demonstrated a beneficial effect of colloidal fluid resuscitation (55–60). Early and sustained increases in CO and oxygen consumption in the colloid groups compared with the crystalloid groups were observed in these studies (55, 56, 59, 60). The colloid was either a dextran polymer or hetastarch dissolved in saline; packed red cells were used for hemoglobin replacement. Albumin solutions may not be as efficacious for shock resuscitation as these glucose polymers.

Restoration of the colloid oncotic pressure may be obtained by the use of whole blood instead of packed red blood cells. Studies by Lowery et al. demonstrated that patients suffering hemorrhagic shock after war wounds could be well resuscitated with crystalloid and whole blood (53). Modified whole blood and crystalloid were used just as successfully by Counts et al. to treat hemorrhagic shock in a civilian setting (65).

Further, a well-conducted study compared crystalloid and packed red blood cells with colloid and packed red cells for the fluid management of patients undergoing elective abdominal aortic surgery (50). Fluid resuscitation was titrated against physiologic endpoints of maintaining pulmonary capillary wedge pressure within ±5 mm Hg of preoperative levels, CO greater than or equal to preoperative values, and urine output ≥50 ml/hr. Both fluid regimens were successful, although twice as much fluid was required in the crystalloid group as in the colloid group. Errors with crystalloid administration tended to be on the side of underresuscitation, and errors with colloid administration tended to be on the side of overhydration and pulmonary edema.

Thus, the advantages of colloid resusci-

tation seem to be rapid restoration of CO and oxygen consumption with smaller administered volumes. Crystalloid diluent for the colloid continues to be necessary to rehydrate the extracellular, extravascular interstitial space; however, it is important to monitor (e.g., pulmonary artery catheter) these patients carefully to prevent overdistension of the vascular tree and hydrostatic pulmonary edema. On the other hand, crystalloids have the advantage of restoring total body water losses because of the large volumes necessary to retain physiologic amounts of blood volume; however, it is important to monitor these patients carefully to prevent underhydration, which will impair their renal function and leave them with an inadequate CO.

A practical approach would be to start shock resuscitation rapidly with 1 to 2 liters of lactated Ringer's solution for all trauma patients. Pediatric patients should receive 20 ml of lactated Ringer's solution per kg as the initial bolus (see Chapter 11). Further fluid administration must be modified according to the patient's injury. The patient with an isolated head injury will require less fluid in the initial bolus and reduced maintenance intravenous therapy (see Chapter 7). Patients with class I and II hemorrhage who stabilize after the initial fluid infusion will need crystalloid given in a volume approximately three times their blood loss followed by maintenance intravenous infusion rates. Patients with class III hemorrhage will need crystalloid replacement approximately three times their blood loss plus blood—either packed red blood cells or whole blood titrated to achieve a hematocrit of about 30% (see Chapter 5). If these patients continue a brisk hemorrhage intraoperatively, packed red blood cells should be supplemented by crystalloid and/or colloid solutions. However, whole blood is adequately supplemented by crystalloid solutions. Patients in severe shock after class IV hemorrhage will require large-volume crystalloid replacement with colloid supplementation to resuscitate them more rapidly. The colloid will refill the vascular space rapidly and restore CO and oxygen consumption more rapidly than will pure crystalloid infusion (Figs. 4.12 and 4.13). Whole-blood transfusions can be used with crystalloid to replace hemorrhagic losses as well as third space edema losses. Colloid supplementation can be used with crystalloids and packed red blood cells to achieve a high postresuscitation CO similar to that achieved with whole blood and crystalloid resuscitation. Hypertonic crystalloid solutions have been used with limited success in experimental shock resuscitation (66).

## Pharmacologic Treatment

The replacement of hemorrhagic blood loss and trauma-induced interstitial water loss is the primary therapy for traumatic shock. However, pharmacologic adjuncts to fluid therapy are occasionally useful. Inotropic support of the heart is frequently necessary to support the patient who has suffered a class IV hemorrhage and significant injury. The use of invasive hemodynamic monitoring will identify a patient who has a failing heart due to progressive shock. A low left ventricular stroke work (LVSW) value with an elevated pulmonary capillary wedge pressure (PCWP) will indicate heart failure. Another indicator for inotropic support is a low mixed venous oxygen tension ($PvO_2$) associated with a low ratio of oxygen delivery ($DO_2$) to oxygen consumption ($\dot{V}O_2$). An appropriate response to inotropic therapy would be an increase in $DO_2$ and $PvO_2$ while the LVSW

TWO PHASES OF
MONITORING IN SHOCK

IMMEDIATE RESTORATION OF OXYGEN DELIVERY          SCREENING FOR ORGAN SYSTEM DYSFUNCTION

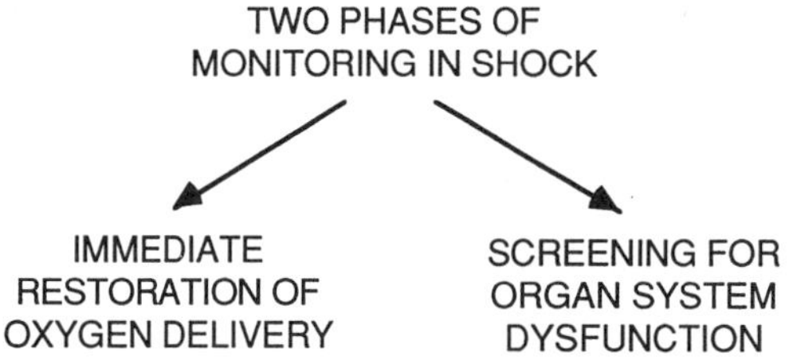

**Figure 4.12. Goals of monitoring patients with posttraumatic shock.** (From Nelson LD: Monitoring and measurement in shock. In Barrett J, Nyhus LM (eds): Treatment of Shock: Principles and Practice. Philadelphia, Lea & Febiger, 1986, p 36.)

increases, with no change or a decrease in PCWP. Dobutamine is probably the most easily controlled inotropic drug to use in this setting.

Many drugs have been used to treat traumatic shock (Table 4.5). Vasopressors have been used to elevate the BP, but they rarely improve the shock state because of the extreme microcirculatory vasoconstriction associated with shock, as mentioned above. However, patients with spinal shock who have a normal blood volume but inadequate endogenous catecholamine secretion will benefit from epinephrine, norepinephrine, or dopamine pressor support. The indirect vasopressors that depend on release of norepinephrine from sympathetic nerve terminals are not useful in the shock state because endogenous catecholamines may be depleted. Similarly, the pure $\alpha$-adrenergic agonists (e.g., phenylephrine) are not as useful in hemorrhagic shock as drugs with strong inotropic $\beta$-adrenergic activity.

From another perspective, microvascular vasoconstriction and obstruction to flow may favorably respond to vasodilator therapy along with fluid replacement. Other pharmacologic therapies used with limited success are listed in Table 4.5. Corticosteroids have not proven efficacious in preventing postresuscitation complications of shock (67). Opioid antagonists such as naloxone may be effective in restoring BP and CO, especially in septic shock, if arterial pH and temperature are controlled (68).

## Monitoring Patients with Traumatic Shock

Traumatologists traditionally have followed the progress of shock resuscitation by monitoring arterial BP and pulse rate. Table 4.6 illustrates approximate correlations of systolic BP with palpable peripheral pulses, which can be used to estimate roughly the patient's BP in the absence of vasodilation (as in spinal shock). Shock causes hypotension and tachycardia, which can be corrected by appropriate fluid resuscitation. The hormonal environment triggered by the shock state may affect both BP and heart rate independently of intravascular filling.

Metabolic Response to Trauma & Sepsis

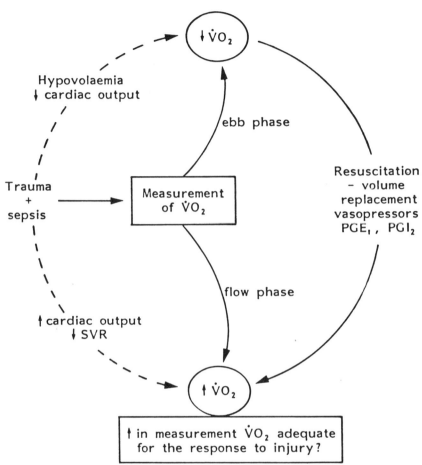

**Figure 4.13. Metabolic response to injury.** The "ebb phase" is associated with depressed oxygen consumption ($\dot{V}O_2$), hypovolemia, and decreased metabolic function. After resuscitation, the patient becomes markedly catabolic in the "flow phase," which is associated with an elevated $\dot{V}O_2$. (From Bihari D: Intensive care. In Westaby S (ed): Trauma Pathogenesis and Treatment. Oxford, England, William Heinemann Medical Books, 1989, p 366.)

Thus, these variables are less than adequate predictors of complete resuscitation. Other variables that correlate well with intravascular volume status are central venous pressure (CVP), usually measured in the superior vena cava, and urinary output. CVP is determined by the intravascular volume and the compliance of the venous/right atrial system. Urinary output is determined by the degree of renal perfusion and water reabsorption, which are both affected by intravascular volume and the inotropic state of the heart. Although restoration of the above variables to normal values may indicate that shock resuscitation is proceeding correctly, $\dot{V}O_2$ is the most sensitive variable to monitor (Fig. 4.13). $\dot{V}O_2$ is determined by the cumulative cellular demand for oxygen and by the cardiopulmonary system's delivery of oxygen to the cells. Because cellular anoxia delivers the "lethal blow" in hemorrhagic shock, the patient is not adequately resuscitated until the cumulative oxygen debt is repaid and oxygen is provided for ongoing metabolic demands. Therefore, the endpoint of shock resuscitation should be to restore $\dot{V}O_2$ to levels adequate to repay the oxygen debt of shock (Fig. 4.4). The utility of

**Table 4.5. Pharmacologic Agents Useful in Traumatic Shock**

Inotropic
  Dobutamine
  Dopamine
  Epinephrine
  Calcium[a]
Chronotropic
  Isoproterenol
  Atropine
Vasopressors
  Epinephrine
  Norepinephrine
  Ephedrine[b]
  Phenylephrine[b]
Buffers[c]
  Bicarbonate
  THAM
Opioid antagonist
  Naloxone
Opioid agonist/antagonist
  Nalbuphine
Steroids[d]
  Methylprednisolone
  Dexamethasone
Mechanical
  Intraaortic balloon pump
  Pacemaker
Experimental
  Fructose 1,6-diphosphate

[a] Guided by $Ca^{++}$ measurements.
[b] Spinal shock.
[c] Guided by blood gases.
[d] Adrenal insufficiency.

**Table 4.6. Correlation of Systolic Blood Pressure with Palpable Pulses**

| Pulse Location | Minimal Systolic BP |
|---|---|
| Radial | 80 |
| Femoral | 70 |
| Carotid | 60 |

this approach has been demonstrated by the fact that hemorrhagic shock is lethal to patients who fail to achieve an elevated $\dot{V}O_2$ during resuscitation (19).

### Restoring Red Cell Mass and Oxygen Carrying Capacity

After blood volume has been restored as the first priority in hemorrhagic shock resuscitation, restoration of hemoglobin is the second priority and treating disorders of hemostasis is the third, although in reality these issues are often addressed simultaneously. (Chapter 5, "Blood Component Therapy for Trauma Patients" covers these topics in depth.) Hemoglobin restoration is critical to the maintenance of an oxygen carrying capacity adequate to meet cellular oxygenation need with a reasonable CO. Traditionally, the hemoglobin concentration associated with a hematocrit of 28 to 30% has been considered to optimize rheologically (in terms of cardiac work, fluid viscosity, and microcirculatory flow while providing adequate oxygen carrying capacity) the mixed venous oxygen content ($CvO_2$). Recent experience in trying to avoid transmission of blood-borne diseases (e.g., acquired immune deficiency syndrome, hepatitis) to surgical patients has demonstrated successful outcomes with lower hemoglobin concentrations. Hemodilution, especially with plasma colloidal solutions, can reduce blood viscosity and erythrocyte stasis in capillaries and postcapillary venules during and immediately after resuscitation from shock (69). Theoretically, tissue oxygen transport from the microcirculation is maximized at a hemoglobin concentration of 10 g/dl with a normal plasma albumin concentration (69). The anecdotal experience in elective surgical patients of one of the authors (J.K.S) has demonstrated that most patients tolerate acute anemia without signs of organ (e.g., heart, kidney) ischemia as long as the hemoglobin remains ≥ 7 g/dl. However, in cases of acute (e.g., cardiac contusion) or chronic (e.g., coronary artery disease) cardiac pathology and/or in elderly trauma patients, it is prudent to opt for higher hemoglobin/hematocrit levels.

The use of blood substitutes in an attempt to provide oxygen carrying capacity without red blood cells has been only partially successful. Perfluorocarbon emulsions such as Fluosol-DA are unsatisfactory as a blood substitute because of toxicity to blood cells and the need for high oxygen ventilation (70, 71). Other blood substitutes, such as stroma-free hemoglobin solutions, are being explored (70) (see Chapter 5). The future of trauma care will partially be devoted to developing a resuscitation fluid that provides both volume resuscitation and oxygen carrying capacity and that is ultimately both easy to use and easy to store.

## Hemostasis/Coagulopathy

Hemostatic elements of blood are lost after severe injury and massive transfusion. Although the platelet count is most seriously depressed after trauma, series of trauma resuscitations have been successful both with and without platelet transfusions (65, 72). All coagulation proteins except factor VIII are preserved in adequate amounts in blood banked at 4°C; therefore, massive transfusion does not seem to decrease in vivo concentrations of coagulation proteins except factor VIII. However, disseminated intravascular coagulation may be triggered by thromboplastins released from injured tissue and hematomas, which consume

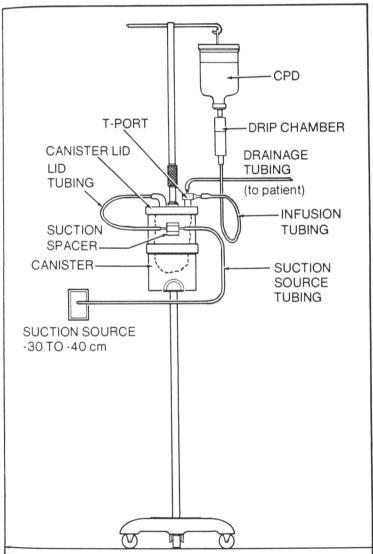

**Figure 4.14.**   **This simple autotransfusion device anticoagulates blood** suctioned from the surgical field, a chest tube, or a wound drain. The anticoagulated shed blood is collected in a plastic bag and can be reinfused through an intravenous infusion set. (From Cardona VD (ed): Trauma Reference Manual. Bowie, MD, Brady Communications Company, 1985, p 117.)

coagulation proteins and platelets (see Chapter 5).

The practice of administering large quantities of fresh frozen plasma to correct pathologic bleeding or abnormal coagulation profiles—prothrombin time and partial thromboplastin time—has been condemned theoretically but works experimentally in animals and is widely practiced in trauma centers (73). Regardless of the theoretical advantage of platelets over fresh frozen plasma, neither should be administered in the absence of a clinically identified coagulopathy or pathologic hemorrhage.

### Blood Conservation/Autotransfusion

Recycling the patient's blood from sites of hemorrhage to the circulatory system is an attractive idea in trauma management (74–76). Using the patient's own blood would avoid many of the problems of blood banking such as correct matching of donor's and recipient's blood types, prevention of disease transmission, and storage of blood

products. However, the practice of reinfusing shed blood (autotransfusion) has its own risks. Among the problems are bacterial contamination of hemorrhaged blood, clotting of the autotransfusion product, and contamination by vasoactive tissue debris (77–79). The simplest autotransfusion devices are sterile containers used with chest tube suction bottles that collect defibrinated blood draining from a hemothorax (74) (Fig. 4.14). These sterile containers are then inverted onto intravenous tubing, and the blood is reinfused. This type of device is also available for orthopedic wound drains.

Modern autotransfusion devices (Fig. 4.15) were developed to collect blood from the surgical field by suction and anticoagulate it. The red cells are washed to remove plasma and cellular debris generated in the wound. The washed red cells are then centrifuged to concentrate them and delivered to infusion bags as packed red blood cells with an approximate hematocrit of 70%. The blood evacuated from fracture

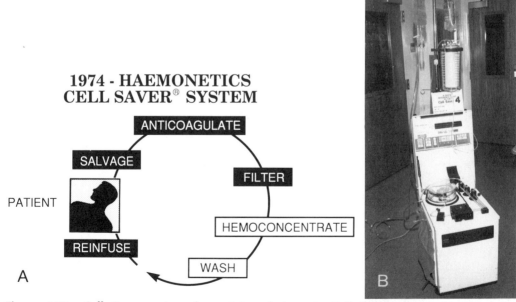

**Figure 4.15. Cell Saver system for autotransfusion. A,** Cell Saver system (designed by Haemonetics, Marshfield, MA) provides washed packed red blood cells from blood salvaged by suctioning from the surgical field. **B,** The Cell Saver IV designed to cycle automatically through the steps outlined in **A.**

sites must be washed carefully to remove bone spicules and red blood cell ghosts formed by hemolysis at the air/blood interface of the fracture (77). Red cell ghosts (red cell membranes that have lost their hemoglobin and cytosol during hemolysis) are toxic to the human circulation; they can cause hypotension, renal failure, and a hemodynamic profile similar to that of septic shock (70, 79, 80). The future of autotransfusion for trauma patients will be ensured if methods are developed to clean vasoactive cellular debris and bacteria from shed blood reliably.

## COMPLICATIONS OF SHOCK RESUSCITATION

### "Shock Lung": The Adult Respiratory Distress Syndrome

It is discouraging for a traumatologist to observe a patient who has been successfully resuscitated from severe trauma and hemorrhagic shock develop ARDS during post-

traumatic intensive care. Among the many causes of ARDS associated with trauma are prolonged hemorrhagic shock, the fat emboli syndrome, and aspiration of gastric contents. Clinically, ARDS is manifested by a patchy interstitial pulmonary infiltrate, marked loss of lung compliance, and severe maldistribution of the pulmonary ventilation to perfusion (V/Q) ratio with combinations of both increased venous admixture and dead space. The decreased compliance reduces functional residual capacity (FRC) of the lung and leads to rapid, shallow spontaneous respirations.

Pathophysiologically, ARDS first develops with an interstitial pulmonary edema, which then organizes with fibrous tissue replacing the edema. The microscopic and macroscopic pulmonary anatomy is lost as the lung becomes grossly hemorrhagic and boggy—grossly appearing more like liver than lung ("red hepatization"). The alveolar architecture is destroyed by the fibrous tissue and a proliferation of type II (cuboidal) alveolar cells. The pulmonary micro-

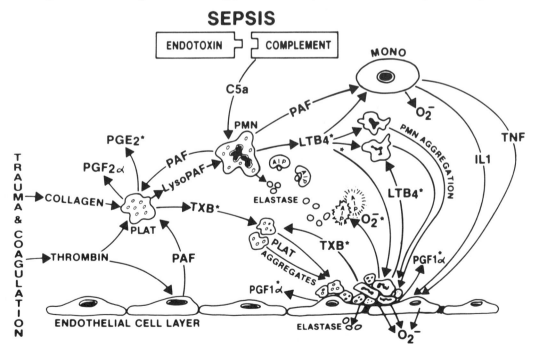

**Figure 4.16.  Pathophysiology of ARDS.** (From Rivkind AI, Siegel JH, Guadalupi P, Littleton M: Sequential patterns of eicosanoid, platelet, and neutrophil interactions in the evolution of the fulminant post-traumatic adult respiratory distress syndrome. Ann Surg 1989;210:355–373.)

vasculature is markedly reduced in cross-sectional area as arteriolar capillary obstruction develops (81). As the microvessels are destroyed, pulmonary vascular resistance increases significantly.

Healing takes place as the type II cells develop into new alveoli lined with type I squamous epithelial cells. The new growth of lung gradually replaces the fibrous tissue, and nearly normal lung structure and function may result. Unfortunately, the mortality rate from ARDS is still so high (≥65%) that many patients' lungs do not get a chance to heal (81).

Endothelial cell damage occurs when white blood cells (polymorphonuclear neutrophils [PMNs]) marginate along the pulmonary vessels in response to an inflammatory condition (53, 62, 82, 83) (Fig. 4.16). Activated complement, especially C5a, attracts the PMNs, which release free radicals of oxygen (e.g., superoxide, hydroxyl radicals) that damage the endothelium, increasing the permeability to water. The interstitial pulmonary edema that occurs with increased endothelial water permeability decreases pulmonary compliance and sets the stage for interstitial fibrosis.

Because chemotactic stimulation is required to cause PMN margination in the lung, interleukin-1 released from tissue macrophages in response to soft tissue trauma or bacterial invasion during sepsis probably stimulates the formation of leukotriene B4, which causes white cell margination in the pulmonary blood vessels (38, 62, 83). Because sepsis usually causes a more profound acute phase response than does tissue trauma, one would expect a strong association between sepsis and ARDS. Indeed, the lung is frequently the first organ to fail, developing ARDS, in the multiorgan failure syndrome that occurs with sepsis (13, 20) (Table 4.7). Among the phagocytic cells of the reticuloendothelial system that release interleukin-1 are the tissue macrophages in the liver and spleen as well as the lung. Prolonged shock, which is frequently associated with postresuscitation ARDS,

**Table 4.7.   Hallmarks of Multiple Organ Failure[a]**

Respiratory
  Early: Tachypnea, hypoxia, congestive atelectasis
  Late: Cyanosis, decrease in compliance, fibrosis
Renal
  Early: Oliguria/polyuria, acute tubular necrosis
  Late: CHF, edema, cortical necrosis
Immune
  Early: Disorientation, fever, leukocytosis
  Late: DIC, hyperglycemia, occult abscesses
Hepatic
  Early: Jaundice, bile stasis
  Late: Encephalopathy, periportal fibrosis
Gastrointestinal
  Early: Ileus, loss of mucosal villi
  Late: Gastrointestinal bleeding, submucosal hemorrhage
Coagulation
  Early: Elevations in PT and PTT, pulmonary microaggregates
  Late: DIC, fibrin split products, interstitial hemorrhage
Cardiovascular
  Early: Dysrhythmias, myocardial edema
  Late: Hypotension/CHF subendocardial infarction
Neurologic
  Early: Disorientation, interstitial edema
  Late: Coma, hemorrhage/infarction

[a] Abbreviations: CHF, congestive heart failure; DIC, disseminated intravascular coagulation: PT, prothrombin time; PTT, partial thromboplastin time.
From Baker CC. Trauma in the 1980's: the "success story" of multiple organ failure. In Maull KI, Cleveland HC, Strauch GO, Wolferth CC (eds): Advances in Trauma. Chicago, Year Book, 1988, vol 3, p 40.

probably stimulates liver phagocytes (Kupffer cells) to release interleukin-1 in response to prolonged local tissue ischemia and intestinal bacteria that have entered the portal circulation from an ischemic gut (14).

If a large number of bacteria enter the circulation, the phagocytes become overwhelmed and sepsis develops. However, if the liver phagocytes clear the bacteria, the patient may develop ARDS and a brief period of hemodynamic instability without bacteremia. Currently, preventing ARDS is more effective than treating it. Rapid and effective shock resuscitation after trauma helps to prevent ARDS (84). Rapid and effective control of sepsis and other posttraumatic inflammatory conditions also prevents ARDS. ARDS that follows long bone fractures responds to early osteosynthesis performed under general anesthesia with mechanical ventilation (85). Delaying extubation until the patient demonstrates that the lungs are efficiently exchanging oxygen prevents postfracture ARDS. Preventing ARDS secondary to long bone fractures also blocks the development of the entire fat emboli syndrome, which follows all too often.

Currently, antinflammatory drug therapy with steroids has been disappointing in the prevention or treatment of ARDS (67). Mechanical ventilation with positive end-expiratory pressure (PEEP) adjusted to allow an adequate arterial $PO_2$ with a nontoxic $FIO_2$ ($\leq$50%) is currently the only effective treatment for ARDS (62, 81). Supportive care of the patient must be aimed at further reducing pulmonary insults such as atelectasis, barotrauma, infection, and starvation.

Other modes of supporting gas exchange such as high-frequency ventilation, independent lung ventilation, and extracorporeal membrane oxygenation may be used in managing individual patients who cannot tolerate standard mechanical ventilation with PEEP at an $FIO_2$ of $\leq$50% (61, 86, 87).

## Renal Failure after Shock Resuscitation

Hemorrhagic shock after trauma overwhelms the compensatory mechanisms in the kidney. The glomerular filtration rate (GFR) decreases acutely and the patient develops oliguria (<500 ml/day) (25, 88). After resuscitation, the majority of patients recover a normal GFR when renal blood flow is restored. Some patients retain a decreased GFR for a prolonged period after resuscitation. The majority of these patients exhibit nonoliguric renal failure with an elevated free water clearance providing high urine flows (several liters per day) with a low GFR. These patients usually recover normal GFR and renal concentrating mechanisms after a few weeks unless they are inappropriately iatrogenically dehydrated (89–91).

A small group of patients who fail to achieve a normal postresuscitation GFR develop oliguric renal failure with failure of renal tubular function (88). These patients have a low GFR, a low urine output, and a high free water clearance. This syndrome is frequently referred to as acute tubular

**Table 4.8.   Common Renal Function Tests[a]**

| Test | Normal Value | Measurements | Effects of Shock |
|---|---|---|---|
| Creatinine clearance (Ccr) | M 110–150 ml/min<br>F 105–132 ml/min | Ccr (ml/min) =<br>(Ucr/Pcr) × V | Decrease with progressive shock. Resuscitation should restore Ccr to normal or higher than normal |
| Fractional excretion of sodium ($FE_{Na}$) | $\leq$1 | $FE_{Na}$ (%) =<br>$\dfrac{UNa/PNa}{Ucr/Pcr} \times 100$ | Very low with shock; will become positive (>3) if posttraumatic renal failure occurs |
| Osmolar clearance (Cosm) | | Cosm (ml/min) =<br>(Uosm/Posm) × V | |
| Free water clearance ($CH_2O$) | Normal varies with $H_2O$ load but is usually around −10 ml/min | $CH_2O$ (ml/min) =<br>V − Cosm | Becomes very negative (<−20 ml/min) with shock; rises to >−10 if posttraumatic renal failure develops |
| Urinary sodium | Normally low but depends on salt ingestion | $U_{Na}$ (mEq/liter) | <20 mEq/liter in shock; >40 mEq/liter in posttraumatic renal failure |

[a] Ucr, urinary creatinine (mg/dl); Pcr, plasma creatinine (mg/dl); V, urinary volume flow (ml/min); UNa, urinary sodium (mEq/liter); PNa, plasma sodium (mEq/liter); Uosm, urinary osmolarity (mosm/liter); Posm, plasma osmolarity (mosm/liter).

necrosis and is associated with obstruction and destruction of renal tubules. These patients will need dialysis or extracorporeal hemoultrafiltration to survive their acute renal failure (90). The mortality rate associated with oliguric posttraumatic renal failure is much higher (70–90%) than that associated with nonoliguric renal failure (23–30%) (88).

The diagnosis of posttraumatic renal failure requires frequent measurement of urine output (V), creatinine clearance (Ccr), urine osmolality (Uosm), urine sodium (UNa), plasma osmolality (Posm), and plasma sodium (PNa). Table 4.8 outlines the formulas for calculating renal function. The Ccr is a very sensitive indicator of posttraumatic renal failure despite the problems equating Ccr to GFR (26, 91). Frequent measurement of Ccr during and after trauma resuscitation will reveal a pattern of prolonged depression of GFR in patients destined to develop posttraumatic renal failure. Evaluation of V at that time will indicate oliguric or nonoliguric renal failure. Measurements of free water clearance and the fractional excretion of sodium can help distinguish prerenal from intrarenal failure (88). If traumatic injury to the kidney or urinary tract is suspected, reontgenographic contrast studies such as an intravenous pyelogram are indicated.

Patients with prerenal failure with a very low V should be treated with an appropriate intravenous fluid challenge. One of the advantages of shock resuscitation with a large volume of crystalloid is inducing a diuresis that maintains a high urinary flow. Intrarenal oliguric renal failure with a low Ccr, a low V, and an elevated urinary sodium should be treated with a diuretic trial in an attempt to change oliguria to nonoliguric renal failure (88). Adequate shock resuscitation is a prerequisite to the avoidance of nonoliguric renal failure as well as to the preservation of normal renal function in patients whose kidneys survive intact after resuscitation from traumatic shock.

## Sepsis

Sepsis is commonly found in severely injured patients maintained in posttraumatic critical care units (37, 39, 63). Traumatic

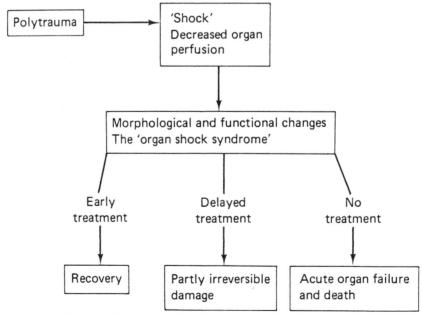

**Figure 4.17.    Flow diagram illustrating the value of early treatment of traumatic shock.** (From Westaby S, Kobayashi K: Shock and blood volume replacement. In Westaby S (ed): Trauma Pathogenesis and Treatment. Oxford, England, William Heinemann Medical Books, 1989, p 42.)

shock leads to breakdown of epithelial barriers (e.g., skin, gut), allowing bacterial invasion. Sepsis develops in response to microorganism release of bacterial toxins (endotoxin) or antigen/antibody complexes (38). The acute phase response to microorganism invasion tends to be more profound and sustained than the response to tissue trauma. Sepsis, which has been called "inflammation of the blood," involves a multiphasic metabolic response, which has been outlined by Siegel and Vary (39).

Initially, oxygen consumption increases as the muscle cells decrease their capacity to utilize glucose and convert to mechanisms that metabolize branched-chain amino acids for energy (37). The hyperdynamic cardiovascular response that is classically associated with sepsis occurs during this initial phase of sepsis, as long as the patient's heart has adequate preload and contractility. Patients who are volume-depleted or have posttraumatic cardiac failure will not exhibit a hyperdynamic response to sepsis but will demonstrate only a decrease in $PvO_2$. As sepsis progresses, a generalized depression of oxygen consumption occurs. Heart failure eventually develops as septic shock becomes irreversible (39).

## SUMMARY

Anesthesiologists who care for severely injured patients must resuscitate them from hemorrhagic shock rapidly and effectively. Untreated hemorrhagic shock kills trauma victims when their cumulative oxygen debt reaches a critical level (Fig. 4.17). Therefore, the goal of shock resuscitation is to restore circulating blood volume rapidly to the point of increasing oxygen consumption enough to repay shock-incurred oxygen debt. Both crystalloid and colloidal fluids can be used effectively for shock resuscitation. Crystalloids must be infused in large quantities to achieve a rapid and sustained restoration of CO and $\dot{V}O_2$. Patients receiving these fluids must be monitored carefully to prevent complications of inadequate intravascular volume, as well as those of overzealous fluid infusion. Colloidal fluids will increase CO and $\dot{V}O_2$ very rapidly and become more useful in cases of massive hemorrhage; however, patients to whom they are administered must also be monitored carefully to prevent intravascular overhydration and hydrostatic pulmonary edema. The oxygen carrying capacity of hemoglobin is a critical factor in the maintenance of oxygen consumption (see Chapter 5). Finally, rapid restoration of circulating blood volume and lost tissue water will minimize the cellular injury caused by shock and reduce the incidence of late complications such as ARDS and renal failure.

## References

1. Trunkey DD. Trauma. Sci Am 1983;249(2): 28–35.
2. American College of Surgeons Committee on Trauma. Advanced Trauma Life Support Program. Chicago, American College of Surgeons, 1989.
3. Trump BF, Berezesky IK, Cowley RA. The cellular and subcellular characteristics of acute and chronic injury with emphasis on the role of calcium. In Cowley RA, Trump BF (eds): Pathophysiology of Shock, Anoxia, and Ischemia. Baltimore, Williams & Wilkins, 1982, pp 6–46.
4. Trump BF, Valigorsky JM, Dees JH Mergner WJ, Kim KM, Jones RT, Pendergrass RE, Garbus J, Cowley RA. Cellular changes in human disease: a new method of pathological analysis. Hum Pathol 1973;4:89–109.
5. McCuskey RS. Microcirculation—basic considerations. In Cowley RA, Trump BF (eds): Pathophysiology of Shock, Anoxia, and Ischemia. Baltimore, Williams & Wilkins, 1982, pp 156–164.
6. Guyton AC, Jones CE, Coleman TG. Circulatory Physiology: Cardiac Output and Its Regulation. Philadelphia, WB Saunders, 1973.
7. Mitzner W, Goldberg HS, Lichtenstein S. Effects of thoracic blood volume changes on steady state cardiac output. Circ Res 1976;38:255–261.
8. Stene JK, Burns B, Permutt S, Caldini P, Shanoff M. Increased cardiac output following occlusion of the descending thoracic aorta in dogs. Am J Physiol 1982;243:R152–R158.
9. Caldini P, Permutt S, Waddell JA, Riley RL. Effect of epinephrine on pressure, flow and volume relationships in the systemic circulation of dogs. Circ Res 1974;34:606–623.
10. Rogers MC, Kirsch JR. Current concepts in brain resuscitation. JAMA 1989;261:3143–3147.
11. Webb WR, Brunswick RA. Microcirculation in

shock—clinical review. In Cowley RA, Trump BF (eds): Pathophysiology of Shock, Anoxia, and Ischemia. Baltimore, Williams & Wilkins, 1982, pp 181–185.

12. Moore FD. The effects of hemorrhage on body composition. N Engl J Med 1965;273:567–577.

13. DeCamp MM, Demling RH. Posttraumatic multisystem organ failure. JAMA 1988;260:530–534.

14. Cerra FB, Holman RT, Bankey PE, Mazuski JE. Nutritional pharmacology: its role in the hypermetabolism-organ failure syndrome. Crit Care Med 1990;18:S154–S158.

15. Crowell JW, Smith EE. Oxygen deficit and irreversible hemorrhagic shock. Am J Physiol 1964;206:313–316.

16. Crowell JW, Guyton AC. Evidence favoring a cardiac mechanism in irreversible hemorrhagic shock. Am J Physiol 1961;201:893–896.

17. Crowell JW, Guyton AC. Further evidence favoring a cardiac mechanism in irreversible hemorrhagic shock. Am J Physiol 1962;203:248–252.

18. Hackel DB, Ratliff NB, Mikat E. The heart in shock. Circ Res 1974;35:805–811.

19. Shoemaker WC, Appel PL, Kram HB. Tissue oxygen debt as a determinant of lethal and nonlethal postoperative organ failure. Crit Care Med 1988;16:1117–1120.

20. Hoff BH. Multisystem failure: a review with special reference to drowning. Crit Care Med 1979;7:310–320.

21. Trunkey DD, Sheldon GF, Collins JA. The treatment of shock. In Zuidema GD, Rutherford RB, Ballinger WF (eds): The Management of Trauma, ed 4. Philadelphia, WB Saunders, 1985, pp 105–125.

22. Peters RM. Fluid resuscitation and oxygen exchange in hypovolemia. In Siegel JH (ed): Trauma: Emergency Surgery and Critical Care. New York, Churchill Livingstone, 1987, pp 157–179.

23. McLaughlin JS, Suddhimondala C, Mech K Jr, Lee Llacer RL, Houston J, Blide R, Attar S, Cowley RA. Pulmonary gas exchange in shock in humans. Ann Surg 1969;169:42–56.

24. McLaughlin JS. Physiologic consideration of hypoxemia in shock and trauma. Ann Surg 1971;173:667–679.

25. Badr KF, Ichikawa I. Prerenal failure: a deleterious shift from renal compensation to decompensation. N Engl J Med 1988;319:623–629.

26. Rose BD. Approach to the patient with renal disease. In Rubenstein E, Federman DD (eds): Scientific American Medicine. New York, Scientific American, 1989, sect 10, ch III, pp 1–11.

27. Campion DS, Lynch LJ, Rector FC Jr, Carter N, Shires GT. The effect of hemorrhagic shock in transmembrane potential. Surgery 1969;66:1051–1059.

28. Shires GT. Principles and management of hemorrhagic shock. In Shires GT (ed): Principles of Trauma Care, ed 3. New York, McGraw-Hill, 1985, pp 3–42.

29. Carrico CJ, Canizaro PC, Shires GT. Fluid resuscitation following injury: rationale for the use of balanced salt solutions. Crit Care Med 1976;4:46–54.

30. Engelbrecht FM, Mattheyse FJ, Mowton WL. Haemorrhagic shock—metabolic parameters for the assessment of damage in lung, liver and kidney tissue. S Afr Med J 1984;65:1042–1044.

31. Gann DS, Lilly MP. The neuroendocrine response to multiple trauma. World J Surg 1983;7:101–118.

32. Elliot MJ, Alberti KGMM. Carbohydrate metabolism—effects of preoperative starvation and trauma. Clin Anaesthesiol 1983;1:527–550.

33. Kehlet H, Brandt MR, Prang-Hansen A, Alberti KGMM. Effect of epidural analgesia on metabolic profiles during and after surgery. Br J Surg 1979;66:543–546.

34. Brown MJ, Brown DC, Murphy MB. Hypokalemia from beta$_2$-receptor stimulation by circulating epinephrine. N Engl J Med 1983;309:1414–1419.

35. Rosa RM, Silva P, Young JB, Landsberg L, Brown RS, Rowe JW, Epstein FH. Adrenergic modulation of extrarenal potassium disposal. N Engl J Med 1980;302:431–434.

36. Williams ME, Rosa RM, Silva P, Brown RS, Epstein FH. Impairment of extrarenal potassium disposal by $\alpha$ adrenergic stimulation. N Engl J Med 1984;311:145–149.

37. Jeevanandam M, Grote-Holman AE, Chikenji T, Askanazi J, Elwyn DH, Kinney JM. Effects of glucose on fuel utilization and glycerol turnover in normal and injured man. Crit Care Med 1990;18:125–135.

38. Dinarello CA. Interleukin-1 and the pathogenesis of the acute phase response. N Engl J Med 1984;311:1413–1418.

39. Siegel JH, Vary TC. Sepsis, abnormal metabolic control, and the multiple organ failure syndrome. In Siegel JH (ed): Trauma: Emergency Surgery and Critical Care. New York, Churchill Livingstone, 1987, pp 411–501.

40. Giesecke AH Jr, Grande CM, Whitten CW. Fluid therapy and the resuscitation of traumatic shock. Crit Care Clin 1990;6:61–72.

41. Arrighi DA, Farnell MB, Mucha P Jr, Ilstrup DM, Anderson DL. Prospective randomized trial of rapid venous access for patients in hypovolemic shock. Ann Emerg Med 1989;18:927–930.

42. Hoelzer MF. Recent advances in intravenous therapy. Emerg Med Clin North Am 1986;4:487–500.

43. Schwab CW, Gore D. MAST: medical antishock trousers. In Nyhus L (ed): Surgery Annual. East Norwalk, CT, Appleton-Century-Crofts, 1983, vol 15, pp 41–59.

44. Mucha P Jr, Welch TJ. Hemorrhage in major pelvic fractures. Surg Clin North Am 1988;68:757–773.

45. Committee on Trauma, American College of Surgeons. Resources for Optimal Care of the Injured Patient. Chicago, American College of Surgeons, 1990.

46. Taylor J, Weil MH. Failure of the Trendelenburg position to improve circulation during clinical shock. Surg Gynecol Obstet 1967;124: 1005–1010.

47. Sibbald WJ, Paterson NAM, Holliday RL, Baskerville J. The Trendelenburg position: hemodynamic effects in hypotensive and normotensive patients. Crit Care Med 1979;7:218–224.

48. Keen RI, Anderton JM. Hazards and changes with positioning. In Nunn JP, Utting JE, Brown BR (eds): General Anaesthesia, ed 5. London, Butterworth, 1989, pp 540–548.

49. Safar P, Bircher NG. Cardiopulmonary Cerebral Resuscitation, ed 3. Philadelphia, WB Saunders, 1988.

50. Virgilio RW, Rice CL, Smith DE, James DR, Zarins CK, Hobelmann CF, Peters RM. Crystalloid vs. colloid resuscitation: is one better? Surgery 1979; 85:129–139.

51. Moore FA, Moore EE. Trauma resuscitation. In Wilmore DW, Brennan MF, Harken AH, Holcroft JW, Meakins JL (eds): American College of Surgeons' Care of the Surgical Patient. New York, Scientific American, 1988–89, vol 1, ch 2, pp 1–15.

52. Poole GV, Meredith JW, Pennell T, Mills SA. Comparison of colloids and crystalloids in resuscitation from hemorrhagic shock. Surg Gynecol Obstet 1982;154:577–586.

53. Lowery BD, Cloutier CT, Carey LC. Electrolyte solutions in resuscitation in human hemorrhagic shock. Surg Gynecol Obstet 1971;133:273–284.

54. Lowe RJ, Moss GS, Jilek J, Levine HD. Crystalloid vs colloid in the etiology of pulmonary failure after trauma: a randomized trial in man. Surgery 1977;81:676–683.

55. Modig J. Effectiveness of dextran 70 versus Ringer's acetate in traumatic shock and adult respiratory distress syndrome. Crit Care Med 1986;14:454–457.

56. Hankeln K, Rädel C, Beez M, Laniewski P, Bohmert F. Comparison of hydroxyethyl starch and lactated Ringer's solution on hemodynamics and oxygen transport of critically ill patients in prospective crossover studies. Crit Care Med 1989;17:133–135.

57. Shatney CH, Deepika K, Militello PR, Majerus TC, Dawson B. Efficacy of hetastarch in the resuscitation of patients with multisystem trauma and shock. Arch Surg 1983;118:804–809.

58. Haupt MT, Rackow EC. Colloid osmotic pressure and fluid resuscitation with hetastarch, albumin, and saline solutions. Crit Care Med 1982;10: 159–162.

59. Shoemaker WC, Schluchter M, Hopkins JA, Appel PL, Schwartz S, Chang PC. Comparison of the relative effectiveness of colloids and crystalloids in emergency resuscitation. Am J Surg 1981;142:73–84.

60. Schött U, Lindom L-O, Sjöstrand U: Hemodynamic effects of colloid concentration in experimental hemorrhagic: a comparison of Ringer's acetate, 3% dextran-60, and 6% dextran-70. Crit Care Med 1988;16:346–352.

61. Snider MT, Cambell DB, Kofke WA, High KM, Russell GB, Keamy MF, Williams DR. Venovenous perfusion of adults and children with severe acute respiratory distress syndrome. Trans Am Soc Artif Intern Organs 1988;34:1014–1020.

62. Rinaldo JE, Rogers RM. Adult respiratory distress syndrome: changing concepts of lung injury and repair. N Engl J Med 1982;306:900–909.

63. Rivkind AI, Siegel JH, Guadalupi P, Littleton M. Sequential patterns of eicosanoid, platelet and neutophil interactions in the evolution of the fulminant post-traumatic adult respiratory distress syndrome. Ann Surg 1989;210:355–373.

64. Demling RH, Duy N, Manohar M, Proctor R. Comparison between lung fluid filtration rate and measured Starling forces after hemorrhagic and endotoxic shock. J Trauma 1980;20:856–860.

65. Counts RB, Haisch C, Simon TL, Maxwell NG, Heimbach DM, Carrico CJ. Hemostasis in massively transfused trauma patients. Ann Surg 1979;190:91–99.

66. Armistead CW Jr, Vincent J-L, Preiser JC, De-Backer D, Le Mink T. Hypertonic saline solution: hetastarch for fluid resuscitation in experimental septic shock. Anesth Analg 1989;69:714–720.

67. Bernard GR, Luce JM, Sprung CL, Rinaldo JE, Tate RM, Sibbald WJ, Kariman K, Higgins S, Bradley R, Metz CA, Harris TR, Brigham KL. High-dose corticosteroids in patients with the adult respiratory distress syndrome. N Engl J Med 1978; 317:1565–1570.

68. Gurll NJ, Reynolds DG, Holaday JW. Evidence for a role of endorphins in the cardiovascular pathophysiology of primate shock. Crit Care Med 1988;16:521–530.

69. Gelin L-E, Dawidson I. Plasma expanders and hemodilution in the treatment of hypovolemic shock. In Cowley RA, Trump BF (eds): Pathophysiology of Shock, Anoxia, and Ischemia. Baltimore, Williams & Wilkins, 1982, pp 454–463.

70. Kahn RA, Allen RW, Baldassare J. Alternate sources and substitutes for therapeutic blood components. Blood 1985;66:1–12.

71. Tremper KK, Friedman AE, Levine EM, Lapin K, Camarillo D. The preoperative treatment of severely anemic patients with a perfluorochemical oxygen-transport fluid, Fluosol-DA. N Engl J Med 1982;307:277–283.

72. Harrigan C, Lucas CE, Ledgerwood AM, Walz DA, Mammen EF. Serial changes in primary hemostasis after massive transfusion. Surgery 1985; 98:836–844.

73. Martin DJ, Lucas CE, Ledgerwood AM, Hoschner J, McGonigal MD, Grabow D. Fresh frozen plasma supplement to massive red blood cell transfusion. Ann Surg 1985;202:505–511.
74. Young GP, Purcell TB. Emergency autotransfusion. Ann Emerg Med 1983;12:180–186.
75. Clifford PC, Kruger AR, Smith A, Chant AD, Webster JH. Salvage autotransfusion in aortic surgery: initial studies using a disposable reservoir. Br J Surg 1987;74:755–757.
76. Hallett JW Jr, Popovsky M, Ilstrup D. Minimizing blood transfusions during abdominal aortic surgery: recent advances in rapid autotransfusion. J Vasc Surg 1987;5:601–606.
77. Sandmann W, Bruster H, Vossberg H, Schier R, Fudicar U. Autotransfusion in der Aneurysmachirurgie. Langenbecks Arch Chir 1985;366:353–358.
78. Watts C. Disseminated intravascular coagulation. Surg Neurol 1977;8:258–262.
79. Stillman RM, Gottlieb BS, Sawyer PN. Alleviation of autotransfusion-induced haemotological damage by corticosteroids. Br J Surg 1980;67:99–100.
80. Goldfinger D. Acute hemolytic transfusion reactions—a fresh look at pathogenesis and considerations regarding therapy. Transfusion 1977;17:85–98.
81. Snider MT. Adult respiratory distress syndrome in the trauma patient. Crit Care Clin 1990;6:103–110.
82. Grande CM, Ramanathan S, Turndorf H. The structural correlates of airway function. In Bishop MJ, Kirby RR, Brown DL. (eds): Problems in Anesthesia, Volume 2, Physiology and Consequences of Tracheal Intubation. Philadelphia, JB Lippincott, 1988, pp 175–190.
83. Sibille Y, Reynolds HY. Macrophages and polymorphonuclear neutrophils in lung defense and injury. Am Rev Respir Dis 1990;141:471–501.
84. Blaisdell FW. Traumatic shock: the search for a toxic factor. Scudder oration on trauma. Am Coll Surg Bull 1983;68(10):2–10.
85. Burgess AR, Mandelbaum BR. Acute orthopedic injuries. In Siegel JH (ed): Trauma: Emergency Surgery and Critical Care. New York, Churchill Livingstone, 1987, pp 1049–1074.
86. Siegel JH, Stoklosa JC, Borg U, Wiles CE III, Sganga G, Geisler FH, Belzberg H, Wedel S, Blevins S, Goh KC. Quantification of asymmetric lung pathophysiology as a guide to the use of simultaneous independent lung ventilation in posttraumatic and septic adult respiratory distress syndrome. Ann Surg 1985;202:425–439.
87. Borg UR, Stoklosa JC, Siegel JH, Wiles CE II, Belzberg H, Blevins S, Cotter K, Laghi F, Rivkind A. Prospective evaluation of combined high-frequency ventilation in post-traumatic patients with adult respiratory distress syndrome refractory to optimized conventional ventilatory management. Crit Care Med 1989;17:1129–1142.
88. Stene JK. Renal failure in the trauma patient. Crit Care Clin 1990;6:111–119.
89. Shin B, Mackenzie CF, McAslan TC, Helrich M, Cowley RA. Postoperative renal failure in trauma patients. Anesthesiology 1979;51:218–221.
90. Baxter CR. Acute renal insufficiency complicating trauma and surgery. In Shires GT (ed): Principles of Trauma Care, ed 3. New York, McGraw-Hill, 1985, pp 502–511.
91. Shin B, Isenhower NN, McAslan TC, Mackenzie CF, Helrich M. Early recognition of renal insufficiency in post-anesthetic trauma victims. Anesthesiology 1979;50:262–265.

# Blood Component Therapy for Trauma Patients

*Bennett Edelman and Meyer R. Heyman*

The purpose of blood component therapy is to replace clinically significant deficits of cells or plasma proteins. Trauma patients most frequently require red cells to maintain an adequate oxygen carrying capacity, platelets, and coagulation factors to treat clinically significant coagulopathies. All of these components obviously contribute to the maintenance of intravascular volume but should not be used only for that purpose (see also Chapter 4).

Ideally, laboratory tests and clinical observation should be used to assess the presence of significant deficits of cells or plasma proteins. Components containing the needed elements should then be selected in quantities sufficient to reach appropriate target levels. The efficacy of therapy should be monitored by clinical response and laboratory tests.

In practice, the approach to blood component therapy in trauma is more empirical for several reasons: target levels (e.g., hematocrit, platelet count, coagulation factors) are approximate; most available blood components contain multiple constituents; and the turnaround time of laboratory results may not keep pace with rapidly changing patient status. Despite these practical constraints, it is important to strive to define the patient's component needs as specifically as possible, to dose rationally, and to monitor therapy frequently.

# RED CELLS

## Composition of Red Cell Components

### WHOLE BLOOD

A unit of whole blood is 450 ml ± 10%, to which is added approximately 60 ml of anticoagulant-preservative solution, most commonly citrate phosphate dextrose (CPD) or citrate phosphate dextrose with adenine (CPDA-1). Although "fresh" (i.e., unrefrigerated) blood has been used effectively as a source of platelets under battlefield conditions, banked blood is always refrigerated, resulting in significantly reduced platelet viability and function (1–3). For practical purposes, whole blood and red cells refrigerated for even short periods (24 hours or less) must be considered devoid of functional platelets.

The plasma in refrigerated whole blood or packed cells supplies all coagulation factors in essentially normal amounts with the exception of factors V and VIII, which are labile at 4°C. Taking the median of several published studies (4–8), there is a rapid initial drop of factor VIII to 51% after 1 day of storage and a slower decline to 38% and 26% after 1 and 3 weeks, respectively. Factor V declines more slowly, with levels of 98%, 85%, and 45% after 1 day, 1 week, and 3 weeks of storage, respectively (4–7).

### RED CELLS

"Packed" red cells are prepared by the centrifugation or sedimentation of a single unit of whole blood to remove most of the plasma. Approximately 180 ml of red cells are contained in a final volume of 250 ml.

Licensed "additive systems" for the preservation of red cells are now in common use. Blood is collected in a primary anticoagulant-preservative solution. After removing about 85% of the plasma, 100 ml of a second preservative solution are added to the red cells from an integrally attached bag, resulting in a final volume of approximately 350 ml. Red cells so prepared are known officially and labeled as "AS-1 Red Cells" (Adsol; Fenwal Laboratories) or "AS-3 Red Cells" (Nutricel; Cutter Laboratories).

Additive systems have the advantage of longer storage (42 days versus 35 days for CPDA-1 and 21 days for CPD), better flow (viscosity of 1.2 relative to whole blood versus 2.6 for CPDA-1), and larger plasma yield for component preparation. Compared to CPDA-1 red cells, each unit of AS-1 or AS-3 red cells contains a larger load of glucose, sodium, and adenine and is somewhat hyperosmolar (9, 10). (See "Special Considerations in Massive Transfusion" for a discussion of concerns regarding the potential for adenine toxicity and preservation of red cell 2,3-diphosphoglycerate [2,3-DPG].)

### LEUKOCYTE-POOR RED CELLS

Leukocyte-poor ("buffy-poor") red cells are prepared by centrifugation, washing, or filtration to reduce the leukocyte number in the final component to less than $5 \times 10^8$ (about 85% of the leukocytes removed) and to retain at least 80% of the red cells (11). The percentage of leukocytes, red cells, and plasma proteins remaining and the final volume and hematocrit depend on the method of preparation. Leukocyte-poor units are usually reserved for patients with a history of multiple or severe febrile reactions.

## WASHED RED CELLS

Washed red cells are prepared by extensive washing with physiologic saline to remove plasma proteins. Depending on the method used, variable numbers of leukocytes may also be removed. This component is intended for patients with a history of allergic (most commonly urticarial) reactions to plasma proteins.

## FROZEN RED CELLS

Red cells may be frozen in the presence of glycerol, a cryoprotective agent, and stored for years. The freezing, thawing, and deglycerolizing process removes nearly all white cells and plasma protein. This component is used mainly for extended storage of selected red cells (e.g., rare blood types).

### Routine Compatibility Testing

Procedures for routine compatibility tests must comply with federal regulations (12), and most hospitals conform voluntarily to standards set by the American Association of Blood Banks (13, 14). Although commonly thought of as synonymous with the cross-match, compatibility testing also includes ABO and Rh type and the antibody screen.

## ABO GROUP

With extremely rare exceptions, all individuals possess isoagglutinins of the ABO system (i.e., anti-A or anti-B) corresponding to the antigens they lack. These antibodies are potent hemolysins capable of fixing complement in vivo and causing rapid intravascular red cell destruction. If red cells of the identical ABO group are not available,

another group compatible with the recipient's isoagglutinins may be selected (e.g., group A red cells for an AB recipient, group O for any recipient). Out-of-group transfusions must be given as red cells, never as whole blood, because ABO isoagglutinins in the *donor's* plasma may hemolyze the *recipient's* red cells (see "Abbreviation of Compatibility Tests in Emergencies"). In the past, group O whole blood selected to contain low titers of isoagglutinins was used extensively with a good safety record (15), but this is no longer standard practice.

## RH TYPE

"Rh type" in casual parlance refers to the presence or absence of the $Rh_0D$ antigen, one of many antigens in the Rh system. Unlike ABO isoagglutinins, anti-D is formed only in response to immunization by red cells through transfusion or pregnancy. The rationale for routine typing of this antigen is its high immunogenicity. Of all Rh-negative recipients, 80% will be immunized by a single unit transfusion of Rh-positive blood (16). Given the frequency of the D antigen (85%), approximately 10% of all recipients would be immunized by a single ABO-compatible transfusion in the absence of Rh typing.

## ANTIBODY SCREEN AND CROSS-MATCH

Of more than 300 known red cell antigens, routine typing is performed for only ABO and D. Approximately 2 to 3% of sera submitted to large transfusion services contains antibodies other than the expected ABO isoagglutinins (17, 18), so-called "unexpected antibodies." Antibodies to most red cell antigens result from transfusion or pregnancy. The risk of alloimmunization from a single unit of ABO- and D-matched red cells is approximately 1% (19). Other unexpected antibodies occur without red cell exposure, as do those of the ABO system, but in only a small proportion of antigen-negative individuals. The "antibody screen" detects unexpected antibodies by mixing the recipient's serum with group O red cells from two or three individuals chosen to express a wide range of antigens.

These cells are usually obtained from commercial suppliers. A reaction with one or more of the screening cells prompts further testing to identify the specificity of the antibody. In the presence of a negative antibody screen, donor units of the appropriate ABO and Rh type are cross-matched for the recipient. The recipient's serum is mixed with donor red cells. In the absence of agglutination or hemolysis, the units are deemed compatible.

Traditionally, the cross-match has used reaction conditions that allow the detection of a wide variety of antibodies, including ABO isoagglutinins and the host of unexpected antibodies described above. The cross-match serves as a final check of ABO compatibility and detects unexpected antibodies that may have been missed by the antibody screen. The latter function has been shown to have a low yield. In the presence of a negative antibody screen, the probability of detecting an unexpected antibody during a single cross-match is less than 0.1% (17, 18). In consideration of such data, the American Association of Blood Banks and the Food and Drug Administration now recognize an abbreviated or "immediate spin" cross-match as acceptable routine practice if the recipient has no unexpected antibodies demonstrable in the antibody screen and has no prior history of such antibodies. The test may be performed very quickly because the reaction conditions are designed to detect only ABO incompatibility. Individual transfusion services may choose whether to abbreviate the routine cross-match.

If an unexpected antibody is present, the appropriate course of action depends on its specificity. Red cell alloantibodies are considered to be clinically significant if they are known to cause marked shortening of red cell survival in vivo or to pose a risk of hemolytic transfusion reaction. In the presence of such an antibody, red cells that lack the corresponding antigen, in addition to being of the appropriate ABO and Rh type, should be selected. The difficulty of this task depends on the antigen frequency. Even if the unexpected antibody is not demonstrable subsequently, the antigen should be withheld in all future transfusions to avoid stimulation of an anamnestic response, which could cause a delayed hemolytic transfusion reaction (see "Delayed Hemolytic Transfusion Reactions").

Some red cell alloantibodies are not clinically significant as judged by expected increment in hematocrit, lack of apparent adverse reaction, and normal short-term survival of red cells labeled with radioactive chromium (e.g., anti-Chido [20]). Although long-term survival may be measurably reduced, transfusion is beneficial and without adverse clinical consequences (21). If the antigen is of high frequency, it may be necessary to transfuse red cells that are incompatible in vitro but can be expected to produce good clinical outcome. This fact illustrates that the cross-match is a reliable, but not infallible, predictor of in vivo red cell survival. The converse situation of markedly reduced in vivo red cell survival in the presence of negative in vitro serologic studies may occur on rare occasions (22). Short-term chromium survival studies are needed only occasionally to assess the safety of transfusion in routine blood banking practice. The requirement for a stable red cell mass obviates their use in patients who are bleeding actively.

## Abbreviation of Compatibility Tests in Emergencies

The extent to which compatibility tests may be abbreviated is determined on a case-by-case basis, considering both the urgency of the red cell requirement and the risk of incomplete testing. The antibody screen and cross-match are the most time-consuming compatibility tests and, hence, the most likely to be incomplete at the time of emergency transfusion. Once the antibody screen is known to be negative, the probability of cross-match incompatibility resulting from undiscovered irregular antibodies is less than 0.1% per unit (17, 18). There is thus little risk in using an abbreviated cross-match. As discussed previously, this procedure is now considered acceptable in nonemergency situations as well. Failure to complete even an abbreviated cross-match eliminates this last check of ABO compatibility. In the authors' experience, this additional risk is extremely small provided that strict guidelines for patient and sample identification are enforced.

Once the patient has received transfusions approximating the total blood volume, it is an accepted and common practice to abbreviate the cross-match for reasons unrelated to time constraint (23). After what is effectively an exchange transfusion, the pretransfusion sample is no longer representative of the circulating blood. An immediate spin cross-match should be performed to confirm ABO compatibility.

Transfusion before completion of the antibody screen incurs the additional risk of missing unexpected antibodies. Although most severe acute hemolytic reactions are caused by ABO incompatibility, other alloantibodies are capable of causing symptomatic and even fatal hemolysis (24). Excluding those not likely to cause hemolysis, the frequency of potentially significant unexpected antibodies is approximately 1% (17, 18, 25). A history of previous transfusion or pregnancy should bring to mind this possibility. In practice, if the requirement for red cells is truly immediate, they are not withheld pending completion of the antibody screen or even when the screen is found to be positive.

ABO compatibility must always be assured. Un-cross-matched ABO-group-specific red cells can be provided with minimal delay because it takes only minutes to determine the recipient's ABO group. Group-specific red cells have an excellent safety record (26, 27) despite the theoretical risks associated with abbreviated compatibility testing. So-called "universal donor" group O red cells may be given if clinical urgency allows no time even for ABO grouping. The risk of clinically significant hemolysis resulting from transfused anti-A and anti-B is minimized by the use of packed cells, although even small amounts of group O plasma may on rare occasions provoke a hemolytic reaction (28). Clinical experience has shown that the administration of group O red cells is quite safe (29, 30). Indiscriminate use should be avoided, however, to conserve limited supplies. A non-group-O recipient may require continued support with group O cells after the initial transfusion because of passively acquired isoagglutinins (31).

With the exception of a small number of previously alloimmunized patients, the risk of transfusing Rh-positive (D-positive) blood to an Rh-negative individual is not that of immediate hemolysis but, rather, of sensitizing the patient. As noted above, this is a likely outcome. The use of Rh-negative blood is limited by the restricted supply. Group O Rh-negative red cells should be used with extreme discretion when transfusing patients of unknown blood type. Such use is usually restricted to women of child-bearing age. The Rh type is performed with about the same rapidity as the ABO group, so the unnecessary transfusion of Rh-negative blood to Rh-positive individuals can be discontinued quickly. Even for patients who are found to be Rh-negative, continued support with Rh-negative blood may be impossible in the face of severe hemorrhage. (See "Special Considerations in Massive Transfusion" for a discussion of immunoprophylaxis of Rh sensitization.)

### Practical Considerations in Obtaining Samples for Compatibility Testing

The single most important consideration is proper identification of the patient and the specimen. Along with administration of blood to the wrong patient, misidentification of the sample is a major cause of fatal transfusion reactions (32). Proper procedures for specimen identification must always be maintained no matter how grave the emergency. It is also imperative to draw a sample for compatibility tests before any blood is administered. Omission of the pretransfusion sample may occur inadvertently if a supply of group O red cells is maintained in an acute care area. A pretransfusion sample is needed to assure accurate compatibility testing uncomplicated by dilution of antibodies or admixture of foreign cells. In an emergency, rapid delivery of the sample to the blood bank will expedite the transfusion of group-specific red cells. The recipient's ABO group may never be assumed from previous records. The sample should be of adequate volume, free of contamination by intravenous fluids, and unhemolyzed. The presence of hemoglobin may mask immune hemolysis during compatibility testing.

A recently transfused patient may be stimulated to form alloantibodies. To detect newly formed alloantibodies, one must obtain pretransfusion samples for subsequent transfusions within a short time of the anticipated transfusion. An arbitrary but functional limit of 2 to 3 days is in common use (33).

## Indications for Red Cell Administration

The primacy of volume replacement over red cell replacement is widely accepted in the management of acute hemorrhage (33–36) (see Chapter 4). Adequate oxygen delivery can be maintained by a variety of compensatory mechanisms after an acute reduction of hemoglobin concentration, including increased tissue oxygen extraction, increased cardiac output, and redistribution of blood flow (37).

Several animal studies provide information that helps to define, albeit imprecisely, the amount of acute hemorrhage requiring red cell replacement (38–42). One hundred per cent survival was obtained in eight splenectomized dogs treated only with buffered saline (fourfold volume replacement) after experimental hemorrhage of 30% of blood volume (38). In the same study, however, identical treatment of larger hemorrhages resulted in reduced survival after 1 week. Five of the eight animals subjected to 50% hemorrhage survived; none of four animals with 66% hemorrhage survived, all dying within 12 hours. In another study, experimental hemorrhage with colloid re-

placement (dextran 40, dextran 75, or hydroxyethyl starch) in nonsplenectomized dogs resulted in no change of oxygen consumption until hemoglobin levels dropped to 5.5 g/dl, corresponding to approximately 60% hemorrhage (39). Survival was 78 to 84% when the hematocrit was reduced to 10%, corresponding to approximately 80% hemorrhage. After exchange transfusion with albumin, anesthetized, ventilated baboons kept their myocardial oxygen delivery and extraction unchanged down to hematocrits of 10% by means of reduced systemic vascular resistance and increased cardiac output (40). There was net production of myocardial lactate only at hematocrits below 10%. Survival was not studied. The total body oxygen extraction ratio increased sharply from 25 to 50% when the hematocrit dropped below 10% (41). Similarly, normovolemic hemodilution of anesthetized, ventilated dogs to hematocrits of 20% resulted in increased cardiac output with no change in mixed venous $PO_2$ (42).

Clinical observations also support the successful replacement of significant blood loss without red cells. In one retrospective review of operative records, there were 100 patients undergoing a variety of major surgical procedures who had surgical blood losses of 1 to 3 liters (86% between 1 and 1.5 liters) replaced successfully with crystalloid solution (43). Patients refusing blood transfusion for religious reasons have undergone major surgery successfully without red cell replacement (44, 45). In one such series (44), 36 individuals underwent successful coronary artery bypass surgery with average hematocrits of 42% before surgery, 34.4% between 1 and 3 hours after, and 27.1% on discharge. In a similar report (45), 5 of 6 patients survived open heart surgery with preoperative hematocrits of 31 to 45%, falling to 22 to 28% on the 1st postoperative day and 17 to 30% on the 6th postoperative day. Postoperative courses were uneventful except for "marked lassitude" in some patients. Clinical experience with preoperative normovolemic hemodilution as a blood conservation measure also supports the safety of replacing moderate acute blood loss without red cells (46). Volumes in the range of 1500 to 2000 ml may be replaced with albumin immediately before surgery without adverse effect, resulting in hematocrits of 25 to 30%.

In a retrospective series of 94 critically ill postoperative patients, hematocrits in the 27 to 33% range were associated with greater survival than both lower and higher hematocrits (47). Pre- and posttransfusion hemodynamic studies demonstrated that transfusions did not result in significant increments of oxygen consumption when the pretransfusion hematocrit was above 32 to 33%. In a recent prospective study, 25 patients with acute injury and hemorrhage were randomized to have their hematocrits maintained at approximately 30% or 40% (48). There was no hemodynamic benefit at the higher hematocrit over the 3-day period of study. Oxygen consumption and cardiac index were not significantly different between the two groups.

The above-mentioned animal and clinical studies suggest than an acute 30% blood volume loss (approximately 1.5 liters) can usually be replaced without red cells, resulting in a functionally adequate hematocrit of 25 to 30%. Minimal hematocrits of 25% (49) and 30% (50) have been recommended. Hemorrhages in excess of 40 to 50% of blood volume usually require at least partial red cell replacement (33, 51). The need for red cells depends on the integrity of the patient's compensatory mechanisms for increasing oxygen delivery and the response to therapy (37, 52).

Similar flexibility is needed in considering the minimal acceptable hematocrit for the induction of anesthesia. Rigid insistence on 30% (10 g of hemoglobin per dl) is frequent (53) but is unsubstantiated by clinical studies. It is clear that surgery may be performed successfully with lower preoperative hematocrits (54–56). Again, consideration must be given to the individual patient's ability to compensate for reduced

oxygen carrying capacity and the state of tissue oxygen delivery.

A recent National Institutes of Health Consensus Development Conference concluded that, on the basis of current experience, perioperative transfusion is rarely required in otherwise healthy patients with a hemoglobin of 10 g/dl or more and is frequently required in those with acute anemia and a hemoglobin of less than 7 g/dl (57). The panel acknowledged that some patients with chronic anemia or chronic renal failure may tolerate hemoglobin values of less than 7 g/dl.

## Ordering Practices to Improve Utilization of Blood Resources

The "type and screen" and maximal surgical blood order schedule (MSBOS) conserve the finite product and manpower resources of the blood bank by reducing the number of units cross-matched but not transfused.

### TYPE AND SCREEN

The "type and screen" may be used as an alternative to the type and cross-match in situations where the use of red cells is not likely. Although most commonly employed in elective surgery, it may be applied to selected trauma patients whose initial evaluations reveal a low probability of red cell usage. The type and screen consists of ABO and Rh typing and an antibody screen. If the antibody screen is negative, no units are cross-matched. As discussed above, the negative screen excludes unexpected antibodies with a high degree of confidence. Cross-matching of subsequently required units can be expected to proceed quickly. If an emergency need develops, transfusion with an abbreviated cross-match or the use of un-cross-matched, type-specific units can be undertaken with little risk. The requesting physician should notify the blood bank as soon as possible of a change in the patient's status that would make transfusion more likely. The type and screen procedure cannot be applied to alloimmunized patients; appropriately selected antigen-negative units should be cross-matched for them.

## MAXIMAL SURGICAL BLOOD ORDER SCHEDULE

A MSBOS protocol is applicable only to elective surgical procedures. It is simply a list by type of procedure of the expected number of red cell units to be transfused per case. The schedule should be based on data from the particular institution, although published data may be helpful as a guideline (58, 59). The intent of the MSBOS is not to dictate surgical blood orders by arbitrary rules, but to discourage routine cross-matching of blood in excess of the usual transfusion requirement shown by experience. Appropriate blood orders will obviously vary with the specifics of the case.

## COMPONENTS FOR COAGULATION DISORDERS

### Composition of Components Used to Treat Coagulation Disorders

#### PLATELET CONCENTRATE

Each unit is prepared from a single unit of whole blood by the centrifugation and resuspension of platelets in approximately 50 ml of plasma. Permissible storage at 22°C is 5 days. Each unit contains a minimum of 5.5 (average of 7) $\times 10^{10}$ platelets and can be expected to raise the platelet count of a 70-kg adult by approximately 5,000 to 10,000/$\mu$l (60).

Less widely appreciated is the fact that platelet concentrates also contain significant levels of coagulation factors despite their storage at room temperature. One study found no significant decline of fibrinogen and factors II, VII, IX, X, XI, and XII in 32 platelet concentrates stored for 72 hours at 22°C. Heat-labile factors V and VIII declined to 47 ± 18% and 68 ± 22% (mean ± SD) of normal, respectively (61). These findings have been confirmed by other investigators (62, 63). Four units of platelet concentrate stored for up to 72 hours thus provide the nonlabile factors found in approximately 1 unit of fresh frozen plasma. The labile factors are present at lower, but still hemostatic, levels. Permissible 22°C platelet storage has been extended from 3 to 5 days since these data were collected. A recent study examined factor levels in platelet concentrates stored at 22°C for up to 7 days (64). After 5 days factors II, VII, IX, X, and XI were somewhat reduced, with mean levels of at least 69%. The labile factors V and VIII were markedly reduced, with mean levels of 26% and 32%, respectively. There was some further deterioration after 7 days. Only fibrinogen levels were stable for the entire study period.

#### FRESH FROZEN PLASMA

Each unit is prepared by centrifugation from a single unit of whole blood. The plasma must be separated and cooled to −18°C within 6 hours and may be stored at this temperature for 1 year. The product should be used within 6 hours after thawing at 37°C. The total volume is 200 to 250 ml.

Freezing preserves normal levels of all coagulation factors, including factors V and VIII, which are labile at room or refrigerator temperatures. Pooled plasma by definition contains 100% (1 unit/ml) of all factors. Thus, an average of about 200 units of each factor should be present. Typical normal ranges for coagulation factors, however, are 50 to 150% (0.5 to 1.5 units/ml), so there may be considerable variation between units. The normal fibrinogen content ranges from 160 to 360 mg/dl, with a mean of 260 mg/dl (in-house data). A unit of fresh frozen plasma is expected to contain an average of 500 mg of fibrinogen, which again is subject to considerable interindividual variation.

Some blood centers are now supplying a product called "plasma frozen within 24 hours" in lieu of fresh frozen plasma. The plasma is refrigerated, then frozen solid at −18°C within 24 hours (instead of 6 hours). The extra time allows more flexibility in transporting blood from outside collection sites. This product contains about two-thirds to three-fourths of the factor VIII in fresh frozen plasma and essentially identical levels of all other coagulation factors (4–8, 65).

## CRYOPRECIPITATE

Each unit consists of the cold-insoluble material remaining when a unit of fresh frozen plasma is allowed to thaw at 4°C. The precipitate is refrozen and stored for up to 1 year at a maximum of −18°C. After thawing at 37°C, it must be infused within 6 hours. The total volume is 10 to 15 ml. Multiple units are usually pooled by the blood bank and dispensed in a single container.

Cryoprecipitate contains both the procoagulant and platelet adhesive (i.e., von Willebrand factor) activities of factor VIII, fibrinogen, and factor XIII. Each unit (i.e., bag) contains an average of 145 units of factor VIII procoagulant activity (minimum of 80 units required) and 265 mg of fibrinogen, although content may vary significantly with the method of preparation (66). Given an average plasma volume and the 50% in vivo recovery of fibrinogen (67), 1 unit is expected to raise the fibrinogen level approximately 5 mg/dl in a 70-kg individual.

## FACTOR CONCENTRATES

Purified factor VIII and prothrombin complex (II, VII, IX, and X) concentrates are manufactured from large plasma pools. The assayed factor VIII or IX content is specified. The concentrates are stored in lyophilized form at 4°C and reconstituted immediately before use. Unlike plasma and cryoprecipitate, factor VIII concentrate does not provide von Willebrand factor activity.

### Antigenic Considerations

Fresh frozen plasma and cryoprecipitate contain ABO isoagglutinins and should be selected to be ABO-compatible with the recipient's red cells whenever possible. In practice, the use of incompatible plasma is limited to emergency requirements that cannot be met by the existing inventory of compatible units. It is less critical that ABO-compatible cryoprecipitate be dis-

pensed because of the much smaller volume. Factor VIII concentrate may also contain ABO isoagglutinins, resulting in rare hemolytic reactions (68, 69). The possibility of hemolysis from passive transfusion of other antibodies in plasma products is minimized by performing an antibody screen on donated units. Those containing unexpected antibodies are processed only into those components containing minimal amounts of plasma.

ABO compatibility is desirable, but not required, for platelet concentrates. There is a small (20–25%), but not clinically significant, reduction in the recovery of ABO-incompatible platelets (70, 71). Only occasionally can refractoriness to platelet transfusions be attributed to recipient ABO isoagglutinins (72, 73). The amount of red cell contamination is ordinarily less than 0.5 ml (74), an amount insufficient to cause a hemolytic reaction. Significant hemolytic reactions provoked by transfused isoagglutinins in platelet concentrates have been reported but are unusual (75). The most significant immunologic consideration in platelet transfusion is the development of refractoriness because of alloimmunization to histocompatibility antigens of the human leukocyte antigen (HLA) system or platelet-specific antigens. Alloimmunization is most likely to occur in chronically transfused patients.

Platelets and plasma products are ordinarily selected without regard for Rh type. Platelets do not express Rh antigens. Anti-D may develop, however, in D-negative recipients of D-positive platelet concentrates (74) because of contaminating red cells and has been reported rarely in D-negative recipients of large volumes of D-positive liquid stored plasma (76). (See "Special Considerations in Massive Transfusion" for a discussion of the administration of Rh-immune globulin.)

## COAGULOPATHY IN THE TRAUMA PATIENT

A trauma patient, like any other patient,

may have underlying inherited or acquired coagulopathies unrelated to injuries sustained. This discussion will be limited to two entities of particular importance in trauma patients, i.e., the dilutional coagulopathy associated with massive transfusion and disseminated intravascular coagulation (DIC) (see also Chapter 4).

## Dilutional Coagulopathy

Massive transfusion is commonly defined as the administration within a 24-hour period of a volume of blood approximating the recipient's total blood volume (approximately 10 units in an average size adult) (77). Massive transfusion for severe hemorrhage represents an exchange transfusion. A reduction is expected in the concentration of all constituents not present at normal levels in transfused blood products. Factors V and VIII are labile in refrigerated red cells and whole blood and are therefore expected to decline on a dilutional basis. All other coagulation factors are stable. Refrigerated whole blood or red cells should also be considered devoid of functional platelets (see "Whole Blood" above). Using a simple model in which the intravascular space is considered to be isolated from other fluid compartments, the decline of unreplaced constituents is an exponential function of the volume exchanged. This model predicts that 37% of unreplaced constituents will remain after a single blood-volume exchange (typically 10 units of whole blood or 10 units of packed cells given with other fluids), 14% after a two-volume exchange (78).

A number of studies have addressed hemostasis in massively transfused patients (4, 29, 79–84). These studies cannot be compared directly because of a number of important differences, including patient selection, average volume transfused, types of components used, and attempts in some (but not in others) to distinguish surgical from nonsurgical bleeding or dilutional from other coagulopathies (e.g., DIC, liver disease). A number of generalities can nevertheless be made.

It is generally agreed that thrombocytopenia occurs in proportion to the volume transfused (4, 29, 79–82) but to a lesser degree than predicted by a simple exponential "washout" (79, 83). Platelet counts lower than 50,000 are unusual in patients transfused with fewer than 15 to 20 units (4, 79, 81, 82). Patients with clinically impaired hemostasis are more likely to have received large transfusions, often in excess of 20 units (4, 79, 81), to have platelet counts of less than $100,000/\mu l$ (83) or 50,000 to $60,000/\mu l$ (79, 84, 85), and to respond clinically to the administration of platelets (4, 7, 9). However, many patients with similar transfusion volumes and platelet counts do not have abnormal bleeding.

Bleeding has also been found in patients with platelet counts higher than those usually associated with significant hemorrhage. In the study by Counts et al., for example, four of eight patients with generalized bleeding had platelet counts of at least 70,000 and hemostatic levels of fibrinogen and factors V and VIII (4). Platelet dysfunction may contribute to impaired hemostasis in such patients (79, 80, 86), but its role is difficult to assess. Although prolonged bleeding times occur in most massively transfused patients, they do not predict clinical bleeding (4, 79, 87). Abnormal platelet aggregation has also been demonstrated in massive transfusion (80, 87) but does not appear to correlate with clinical bleeding (87).

A significant relationship between the volume transfused and prolongation of the prothrombin time (PT) or partial thromboplastin time (PTT) has been found in some studies (79, 81, 82) but not in others (29, 80). Unless marked, prolongation of the PT or PTT is not helpful in predicting microvascular bleeding. Levels of 1.5 (4) and 1.8 (85) times the control value have been reported to be predictive of bleeding.

Neither factor V nor factor VIII deficiency is likely to be the cause of a hemorrhagic diathesis in the massively transfused patient on the basis of dilutional coagulopathy alone. Levels of both factors seem to be adequate for hemostasis in the vast majority of cases (4, 80, 85). A statistically significant correlation between factor V and VIII levels and the volume transfused was demonstrated in one study (4) but not in another (80). Even in the former study, however, the correlation coefficient was low and neither factor level could be predicted reliably from the volume transfused in an individual patient. Eighty-five per cent of the total variance in factor VIII levels in this study was attributable to factors other than the transfusion volume. Mobilization of endogenous factor VIII stores may account for the higher than expected factor VIII levels in massively transfused patients. The presence or absence of DIC is also an important determinant of factor VIII levels (80). The lack of clinically significant factor V deficiency in massively transfused patients is probably explained by the maintenance of reduced, but hemostatic, levels of factor V in whole blood or red cells even after 21 days of refrigerated storage (4–7).

In summary, thrombocytopenia is the most reproducible manifestation of dilutional coagulopathy in the massively transfused patient and is the most likely cause of bleeding. Clinically significant thrombocytopenia is more likely at transfusion volumes in excess of 15 to 20 units. Functional platelet abnormalities may also contribute to the hemorrhagic diathesis in at least some instances. Although a reduction of the levels of the labile clotting factors V and VIII may occur with very large transfusion volumes, deficiencies of these factors are rarely severe enough to account for clinical bleeding in the absence of DIC.

The exponential decline of platelets and labile coagulation factors predicted by the one-compartment exchange transfusion model is probably mitigated by a number of mechanisms, including mobilization of extravascular stores and administration of some functional platelets and coagulation factors in refrigerated whole blood and red cells. The lack of consistent correlation

between transfusion volume and bleeding is most likely related to the variable occurrence of DIC (the latter consequent to severe tissue injury and shock). In many cases, bleeding more probably results from DIC than from the dilutional effects of massive transfusion per se (4, 81, 83, 84, 88, 89).

## Disseminated Intravascular Coagulation

### ETIOLOGY AND PATHOGENESIS

DIC is a pathologic process resulting from overwhelming activation of the coagulation mechanism via either intrinsic (Hageman factor-activated) or extrinsic (tissue thromboplastin-activated) pathways (90–92). Central to this process is the generation of thrombin, which results in consumption of fibrinogen and other coagulation factors (V, VIII) as well as platelets. Invariably, there is simultaneous activation of the fibrinolytic system with generation of active plasmin, which results not only in the lysis of fibrin clots, but also in the degradation of native fibrinogen and other coagulation factors, further aggravating the consumptive process. Although activation of the fibrinolytic mechanism may be compensatory in terms of lysing fibrin deposited in the microcirculation and thus restoring tissue perfusion, the fibrin-fibrinogen split products (FSPs) that result from the action of plasmin on fibrin and native fibrinogen may interfere not only with fibrin monomer polymerization but also with platelet function (90, 91). The net result is a hemorrhagic diathesis consequent to hypofibrinogenemia (and other coagulation factor depletion) and thrombocytopenia aggravated by the circulating anticoagulant-like effects of the FSPs. Despite the fact that the initial event in DIC is thrombotic in nature (i.e., the deposition of fibrin in the microcirculation), the syndrome is almost always recognized clinically as a diffuse bleeding tendency (90–93). Many different stimuli may result in the development of DIC in the critical care setting, including infection, obstetric disasters (placental abruption, amniotic fluid embolism), malignancy (acute leukemia), penetrating head injury (gunshot wounds), and incompatible blood transfusions, to name but a few. A number of exhaustive lists of clinical conditions associated with DIC have been published previously (93–96). In the setting of massive trauma, however, DIC results from the occurrence of extensive tissue injury, with resultant thromboplastin release, in the face of hypotension and acidosis (90, 94, 97).

## CLINICAL FINDINGS

The trauma surgeon or critical care specialist should first be alerted to the possibility of the development of DIC when a diffuse bleeding tendency is noted. In addition to often uncontrollable bleeding at sites of major injury or in surgical fields, bleeding may occur at sites of arterial puncture and central venous lines and via Foley catheters and nasogastric tubes. Due to excessive fibrinolysis, bleeding may occur at incision sites where hemostasis previously seemed adequate. Although signs of cerebral, pulmonary, and renal dysfunction (coma, adult respiratory distress syndrome, oliguria) have been attributed to fibrin deposition in the microcirculation (91, 97), such clinical findings may in large part be related to hypotension and tissue ischemia resulting from major blood loss or sepsis (98). Although thrombotic events are less frequently recognized clinically (90, 91, 97), cutaneous infarction, acral gangrene, and major arterial and venous thromboses do occur (93, 96, 97).

## LABORATORY DIAGNOSIS

Unfortunately, no single laboratory parameter allows one to make the diagnosis of DIC with certainty (90, 96, 99). A number of combinations of abnormal laboratory values have been touted as being diagnostic of this syndrome. Regardless of what combination of laboratory tests one uses to confirm the clinical suspicion of DIC, the laboratory values must be interpreted in light of the patient's underlying disease (e.g., liver or bone marrow dysfunction) and the extent of recent transfusion.

The commonly used screening tests of coagulation, the PTT (which measures the intrinsic coagulation system) and the PT (which measures the extrinsic system) are most often prolonged in patients with DIC as a result of deficiencies of fibrinogen as well as other coagulation factors. Although some investigators have suggested that the PTT is more sensitive to the presence of DIC than the PT (90), such differences have not been present in other series (91). The PTT is quite sensitive to the presence of heparin, and trace amounts of heparin in heparinized venous or arterial lines may falsely prolong the PTT. Although deficiencies of multiple coagulation factors can be demonstrated by specific factor assay, such assays are time-consuming, are not readily available on an urgent basis, and probably add little to diagnostic accuracy (93, 96).

Fibrinogen levels are typically low in patients with acute DIC. One must remember, however, that fibrinogen is an acute phase reactant, increasing after many stimuli (e.g., trauma and infection) (100, 101). Fibrinogen may be substantially elevated before the onset of coagulopathy, so that a normal fibrinogen value does not rule out the presence of DIC.

The platelet count is typically decreased in the patient with DIC. The thrombocytopenia may be of considerable magnitude, as evidenced by the finding of petechiae and purpura. Preexisting infections and inflammatory states, as well as acute blood loss, may be associated with significant thrombocytosis; therefore, a precipitous fall in the platelet count consequent to DIC may result in an apparent "normal" value. Moreover, the possibility of impaired marrow function contributing to the thrombocytopenia must be considered when DIC is suspected in situations where impaired thrombopoiesis may be present (folate or $B_{12}$ deficiency, marrow infiltration with tumor, leukemia, and chronic alcoholism). Also, the precipitous development of marked thrombocytopenia frequently accompanies septicemia, even in the absence of other evidence of DIC (102).

Because of the invariable activation of the

fibrinolytic system, FSPs are typically increased in the serum of patients with DIC (91, 103). Rapid semiquantitative assays are widely available. The presence of FSPs at levels of less than 40 μg/ml occur in a number of situations unassociated with DIC, such as the presence of extravascular hematomas, large intravascular thrombi, and liver disease. Levels above 40 μg/ml are more likely to be associated with DIC (91).

The simple observation of rapid dissolution of a clot formed in a glass tube may also alert one to the possibility of excessive fibrinolysis in DIC (90). A more standardized assay, such as the euglobulin lysis time, has also been used to demonstrate the presence of excess fibrinolysis, but this test may be normal in the presence of DIC, is time-consuming, is not usually available on an emergency basis, and adds nothing to diagnostic accuracy (90, 91, 93).

Because thrombin activation is central to the development of DIC, a number of laboratory procedures have been developed to demonstrate the presence of products resulting from thrombin-specific cleavage of fibrinogen. So-called "paracoagulation" tests, such as the ethanol gelation and protamine sulfate precipitation tests, which demonstrate the presence of unpolymerized fibrin monomer forming complexes with fibrinogen, are either too insensitive or too nonspecific to be of diagnostic value in DIC (90, 91, 99). Assays are also available to measure the presence of fibrinopeptide A released by the specific action of thrombin on fibrinogen, but elevations are not specific for DIC (91). Although antithrombin III levels are frequently decreased in DIC (91, 103), such decreases may be found in other conditions (hepatic failure, thromboembolism congenital deficiency) and are not specific for DIC.

Despite the difficulties of interpreting the laboratory data, the presence of hypofibrinogenemia, thrombocytopenia, and marked elevation of the FSPs in a patient with a known precipitating cause of DIC and clinical evidence of a diffuse hemorrhagic diathesis provides convincing evidence for the presence of DIC and should warrant therapy. Colman et al. presented evidence that, in the absence of severe liver disease or dilutional coagulopathy consequent to massive transfusion, the finding of hypofibrinogenemia, a prolonged PT, and thrombocytopenia was diagnostic of DIC (91). Laboratory evidence for elevated FSPs was invariably present when all three of these screening tests were abnormal.

In the presence of advanced liver disease, one must be particularly careful in evaluating many of the aforementioned tests when attempting to establish the diagnosis of DIC. Indeed, hypofibrinogenemia, a prolonged PT, and low levels of a number of coagulation factors (II, V, VII, IX, X) may result from inadequate hepatic synthesis and may be misinterpreted as being due to DIC. Moderate thrombocytopenia (due to congestive splenomegaly) and elevated FSPs may be found as well. To confuse the issue further, patients with liver disease are at increased risk of developing DIC, given the proper stimulus, because of inadequate synthesis of inhibitors of coagulation and fibrinolysis such as antithrombin III, protein C, and $\alpha_2$-antiplasmin. Impairment of the normal reticuloendothelial clearance of activated procoagulants and FSPs further predisposes to the development of DIC.

The potential for dilutional coagulopathy must be taken into consideration when attempting to establish the diagnosis of DIC in massively transfused patients. Patients with massive trauma and shock who are at the greatest risk for DIC are also those who are likely to require replacement with large volumes of blood. Significant hypofibrinogenemia should not occur in the massively transfused patient receiving whole blood because fibrinogen is quite stable under conditions of refrigeration. It is possible that significant hypofibrinogenemia could occur in patients whose blood loss has been replaced with packed cells and volume expanders (colloids or crystalloids) devoid of coagulation factors. No firm data exist, however, to confirm that this is the case. Although moderate degrees of thrombocytopenia are often seen after the transfusion of 15 to 20 units of packed cells (4), the finding of severe thrombocytopenia (less than 50,000) in a patient who has received fewer than 10 units of blood is distinctly unusual in the absence of DIC (4, 79, 81, 82).

## Practical Diagnosis and Management

It is apparent that no single strategy for coagulation factor replacement is applicable to all massively transfused individuals. Each patient must be evaluated individually with close attention to the extent of injuries, the volume of blood transfused, the presence or absence of shock, the presence or absence of continued bleeding, and the type of fluids used for volume resuscitation. Prompt restoration of circulatory volume with prevention or reversal of hypoxia, acidosis, and resultant DIC is of far greater importance in preventing uncontrolled bleeding in the massively transfused patient than is the prophylactic administration of fresh frozen plasma and platelet concentrates. The surgeon or traumatologist must be careful to distinguish bleeding due to inadequate surgical hemostasis from a diffuse hemorrhagic diathesis. In the latter instance, bleeding will be noted from multiple sites, such as indwelling venous lines, nasogastric tubes, and endotracheal tubes, as well as from operative sites. In patients with extensive soft tissue and visceral injury, such a distinction may be difficult if not impossible. The decision to administer fresh frozen plasma, cryoprecipitate, or platelets should not be based only on the volume transfused but rather on the surgeon's estimate of the presence or absence of diffuse microvascular bleeding and supporting laboratory data when available.

## MANAGEMENT OF DILUTIONAL COAGULOPATHY

Immediately upon the patient's arrival at the trauma center, a PT, PTT, fibrinogen, and platelet count should be obtained. The finding of hypofibrinogenemia and thrombocytopenia in a diffusely bleeding patient early in the posttrauma period before a significant amount of blood has been transfused is indicative of the presence of DIC and should be treated as discussed below. Although empiric prophylactic administration of fresh frozen plasma and platelet concentrates has been recommended to prevent bleeding from dilutional coagulopathy in the massively transfused patient (49, 52), there is no convincing clinical (29, 82, 83, 104, 105) or experimental (106) evidence that such therapy is beneficial. The use of fresh frozen plasma solely for the purpose of volume expansion is unnecessary and potentially harmful. Volume expansion can be accomplished just as effectively with alternative products such as albumin and plasma protein fraction (105), which do not carry the risk of infectious disease transmission.

If diffuse microvascular bleeding becomes apparent during the course of massive transfusion, the empiric administration of platelet concentrate (6 to 8 units) is justified as an initial maneuver. This is especially true if the patient has received more than 15 to 20 units of blood—an amount at which thrombocytopenia is likely to be the cause of bleeding (4, 79). Ideally, the presence of thrombocytopenia should be documented with a platelet count before platelet administration, but platelets should not be withheld from a patient with diffuse bleeding pending the availability of lab results. A platelet count should be obtained immediately before and 10 minutes after platelet infusion to document that an increment has indeed occurred. One unit of platelet concentrate is expected to raise the platelet count 5,000 to 10,000/µl in a 70-kg adult. Continued bleeding, ongoing DIC, or active sepsis may severely blunt the response to platelet transfusion. These conditions must be considered in any patient not achieving a sustained rise in platelet count after platelet transfusion. Although spontaneous hemorrhage rarely occurs with platelet counts above 50,000/µl, a count of 75,000/µl is generally considered to be adequate for surgical hemostasis in most instances (107, 108). Because platelet functional abnormalities and other coagulation disturbances may be present in the massively transfused patient, it is conceivable that higher platelet counts may be necessary for adequate hemostasis in some patients. At the Shock Trauma Center, platelet counts are maintained at 100,000/µl in situations where diffuse microvascular bleeding could be particularly catastrophic (e.g., head trauma). Admittedly, there are no systematic data to support this practice.

If bleeding is uncontrolled after platelet transfusion, the decision to administer fresh frozen plasma should be based on the results of coagulation studies whenever feasible. PT and PTT values greater than 1.5 times control are more likely to be associated with generalized bleeding (4, 29) and may warrant therapy with fresh frozen plasma.

The optimal dose of fresh frozen plasma in this setting has not been determined. Rapid administration of 800 ml to a 70-kg individual has been suggested (109). Similar doses, approximately 10 to 15 ml/kg, have been recommended to treat multiple factor deficiencies in other clinical settings (e.g., liver disease and bleeding associated with coumarin therapy (110, 111). Assuming a plasma volume of 40 ml/kg, 100% activity of all factors in fresh frozen plasma, and 80% in vivo recovery, a dose of 15 ml/kg is expected to raise all factor levels by about 20%. In practice, administration of fresh frozen plasma to patients with multiple factor deficiencies results in quite variable increments of factor levels (112, 113).

It is important to recognize that the infusion of 6 units of platelet concentrate provides approximately 300 ml of plasma (stored for 5 days or less at room temperature) containing significant amounts of all the coagulation factors (see "Platelet Concentrate" above). Thus, patients who receive large amounts of platelet concentrate are at the same time receiving significant coagulation factor replacement, which should be taken into account when assessing the requirement for fresh frozen plasma.

The failure of fresh frozen plasma administration to improve the PT and PTT and to decrease bleeding suggests ongoing consumption secondary to DIC. A prolonged PTT and PT may reflect hypofibrinogenemia associated with DIC, in which case administration of cryoprecipitate as a concentrated source of fibrinogen may be indicated. A unit of cryoprecipitate (10 to 15 ml) contains approximately 250 mg of fibrinogen and can be expected to raise the fibrinogen level about 5 mg/dl in a 70-kg individual. Fibrinogen concentrations of 100 mg/dl should be adequate for hemostasis (114).

If bleeding from a particular site persists despite laboratory-documented correction of platelet count and coagulation factor repletion, a surgically correctable source of bleeding must be sought vigorously.

Virtually all of the studies addressing the need for plasma in massive transfusion (4, 79, 83) have included patients transfused predominantly with whole blood or modified whole blood (blood from which cryoprecipitate and/or platelets have been removed). Trauma victims whose blood loss has been replaced with packed red cells and colloid or crystalloid solutions devoid of coagulation factors could conceivably require more support with plasma products (e.g., fresh frozen plasma and cryoprecipitate). For this reason, some authors have recommended that whole blood or modified whole blood be used for at least a portion of the red cell replacement in patients receiving massive transfusion (4). Little whole blood is available at the Shock Trauma Center—a common situation because of the practice of processing most whole blood into components. The transfusion of nearly equal quantities of red cells and fresh frozen plasma in some cases indicates a perceived need to administer the equivalent of whole blood to at least selected patients (115).

The optimal coagulation factor therapy for the massively transfused patient remains to be established. Ideally, such therapy should maintain hemostasis, avoid unnecessary plasma exposure (with the attendant risks of allergic reactions and infectious disease transmission), minimize the number of donor exposures, and make the most efficient use of blood resources. Further studies are required to define more accurately (a) the need for coagulation factor replacement in patients receiving massive transfusions with packed cells and colloid or crystalloid solutions and (b) the role of whole blood or modified whole blood. If routine replacement of stable coagulation factors is necessary, it would be preferable to use whole instead of packed cells and fresh frozen plasma. The reduced number of donor exposures may result in reduced infectious disease transmission. Modified whole blood makes more efficient use of donor resources because platelets and cryoprecipitate (containing factor VIII and fibrinogen) can be removed and made available as separate components. The therapeutic efficacy of modified whole blood is likely to be similar to that of whole blood because platelets and factor VIII are lost rapidly from the latter on refrigerated storage and only about half of the fibrinogen is removed by separation of platelet concentrate and cryoprecipitate.

## MANAGEMENT OF DIC

Vigorous and immediate correction of the precipitating stimulus remains the cornerstone of therapy for DIC. In patients with severe trauma and tissue injury, prompt volume repletion and reversal of hypotension, hypoxia, and acidosis are of paramount importance in arresting the acute consumptive process. Failure to pay strict attention to maintaining tissue perfusion will result in failure to control the coagulopathy, regardless of what other measures are used, and will invariably result in the patient's demise. In patients with overwhelming sepsis, appropriate antibiotic treatment is equally critical if the coagulopathy is to be controlled and the patient is to survive.

Once the provocative stimulus has been treated appropriately, repletion of the depleted platelets and coagulation factors with platelet concentrates, fresh frozen plasma,

and/or cryoprecipitate (rich in fibrinogen and factor VIII) should be undertaken to control any ongoing bleeding. Although it has been argued that administration of clotting factors may only serve to "fuel the fire" and result in the generation of more thrombin to perpetuate the process, there are few data to suggest that this in fact occurs (90, 99). In the bleeding patient in whom DIC is self-limited or has been stopped with appropriate therapy, repletion of platelets and clotting factors may in fact be all that is necessary to promote hemostasis (99). Persistent local bleeding in a patient in whom platelet and fibrinogen levels have been corrected with component transfusion should alert one to the possibility of a surgical bleeding site.

The use of heparin has been advocated for persistently bleeding patients when vigorous treatment of their precipitating process and component therapy have failed to result in a sustained rise in platelet count and fibrinogen level. Theoretically, the antithrombin effect of heparin should halt the consumptive process if adequate amounts of antithrombin III (heparin cofactor) are available. Considerable controversy, however, exists as to the appropriateness of heparin therapy in acute DIC (90, 91, 95–97, 99, 103). Although some studies have shown better control of bleeding and improved survival in patients treated with heparin, these studies are nonrandomized and uncontrolled (91, 93, 95, 103). Although heparin seems to have benefit in the more indolent chronic DIC states, such as those associated with a retained dead fetus and mucus-producing adenocarcinomas (91, 93), the benefits of heparin in acute DIC are much less certain (98, 116, 117). Although heparin could conceivably improve tissue perfusion by preventing further deposition of fibrin in the microcirculation, clinically apparent organ dysfunction often attributed to DIC may, as previously noted, be more often a result of the derangement that precipitated the DIC initially.

It is the authors' opinion that heparin has little or no place in the management of acute

DIC associated with massive trauma. Initial management should include prompt correction of the metabolic and hemodynamic derangements of the shock state (see Chapter 4) followed by platelet and clotting factor (fresh frozen plasma/cryoprecipitate) repletion to control bleeding. Patients who fail to respond to these maneuvers are likely to succumb to their underlying disorder rather than to the complications of the coagulopathy. Heparin may aggravate established hemorrhage in acute DIC. Its use is especially dangerous in situations such as gunshot wounds of the brain, where DIC is most often self-limited and bleeding aggravated by heparin could be catastrophic.

Antifibrinolytic agents (e.g., $\epsilon$-aminocaproic acid) theoretically should stabilize existing thrombi to promote hemostasis and prevent further generation of potentially deleterious FSPs. However, the use of antifibrinolytic agents without antecedent heparinization is to be avoided because it may allow the development of progressive tissue ischemia resulting from unopposed fibrin deposition (92, 93).

Studies of Gram-negative sepsis in animal models have demonstrated an improvement of coagulation parameters, metabolic derangements, and organ damage associated with DIC when antithrombin III concentrates are given prophylactically (118). The results of human studies of antithrombin III in preventing the morbidity and mortality associated with DIC remain conflicting. Most reports of a beneficial effect of antithrombin III in DIC are uncontrolled and include only a small number of patients with different provocative illnesses of variable severity (119, 120). In some instances, the use of antithrombin III has resulted in improvement of the coagulation profile without a definite corresponding improvement of survival (121–123). Such an outcome is not surprising because the morbidity and mortality of DIC largely reflect the nature, severity, and adequacy of treatment of the precipitating illness.

In a randomized study comparing heparin, antithrombin III alone, and the combination of antithrombin III and heparin in 51 patients with shock and DIC, Blauhut et al. found that antithrombin III alone was as effective in facilitating improvement in the coagulation abnormalities as was the combination of heparin and antithrombin III. Moreover, the addition of heparin resulted in aggravation of hemorrhage (122). No significant difference in mortality could be demonstrated among the three treatment groups. A Japanese study comparing the use of antithrombin III and a synthetic protease inhibitor in 77 women with DIC related to obstetric problems found antithrombin III (without heparin) to be superior in terms of clinical improvement and reversal of coagulopathy. Unfortunately, no untreated control group was included. Among 77 patients only 3 deaths occurred, and these 3 patients had the most severe disease by the scoring system used (123).

At present, the efficacy of antithrombin III administration to severely ill patients with DIC remains uncertain. Larger and better controlled studies including more homogeneous populations and using survival as an endpoint are necessary to determine whether antithrombin III is truly of benefit in DIC. Although antithrombin III concentrates of high purity and safety have been developed, they are not currently licensed in the United States (124).

## SPECIAL CONSIDERATIONS IN MASSIVE TRANSFUSION

### Mechanics of Administration

#### INFUSION DEVICES

The diameter of the needle is the rate-limiting component of the standard blood infusion set and becomes more restrictive as the infusion pressure increases (125). Maximal gravity-driven flow with a 3-foot elevation of the blood container is approximately 40 ml/min with a 17 gauge needle and approximately 80 ml/min with a 15 gauge needle (125, 126). External compression bags increase flow without causing unacceptable hemolysis (127, 128). Flow rates of 150 to 200 ml/min have been reported for whole blood transfused through a 15 gauge needle at 300 mm Hg (127). Higher pressures are not recommended (128) (see Chapter 4).

Higher flow rates may be achieved using large bore catheters or introducers instead of needles. Rates of 300 to 400 ml/min have been reported for whole blood or diluted packed cells (hematocrit, approximately 45) administered under 200 to 300 mm Hg pressure through a 10 gauge Angiocath or 8 French catheter introducer (129, 130). Large bore intravenous tubing has been recommended by some investigators because the tubing diameter may become rate-limiting when large bore catheters are used (131).

Even higher flow rates may be achieved with specially designed rapid administration systems and large bore catheters. Flow rates up to 2000 ml/min were reported for diluted blood (hematocrit, 28%) administered through two 10 gauge catheters with a pump-driven system developed for transplant surgery (132). Flows up to 1600 ml/min were obtained for packed cells diluted with an equal volume of crystalloid (expected hematocrit, about 35%) administered at 300 mm Hg pressure with a special high-flow administration set through a single 8.5 French catheter (133).

There is an approximately exponential decline in flow rate as the concentration of red cells increases from that of whole blood to that of packed cells (126). The addition of 100 to 200 ml of physiologic saline to a unit of red cells results in a net reduction in the time required for transfusion by increasing flow rate disproportionately to the added volume. Red cells collected in the newer additive systems (i.e., AS-1 and AS-3) already have a relative viscosity similar to that of whole blood (10). Flow rates of AS-1 red cells and CPDA-1 whole blood are similar, resulting in shorter flow times per unit for AS-1 because of the smaller volume (approximately 320 ml versus 520 ml) (134).

## WARMERS

The rapid infusion of even 4 to 5 units of cold blood may result in a significant lowering of core temperature as measured with an esophageal probe at the level of the cardiac atria. Cardiac arrhythmias and cardiac arrest, as well as generalized vasoconstriction and prolonged recovery from anesthesia, may result (135, 136) (see Chapter 13). Use of warmed blood results in a significantly reduced frequency of cardiac arrest in patients receiving 3 liters or more of banked blood at a rate of at least 50 ml/min (137). Blood must be warmed to no more than 38°C (138). Warming should be accomplished distal to the blood container by means of a temperature-controlled water bath or plate warmer (138). Rapid infusion systems usually incorporate high-efficiency warmers to prevent hypothermia at high flow rates (132, 133). To prevent overheating (with resultant hemolysis), warmers must be equipped with a visual temperature monitor and be subject to regular quality control. An audible alarm is desirable (138, 139).

Preliminary in vitro studies suggest that 70°C saline may be added directly to red cells to produce rapid warming without hemolysis or a change in osmotic fragility (140). In vivo studies have not been published. This method of warming is not currently considered acceptable practice.

## COMPATIBLE INTRAVENOUS SOLUTIONS

Only physiologic (0.9%) saline may be added to blood products (138). Calcium-containing solutions (e.g., Ringer's lactate) may antagonize the effects of citrate and result in clot formation. Dextrose solutions, including 5% dextrose and 5% dextrose in 0.225% saline, may result in red cell clumping and hemolysis (141). The use of incompatible solutions to prime the blood infusion set (via a "Y" connector) should be avoided. "Washout" of the priming solution may require several hundred milliliters of blood, resulting in prolonged contact of the incompatible fluid with red cells and possible hemolysis (141).

## FILTERS

A standard blood filter with a 170- to

260-μm pore size is required for all transfusions (142). These filters do not remove smaller particles (microaggregates) that form in stored blood and red cells. Small quantities of microaggregates form during approximately the 2nd to 5th day of storage of citrated blood. These consist primarily of platelet aggregates in which are admixed small numbers of leukocytes (143–145). An accelerated rate of microaggregate formation occurs after about the 7th day of storage, coinciding with the incorporation of increasing quantities of fibrin (144, 145). There are no reported studies of microaggregate formation in AS-1 red cells, but indirect evidence suggests that their formation may be impaired. Successful preparation of leukocyte-poor red cells by centrifugation and microaggregate filtration ("spin, cool, filter" method) requires AS-1 units that are at least 2 weeks old versus 4 days for CPD or CPDA-1 (146). This suggests that microaggregates in AS-1 are perhaps slower to form, smaller, or less stable.

Several microaggregate filters are commercially available, but their use is controversial. A number of clinical and experimental studies (reviewed by Snyder and Bookbinder [147]) support or refute the deleterious effects of microaggregates on pulmonary function. Some of the clinical studies are confounded by such factors as differences in the extent and type of injury and in the volume transfused between control (standard filter) and treatment (microaggregate filter) groups. Current consensus is that there is inadequate evidence supporting the routine use of microaggregate filters in massive transfusion (147–151), which is acknowledged even by those authorities preferring their use (152, 153).

Although microaggregate filters remove variable numbers of platelets from fresh or stored blood (154–156), both screen and depth filters pass the platelets in platelet concentrates. Large volumes of saline, however, may be required to elute platelets remaining in the residual volume (up to 500 ml, depending on the filter) (156). Granulo-cyte concentrates should not be transfused through microaggregate filters. (157)

## Metabolic Consequences of Massive Transfusion

Massive transfusion may result in a number of potential metabolic disturbances related to the administration of large amounts of citrate-containing anticoagulants and potentially toxic metabolites (potassium and lactate), which accumulate in stored blood. Such potential metabolic disturbances include citrate intoxication (hypocalcemia), acidosis, and hyperkalemia.

### CITRATE INTOXICATION (HYPOCALCEMIA)

Citrate anticoagulants exert their effects by chelating the ionized calcium that is necessary for coagulation. The transfusion of large volumes of stored blood containing excess citrate may result in measurable increases in the serum citrate level (158) and decreases in the serum ionized calcium (159, 160). Such changes can be compensated for by the rapid metabolism of citrate via the Krebs tricarboxylic acid cycle and the rapid mobilization of ionized calcium from bone by parathormone (161). Citrate metabolism is so rapid that only with extraordinarily high rates of transfusion (greater than 1 unit of blood every 5 minutes in a 70-kg adult) do citrate levels rise dramatically (161, 162). Indeed, 30 years ago Howland et al. failed to observe citrate toxicity (tetany or hypotension) with rates of administration of acid citrate dextrose (ACD) solution as high as 8.6 mg/kg/min over a period of 20 to 30 minutes despite reaching serum citrate levels as high as 79.6 mg/100 dl (163). It is clear that the amount of citrate infused is less important than the rate at which it is administered. Hypotension, hepatic impairment, and hypothermia may slow the rate of citrate metabolism and potentially increase the risk of citrate toxicity (158, 163). Inadequate circulation to bone consequent to hypotension may also impair parathormone-induced calcium mobilization and thus predispose to citrate toxicity (161, 163). Although an early study (162) reported myocardial functional impairment related to decreases in serum-ionized calcium, the ionized calcium in this study was calculated and not measured directly. More recently, Howland et al. (159) carefully monitored cardiac output by Swan-Ganz catheters and directly measured the ionized calcium in massively transfused patients. Although they found a significant and sometimes marked fall in the serum-ionized calcium, there was no significant change in blood pressure or in cardiac performance despite a significant prolongation of the Q–Tc interval on the electrocardiogram. As might be expected, the fall in the serum-ionized calcium was related to the rate of transfusion rather than to the total volume of blood administered.

Although a fall in serum-ionized calcium can be expected during massive transfusion with citrated blood, there is no convincing evidence that myocardial performance is significantly impaired to warrant routine replacement with calcium salts (160, 164). On the contrary, transient and severe elevations of the serum-ionized calcium associated with life-threatening cardiac arrhythmias have followed the administration of calcium salts (165, 166). Episodes of ventricular fibrillation previously attributed to hypocalcemia may well have been related to hypothermia and may be minimized by the use of blood warmers (167, 168).

## ACIDOSIS

The administration of large amounts of stored blood presents the recipient with an acid load (as high as 30 to 40 mEq/liter in 3-week-old blood) consequent to both the citric acid anticoagulant and the lactic acid produced by red cell metabolism (161). Blood anticoagulated with citrate phosphate dextrose has a lower hydrogen ion concentration than blood anticoagulated with acid citrate dextrose and thus a potentially lower risk of producing metabolic acidosis with massive transfusion (167). Although one might expect that massive transfusion with stored blood would often be associated with significant metabolic acidosis, studies of massively transfused combat casualties in Viet Nam have shown that massive transfusion resulted in the reversal of preexisting metabolic acidosis when hemorrhage could be controlled and tissue perfusion was reestablished with transfusion (169). In contrast, progressive acidosis developed in those patients with uncontrollable hemorrhage and persistent hypotension.

Although the routine use of sodium bicarbonate (44.6 mEq/5 units of blood) has been recommended (170), it seems to be unnecessary even in massively transfused patients if adequate tissue perfusion is restored, allowing rapid metabolism of both lactate and citrate. Miller et al., in a study of 20 battle casualties in Viet Nam, were unable to demonstrate any relationship between the degree of base deficit and the volume of stored ACD blood transfused (171). They suggested that routine bicarbonate administration should be avoided in view of the marked variability of an individual's acid-base response to transfusion.

Alkalosis resulting from the injudicious administration of sodium bicarbonate to massively transfused patients could potentially result in a number of undesirable consequences. Metabolic alkalosis increases the affinity of hemoglobin for oxygen, potentially resulting in decreased availability of oxygen to the tissues (161, 169, 171). Alkalosis may further aggravate the decrease in serum-ionized calcium consequent to massive transfusion by increasing the binding of ionized calcium to albumin (161). Moreover, the excess sodium load resulting from bicarbonate administration may be problematic in trauma patients whose renal function may be limited (161).

Judging from the data at hand, it is clearly more prudent to administer sodium bicarbonate based upon direct arterial pH measurement when available, rather than administering it routinely by some arbitrary formula (168, 169, 171). When appropriate transfusion has failed to correct tissue hypoxia adequately, continued lactate production (due to anaerobic glycolysis) and impaired lactate metabolism (due to inadequate hepatic perfusion) may result in acidosis requiring bicarbonate administration. If, however, hemorrhage remains uncontrollable and tissue perfusion remains inadequate, bicarbonate administration will not alter the ultimately fatal outcome (161, 169).

### HYPERKALEMIA

Although potassium is lost from the red cells into the surrounding plasma during storage, the potential potassium load resulting from massive transfusion seems to be, at most, modest in amount. Indeed, Howland has determined that the potassium load in 1-week-old CPD-preserved whole blood is approximately 4.5 to 4.8 mEq/unit (167); therefore, the isovolumetric replacement of a 20-unit blood loss with 1-week-old CPD-stored blood would result in a total potassium load of only 60 mEq, presuming no urinary loss was taking place simultaneously (167). Even if this replacement was with units stored for 21 days, the potassium load would be only 110 mEq (172).

With the possible exception of patients in whom blood replacement fails to restore tissue perfusion and reverse acidosis, hyperkalemia does not result from massive transfusion. A number of factors serve to prevent the development of hyperkalemia with massive transfusion, including renal excretion and reentry of potassium into the transfused cells as they are rejuvenated in the circulation (161, 167, 173). Most importantly, however, the large amount of citrate administered with the stored blood is ultimately metabolized to bicarbonate, resulting in metabolic alkalosis (167, 171, 174). This alkalosis results in further movement of potassium from the plasma into the red cells. Howland has shown that there is, in fact, a progressive fall in serum potassium in massively transfused patients that is directly related to the volume of blood transfused. In extreme cases, replacement of potassium may be required (167), which is yet another reason to avoid routine administration of sodium bicarbonate to massively transfused

patients because it could result in worsening metabolic alkalosis and hypokalemia.

### Increased Oxygen Affinity of Hemoglobin

The oxygen affinity of hemoglobin increases in stored blood correlating with a decline in red cell 2,3-DPG (175), an important physiologic regulator of hemoglobin function. The reduction of 2,3-DPG occurs in all currently licensed blood preservatives. Figures vary considerably in different studies. Representative values (percentage of initial level) after 1 and 2 weeks of storage in CPDA-1 are 80 and 40%, respectively (176, 177); representative values in AS-1 are 50 and 10 to 20%, respectively (178).

Reduction of the recipient's circulating red cell 2,3-DPG does occur with large transfusions of stored blood. A number of experimental and clinical studies have addressed the physiologic significance of this phenomenon; Sohmer and Dawson have reviewed these studies in detail (179). Although the increased affinity of hemoglobin for oxygen could theoretically result in reduced oxygen delivery and tissue hypoxia, these potentially deleterious effects are mitigated by the rapid in vivo regeneration of 2,3-DPG and compensatory mechanisms that increase oxygen delivery. Levels are usually one-half to two-thirds of normal within 24 hours (180–182). During the period of reduced 2,3-DPG concentration, oxygen delivery can be maintained by increased cardiac output and increased oxygen extraction. Acidosis resulting from tissue hypoxia serves to reduce the oxygen affinity of hemoglobin. Authorities agree that the vast majority of patients, even those massively transfused, suffer no clinically significant ill effects attributable to low 2,3-DPG (179, 183–186). They do acknowledge, however, that selected patients with impaired compensatory mechanisms (e.g., markedly impaired cardiac reserve or stenotic coronary arteries) might benefit from transfusion with 2,3-DPG-replete blood. There are no rules of thumb to guide the selection of such patients. Minimal criteria would seem to be the presence, in a massively transfused patient, of end organ dysfunction attributable to hypoxia which does not respond to the usual therapeutic maneuvers.

The decision to administer blood with normal levels of 2,3-DPG must be tempered by its limited availability. Refrigerated blood should be less than 7 to 10 days old if collected in CPD or CPDA-1 and less than 5 to 7 days old if collected in AS-1 or AS-3. Frozen red cells preserve 2,3-DPG levels as they are at the time of freezing (187). These cells are of limited availability for urgent transfusion, however, because they must be thawed and washed to remove the cryoprotective agent. 2,3-DPG in refrigerated red cells at the end of their dating period may be raised to levels approximately 150% of normal by incubating for 1 hour with a "rejuvenating" solution containing pyruvate, adenine, phosphate, and inosine (188). The cells must be either washed or frozen (and subsequently washed) before administration. In either case, availability for urgent transfusion is restricted. In addition, deglycerolized frozen cells and rejuvenated liquid cells become out of date in 24 hours because the container must be opened during washing. Additives to enhance 2,3-DPG maintenance in liquid stored red cells are under development (189).

## Adenine Toxicity

Adenine, a component of the commonly used CPDA-1, AS-1, and AS-3 preservatives, is nephrotoxic. This is thought to result from its metabolism (2 to 5%) to the poorly soluble compound 2,8-dioxyadenine, which can precipitate in the urinary tract (190). Each unit of CPDA-1 contains 17 mg of adenine, which equilibrates rapidly between red cells and plasma (191). Assuming partition on the basis of volume, the adenine is distributed as follows: red cells, 8.5 mg; platelet concentrate, 1.7 mg; plasma, 6.8 mg. In additive systems, either 27 mg (AS-1) or 30 mg (AS-3) of adenine is added only to the

red cells after the separation of plasma and platelets. Adenine in whole blood or red cells is metabolized; approximately 70% remains after 1 week, 50% after 2 weeks (191).

Adenine toxicity has been studied extensively and reviewed (190, 192). Acute administration of 15 mg/kg is clearly without toxicity in humans and animals. Systematic study of higher doses has been conducted only in animals. Doses of 25 mg/kg and of up to 50 to 70 mg/kg are well tolerated, although they may be associated with crystalluria or transient renal function abnormalities. Large numbers of crystals and significant toxicity appear at doses over approximately 100 mg/kg. The $LD_{50}$ in rats and mice is 200 to 350 mg/kg. Chronic doses of 10 mg/kg are well tolerated for up to 30 days. For comparison, an adenine dose of 25 mg/kg in a 70-kg man corresponds to transfusion with 65 units of AS-1 red cells or all the components made from 103 units of CPDA-1 whole blood (assuming that no in vitro adenine metabolism occurs during red cell storage).

Only one case of adenine nephrotoxicity in humans has been well documented. In 1948, a patient developed oliguric renal failure after a total dose of 460 mg/kg given over 5 days for the treatment of pernicious anemia. He recovered with only a mild residual elevation of urea nitrogen (193). Another reported case that is less clear-cut involved a massively transfused patient who underwent operation for a dissecting aortic aneurysm (194). He received 95 mg of adenine per kg, developed an increased serum creatinine, and died on the 7th postoperative day from hemorrhagic shock. Moderate numbers of 2,8-dioxyadenine crystals were noted in the renal tubules at autopsy. In the 1930s patients treated for agranulocytosis with oral adenine sulfate received up to 6.2 g of adenine (89 mg/kg, assuming a body weight of 70 kg) without apparent ill effects (195).

Clinical experience with high-adenine preservative solutions (e.g., AS-1) has been favorable despite initial concerns about toxicity. Blood loss and in vitro metabolism reduce the actual dosage in massively transfused patients.

## Rhesus Immunization

Massive transfusion is the usual setting in which limited supply may necessitate the transfusion of Rh-positive (D-positive) red cells to an Rh-negative recipient. Approximately 80% of D-negative recipients will be sensitized by 1 unit of D-positive cells, but this sensitization can be prevented by the administration of 20 µg of Rh immune globulin for every 1 ml of red cells transfused (16). Adverse effects are generally mild and may include fever, myalgia, splenomegaly, and modest hyperbilirubinemia. Rh immunoprophylaxis need not be undertaken in every patient at risk but should be considered for women of child-bearing age. The development of anti-D is usually of little consequence in patients not likely to become pregnant. D-negative individuals requiring future transfusion will ordinarily receive D-negative red cells unless they once again require urgent massive blood replacement. Primary immunization typically requires 4 to 6 weeks and will not affect the immediate survival of Rh-positive cells (196).

One vial (1 ml) of standard dose Rh immune globulin contains 300 µg, sufficient for the immunoprophylaxis of 15 ml of red cells. Taking a nominal value of 180 ml of red cells per unit, prophylaxis requires 12 ml of Rh immune globulin. Administration is uncomfortable as only an intramuscular preparation is available in the United States. Injections may be spaced over 72 hours, usually limited to 5 ml in each buttock at one time (197).

It may be possible to return to Rh-negative red cell support as the rate of hemorrhage subsides, effecting an exchange transfusion of Rh-negative for previously transfused Rh-positive cells. Ideally, immunoprophylaxis in such a case should be based on the number of remaining Rh-positive red cells rather than on the number transfused. Commercially available "rosette" screening tests are likely to be unhelpful because they are designed for obstetric practice to detect 15 ml of D-positive cells in the circulation of a D-negative individual (198). Accurate quantitative tests have been reported (199, 200) but are not widely available.

Consideration should also be given to immunoprophylaxis of Rh-negative (D-negative) recipients of platelet concentrates. Platelet concentrates are ordinarily selected without regard for Rh type; 85% are expected to be Rh-positive. Red cell contamination is approximately 0.5 ml/unit (74), an amount sufficient to provoke primary immunization. One milliliter of Rh immune globulin should suffice for each 30 units of platelets.

## ADVERSE REACTIONS TO TRANSFUSION

### Acute Hemolytic Transfusion Reactions

#### CLINICAL MANIFESTATIONS

Major acute hemolytic transfusion reactions, the majority of which are due to ABO incompatibility, are almost invariably the result of clerical rather than technical errors (32, 201). Inadvertent administration of appropriately labeled and cross-matched blood to an unintended recipient accounts for most of such reactions (32, 201). Symptoms may begin quickly after the start of the transfusion, often after the administration of only a few milliliters of incompatible blood. A patient often notices one or more of the following symptoms: chills, fever, pain at the infusion site, substernal discomfort, dyspnea, back pain, vomiting, and diarrhea (202, 203). Hemoglobinuria may become rapidly apparent, especially if a Foley catheter is in place. Occasionally, patients may have remarkably mild reactions, with symptoms limited to chills and fever (203). Hypotension, vascular collapse, and renal failure may occur when reactions are particularly severe. Generalized bleeding, consequent to DIC, may also occur and may be especially apparent in the trauma patient or during operation. General anesthesia will mask most of the signs and symptoms of the acute hemolytic transfusion reaction and, in this situation, unexplained hypotension, generalized bleeding, or hemoglobinuria may be the only evidence that a reaction has occurred (24, 202, 204).

## PATHOPHYSIOLOGY

Most, if not all, of the manifestations of acute hemolytic transfusion reactions result from the interaction of antibody with incompatible red cell membrane antigens (203, 205). The antigen-antibody complexes formed result in complement activation and liberation of anaphylatoxins, which in turn cause histamine and serotonin to be released from mast cells. Antigen-antibody complexes may also activate the Hageman factor, resulting in bradykinin generation as well as activation of the coagulation system (the former contributing to the hypotension and the latter to the DIC seen with hemolytic transfusion reactions) (203, 205). There is considerable evidence that hemoglobinuria, in and of itself, is not the cause of renal failure associated with major hemolytic transfusion reactions. Some studies suggest that hemoglobin is not inherently toxic to the renal tubules, nor is hemoglobin deposition with consequent tubular obstruction the sole cause of acute oliguric renal failure after hemolytic transfusion reactions (206, 207). In a recent clinical trial using stroma-free hemoglobin as a red cell substitute, however, transient decreases in urine output and endogenous creatinine clearance were noted (208). Nevertheless, acute renal failure has been produced in the absence of intravascular hemolysis or hemoglobinuria after the infusion of hemoglobin-free incompatible red blood cell stroma, indicating that the reaction of antibody with incompatible red cell membrane antigens is the primary mechanism responsible for the development of acute renal failure (209). Renal failure complicating acute hemolytic transfusion reactions occurs as the result of renal ischemia brought about by hypotension (resulting from vasoactive complement

components and kinins) and compensatory renal vasoconstriction. These processes may potentially be aggravated by fibrin deposition in the renal microcirculation consequent to the DIC that may accompany major hemolytic transfusion reactions (203, 206).

## MANAGEMENT

When an acute hemolytic transfusion reaction is suspected, the transfusion should be stopped immediately. Frequently, the incompatibility is apparent immediately after checking the patient's identification band against the label on the offending unit of blood. Although the vast majority of transfusion-associated fevers are unrelated to hemolysis, the onset of chills and fever should alert the clinician to the possibility of an acute hemolytic event and should warrant immediate discontinuation of the transfusion. Chills and fever are commonly the initial symptoms of an acute hemolytic reaction (24) and, as noted previously, may occasionally be the only sign that such a reaction has occurred. Allowing the transfusion to continue until there are convincing signs of hemolysis may be disastrous and even fatal. Indeed, the morbidity and mortality of acute hemolytic transfusion reactions are directly related to the volume of incompatible blood transfused (202).

After the transfusion is stopped, the blood remaining in the bag should be returned to the blood bank. If necessary, this blood may be used for repeat ABO typing and re-cross-matching against the recipient's serum. It may also be checked for bacterial contamination if a septic transfusion reaction is suspected. Such a reaction may mimic a hemolytic event. A specimen should be drawn immediately from the patient for performance of the direct antiglobulin (Coombs) test. If positive, the Coombs test indicates the presence of red cells sensitized with antibody or complement in the recipient's circulation. The patient's serum and urine both should be examined for the presence of free hemoglobin. Although serum haptoglobin will fall precipitously after a hemolytic transfusion reaction and indirect reacting bilirubin will rapidly appear in the serum, such tests are not immediately available and are of little or no diagnostic value in the acute situation. A platelet count, PTT, PT, and fibrinogen level should be obtained to look for evidence of DIC when a hemolytic reaction is suspected.

After discontinuation of the incompatible blood transfusion, the cornerstone of the management of acute hemolytic transfusion reactions is the prompt and immediate restoration of blood pressure and tissue perfusion if they are impaired (205). Volume expansion with normal saline should be undertaken to maintain a urine flow rate of greater than 100 ml/hr (202). Adequate volume restoration should be ensured even if invasive monitoring (Swan-Ganz) is required. If at all possible, pressors that induce renal vasoconstriction should be avoided because they may further impair renal blood flow and increase the risk of renal failure (202). The administration of the osmotic diuretic mannitol has been recommended to prevent or reverse oliguric failure (203, 210). Clinical and experimental data suggest, however, that this is of little or no benefit (202, 204, 205). Moreover, if urine output is not restored, mannitol also has the added disadvantage of promoting hypervolemia and potentially inducing pulmonary edema (202). To promote urine output, the loop diuretics furosemide and ethacrynic acid are recommended. These agents not only produce diuresis, but also may improve renal cortical blood flow and thus may have the added advantage of reversing the renal ischemia critical to the development of renal failure in patients with acute hemolytic transfusion reactions (202, 204, 205). The use of heparin both as a prophylactic measure and to treat established DIC (203, 211) has been suggested. Theoretically, the prophylactic administration of heparin could prevent fibrin deposition in the renal microvasculature and subsequent renal ischemia. The routine use of prophylactic heparin cannot be justified because the majority of patients with hemolytic transfusion reactions do not develop severe or irreversible impairment of renal function that could be attributed to DIC (24, 203, 205). Certainly, heparin can increase the risk of bleeding in posttraumatic or perioperative patients. If heparin therapy is to be considered at all, it should be reserved for patients with the most severe reactions who have received more than 200 ml of incompatible blood and in whom no significant contraindications to anticoagulation are present (202, 205). If heparin therapy is used, it should be given by continuous infusion (202, 205), preferably after consultation with a hematologist.

## Delayed Hemolytic Transfusion Reactions

Delayed hemolysis of transfused red cells occurring a few days to 2 weeks after the administration of apparently compatible blood occurs as the result of a rapidly developing immune response to red cell alloantigens to which the patient has been sensitized by previous transfusion or pregnancy. Sensitization may have occurred in the remote past, and sufficient time may have elapsed to allow the antibody titer to fall to levels undetectable by the routine antibody screen. Reexposure to these antigens may produce a rapid rise in antibody titer (an anamnestic response) and subsequent immune destruction of the transfused cells (212, 213). The clinical manifestations of delayed hemolysis are quite variable. Some reactions are signaled only by an unexpected and otherwise unexplained fall in the hematocrit or the occurrence of fever or unexplained jaundice (212, 213). Symptoms and signs such as these are often initially attributed to other causes, delaying diagnosis. Uncommonly, reactions may be quite abrupt in onset with chills, fever, hemoglobinemia, and hemoglobinuria, not unlike those associated with acute hemolytic reactions due to ABO incompatibility (202). The red cell antibodies most frequently responsible for delayed hemolytic transfusion reactions include those directed against the Kidd (Jk[a], Jk[b]), Rh (particularly D, E, c), Duffy (Fy[a], Fy[b]), and Kell (K) antigens (212).

A high index of suspicion must be maintained when one encounters findings of fever, jaundice, or an unexplained fall in hematocrit after transfusion of patients who may have been previously sensitized to red cell antigens. The presence of a delayed hemolytic event can be documented by the presence of sensitized red cells in the recipient's circulation (as indicated by a positive direct antiglobulin test) or the demonstration of a red cell alloantibody that was not present on initial screening. Often delayed hemolysis is not considered as a potential cause for a falling hematocrit in a recently transfused patient until a specimen is sent to the blood bank for further cross-matching. The finding of a positive antibody screen in a previously negative individual may first alert the clinician that a delayed hemolytic reaction has occurred. Patients who have become alloimmunized to one red cell antigen may become sensitized to another after further transfusion and should be observed closely for occult delayed hemolytic events (214).

Most delayed hemolytic transfusion reactions require no treatment. If further transfusion support is necessary, transfusion can be carried out safely with red cells lacking the antigen to which the patient has been previously sensitized. For the small number of patients who have severe hemolytic events, management is no different from that of acute hemolytic reactions.

### Nonhemolytic Febrile Reactions

Nonhemolytic febrile transfusion reactions (NHFTRs) are among the most common adverse reactions to transfusion, occurring in 2 to 3% of recipients (215, 216). NHFTR refers to an elevation in temperature (usually specified as at least 1°C) attributed to a transfusion in the absence of hemolysis and other causes of fever unrelated to transfusion. NHFTRs are usually associated with the presence of antileukocyte antibodies (granulocyte-specific and HLA) in the recipient that are stimulated by previous transfusion or pregnancy

(217–219). Granulocytes are the usual target cell (220), rarely lymphocytes (221) or platelets (222). Some NHFTRs result from passively transfused antibodies (223).

The clinical features are as follows (224–227). Fever usually begins between 0.5 and 2 hours after the start of transfusion but may not occur until after the transfusion is complete. Defervescence usually occurs in about an hour but may require up to 8 to 10 hours. Fever is usually preceded by a chilly feeling or true rigors. Other features (e.g., flushing, headache, backache, and nausea) may be associated; hypotension and pulmonary infiltrates are rarely associated. In the vast majority of cases, the febrile reaction produces no sequelae, although it may be rather uncomfortable for the patient.

The diagnosis of NHFTR is one of exclusion. All causes of fever should be considered, including those unrelated to transfusion. It is most important to exclude a hemolytic transfusion reaction. Although the vast majority of transfusion-associated fevers are ultimately attributed to NHFTRs or non-transfusion-related causes, fever is the most common presenting sign of a hemolytic reaction (228). The transfusion should be discontinued, the line kept open with physiologic saline, and the appropriate investigations performed to exclude hemolysis (see sections on hemolytic transfusion reactions). Although extremely rare, bacterial contamination should be considered. If suspected, Gram stain and culture of the offending unit should be performed.

NHFTRs can usually be prevented by premedicating the patient with an antipyretic (e.g., acetaminophen) or by administering leukocyte-depleted red cells (220, 224). One febrile reaction does not necessarily predict the occurrence of subsequent reactions (215, 229). For this reason, it is a common policy to recommend premedication with an antipyretic and continue the use of ordinary red cells after the first NHFTR. The use of leukocyte-depleted red cells is usually reserved for patients with multiple (two or more) or severe NHFTRs not prevented by antipyretics.

## Noncardiac Pulmonary Edema

Noncardiac pulmonary edema is a rare but potentially life-threatening complication of transfusion thought to be caused by complement-mediated endothelial cell injury by antileukocyte antibodies. In a recent series of 36 cases (230), the incidence was 0.02%/unit and 0.16%/patient transfused. Most of the cases were associated with passively transfused rather than recipient antileukocyte antibodies. The clinical presentation was typically respiratory distress with hypoxemia, hypotension, and bilateral pulmonary infiltrates occurring usually within 1 to 2 hours of transfusion. The patients responded to supportive measures, including oxygen and mechanical ventilation, in most cases with marked improvement within 48 hours. However, some patients had persisting infiltrates. In 2 cases, the reactions were believed to contribute to the patients' death. Diuretic therapy was detrimental in 1 reported case (231). There is no specific treatment. The reaction must be distinguished from volume overload.

## Allergic Reactions

The most common allergic reaction is urticaria. Hives occur with an incidence of approximately 1% (215, 216). The etiology of individual reactions is usually not defined, but as a group the reactions are thought to result most often from recipient antibodies against donor immunoglobulin allotypes or allergens in transfused plasma (232). Some cases have been attributed to passively transfused antibodies against substances in the recipient's plasma (232).

Urticaria alone does not represent a danger to the recipient, nor do hives constitute the sole presenting sign of a hemolytic reaction. After treatment with an antihistamine, the transfusion may be resumed. There is no need to exclude hemolysis with the usual diagnostic studies.

Most urticarial reactions can be prevented by premedicating the recipient with an antihistamine (216). If this is ineffective, washed red cells may be required.

The most severe, and fortunately rare, allergic reaction is frank anaphylaxis. Again, the etiology is not always apparent, but many of these reactions have been associated with the presence of class-specific anti-immunoglobulin A (IgA) antibodies (i.e., those reacting with all IgAs) in IgA-deficient recipients (233–235). The prevalence of IgA deficiency (usually defined as less than 1 to 2 mg of IgA per dl) varies in different studies but is approximately 1 in 1000 (236). Class-specific anti-IgA, usually unrelated to prior transfusion, is found in approximately 25% of deficient individuals, but about one-third of these antibodies are of low enough titer to make serious reactions unlikely (237, 238). The frequency of anti-IgA-mediated reactions was estimated at only 1.3/million transfusions in one large study (234).

Anaphylactic reactions to IgA in blood products may occur with minimal transfusion volumes (e.g., 10 ml). The most common manifestations are hypotension and respiratory distress. Flushing, nausea, vomiting, disorientation, and substernal or abdominal pain may be seen. Treatment, as for other types of anaphylaxis, is epinephrine and supportive measures. Prevention of subsequent reactions requires administration of IgA-deficient products. This can be accomplished for red cells by more extensive saline washing than customary in the production of routine washed red cells. Plasma products must be obtained from IgA-deficient donors. Registries of such individuals are maintained by blood banking organizations.

The term "anaphylactoid" is sometimes applied to allergic reactions intermediate in severity between urticaria and frank anaphylactic shock (239). Manifestations may include angioedema, swollen tongue, wheezing, and dyspnea. Urticaria may also be present. The etiology in most cases is unknown. Occasional reactions of this type have been attributed to anti-IgA of limited specificity (233). Unlike the class-specific anti-IgAs described above, these antibodies react with some, but not all, IgAs. They are encountered regularly in normal individuals (e.g., 6% in one recent study [240]) but their presence does not correlate with the occurrence of transfusion reactions (241). Prophylaxis can be attempted with antihistamines and washed cells.

In the authors' experience, anaphylactoid reactions tend to be idiosyncratic and frequently do not recur with subsequent exposure to plasma proteins. Patients should be evaluated for IgA deficiency. Those shown to be deficient should be managed as previously discussed. Those not IgA-deficient should be managed on an individual basis. Epinephrine should be considered for clinically significant bronchospasm or angioedema.

## Infectious Disease Transmission

Although cytomegalovirus (CMV) may produce clinically important infections in immunodepressed patients, viral hepatitis remains the most common, clinically significant transfusion-transmitted infection. The acquired immunodeficiency syndrome (AIDS) is an infrequent complication of transfusion but one that has received much public attention because of its almost uniform fatality and attendant social issues.

### INCIDENCE AND MANIFESTATIONS OF POSTTRANSFUSION HEPATITIS

The incidence of posttransfusion hepatitis is approximately 10% in prospective studies using volunteer donors screened for hepatitis B surface antigen (242, 243). Posttransfusion hepatitis is defined by exclusion in such studies on the basis of alanine aminotransferase (ALT) elevations not attributable to other causes occurring within the appropriate incubation period. The background incidence of ALT elevation in nontransfused control patients tested at the same intervals has been reported as 0.5% (243) and 0.7 to 3.8% (244) in different centers. According to a recent review, the corrected incidence of transfusion-associated hepatitis based on prospective data from the late 1970s and early 1980s can be estimated at 0.5 to 1.0% per unit transfused

(245). The current incidence is likely to be lower because of newly implemented screening procedures (see "Prevention of Posttransfusion Hepatitis").

On the basis of viral antibody measurements, hepatitis B accounts for about 10% of posttransfusion hepatitis cases; hepatitis A and Epstein-Barr virus hepatitis are extremely rare (242, 243). CMV seroconversion is common after transfusion (246), but the extent to which this agent causes posttransfusion hepatitis is unclear (247). So-called "non-A, non-B" (NANB) hepatitis is diagnosed by exclusion in approximately 90% of the cases (242, 243). Positive diagnosis has been impossible because serologic markers have been unavailable (248). A specific assay has been developed recently, however, for antibody against a major agent of NANB hepatitis (249) and is under commercial development (250).

Most cases of posttransfusion hepatitis are not clinically apparent. Approximately 25% of NANB and 50% of hepatitis B cases are icteric (247). Fulminant acute hepatitis is unusual but may result in serious morbidity and mortality. Chronic active hepatitis develops in 1 to 3% of patients with hepatitis B (251).

Chronicity is more common in posttransfusion NANB hepatitis. Reviews of its natural course (247, 252, 253) report ALT elevations lasting more than 6 months in about 50% of cases. Of these, approximately one-third have biopsy findings of chronic persistent hepatitis and two-thirds have chronic active hepatitis. Of the latter, approximately one-quarter have histologic evidence of cirrhosis, representing 8% of those infected. Estimates of the frequency of clinical chronic liver failure are more variable. Of 83 patients with chronic posttransfusion NANB hepatitis in five studies (254–258), 5 developed clinical signs of hepatic failure (6%), corresponding to approximately 3% of those initially infected. There may also be additional morbidity in a proportion of those individuals with chronic persistent hepatitis. Interestingly, some studies demonstrate a lower rate of chronicity, similar to that of hepatitis B, in NANB hepatitis that is not transfusion-related (247). The reason for the difference in natural history is speculative and may relate to the dose of infectious agent, route of administration, or immunosuppressive effect of transfusion.

## PREVENTION OF POSTTRANSFUSION HEPATITIS

Major reductions in the incidence of posttransfusion hepatitis have resulted from the use of volunteer donors and screening for hepatitis B surface antigen (242, 244, 259). The incidence of NANB hepatitis may be reduced an additional 30 to 40% by excluding donors with either elevated ALT or positivity for hepatitis B core antibody (242, 243, 260). Growing concern about transfusion-transmitted infection among blood bankers and the public alike has led to the universal adoption of both screening tests in the United States, although neither one is sensitive or specific for the presence of NANB infectivity in the donor (242, 243). The estimated reduction of posttransfusion NANB hepatitis using both tests is 50 to 60%, with a loss of 5 to 6% of the donor pool (243). The incidence of posttransfusion hepatitis may be reduced further by screening procedurees designed to prevent transfusion-transmitted AIDS (261, 262).

A newly discovered assay for antibodies to a major agent of NANB hepatitis holds great promise as a screening test for blood donors (249, 250). Preliminary data indicate that it may not be effective when used alone because of less than optimal sensitivity, a prolonged period for seroconversion, and the possibility of other NANB agents (250). More extensive experience will be necessary to determine the final role of this test in donor screening. It is not yet commercially available.

What can the clinician do to reduce the incidence of posttransfusion hepatitis? As the most commonly transfused components represent "average risk" products (i.e., red cells, plasma, platelets, cryoprecipitate), the main duty of the clinician is to avoid unnecessary transfusion and use autologous blood when possible (see "Autologous Donation" below).

Attempts to reduce the incidence of posttransfusion NANB hepatitis by prophylactic administration of immune serum globulin (ISG) have yielded equivocal and conflicting results but have suggested that ISG might reduce the number of icteric cases (263–265). Use, in part, of paid donors (263, 265) and less advanced screening tests (263–265) in these studies make them difficult to apply to today's transfusion practice. A recent study from Spain found that ISG reduced the incidence of posttransfusion NANB hepatitis but was not placebo-controlled and did not use donors screened for ALT and hepatitis B core antibody (266). It has been suggested (267) that studies in which ISG was administered before transfusion (263, 266) demonstrate a greater protective effect than those in which it was given up to a week afterward (263, 265). In the absence of conclusive data, ISG is not currently used for prophylaxis of posttransfusion NANB hepatitis (268, 269).

### AIDS

AIDS is caused by a retrovirus known as human T cell lymphotropic virus (HTLV-III), lymphadenopathy-associated virus (LAV), or, more recently, human immunodeficiency virus (HIV) (270). There is ample epidemiologic, serologic, and virologic evidence that AIDS may be transmitted by transfusion (271, 272). Of the AIDS cases reported to the Centers for Disease Control, approximately 2% are related to the transfusion of blood components to nonhemophiliacs and an additional 1% to the transfusion of hemophiliacs (273). Among children less than 13 years old, the corresponding percentages are 11 and 7%, respectively (273). All blood products, with the apparent exception of ISG, albumin, and plasma protein fraction, may transmit AIDS, (274, 275). Factor concentrates, formerly considered high-risk products because of their preparation from plasma pools, are now safer than single donor products because they are subjected to one or more of several available virucidal treatments including heating, affinity purification, and solvent-detergent extraction (276, 277).

The observed median incubation period of transfusion-transmitted AIDS is approximately 30 months in adults and 14 months in children under 13 years but may extend as long as 7 years (271). Based on mathematical extrapolations, estimates of the true mean incubation period have ranged from 4.5 (278) to as long as 15 (279) years.

The risk of transfusion-transmitted AIDS has been reduced substantially by a combination of (a) improved historical screening of potential blood donors designed to identify individuals at high risk of transmitting AIDS; (b) confidential postdonation exclusion (i.e., each donor is given an additional opportunity *after* donating to indicate that the blood should not be transfused); and (c) mandatory screening of all donors for antibodies against HIV. Antibody screening is performed using enzyme-linked immunosorbent assay (ELISA) tests that have been commercially available since the spring of 1985. Early data collected nationwide showed approximately 0.3% of blood donors to be repeatably positive by ELISA, i.e., positive in replicate testing on the same specimen (280). The prevalence of HIV seropositivity in donors in declining (281) and is now closer to 0.012% nationwide (282). As a consequence of the low prevalence of HIV positivity among blood donors, only approximately 10 to 25% of positive donor ELISA tests can be confirmed by the more specific Western blot assay (283, 284). The remainder are thought to be false-positives. Infectivity of blood is strongly correlated with Western blot positivity (285). Current policies are conservative, however, and the blood of ELISA-positive, Western blot-negative individuals is not transfused (275).

The commercially available ELISA tests for HIV antibody are quite sensitive (284, 286, 287), with a false-negative rate believed to be less than 1% (284, 286). "Silent" HIV infection with a negative anti-HIV

ELISA test, however, remains a concern. This may occur in a newly infected individual during the 6 to 8 week "window" period during which seropositivity usually develops or less commonly when antibody disappears from the serum of an individual with an established infection (288). Prolonged seronegativity may occur in certain high-risk individuals before the appearance of antibody (289). Although infrequent, transmission of HIV by blood transfusions screened as negative for HIV antibody has been documented (282). The risk of transmitting HIV by an ELISA-negative transfusion is not known with certainty and is probably decreasing as the prevalence of HIV in the donor population becomes lower and donor screening methods are improved (261). Typically, risk estimates for single donor products have been calculated simply by multiplying the prevalence of donor Western blot positivity (presumed true infection) by the false-negative rate of the ELISA screening test (290). Estimates have ranged from approximately 1:40,000 to 1:1,000,000 per transfusion (57). The observed rate of transfusion-transmitted HIV infection in a prospective study of cardiac surgery patients receiving HIV antibody-negative blood products was approximately 1:36,000 per component transfused (291). However, the calculated 95% confidence interval extends from 1:7500 to 1:625,000 (292).

Efforts to further reduce the incidence of transfusion-transmitted HIV infection include the development of more effective communication with donors to eliminate high-risk individuals and more sensitive screening tests. Despite detailed and explicit procedures for donor education and screening, most Western blot-confirmed antibody-positive donors are members of high-risk groups (284, 293). More effective communication of risk group information is needed. Direct detection of HIV (e.g., proteins, nuclei acid) has been viewed as the most promising new approach (287) to laboratory screening but has not yet been applied successfully to donor blood. The possible utility of HIV p24 *antigen* testing was recently examined in a collaborative study of 475,501 donors nationwide (294). No donor was found to have a positive test for antigen in the absence of antibody to HIV. Others have also found HIV antigen screening of donors to be unproductive (295, 296). Perhaps other types of direct assay will be helpful (297).

Another retrovirus called HIV-2 has also been associated with AIDS (298, 299), predominantly in Africa and more recently in Europe. Although related to HIV (now HIV-1), antibodies against HIV-2 react poorly in ELISA assays for anti-HIV-1 (298, 300). Although cases have been reported in immigrants to the United States (301, 302), no antibody to HIV-2 was found in a survey of serum samples from 22,699 individuals in the United States, including 8503 blood donors (301). In consideration of these data, the Food and Drug Administration has recommended exclusion of all donors from sub-Saharan Africa and the adjacent islands but has not recommended additional laboratory tests for HIV-2 (303).

### HUMAN T CELL LYMPHOTROPIC VIRUS TYPE 1 (HTLV-1)

This retrovirus, endemic largely in Japan and the Carribean, is found in the United States mainly in intravenous drug abusers (304). The virus does not cause AIDS. It is associated with adult T cell leukemia/lymphoma (ATL), a rare hematologic malignancy, and with a degenerative neurologic disease known as tropical spastic paraparesis (TSP) or HTLV-1-associated myelopathy (HAM) (304, 305). The virus is transmitted efficiently by cellular blood products, with an approximately 70% seroconversion rate in recipients of seropositive units (306). The lifetime risk of ATL in HTLV-1-infected individuals is thought to be about 2%, with a latency period of years to decades. There are no documented cases of transfusion-induced ATL (304, 305). The lifetime risk of TSP/HAM in HTLV-1-infected individuals is not known but is thought to be low, with a shorter incubation period of several years (304). Transfusion-induced TSP/HAM is thought to occur (304, 307).

All donor blood must now be screened for antibody to HTLV-1 (304). Antibody prevalence was 0.025% in a recent multicenter study of nearly 40,000 donors (308). Positive ELISA screening tests are confirmed by Western blot or radioimmunoprecipitation assay. Currently available tests do not allow the differentiation of antibodies against HTLV-1 from those to a closely related retrovirus, HTLV-2. Although originally isolated from a patient with hairy cell leukemia, the disease associations of the latter virus are unclear (304, 305).

### OTHER INFECTIONS

CMV seroconversion is noted in approximately 30% of CMV-negative transfusion recipients, but it is clinically apparent in only about 10% of cases, usually producing an infectious mononucleosis-like syndrome that resolves completely (246). Although routine use of CMV-negative blood (i.e., lacking antibody to CMV) is not indicated, its administration may prevent clinically serious infection and death in certain groups of patients, most notably low-birth-weight, CMV-negative infants (309). CMV-negative blood has also been recommended for CMV-negative pregnant women and CMV-negative recipients of organ transplants from CMV-negative donors (246).

Other transfusion-transmitted infections (e.g., Epstein-Barr virus, hepatitis A, syphilis, malaria) are extremely uncommon and have been reviewed (310). No case of transfusion-associated Lyme disease has been reported, although transmission by transfusion is theoretically possible (311).

## Other Adverse Effects of Transfusion

See "Special Considerations in Massive Transfusion" for discussions of electrolyte imbalance, citrate excess, microaggregate effects, hypothermia, adenine toxicity, and alteration of hemoglobin function.

## AUTOLOGOUS AND DIRECTED DONATIONS

### Autologous Donation

Autologous blood may be obtained by intraoperative salvage (discussed in a separate section) and predeposit autologous donation. The latter refers to the patient donating blood for later use, usually during an elective surgical procedure. Although obviously not applicable to the initial management of trauma patients, this source should be considered for follow-up surgery occurring perhaps during subsequent admissions. Autologous blood is the safest for any patient to receive, not only with respect to infectious disease transmission but also because the risk of adverse reactions caused by alloantigens (on red cells, white cells, and proteins) is minimized (312). Individuals may be suitable autologous donors even if they do not meet the criteria for ordinary volunteer donation. Autologous donation has been accomplished safely in elderly individuals, children, pregnant women, and patients with heart disease (313, 314).

### Directed Donation

Increased public awareness of transfusion-transmitted infections, especially AIDS, has resulted in requests for so-called "directed" or "designated" donations (i.e., blood provided by individuals known to the recipient, usually family and friends). Directed donations remain a controversial and emotionally charged topic. Opposing viewpoints are well summarized in a pair of recent editorials (315, 316).

The following arguments are frequently presented against directed donations: (a) they encourage people to "hoard" their blood, creating an overall shortage and a "two-class" system in which patients without directed donors would have even more limited blood resources; (b) they do not prevent disease transmission; (c) blood so procured is not available on an urgent basis and may discourage timely transfusion; (d) there are pressures brought by family and friends on directed donors that may overcome their obligation to divulge relevant medical or social history; (e) directed donors effectively lose their anonymity and may risk potential lawsuits in the event of transfusion-transmitted infection; and (f) current screening techniques, although not infallible, have reduced the risk of transfusion-transmitted AIDS to very low levels.

Proponents of directed donations are of the opinion that they are, at worst, no less safe than ordinary volunteer donations, that the practice does not compromise the blood supply, and that patients have a "right" to receive them.

Facts are less available than opinions in this controversy. One study compared directed with volunteer donations and found no significant difference in the rate of deferral or of positivity for hepatitis and AIDS screening tests (317). Another study, conducted by the Washington State Health Department (318), reported a statistically higher rate of hepatitis B surface antigen positivity in programs encouraging directed donation compared to random volunteer donations. No such difference was found in programs accepting, but not encouraging, directed donation. There were no statistically significant differences in HIV seropositivity between directed and volunteer donors regardless of whether the former were "encouraged" or "accepted." Several other studies, reported only in abstract form, have found directed donors to have a higher (319) or indistinguishable (320, 321) frequency of positivity for infectious disease markers. No studies have been conducted to compare directly the incidence of transfusion-transmitted infections in recipients of volunteer and directed blood donations. There are also no available data measuring the effect of directed donations on the blood supply.

Clinicians are often the recipients of requests for directed donations. Several practical considerations should be noted. It is important to check with the transfusion service regarding local policy before indicating to a patient or family that the donation can be arranged. Granted that the basis for such policies is subject to argument, it is important from a legal and ethical standpoint for institutions to be consistent in their approach. In addition, some jurisdictions have passed laws affecting directed donations. Directed donors must undergo all of the same screening tests required of volunteer donors. Availability of units for transfusion may be delayed up to several days depending on the frequency with which the necessary tests are performed.

## ALTERNATIVES TO BLOOD COMPONENT THERAPY

### Blood Product Substitutes

There are no red cell substitutes currently licensed for routine use. Most research and development has been directed toward fluorocarbons and hemoglobin solutions (322–326). In brief, fluorocarbon emulsions carry oxygen in solution (see Chapter 4). Their principle disadvantage is the requirement for high inspired oxygen concentrations to achieve meaningful increments in oxygen carrying capacity. A recent study of patients with acute anemia who refused blood transfusion on religious grounds concluded that Fluosol-DA, a fluorocarbon emulsion, was unnecessary in moderate anemia and ineffective in severe anemia (327). Fluorocarbon emulsions also have several adverse effects, including activation of the complement system and interference with granulocyte and monocyte function, which may be toxic effects of the emulsifier rather than of the fluorocarbon itself (322, 325). Second generation products are under development (325).

Unmodified hemoglobin solutions are limited in their effectiveness by their short in vivo half-life, considerable oncotic effect (limiting total concentration), markedly elevated oxygen affinity, and possible nephrotoxicity (322–324). The most successful derivative is modified by both polymerization to reduce clearance and pyridoxalation to improve oxygen unloading (322–324).

Animal studies have been encouraging, but no human trials have been conducted in the face of unresolved questions about nephrotoxicity (323).

Improvements in liposome technology have allowed the production of "synthetic erythrocytes"—membrane-encapsulated hemoglobin solutions. Products with good in vitro and in vivo function have been developed, but reticuloendothelial toxicity with predisposition of the recipient to infection remains a concern (326). No human trials have been conducted.

Perhaps closer on the horizon are plasma proteins produced by recombinant DNA technology. The genes for albumin and many coagulation factors have been cloned, and large scale production is possible (328). Preliminary clinical trials of recombinant factor VIII have been reported (329).

### Erythropoietin

Recombinant human erythropoietin (rHuEPO) has clearly been demonstrated to increase significantly the hematocrit and red cell mass in patients with chronic renal failure, both dialysis- and nondialysis-dependent (330–332). Similar rises in hematocrit have been reported in patients with rheumatoid arthritis and the anemia of chronic disease (333). It is conceivable that rHuEPO administration could decrease the postoperative transfusion requirements of patients who have experienced multiple trauma and also allow autologous donation for any subsequent elective surgery (334). Large-scale trials of rHuEPO no doubt will address these issues.

### SUMMARY

Transfusion therapy is an extremely important component of shock resuscitation for the trauma patient. The principles outlined in this chapter are necessary for the trauma anesthesiologist/critical care specialist (TA/CCS) to use blood components intelligently to supplement shock resuscitation (outlined in Chapter 4).

## References

1. Murphy S, Gardner FH. Platelet preservation: effect of storage temperature on maintenance of platelet viability—deleterious effect of refrigerated storage. N Engl J Med 1969;280:1094–1098.
2. Baldini M, Costeau N, Dameshek W. The viability of stored human platelets. Blood 1960; 16:1669–1692.
3. Slichter SJ, Harker LA. Preparation and storage of platelet concentrates: II. Storage variables influencing platelet viability and function. Br J Haematol 1976;34:403–419.
4. Counts RB, Haisch C, Simon TL, Maxwell NG, Heimbach DS. Hemostasis in massively transfused trauma patients. Ann Surg 1979;190: 91–99.
5. Nilsson L, Hedner U, Nilsson IM, Robertson B. Shelf-life of bank blood and stored plasma with special reference to coagulation factors. Transfusion 1983;23:377–381.
6. Bowie EJW, Thompson JH, Owen CA. The stability of antihemophilic globulin and labile factor in human blood. Mayo Clin Proc 1964; 39:144–151.
7. Hondow JA, Russell WJ, Duncan BM, Lloyd JV. The stability of coagulation factors in stored blood. Aust NZ J Surg 1982;52:265–269.
8. Pepper MD, Learoyd PA, Rajah SM. Plasma factor VIII: variables affecting stability under standard blood bank conditions and correlation with recovery in concentrates. Transfusion 1978;18:756–760.
9. Heaton A, Miripol J, Aster R, Hartman P, Dehart D, Rzad L, Grapka B, Davisson W, Buchholz DH. Use of Adsol preservation solution for prolonged storage of low viscosity AS-1 red blood cells. Br J Haematol 1984;57:467–478.
10. Simon TL, Marcus CS, Myhre BA, Nelson EJ. Effects of AS-3 nutrient-additive solution on 42 and 49 days of storage of red cells. Transfusion 1987;27:178–182.
11. Holland PV (ed). Standards for Blood Banks and Transfusion Services, ed 13. Arlington, VA, American Association of Blood Banks, 1989, p 12.
12. Food and Drug Administration. Code of Federal Regulations, revised as of April 1, 1986. Washington, DC, Government Printing Office, 1986, vol 21 (parts 600 to 799), ch 1, p 37.
13. Widmann FK (ed). Technical Manual, ed 9. Arlington, VA, American Association of Blood Banks, 1985, pp 195–220.
14. Holland PV (ed). Standards for Blood Banks and Transfusion Services, ed 13. Arlington, VA, American Association of Blood Banks, 1989, pp 28–29.
15. Barnes A Jr. Status of the use of universal donor blood transfusion. CRC Crit Rev Clin Lab Sci 1973;4:147–161.
16. Pollack W, Ascari WQ, Crispen JF, O'Connor RR, Ho TY. Studies on Rh prophylaxis II: Rh immune prophylaxis after transfusion with Rh positive blood. Transfusion 1971;11:340–344.
17. Boral LI, Henry JB. The type and screen—a safe alternative and supplement in selected surgical procedures. Transfusion 1977;17:163–168.
18. Schulman IA, Nelson JM, Saxena S, Thompson JC, Okamoto M, Kent DR, Nakayama RK. Experience with the routine use of an abbreviated crossmatch. Am J Clin Pathol 1984;82: 178–181.
19. Lostumbo MM, Holland PV, Schmidt PJ. Isoimmunization after multiple transfusions. N Engl J Med 1966;275:141–144.
20. Moore HC, Issitt PD, Pavone BG. Successful transfusion of Chido-positive blood to two patients with anti-Chido. Transfusion 1965; 15:266–269.
21. Baldwin ML, Ness PM, Barrasso C, Kickler TS, Drew H, Tsan M-F, Shirey RS. In vivo studies of the long term $^{51}$Cr red cell survival of serologically incompatible red cell units. Transfusion 1985;25:34–38.
22. Baldwin ML, Barrasso C, Ness PM, Garratty G. A clinically significant erythrocyte antibody detectable only by $^{51}$Cr survival studies. Transfusion 1983;23:40–44.
23. Widmann FK (ed). Technical Manual, ed 9. Arlington, VA, American Association of Blood Banks, 1985, p 216.
24. Taswell HF, Pineda AA, Moore SB. Hemolytic transfusion reactions—frequency and clinical and laboratory aspects. In Bell CA (ed). A Seminar on Immune-mediated Cell Destruction. Chicago, American Association of Blood Banks, 1981, pp 71–92.
25. Giblett ER. Blood group alloantibodies: an assessment of some laboratory practices. Transfusion 1977;17:299–308.
26. Gervin AS, Fischer RP. Resuscitation of trauma patients with type specific uncrossmatched blood. J Trauma 1984;24:327–331.
27. Blumberg N, Bove JR. Un-crossmatched blood for emergency transfusion: one year's experience in a civilian setting. JAMA 1978;240: 2057–2059.
28. Inwood MJ, Zuliani B. Anti-A hemolytic transfusion with packed O cells. Ann Intern Med 1978;89:515–516.
29. Sohmer PR, Scott RL. Massive transfusion. Clin Lab Med 1982;2:21–34.
30. Lefebre J, McLellan BA, Coovadia AS. Seven years experience with group O unmatched packed red cells in a regional trauma unit. Ann Emerg Med 1987;16:344–349.
31. Barnes A, Allen TE. Transfusions subsequent to administration of universal donor blood in Vietnam. JAMA 1968;204:695–697.
32. Honig CL, Bove JR. Transfusion associated

fatalities: review of Bureau of Biologics reports 1976–1978. Transfusion 1980;20:653–661.

33. Masouredis SP. Preservation and clinical use of erythrocytes and whole blood. In Williams WJ, Beutler E, Erslev AJ, Lichtman MA (eds): Hematology, ed 3. New York, McGraw-Hill, 1983, pp 1529–1549.

34. Wintrobe MM, Lee GR, Boggs DR, Bithell TC, Foerster J, Athens JW, Lukens JN. Clinical Hematology, ed 8. Philadelphia, Lea & Febiger, 1981, pp 677–697.

35. Collins JA. Hemorrhage, shock, and burns: pathophysiology and treatment. In Petz LD, Swisher SN (eds): Clinical Practice of Blood Transfusion. New York, Churchill Livingstone, 1981, pp 425–453.

36. Oberman H, Chaplin H, Polesky H, Schmidt PJ, Widmann FK (eds). General Principles of Blood Transfusion. Chicago, American Medical Association, 1985, pp 43–47.

37. Finch C, Lenfant C. Oxygen transport in man. N Engl J Med 1972;286:407–415.

38. Rush B. Limits of non-colloid solution replacement in experimental hemorrhagic shock. Ann Surg 1967;165:977–984.

39. Takaori M, Safar P. Treatment of massive hemorrhage with colloid and crystalloid solutions. JAMA 1967;199:297–302.

40. Wilkerson DK, Rosen AL, Sehgal LR, Gould SA, Sehgal HL, Moss GS. Limits of cardiac compensation in anemic baboons. Surgery 1988;103:665–701.

41. Wilkerson DK, Rosen AL, Gould SA, Sehgal LR, Sehgal HL, Moss GS. Whole body oxygen extraction ratio as an indicator of cardiac status in anemia. Curr Surg 1988;45:214–217.

42. Mesmer K, Sunder-Plassman L, Jesch F, Gornandt L, Sibnagowitz E, Kessler M, Pfeiffer R, Horn E, Hoper J, Joachimsmeir K. Oxygen supply to the tissues during limited normovolemic hemodilution. Res Exp Med (Berl) 1973;159:152–166.

43. Rigor B, Bosomworth P, Rush RF. Replacement of operative blood loss of more than 1 liter with Hartmann's solution. JAMA 1968;203:399–402.

44. Sandiford FM, Chiariello L, Hallman GL, Cooley DA. Aorto-coronary bypass in Jehovah's Witnesses. J Thorac Cardiovasc Surg 1974;68:1–7.

45. Gollub S, Bailey CP. Management of major surgical blood loss without transfusion. JAMA 1966;198:1171–1174.

46. Mesmer K, Sunder-Plassman L. Hemodilution. Progr Surg 1974;13:208–245.

47. Czer LSC, Shoemaker WC. Optimal hematocrit value in critically ill postoperative patients. Surg Gynecol Obstet 1978;147:363–368.

48. Fortune JB, Feustel PJ, Saifi J, Stratton HH, Newell JC, Shah DM. Influence of hematocrit on cardiopulmonary function after acute hemorrhage. J Trauma 1987;27:243–247.

49. Gill W, Champion HR. Volume resuscitation in critical major trauma. In Dawson RB (ed): Transfusion Therapy. Arlington, VA, American Association of Blood Banks, 1974, pp 77–88.

50. Rush BF Jr: Volume replacement. when, what and how much? In Schumer W, Nyhus LM (eds): Treatment of Shock: Principles and Practice. Philadelphia, Lea & Febiger, 1974, pp 23–36.

51. Oberman H, Chaplin H, Polesky H, Schmidt PJ, Widmann FK (eds). General Principles of Blood Transfusion. Chicago, American Medical Association, 1985, p 14.

52. Sohmer PR, Dawson RB. Transfusion therapy in trauma: a review of the principles and techniques used in the MIEMSS program. Am Surg 1979;45:109–125.

53. Stehling LC, Ellison N, Faust RJ, Girotta AW, Moyers JR. A survey of transfusion practices among anesthesiologists. Vox Sang 1987;52:60–62.

54. Graves CL, Allen RM. Anesthesia in the presence of severe anemia. Rocky Mountain Med J 1970;67:35–40.

55. Lorhan PH, Burch J. Anesthesia for a Jehovah's Witness with a low hematocrit. Anesthesiology 1968;29:847–848.

56. Carson JL, Spence RK, Poses RM, Bonavita G. Severity of anemia and operative mortality and morbidity. Lancet 1988;1:727–729.

57. National Institutes of Health Consensus Development Conference. Perioperative red cell transfusion. Transfusion Med Rev 1989;3:63–68.

58. Friedman BA. An analysis of surgical blood use in United States hospitals with application to the maximum surgical blood order schedule. Transfusion 1979;19:268–278.

59. Mintz PD, Nordine RB, Henry JB, Webb WR. Expected hemotherapy in elective surgery. NY State J Med 1976;76:532–537.

60. Schiffer CA, Lee EJ, Ness PM, Reilly J. Clinical evaluation of platelet concentrates stored for one to five days. Blood 1986;67:1591–1594.

61. Simon TL, Henderson R. Coagulation factor activity in platelet concentrates. Transfusion 1979;19:186–189.

62. Murphy S, Martinez J, Holburn R. Stability of plasma fibrinogen during storage of platelet concentrates at 22°C. Transfusion 1983;23:480–483.

63. Hymas PG, Perkins HA. Plasma in platelet concentrates. Transfusion 1981;21:471 (letter).

64. Ciavarella D, Lavallo E, Reiss RF. Coagulation factor activity in platelet concentrates stored up to 7 days: an in vitro and in vivo study. Clin Lab Haematol 1986;8:233–242.

65. Hughes C, Thomas KB, Schiff P, Herrington RW, Polacsek EE, McGrath KM. Effect of delayed blood processing on the yield of factor VIII in cryoprecipitate and factor VIII concentrate. Transfusion 1988;28:566–570.

66. Ness PM, Perkins HA. Cryoprecipitate as a reliable source of fibrinogen replacement. JAMA 1979;241:1690-1691.
67. Wintrobe MM, Lee GR, Boggs DR, Bithell TC, Foerster J, Athens JW, Lukens JN. Clinical Hematology, ed 8. Philadelphia, Lea & Febiger, 1981, p 1185.
68. Tamagnini GP, Dormandy KM, Ellis D, Maycock WD'A. Factor-VIII concentrate in haemophilia. Lancet 2:188, 1975 (letter).
69. Rosati LA, Barnes B, Oberman HA, Penner JA. Hemolytic anemia due to anti-A in concentrated antihemophilic factor preparations. Transfusion 1971;10:139-141.
70. Duquesnoy RJ, Anderson AJ, Tomasulo PA, Aster RH. ABO compatibility and platelet transfusions of alloimmunized thrombocytopenic patients. Blood 1979;54:595-599.
71. Tosato G, Applebaum FR, Deisseroth AB. HLA-matched platelet transfusion therapy of severe aplastic anemia. Blood 1978;52:846-854.
72. Brand A, Sintnicolaas K, Claas FHJ, Eernisse JG. ABH antibodies causing platelet transfusion refractoriness. Transfusion 1986;26:463-466.
73. Lee EJ, Schiffer CA. ABO compatibility can influence the results of platelet transfusion: results of a randomized trial. Transfusion 1989;29:384-389.
74. Goldfinger D, McGinniss MH. Rh-incompatible platelet transfusions—risks and consequences of sensitizing immunosuppressed patients. N Engl J Med 1971;284:942-944.
75. Pierce RN, Reich LM, Mayer K. Hemolysis following platelet transfusion from ABO-incompatible donors. Transfusion 1985;25:60-62.
76. McBride JA, O'Hoski P, Barnes CC, Spiak C, Blajchman MA. Rhesus alloimmunization following intensive plasma exchange. Transfusion 1983;23:352-354.
77. Widmann FK (ed). Technical Manual, ed 9. Arlington, VA, American Association of Blood Banks, 1985, p 216.
78. Chopek M, McCullough J. Protein and biochemical changes during plasma exchange. In Berkman EM, Umlas J (eds): Therapeutic Hemapheresis—A Technical Workshop. Washington, DC, American Association of Blood Banks, 1980, pp 15-17.
79. Miller RD, Robbins TO, Tong M, Barton SL. Coagulation defects associated with massive blood transfusion. Ann Surg 1971;174:794-801.
80. Lim RC, Olcott C, Robinson AJ, Blaisdell FW. Platelet response and coagulation changes following massive blood replacement. J Trauma 1973;13:577-582.
81. Lucas CE, Ledgerwood AM. Clinical significance of altered coagulation tests after massive transfusion for trauma. Am Surg 1981;47:125-130.
82. Mannucci PM, Federici AB, Sirchia G. Hemostasis testing during massive blood replace-ment—a study of 172 cases. Vox Sang 1982;42:113-123.
83. Reed RL, Ciavarela D, Heimbach DM, Baron L, Pavlin E, Counts RB, Carrico CJ. Prophylactic platelet administration during massive transfusion. Ann Surg 1986;203:40-48.
84. Wilson RF, Mammen E, Walt AJ. Eight years experience with massive blood transfusions. J Trauma 1971;11:275-285.
85. Ciavarella D, Reed RL, Counts RB, Baron L, Pavlin E, Heimbach DM, Carrico CJ. Clotting factor levels and the risk of diffuse microvascular bleeding in the massively transfused patient. Br J Haematol 1987;67:365-368.
86. Slichter SJ. Identification and management of defects in platelet hemostatis in massively trans-fused patients. In Massive Transfusion in Surgery and Trauma. New York, Alan R Liss, 1982, pp 225-258.
87. Harrigan C, Lucas CE, Ledgerwood AM, Waltz DA, Mamman EF. Serial changes in primary hemostasis after massive transfusion. Surgery 1985;98:836-842.
88. McNamara JJ, Burran EL, Stremple JF, Molot MD. Coagulopathy after major combat injury: occur-rence, management, and pathophysiology. Ann Surg 1972;20:243-246.
89. Harke H, Rahman S. Haemostatic disorders in massive transfusion. Bibl Haematol 1980;46:179-188.
90. Bell WR. Disseminated intravascular coagula-tion. Johns Hopkins Med J 1980;146:289-299.
91. Colman RW, Robboy SJ, Minna JD. Dissemi-nated intravascular coagulation: a reappraisal. Annu Rev Med 1979;30:359-374.
92. Marder VJ. Consumptive thrombohemorrhagic disorders. In Williams WJ, Beutler E, Erslev AJ, Lichtman MA (eds): Hematology. New York, McGraw-Hill, 1983, pp 1433-1461.
93. Sharp AA. Diagnosis and management of dis-seminated intravascular coagulation. Br Med Bull 1977;33:265-272.
94. Feinstein DI, Counts R, Harker LA, Hultin M, Kasper C, Shapiro S: Inhibitors, D.I.C., and hemostatic defects associated with massive transfusion and cardiopulmonary bypass. In Hematology 1982. Washington, DC, Education-Program, American Society of Hematology, 1982, p 28.
95. Schmaier AH, Colman RW. Disseminated intra-vascular coagulation. In Brain MC, McCulloch PB (eds): Current Therapy in Hematology-Oncology. Philadelphia, BC Decker, 1983, pp 164-169.
96. Colman RW, Robboy SJ, Minna JD. Dissemi-nated intravascular coagulation (DIC): an ap-proach. Am J Med 1972;52:679-689.
97. Siegal T, Seligsohn U, Aghai E, Modan M. Clinical and laboratory aspects of disseminated

intravascular coagulation (DIC): a study of 118 cases. Thromb Haemost 1978;39:122–134.

98. Mant MJ, King EG. Severe, acute disseminated intravascular coagulation: a reappraisal of its pathophysiology, clinical significance and therapy based on 47 patients. Am J Med 1979; 67:557–563.

99. Feinstein DI. Diagnosis and management of disseminated intravascular coagulation: the role of heparin therapy. Blood 1982;60:284–287.

100. Owen JA. Effect of injury on plasma proteins. Adv Clin Chem 1976;9:1–41.

101. Aronsen KF, Ekelund G, Kindmark EO, Laurell CB. Sequential changes of plasma proteins after surgical trauma. Scand J Clin Lab Invest 1972; 29(suppl 124):127–136.

102. Neame PB, Kelton JG, Walker IR, Stewart IO, Nossel HL, Hirsch J: Thrombocytopenia in septicemia. the role of disseminated intravascular coagulation. Blood 1980;56:88–92.

103. Spero JA, Lewis JH, Hasiba U. Disseminated intravascular coagulation. Thromb Haemost 1980;38:28–33.

104. National Institutes of Health Consensus Development Conference. Fresh frozen plasma: indications and risks. JAMA 1985;253:551–553.

105. National Institutes of Health Consensus Development Conference. Platelet transfusion therapy. JAMA 1987;257:1777–1780.

106. Martin DJ, Lucas CE, Ledgerwood AM, Hoschner J, McGonigal MD, Grabow D. Fresh frozen plasma supplement to massive red blood cell transfusion. Ann Surg 1985;202:505–511.

107. Reiner A, Kickler TS, Bell WR. How to administer massive transfusions effectively: guidelines for selecting blood components and monitoring reactions. J Crit Ill 1987;20:15–24.

108. Edmunds LH, Addonizio VP. Massive transfusion. In Colman RW, Hirsch J, Marder VJ, Salzman EW (eds): Hemostasis and Thrombosis—Basic Principles and Clinical Practice, ed 2. Philadelphia, JB Lippincott, 1987, pp 913–919.

109. Wolff G. Fresh frozen plasma: effects and side effects. Bibl Haematol 1980;46:189–206.

110. Ratnoff OD. Some therapeutic agents influencing hemostasis. In Colman RW, Hirsch J, Marder VJ, Salzman EW (eds): Hemostasis and Thrombosis—Basic Principles and Clinical Practice, ed 2. Philadelphia, JB Lippincott, 1987, pp 1026–1047.

111. American Medical Association. General Principles of Blood Transfusion, ed 2. Chicago, American Medical Association, 1985, pp 32–33.

112. Spector I, Corn M, Ticktin HE. Effect of plasma transfusions on the prothrombin time and clotting factors in liver disease. N Engl J Med 1966;275:1032–1037.

113. Manmucci DM, Franchi F, Dioguardi N. Correction of abnormal coagulation in chronic liver disease by combined use of fresh-frozen plasma and prothrombin complex concentrates. Lancet 1976;2:542–545.

114. Salzman W. Hemostatic problems in surgical patients. In Coleman RW, Hirsh J, Marder VJ, Salzman EW (eds): Hemostasis and Thrombosis—Basic Principles and Clinical Practice, ed 2. Philadelphia, JB Lippincott, 1987, pp 1026–1047.

115. Blumberg N, Laczin J, McMican A, Heal J, Awan D. A critical survey of fresh frozen plasma use. Transfusion 1986;26:511–513.

116. Lasch HG, Heene DH. Heparin therapy of diffuse intravascular coagulation (DIC). Thromb Diathes Haemorrh 1974;33:105–106.

117. Straub PW. A case against heparin therapy of intravascular coagulation. Thromb Diathes Haemorrh 1974;33:107–112.

118. Emerson TE, Fournel MA, Redens TB, Taylor FB Jr. Efficacy of antithrombin III supplementation in animal models of fulminant Escherichia coli endotoxemia or bacteremia. Am J Med 1989; 87(3b):27s–33s.

119. vonKries R, Stannigel H, Gobel U. Anticoagulant therapy by continuous heparin-antithrombin III infusion in newborns with disseminated intravascular coagulation. Eur J Pediatr 1985;144: 191–194.

120. Schipper HG, Kahle LH, Jenkins CSP, Ten Cate JW. Antithrombin III transfusion in disseminated intravascular coagulation. Lancet 1978; 1:854–856.

121. Hellgren M, Javelin L, Hagnevik K, Blomback M, Meden-Britth G. Antithrombin III concentrate as adjuvant in DIC treatment: a pilot study in 9 severely ill patients. Thromb Res 1984;35: 459–466.

122. Blauhut B, Kramar H, Vinazzer H, Bergmann H. Substitution of antithrombin III in shock and DIC: a randomized study. Thromb Res 1985; 39:81–89.

123. Maki M, Terao T, Ikenoue T, Takemura T, Sekiba K, Shirakawa K, Soma H. Clinical evaluation of antithrombin III concentrate (BI 6.013) for disseminated intravascular coagulation in obstetrics. Gynecol Obstet Invest 1987; 23:230–240.

124. Hoffman DL, Berkeley BA. Purification and large-scale preparation of antithrombin III. Am J Med 1989;87(3B):3B-23S–3B-26S.

125. Walter CW, Bellamy D, Murphy WP. The mechanical factors responsible for rapid infusion of blood. Surg Gynecol Obstet 1955; 101:115–118.

126. Chaplin H, Chang BA. In vitro comparison of the effects of four different preservative solutions on single donor blood with special emphasis on rate of flow. J Lab Clin Med 1955;46:234–244.

127. Du Plessis JME, Bull AB. Haemolysis occurring during pressure transfusion of stored blood. S Afr Med J 1966;40:479–483.

128. Widmann FK (ed). Technical Manual, ed 9. Arlington, VA, American Association of Blood Banks, 1985, p 290.
129. Millikan JS, Cain TL, Hansbrough JH. Rapid volume replacement for hypovolemic shock: a comparison of techniques and equipment. J Trauma 1984;24:428–431.
130. Mateer JR, Thompson BM, Aprahamian C, Darin JC. Rapid fluid resuscitation with central venous catheters. Ann Emerg Med 1983;12:149–152.
131. Iserson KV, Reeter AK, Criss E. Comparison of flow rates for standard and large-bore blood tubing. West J Med 1985;143:183–185.
132. Sassano JJ. The rapid infusion system. In Winter PM, Kang YG (eds): Hepatic Transplantation—Anesthetic and Perioperative Management. New York, Prager, 1986, pp 120–134.
133. Fried SJ, Satiani B, Zeeb P. Normothermic rapid volume replacement for hypovolemic shock: an in vivo and in vitro study utilizing a new technique. J Trauma 1986;26:183–188.
134. Pineda AA, Rippeteau ND, Clare DE, Bunkowske BM. Infusion flow rates of whole blood and AS-1 preserved erythrocytes: a comparison. Mayo Clin Proc 1987;62:199–202.
135. Boyan CP, Howland WS. Blood temperature: a critical factor in massive transfusion. Anesthesiology 1961;22:559–563.
136. Boyan CP, Howland WS. Cardiac arrest and temperature of bank blood. JAMA 1963;183:58–60.
137. Boyan CP. Cold or warmed blood for massive transfusions. Ann Surg 1964;160:282–286.
138. Holland PV (ed). Standards for Blood Banks and Transfusion Services, ed 13. Arlington, VA, American Association of Blood Banks, 1989, pp 34–35.
139. Klein RE (ed). Accreditation Requirements Manual of the American Association of Blood Banks. Arlington, VA, American Association of Blood Banks, 1986, pp 12–13.
140. Wilson EB, Knauf MA, Iverson KV. Red cell tolerance of admixture with heated saline. Transfusion 1988;28:170–172.
141. Ryden SE, Oberman HA. Compatibility of common intravenous solutions with CPD blood. Transfusion 1975;15:250–255.
142. Klein RE (ed). Accreditation Requirements Manual of the American Association of Blood Banks. Arlington, VA, American Association of Blood Banks, 1986, p 137.
143. Swank RL. Alteration of blood on storage: measurement of adhesiveness of "aging" platelets and leukocytes and their removal by filtration. N Engl J Med 1961;265:728–733.
144. Arrington P, McNamara JJ. Mechanisms of microaggregate formation in stored blood. Ann Surg 1974;179:146–148.
145. Harp JR, Wyche MQ, Marshall BE, Wurzel HA. Some factors determining rate of microag-gregate formation in stored blood. Anesthesiology 40:398–400, 1974.
146. Wenz B. Leukocyte-poor blood. CRC Crit Rev Clin Lab Sci 1986;24:1–20.
147. Snyder EL, Bookbinder M. Role of microaggregate blood filtration in clinical medicine. Transfusion 1983;23:460–467.
148. Oberman HA. Microaggregate filtration. Transfusion 1983;23:89, (editorial).
149. American Medical Association. General Principles of Blood Transfusion, ed 2. Chicago, American Medical Association, 1985, p 67.
150. Collins JA. Surgical problems of transfusion therapy, including cardiopulmonary bypass. In Petz LD, Swisher SN (eds): Clinical Practice of Blood Transfusion. New York, Churchill Livingstone, 1981, pp 462–464.
151. Perkins HA. Strategies for massive transfusion. In Petz LD, Swisher SN (eds): Clinical Practice of Blood Transfusion. New York, Churchill Livingstone, 1981, pp 485–499.
152. Miller RD, Brzica SM. Blood, blood components, colloids and autotransfusion therapy. In Miller RD (ed): Anesthesia, ed 2. New York, Churchill Livingstone, 1986, vol 2, pp 1329–1362.
153. Howland WS. Anesthesiologic perspectives of blood transfusion. In Petz LD, Swisher SN (eds): Clinical Practice of Blood Transfusion. New York, Churchill Livingstone, 1981, pp 471–484.
154. Marshall BE, Wurzel HA, Ellison N, Neufeld GR, Soma LR. Microaggregate formation in stored blood: III. Comparison of Bentley, Fenwal, Pall, and Swank micropore filtration. Circ Shock 1975;2:249–263.
155. Mason KG, Hall LE, Lamoy RE, Wright CB. Evaluation of blood filters: dynamics of platelets and platelet aggregates. Surgery 1975;77:235–240.
156. Snyder EL, Hezzey A, Cooper-Smith M, James R. Effect of microaggregate blood filtration on platelet concentrates in vitro. Transfusion 1981;21:427–434.
157. Klein RE (ed). Accreditation Requirements Manual of the American Association of Blood Banks. Arlington, VA, American Association of Blood Banks, 1986, pp 137–138.
158. Bunker JP, Stetson JB, Coe RC, Grillo HC, Murphy AJ. Citric acid intoxication. JAMA 1955;157:1361–1367.
159. Howland WS, Schweizer O, Carlon GC, Goldiner PL. The cardiovascular effects of low levels of ionized calcium during massive transfusion. Surg Gynecol Obstet 1977;145:581–586.
160. Howland WS, Schweizer O, Jascott D, Ragasa J. Factors influencing the ionization of calcium during major surgical procedures. Surg Gynecol Obstet 1976;143:895–900.
161. Collins JA. Massive blood transfusion. Clin Haematol 1976;5:201–222.
162. Bunker JP, Bendixen HH, Murphy AJ. Hemody-

namic effects of intravenously administered sodium citrate. N Engl J Med 1962;266:372–377.

163. Howland WS, Bellville JW, Zucker MB, Boyan P, Ciffton EE: Massive blood replacement. V. Failure to observe citrate intoxication. Surg Gynecol Obstet 1957;105:529–540.

164. Perkins HA, Synder M, Thacher C, Rolfs MR. Calcium ion activity during rapid exchange transfusion with citrated blood. Transfusion 1971;11:204–212.

165. Carlon GC, Howland WS, Goldiner PL, Kahn RC, Bertoni G, Turnbull AD. Adverse effects of calcium administration. Arch Surg 1978;113:882–885.

166. Wolf PL, McCarthy LJ, Hafleigh B. Extreme hypercalcemia following blood transfusion combined with intravenous calcium. Vox Sang 1970;19:544–545.

167. Howland WS. Calcium, potassium and pH changes during massive transfusion. In Nusbacher J (ed): Massive Transfusion. Washington, DC, American Association of Blood Banks, 1978, pp 17–24.

168. Howland WS. Anesthesiologic perspectives of blood transfusion. In Petz LD, Swisher SN (eds): Clinical Practice of Blood Transfusion. New York, Churchill Livingstone, 1981, pp 471–484.

169. Collins JA, Simmons RL, James PM, Bredenberg CE, Anderson RW, Heisterkamp CA III. Acid-base status of seriously wounded combat casualties: II. Resuscitation with stored blood. Ann Surg 1971;173:6–18.

170. Schweizer O, Howland WS. Significance of lactate and pyruvate according to volume of blood transfusion in man: effect of exogenous bicarbonate buffer on lactic acidemia. Ann Surg 1965;162:1017–1027.

171. Miller RD, Tong MJ, Robbins TO. Effects of massive transfusion of blood on acid-base balance. JAMA 1971;216:1762–1765.

172. Michael JM, Dorner I, Bruns D, Ladenson JH, Sherman LA. Potassium load in CPD-preserved whole blood and two types of packed red blood cells. Transfusion 1975;15(2):144–149.

173. Bunker JP. Metabolic effects of blood transfusion. Anesthesiology 1966;27:446–455.

174. Litwin MS, Smith LL, Moore FD. Metabolic alkalosis following massive transfusion. Surgery 1959;45(5):805–813.

175. Shafer AW, Tague LL, Welch MH, Guenter CA. 2,3-Diphosphoglycerate in red cells stored in acid-citrate-dextrose and citrate-phosphate-dextrose: implications regarding delivery of oxygen. J Lab Clin Med 1974;77:430–437.

176. Moroff G, Dende D. Characterization of biochemical changes occurring during storage of red cells—comparative studies with CPD and CPDA-1 anticoagulant-preservative solutions. Transfusion 1983;23:484–489.

177. Dawson RB, Fagan DS, Meyer DR. Dihydrozyac-etone, pyruvate and phosphate effects on 2,3-DPG and ATP in citrate-phosphate-dextrose-adenine blood preservation. Transfusion 1984;24:327–329.

178. Valeri CR, Pivacek LE, Ragno G, Dennis RC, Palter M, Yeston N, Emerson CP, Altschule MD. A Clinical Experience with Adsol-preserved Red Blood Cells, Technical Report 85-03. Boston, Naval Blood Research Laboratory, Boston University School of Medicine and Surgical Critical Care and Surgical Departments, Boston University Medical Center, 1985, p 31.

179. Sohmer PR, Dawson RB. The significance of 2,3-DPG in red blood cell transfusions. CRC Crit Rev Clin Lab Sci 1979;11:107–174.

180. Valeri CR, Hirsch NM, French M, Gildea S, Livacek L, Herdegen C, Patti K. Restoration in vivo of erythrocyte adenosine triphosphate, 2,3-diphosphoglycerate, potassium ion, and sodium ion concentrations following the transfusion of acid-citrate-dextrose-stored human red blood cells. J Lab Clin Med 1969;73:722–733.

181. Beutler E, Wood L. The in vivo regeneration of red cell 2,3 diphosphoglyceric acid (DPG) after transfusion of stored blood. J Lab Clin Med 1969;74:300–304.

182. Heaton A, Keegan T, Holme S. In vivo regeneration of red cell 2,3-diphosphoglycerate following transfusion of DPG-depleted AS-1, AS-3 and CPDA-1 red cells. Br J Haematol 1989;71:131–136.

183. Howland WS. Anesthesiologic perspectives of blood transfusion. In Petz LD, Swisher SN (eds): Clinical Practice of Blood Transfusion. New York, Churchill Livingstone, 1981, pp 471–484.

184. Collins JA. Surgical problems of transfusion therapy, including cardiopulmonary bypass. In Petz LD, Swisher SN (eds): Clinical Practice of Blood Transfusion. New York, Churchill Livingstone, 1981, pp 457–459.

185. Miller RD, Brzica SM. Blood, blood components, colloids and autotransfusion therapy. In Miller RD (ed): Anesthesia, ed 2. New York, Churchill Livingstone, 1986, vol 2, pp 1329–1362.

186. American Medical Association. General Principles of Blood Transfusion, ed 2. Chicago, American Medical Association, 1985, p 39.

187. Valeri CR. Biochemical modification of red blood cells prior to cryopreservation. In Dawson RB, Barnes A (eds): Clinical and Practical Aspects of the Use of Frozen Blood. Washington, DC, American Association of Blood Banks, 1977, pp 61–76.

188. Valeri CR. Use of rejuvenation solutions in blood preservation. CRC Crit Rev Clin Lab Sci 1982;17:299–374.

189. Heaton WAL. Enhancement of cellular elements. In Wallas CH, McCarthy LJ (eds): New Frontiers in Blood Banking. Arlington, VA, Amer-

ican Association of Blood Banks, 1986, pp 108, 114–116.

190. Peck CC, Moore GL, Bolin RB. Adenine in blood preservation. CRC Crit Rev Clin Lab Sci 1981; 13:173–212.

191. Moore GL, Ledford ME. The uptake and egress of adenine from human red blood cells in vitro. Transfusion 1977;17:38–43.

192. Warner WL. Toxicology and pharmacology of adenine in animals and man. Transfusion 1977; 17:326–332.

193. Stone RE, Spies TD. Adenine: its failure to stimulate hemopoiesis or to produce pellagra in a case of pernicious anemia. Am J Med Sci 1948;215:411–414.

194. Falk JS, Lindblad GTO, Westman BJM. Histopathological studies from patients treated with large amounts of blood preserved with ACD-adenine. Transfusion 1972;12:376–381.

195. Reznikoff P. The treatment of agranulocytosis with adenine sulfate. J Clin Invest 1933;12: 45–53.

196. Mollison PL. Blood Transfusion in Clinical Medicine, ed 7. Oxford, England, Blackwell Scientific Publications, 1983, p 360.

197. Widmann FK (ed). Technical Manual, ed 9. Arlington, VA, American Association of Blood Banks, 1985, p 322.

198. Taswell HF, Reisner RK. Prevention of $Rh_0$ hemolytic disease of the newborn: the rosette method—a rapid, sensitive screening test. Mayo Clin Proc 1983;58:324–343.

199. Riley JZ, Ness PM, Taddie SJ, Barrasso C, Baldwin ML. Detection and quantitation of fetal maternal hemorrhage utilizing an enzyme-linked antiglobulin test. Transfusion 1982;22:472–474.

200. Nance SJ, Nelson JM, Arndt PA, Lam HTC, Garratty G. Quantitation of fetal-maternal hemorrhage by flow cytometry: a simple and accurate method. Am J Clin Pathol 1989;91:288–292.

201. Myhre BA. Fatalities from blood transfusion. JAMA 1980;244:1333–1335.

202. Holland PV. Other adverse effects of transfusion. In Petz LD, Swisher SN (eds): Clinical Practice of Blood Transfusion. New York, Churchill Livingstone, 1981, pp 783–803.

203. Greenwalt TJ. Pathogenesis and management of hemolytic transfusion reactions. Semin Hematol 1981;18:84–94.

204. Weisz-Carrington P. Transfusion reactions. In Principles of Clinical Immunohematology. Chicago, Year Book, 1986, pp 325–354.

205. Goldfinger D. Acute hemolytic transfusion reactions—a fresh look at pathogenesis and considerations regarding therapy. Transfusion 1977; 17:85–98.

206. Mollison PL. Blood Transfusion in Clinical Medicine, ed 7. Oxford, England, Blackwell Scientific Publications, 1983, pp 627–674.

207. Relihan M, Olsen RE, Liturn MS. Clearance rate and effect on renal function of stroma-free hemoglobin following renal ischemia. Ann Surg 1971;176:700–704.

208. Savitsky JP, Doczi J, Black J, Arnold JD. A clinical safety trial of stroma free hemoglobin. Clin Pharmacol Ther 1978;23(1):73–80.

209. Schmidt PJ, Holland PV. Pathogenesis of the acute renal failure associated with incompatible transfusion. Lancet 1967;1169–1172.

210. Barry KG, Crosby WH. The prevention and treatment of renal failure following transfusion reactions. Transfusion 1963;3:34–36.

211. Rock RC, Bove JR, Nemerson Y. Heparin treatment of intravascular coagulation accompanying hemolytic transfusion reactions. Transfusion 1969;9:57–61.

212. Pineda AA, Taswell HF, Brzica SM Jr. Delayed hemolytic transfusion reaction, an immunologic hazard of blood transfusion. Transfusion 1978; 18:1–7.

213. Woodfield DG. Delayed blood transfusion reactions. NZ Med J 1979;90:496–498.

214. Sarnaik S, Schornack J, Lusher JM. The incidence of development of irregular red cell antibodies in patients with sickle cell anemia. Transfusion 1986;26:249–252.

215. Kevy SV, Schmidt PJ, McGinniss AB, Workman WG. Febrile, nonhemolytic transfusion reactions and the limited role of leukoagglutinins in their etiology. Transfusion 1962;2:7–16.

216. Wilhelm RE, Nutting HM, Devlin HB, Jennings ER, Brines OA. Antihistaminics for allergic and pyrogenic transfusion reactions. JAMA 1955; 158:529–531.

217. Payne R. The association of febrile transfusion reactions with leukoagglutinins. Vox Sang 1957; 2:233–241.

218. deRie MA, van der Plas-van Dalen CM, Engelfriet CP, von dem Borne AEGK. The serology of febrile transfusion reactions. Vox Sang 1985; 49:126–134.

219. Heinrich D, Mueller-Eckhardt C, Stier W. The specificity of leukocyte and platelet alloantibodies in sera of patients with nonhemolytic transfusion reactions—absorptions and elution studies. Vox Sang 1973;25:442–456.

220. Greenwalt TJ, Gajewski M, McKenna JL. A new method of preparing buffy coat-poor blood. Transfusion 1962;2:221–229.

221. Perkins HA, Payne R, Ferguson J, Wood M. Nonhemolytic febrile transfusion reactions—quantitative effects of blood components with emphasis on isoantigenic incompatibility of leukocytes. Vox Sang 1966;11:578–600.

222. Aster RH, Jandl JH. Platelet sequestration in man: II. Immunological and clinical studies. J Clin Invest 1964;43:856–869.

223. Ahrons S, Kissmeyer-Nielsen F. Febrile transfusion reaction caused by minor specific (LA1)

leukocyte incompatibility—a case. Dan Med Bull 1968;15:257–258.

224. Brittingham TE, Chaplin H Jr. Febrile transfusion reactions caused by sensitivity to donor leukocytes and platelets. JAMA 1957;165:819–827.

225. Thulstrup H. The influence of leukocyte and thrombocyte incompatibility on non-hemolytic transfusion reactions: I. A retrospective study. Vox Sang 1971;21:233–250.

226. Mollison PL. Blood Transfusion in Clinical Medicine, ed 7. Oxford, England, Blackwell Scientific Publications, 1983, pp 731–732, 761–762.

227. Huestis DW, Bove JR, Case J. Practical Blood Transfusion, ed 4. Boston, Little, Brown & Co, 1988.

228. Pineda AA, Brzica SM, Taswell HF: Hemolytic transfusion reaction—recent experience in a large blood bank. Mayo Clin Proc 1978;53: 378–390.

229. Menitove JE, McElligott MC, Aster RH. Febrile transfusion reaction: what blood component should be given next? Vox Sang 1982;42: 318–321.

230. Popovsky MA, Moore SB. Diagnostic and pathogenetic considerations in transfusion-related acute lung injury. Transfusion 1985;25:573–577.

231. Levy GJ, Shabot MM, Hart ME, Mya WW, Goldfinger D. Transfusion-associated noncardiogenic pulmonary edema—report of a case and a warning regarding treatment. Transfusion 1986;26:278–281.

232. Mollison PL. Blood Transfusion in Clinical Medicine, ed 7. Oxford, England, Blackwell Scientific Publications, 1983, pp 741–745.

233. Vyas GN, Perkins HA, Fudenberg HH. Anaphylactoid transfusion reactions associated with anti-IgA. Lancet 1968;2:312–315.

234. Laschinger C, Shepherd FA, Naylor DH. Anti-IgA-mediated transfusion reactions in Canada. Can Med Assoc J 1984;130:141–144.

235. Leikola J, Koistinen J, Lehtinen M, Virolainen M. IgA induced anaphylactic transfusion reactions—a report of four cases. Blood 1973; 42:111–119.

236. Ropars C, Muller A, Paint N, Beige D, Avernard G. Large scale detection of IgA deficient blood donors. J Immunol Methods 1982;54:183–189.

237. Vyas GN, Perkins HA, Yang Y-M, Basantani GK. Healthy blood donors with selective absence of immunoglobulin A: prevention of anaphylactic transfusion reactions caused by antibodies to IgA. J Lab Clin Med 1975;85:838–842.

238. Vyas GN, Perkins HA. Anti-IgA in blood donors. Transfusion 1976;16:289–290 (letter).

239. Mollison PL. Blood Transfusion in Clinical Medicine, ed 7. Oxford, England, Blackwell Scientific Publications, 1983, p 740.

240. Petty RE, Sherry DD, Johannson J. Anti-IgA antibodies in pregnancy. N Engl J Med 1985; 313:1620–1625.

241. Rivat L, Rivat C, Daveau M, Ropartz C. Comparative frequencies of anti-IgA antibodies in patients with anaphylactic transfusion reactions and among normal blood donors. Clin Immunol Immunopathol 1977;7:340–348.

242. Aach RD, Szmuness W, Mosley JW, Hollinger FB, Kahn RA, Stevens CE, Edwards VM, Werch J. Serum alanine aminotransferase of donors in relation to the risk of non-A, non-B hepatitis in recipients—the transfusion-transmitted viruses study. N Engl J Med 1981;304:989–994.

243. Koziol DE, Holland PV, Alling DW, Melpolder JC, Solomon RE, Purcell RH, Hudson LM, Shoup F, Krakauer H, Alter HJ. Antibody to hepatitis B core antigen as a paradoxical marker for non-A, non-B hepatitis agents in donated blood. Ann Intern Med 1986;104:488–495.

244. Aach RD, Lander JJ, Sherman LA, Miller WV, Kahn RA, Gitnick GL, Hollinger FB, Werch J, Szmuness W, Stevens CE, Kellner A, Weiner JM, Mosley JW. Transfusion-transmitted viruses: interim analysis of hepatitis among transfused and nontransfused patients. In Vyas GN, Cohen SN, Schmid R (eds): Viral Hepatitis—A Contemporary Assessment of Etiology, Epidemiology, Pathogenesis and Prevention. Philadelphia, Franklin Institute Press, 1978, pp 383–396.

245. Holland PV. Informing the transfusion recipient: how much is enough? In Smith DM Jr, Carlson KB (eds): Current Scientific/Ethical Dilemmas in Blood Banking. Arlington, VA, American Association of Blood Banks, 1987, pp 15–28.

246. Adler SP. Transfusion-associated cytomegalovirus infections. Rev Infect Dis 1983;5:977–993.

247. Dienstag JL. Non-A, non-B hepatitis: I. Recognition, epidemiology and clinical features. Gastroenterology 1983;85:439–462.

248. Wick MR, Moore S, Taswell HF. Non-A, non-B hepatitis associated with blood transfusion. Transfusion 1985;25:93–101.

249. Kuo G, Choo Q-L, Alter HJ, Gitnick GL, Redeker AG, Purcell RH, Miyamura T, Dienstag JL, Alter MJ, Stevens CE, Tegtmeier GE, Bonino F, Colombo M, Lee W-S, Kuo C, Berger K, Shuster JR, Overby LR, Bradley DW, Houghton M. An assay for circulating antibodies to a major etiologic virus of human non-A, non-B hepatitis. Science 1989;244:362–364.

250. Alter HJ. Discovery of the non-A, non-B hepatitis virus: the end of the beginning or the beginning of the end. Transfusion Med Rev 1989;3:77–81, (editorial).

251. Dienstag JL, Wands JR, Koff RS. Acute hepatitis. In Braunwald E, Isselbacher KJ, Petersdorf RG, Wilson JD, Martin JB, Fauci AS (eds): Harrison's Principles of Internal Medicine, ed 11. New York, McGraw-Hill, 1987, pp 1325–1338.

252. Hornbrook MC, Dodd RY, Jacobs P, Friedman LI, Sherman KE. Reducing the incidence of non-A, non-B post-transfusion hepatitis by test-

ing donor blood for alanine aminotransferase—economic considerations. N Engl J Med 1982; 307:1315–1321.

253. Silverstein MD, Mulley AG, Dienstag JL. Should donor blood be screened for elevated aminotransferase levels? JAMA 1984;252:2839–2845.

254. Koretz RL, Stone O, Gitnick GL. The long-term course of non-A, non-B post transfusion hepatitis. Gastroenterology 1980;79:893–898.

255. Knodell RG, Conrad ME, Ishak KG. Development of chronic liver disease after acute non-A non-B post-transfusion hepatitis. Gastroenterology 1977;72:902–909.

256. Rakela J, Redeker AG. Chronic liver disease after acute non-A non-B viral hepatitis. Gastroenterology 1979;77:1200–1202.

257. Berman M, Alter HJ, Ishak KG, Purcell RH, Jones EA: The chronic sequelae of non-A, non-B hepatitis. Ann Intern Med 1979;91:1–6.

258. Realdi G, Alberti A, Rugge M, Rigoli AM, Tremolada F. Long term follow-up of acute and chronic non-A, non-B post-transfusion hepatitis: evidence of progression to liver cirrhosis. Gut 1982;23:270–275.

259. Grady GF, Bennett AJE. Risk of posttransfusion hepatitis in the United States: a prospective cooperative study. JAMA 1972;220:692–701.

260. Sugg U, Schenzle D, Hess G. Antibodies to hepatitis B core antigen in blood donors screened for alanine aminotransferase level and hepatitis non-A, non-B in recipients. Transfusion 1988;28:386–388.

261. Bove JR. Transfusion-associated hepatitis and AIDS—what is the risk? N Engl J Med 1987; 317:242–245.

262. Mattsson L, Aberg B, Weiland O, Sellman M, Davilen J. Non-A, non-B hepatitis after open-heart surgery in Stockholm: declining incidence after introduction of restrictions for blood donations due to the human immunodeficiency virus. Scand J Infect Dis 1988;20:371–376.

263. Kuhns WJ, Prince AM, Brotman B, Hazzi C, Grady GF. A clinical and laboratory evaluation of immune serum globulin from donors with a history of hepatitis: attempted prevention of post-transfusion hepatitis. Am J Med Sci 1976; 272:255–261.

264. Knodell RG, Ginsberg AL, Conrad ME, Bell CJ, Flannery EP. Efficacy of prophylactic gamma-globulin in preventing non-A, non-B post-transfusion hepatitis. Lancet 1976;1:557–561.

265. Seeff LB, Zimmerman HJ, Wright EC, Finkelstin JD, Garcia-Pont P, Greenlee HB, Dietz AA, Leevy CM, Tamburro CH, Schiff ER, Schimmel EM, Zemel R, Zimmon DS, McCollum RW. A randomized, double blind controlled trial of the efficacy of immune serum globulin for the prevention of post-transfusion hepatitis: a Veterans Administration cooperative study. Gastroenterology 1977;72:111–121.

266. Sanchez-Quijano A, Lissen E, Diaz-Torres MA, Rivera F, Pineda JA, Leal M, Garcia de Pesquera F, Castro R, Munoz J. Prevention of post-transfusion non-A, non-B hepatitis by non-specific immunoglobulin in heart surgery patients. Lancet 1988;1:1245–1249.

267. Conrad ME. Preventing post-transfusion hepatitis. Lancet 1988;2:217, (letter).

268. Immunization Practices Advisory Committee. Recommendations for protection against viral hepatitis. MMWR 1985;34:313–335.

269. Barker LF, Dodd RY. Viral hepatitis, acquired immunodeficiency syndrome, and other infections transmitted by transfusion. In Petz LD, Swisher SN (eds): Clinical Practice of Transfusion Medicine, ed 2. New York, Churchill Livingstone, 1989, pp 683–684.

270. Broder S, Gallo RC. A pathogenic retrovirus (HTLV-III) linked to AIDS. N Engl J Med 1984;311:1292–1297.

271. Peterman TA, Jaffe HW, Feorino PM, Getchell JP, Warfield D, Haverkos HW, Stoneburner RL, Curran JW. Transfusion-associated acquired immunodeficiency syndrome in the United States. JAMA 1985;254:2913–2917.

272. Feorino PM, Jaffe H, Palmer E, Peterman TA, Francis DP, Kalyanaraman VS, Weinstein RA, Stoneburner RL, Alexander WJ, Raevsky C, Getchell JP, Warfield D, Haverkos HW, Kilbourne BW, Nicholson JKA, Curran JW. Transfusion-associated acquired immunodeficiency syndrome—evidence for persistent infection in blood donors. N Engl J Med 1985; 312:1293–1296.

273. Centers for Disease Control. AIDS and human immunodeficiency virus infection in the United States: 1988 update. MMWR 1988;38(suppl 4):1–38.

274. Department of Health and Human Services/Public Health Service/Federal Drug Administration. FDA Drug Bull 1986;16(1):3.

275. Centers for Disease Control. Provisional public health service inter-agency recommendations for screening donated blood and plasma for antibody to the virus causing acquired immunodeficiency syndrome. MMWR 1985;34:13–16.

276. Pierce GF, Lusher JM, Brownstein AP, Goldsmith JC, Kessler CM. The use of purified clotting factor concentrates in hemophilia—influence of viral safety, cost, and supply on therapy. JAMA 1989;261:3434–3438.

277. Brettler DB, Levine PH. Factor concentrates for treatment of hemophilia: which one to choose? Blood 1989;73:2067–2073.

278. Lui K-J, Lawrence DN, Morgan WM, Peterman TA, Haverkos HW, Bregman DJ. A model-based approach for estimating the mean incubation period of transfusion-associated acquired immunodeficiency syndrome. Proc Natl Acad Sci USA 1986;83:3051–3055.

279. Rees M. The sombre view of AIDS. Nature 1987;326:343–345.
280. Kuritsky JN, Rastogi SC, Faich GA, Schorr JB, Menitov JE, Reilly RW, Bove JR. Results of nationwide screening of blood and plasma for antibodies to human T-cell lymphotrophic virus, type III. Transfusion 1986;26:205–207.
281. Ness PM, Douglas DK, Harper M, Polk BF. Declining prevalence of HIV-seropositive blood donors. N Engl J Med 1989;321:615, (letter).
282. Ward JW, Holmberg SD, Allen JR, Cohn DL, Critchley SE, Kleinman SH, Lenes BA, Ravenholt O, Davis JR, Quinn MG, Jaffe HW. Transmission of human immunodeficiency virus (HIV) by blood transfusions screened as negative for HIV antibody. N Engl J Med 1988;318:473–478.
283. Schorr JB, Berkowitz A, Cumming PD, Katz A, Sandler S. Prevalence of HTLV-III antibody in American blood donors. N Engl J Med 1985; 313:384–385, (letter).
284. Ward JW, Grindon AJ, Feorino PM, Schable C, Porvin M, Allen JR. Laboratory and epidemiologic evaluation of an enzyme immunoassay for antibodies to HTLV-III. JAMA 1986; 256:357–361.
285. Esteban JL, Tai C-C, Kay JWD, Shih JW-K, Bodner A, Alter HJ. Importance of Western blot analysis in predicting ineffectivity of anti-HTLV-III/LAV positive blood. Lancet 1985; 2:1083–1086.
286. Petricciani JC. Licensed tests for antibody to human T-lymphotropic virus type III: sensitivity and specificity. Ann Intern Med 1985;103: 726–729.
287. National Institutes of Health Consensus Development Panel. The impact of routine HTLV-III antibody testing of blood and plasma donors on public health. JAMA 1986;256:1778–1783.
288. Haseltine WA. Silent HIV infections. N Engl J Med 1989;320:1487–1489, (editorial).
289. Imagawa DT, Lee MH, Wolinsky SM, Sano K, Morales F, Kwok S, Sninsky JJ, Nishanian PG, Giorgi J, Fahey JL, Dudley J, Visscher BR, Detels R. Human immunodeficiency virus type 1 infection in homosexual men who remain seronegative for prolonged periods. N Engl J Med 1989;320:1458–1462.
290. Kolins J. The continued risk of transfusion-transmitted AIDS. Pathologist 1986;40:9–10.
291. Cohen ND, Munoz A, Reitz BA, Ness PK, Frazier OH, Yawn DH, Lee H, Blattner W, Donahue JG, Nelson KE, Polk BF. Transmission of retroviruses by transfusion of screened blood in patients undergoing cardiac surgery. N Engl J Med 1989;320:1172–1176.
292. Lentner C, Dliem K (eds). Scientific Tables, ed 7. Basle, Ciby-Geigy, 1970, p 186.
293. Ward JW, Kleinman SH, Douglas DK, Grindon AJJ, Holmberg SD. Epidemiologic characteristic of blood donors with antibody to human immunodeficiency virus. Transfusion 1988;28: 298–301.
294. Alter HJ, Epstein JS, Swenson SG, Menitove JE, Ward JW, Kaslow RA, Van Raden M, Klein HG, Sandler SG, Sayers MH, Chernoff AI and the HIV-Antigen Study Group. Collaborative study to evaluate HIV-antigen (HIV-Ag) screening of blood donors. Transfusion 1989;29(Suppl):56s (abstract).
295. Backer U, Weinhauer F, Gathof G, Eberle J. HIV antigen screening in blood donors. Lancet 1987;2:1213–1214.
296. Peitrequin R, Graf I, Lantin J-P, Frei P-C. Routine tests for HIV antigen. Lancet 1987;2:916–917.
297. Hjelle B, Busch M. Direct methods for detection of HIV-1 infection. Arch Pathol Lab Med 1989; 113:975–980.
298. Clavel F, Mansinho K, Chamaret S, Guetard D, Favier V, Nina J, Santos-Ferreira M-O, Champalimaud J-L, Montagnier L. Human immunodeficiency virus type 2 infection associated with AIDS in West Africa. N Engl J Med 1987; 316:1180–1185.
299. Horsburgh CR, Holmberg SD. The global distribution of human immunodeficiency virus type 2 (HIV-2) infection. Transfusion 1988;28:192–195.
300. Brun-Vezinet F, Katlama CJ, Doulot D, Lonoble L, Alizon M, Madjar JJ, Rey MA, Girard PM, Yeni P, Clavel F, Gadelle S, Harzic M. Lymphadenopathy-associated virus type 2 in AIDS and AIDS-related complex: clinical and virological features in four patients. Lancet 1987; 1:128–132.
301. Centers for Disease Control. AIDS due to HIV-2 infection—New Jersey. MMWR 1988;37:33–35.
302. Ayanian JZ, Maguire JH, Marlink RG, Essex M, Kanki P. HIV-2 infection in the United States. N Engl J Med 1989;320:1422–1423, (letter).
303. Esber EC. Recommendations concerning persons at increased risk of HIV-1 and HIV-2 infection: memo to all registered blood establishments, Food and Drug Administration, 4/6/88.
304. Centers for Disease Control. Licensure of screening tests for antibody to human T-lymphotropic virus type I. MMWR 1988;37: 736–747.
305. Rosenblatt JD, Chen ISY, Wachsman W. Infection with HTLV-I and HTLV-II: evolving concepts. Semin Hematol 1988;25:230–246.
306. Anonymous. HTLV-1 comes of age. Lancet 1988;1:217–219.
307. Petz LD, Szxton E, Lee H, Chen ISY, Chin E, Delamarter R, Rosenblatt JD, Harper M, Ness PM. A case of transfusion-transmitted HTLV-I associated myelopathy. Transfusion 1989; 29(Suppl):55S, (abstract).
308. Williams AE, Fang CT, Slamon DJ, Poiesz BJ, Sandler G, Darr F, Shulman G, McGowan EI, Douglas DK, Bowman RJ, Peetoom F, Kleinman

SH, Lenes B, Dodd RY. Seroprevalence and epidemiological correlates of HTLV-I infection in U.S. blood donors. Science 1988; 240:643–646.

309. Yeager AS, Grumet FC, Hafleigh EB, Arvin AM, Bradley JS,

319. Collins AJ, Baudin JC, Cooper ES. Comparison of donor unit exclusion percentages of designated donors vs. volunteer donors. Transfusion 1987; 27:575 (abstract).

320. Fisher A, Pura L, Smith L, Goldfinger D. Safety and effectiveness of directed blood donation in a large teaching hospital. Transfusion 1986; 26:600 (abstract).

321. Shah VP, Molstad JR, Segall SL, Strand CL. A hospital donor room's three year experience with directed donations. Transfusion 1986;26: 599 (abstract).

322. Allen RW, Kahn RA, Baldassare JJ. Advances in the production of blood cell substitutes with alternate technologies. In Wallas CH, McCarthy LJ (eds): New Frontiers in Blood Banking. Arlington, VA, American Association of Blood Banks, 1986, pp 21–50.

323. Moss GS, Gould SA, Sehgal LR, Rosen A, Sehgal HL. Polyhemoglobin and fluorocarbon as blood substitutes. Biomater Artif Cells Artif Organs 1987;15:333–336.

324. Chang TMS. The use of modified hemoglobin as an oxygen carrying blood substitute. Transfusion Med Rev 1989;3:213–218.

325. Riess JG. Blood substitutes: where do we stand with the fluorocarbon approach? Curr Surg 1988;45:365–370.

326. Djordjevich L, Ivankovich AD. Progress in development of synthetic erythrocytes made by encapsulation of hemoglobin. Adv Exp Med Biol 1986;238:171–197.

327. Gould SA, Rosen AL, Sehgal LR, Sehgal HL, Langdale LA, Krause LM, Rice CL, Chamberlin

WH, Moss GS. Fluosol-DA as a red-cell substitute in acute anemia. N Engl J Med 1986; 314:1653–1656.

328. Rock G. Production of plasma products and derivatives. In Wallas CH, McCarthy LJ (eds): New Frontiers in Blood Banking. Arlington, VA, American Association of Blood Banks, 1986, pp 51–88.

329. White GC, McMillan CW, Kingdon HS, Shoemaker C. Use of recombinant antihemophilic factor in the treatment of two patients with classic hemophilia. N Engl J Med 1989;320: 166–170.

330. Winearls CG, Pippard MJ, Downing MR, Oliver DO, Reid C, Cotes PM. Effect of human erythropoietin derived from recombinant DNA on the anaemia of patients maintained by chronic haemodialysis. Lancet 1986; 2:1175–1178.

331. Stone WJ, Graber SE, Krantz SB, Dessypris EN, O'Neil VL, Olsen NJ, Pincus TP. Treatment of the anemia of predialysis patients with recombinant human erythropoietin: a randomized, placebo-controlled trial. Am J Med Sci 1988; 296(3):171–179.

332. Eschbach JW, Egrie JC, Downing MR, Browne JK, Adamson JW. Correction of the anemia of end-stage renal disease with recombinant human erythropoietin: results of a combined phase I and II trial. N Engl J Med 1987;316:73–78.

333. Means RT, Olsen NJ, Krantz SB, Dessypris EN, Graber SE, Stone WJ, O'Neil VL, Pincus T. Treatment of the anemia of rheumatoid arthritis with recombinant human erythropoietin: clinical and in vitro studies. Arthritis Rheum 1989; 32(5):638–642.

334. Goodnough LT, Wasman J, Corlucci K, Chernosky A. Limitations to donating adequate autologous blood prior to elective orthopedic surgery. Arch Surg 1989;124:494–496.

# 6

# Perioperative Anesthetic Management of the Trauma Patient: Thoracoabdominal and Orthopaedic Injuries

*John K. Stene, Christopher M. Grande, William N. Bernhard, and Charles R. Barton*

This multipartite chapter is pivotal to the thrust of this book: it not only ties together the essentials of preoperative anesthetic management (i.e., the role of the anesthesia care provider, initial evaluation procedures, airway management, and resuscitation), but also focuses on the issues of concern during the immediate preinduction (e.g., choices of monitoring equipment) and intraoperative (e.g., pharmacology) periods. In addition, the reader is provided with a treatment of issues germane to two of the major and often most important organ systems that sustain injury. Thoracoabdominal injuries do not commonly require immediate surgery but can present the most life-threatening situations (e.g., pericardial tamponade). In the majority of these cases, the well-trained trauma anesthesia/critical care specialist (TA/CCS) possesses the knowledge and expertise to restore homeostasis rapidly and decisively, with or without the assistance of other medical specialists. Conversely, orthopaedic injuries are among the most common requiring operative intervention during the immediate postadmission period. A majority of the TA/CCS's time in the operating room (OR) is spent providing anesthetic care for patients with musculoskeletal injuries. Further, as will be discussed, orthopaedic injuries are increasingly thought to be responsible for much of the morbidity and mortality seen in follow-up trauma care (i.e., beyond the first few days).

When discussing these issues, we must repeat some material covered elsewhere in the book to present information in a congruous fashion. We have attempted to minimize this repetition as much as possible.

## INTRODUCTION TO PERIOPERATIVE CONSIDERATIONS FOR TRAUMA ANESTHESIA

Titrated care is the hallmark of sophisticated trauma care, just as it is the hallmark of good anesthetic care. The priorities of anesthesia care for the trauma patient are different from the priorities for either elective or nontraumatic, emergency surgical patients. During the initial phases of medical care of the trauma patient, examination and treatment must proceed simultaneously, often guided by preexisting protocols rather than by formal diagnosis (1, 2). Table 6.1 describes the "primary survey" and treatment for trauma patients, as suggested by the American College of Surgeons' Advanced Trauma Life Support (ATLS) protocols (3).

Most anesthesiologists consider it axiomatic that a thorough preoperative anesthetic history and physical, which lead to a sound diagnosis and an appropriate anesthetic prescription, improve anesthesia patient care. However, many otherwise compulsive anesthesiologists are conversely willing to forego preoperative evaluation before emergency trauma surgery. For example, by not being present in the emergency room at the earliest opportunity, the anesthesiologist who waits for the trauma patient in the OR will be forced to rapidly anesthetize an unfamiliar patient who requires life-saving surgery. In the emergency situation, the value of preoperative preparation is especially critical, as is the value of written documentation of such, from both a clinical and a medicolegal standpoint (see Chapter 18).

**Table 6.1.    Resuscitation Protocols**[a]

*Primary Survey*

Overview (15-20 sec) *Scan* the patient for obvious injuries.
Listen to EMS providers' history.
*Ask* the patient to describe his/her injuries.
*Ascertain* the following;
Airway—Does the patient have a patent airway?
   Look—Chest wall movements—retraction nasal flaring
   Listen—Breath sounds—stridor, stertorous respirations
   Feel—Air movement
   *Correct* any obstruction—may require intubation
Breathing—Can the patient sustain adequate spontaneous ventilation?
   *Inspect* thoracic cage for symmetric chest movement
   Open pneumothorax (sucking chest wound)
   Flail segments
   *Auscultation*—for bilateral air movement
   *Correct* ventilatory failure by mechanical ventilatory assist
Circulation—Is the patient perfusing adequately?
   Peripheral pulses, capillary refill, arterial blood pressure, ECG, grade shock by vital signs, etc.
Correct—circulatory shock—start IVs
Draw blood sample for crossmatch and diagnostic laboratory parameters
Disability—*Ascertain* neurologic injury,
   *Evaluate* central function:
   A—alert
   V—responds to vocal stimuli
   P—responds to painful stimuli
   U—unresponsive
   *Evaluate:* pupil size and light responses,
      motor function in all four extremities, reflexes,
      Glasgow Coma Scale (see Chapter 7)
      Remember: *Treat a problem when it is identified.*
      *Do not wait for primary survey to be completed.*

Secondary Survey—For Complete Surgical/Anesthesia Diagnosis—More Formal History and Physical Exam.

[a] Based on elements of the Advanced Trauma Life Support (ATLS) Course, American College of Surgeons, Committee on Trauma, Chicago, IL.

This chapter discusses the logical approach to the perioperative anesthetic care of the trauma patient. With appropriate focus on the necessary and desirable components of the preoperative visit, an anesthesiologist can efficiently use available time to maximize his/her preanesthetic appreciation and preparation for the emergent trauma patient.

As described in Chapter 1, the establishment of trauma centers and trauma systems undoubtedly affects the anesthetic care of the trauma patient. A by-product of this regionalization of trauma care into trauma centers is that it allows efficient utilization of increasingly scarce hospital resources (4).

Trauma centers (including "accident hospitals") also provide adequate case experience to hone the skills of the surgical and anesthesia staff. The American College of Surgeons' guide for trauma center organization recognizes trauma as a surgical illness that requires highly skilled anesthesia care for optimal outcome (4). Within the United States the trauma surgeon concentrates on surgical diagnosis and treatment, whereas the TA/CCS provides not only a secure airway, adequate ventilation, appropriate intravenous fluid management (ABCs), but also the required sedation, analgesia, or anesthesia to facilitate both diagnosis and the surgical therapy, as well as overseeing general management (5). The TA/CCS's mission outside the United States is expanded to provide optimum care for the trauma patient in the ambulance or helicopter, in the emergency room, and in the critical care unit, as well as in the OR. In some countries, anesthesiologists are involved in the organization of prehospital (emergency medical services) care and transportation of trauma patients (2). By virtue of sheer numbers of trauma patients (trauma is the primary cause of death among individuals younger than 40 years old and is third overall), however, anesthesiologists working in hospitals not designated as trauma centers will find their expertise in airway management and monitoring the critically ill to be invaluable in the optimal care of an occasional (or not-so-occasional) trauma patient.

Early involvement of anesthesia care providers, both anesthesiologists and certified registered nurse anesthetists (CRNA), as part of the "trauma team" is incorporated in the trauma center concept. The anesthesia care provider derives several benefits from early involvement in trauma patient care.

1. He/she has the opportunity to perform a history and physical examination of the patient simultaneously with the surgeon. Therefore, if the patient requires early transport to the OR, the TA/CCS is just as aware of the patient's condition as are the surgeons. It is absolutely vital in trauma care not to lose valuable time while the anesthesia care provider attempts to become familiar with the trauma patient in the OR.

2. The anesthesia care provider will be able to take early steps to ensure that the trauma patient is properly prepared for the operation, before moving into the OR (Table 6.2). Frequently, the transfer of a trauma patient to the OR becomes extremely chaotic as soon as the decision is made to operate. Preparing the patient includes not only establishing vascular access for intravenous fluids, but also having instrumentation available to monitor appropriate cardiovascular parameters. Figures 6.1 and 6.2 illustrate appropriate OR facilities in a modern

**Table 6.2.   Preoperative Checklist for Trauma Anesthesia**

\_\_\_\_ History of present illness and mechanism of injury
\_\_\_\_ History of allergies,
     drug use,
     preexisting diseases—coronary artery disease,
     diabetes mellitus,
     asthma,
     COPD,
     cirrhosis,
     renal disease,
     endocrinopathies,
     coagulation defects,
     neurologic disease
\_\_\_\_ At least two large-bore intravenous lines (one above diaphragm, one below diaphragm for injuries to the trunk)
\_\_\_\_ Airway management and intubation equipment
\_\_\_\_ Adequate level of monitoring equipment
\_\_\_\_ Physical examination (via primary and secondary surveys)
\_\_\_\_ Adequate diagnostic studies (circumstances permitting)
\_\_\_\_ Surgical diagnosis and plan
\_\_\_\_ Anesthesia diagnosis and plan
\_\_\_\_ Anesthesia machine, ventilator equipment "checked-out" and on "stand by"
\_\_\_\_ All pharmacologic agents (anesthestic and emergency) ready
\_\_\_\_ Special equipment
     Autotransfusion device
     Oxygenator (pump)
     High-volume, rapid fluid infusion system

trauma center, with the equipment needed by the TA/CCS to anesthetize the trauma patient safely.

3. The Maryland Institute for Emergency Medical Services Systems (MIEMSS) Shock Trauma Center experience is that having an anesthesia care provider participate in the admission process reduces the requirement for tracheostomies. As described in Chapter 3, the TA/CCS can usually achieve control of the trauma patient's airway through endotracheal intubation by an oral or nasal route, which reduces the need for emergency tracheostomies. Conversely, patients who do require a tracheostomy to facilitate surgical repair of facial trauma can have a secure endotracheal tube airway placed before the tracheostomy is created, which is usually desirable (see Chapter 3).

## PREANESTHETIC DIAGNOSIS AND TREATMENT

As stated above, treatment must often be concurrent with diagnosis to optimize resuscitation of the critically injured trauma patient (2). Thus, anesthetic diagnosis also must occur simultaneously with treatment of the trauma patient. The anesthesia care provider works in cooperation with the surgical team. The preanesthetic workup begins with the initial evaluation protocols outlined in the ATLS Course of the American College of Surgeons (Table 6.1). Thus, the patient is scrutinized quickly to rule out cardiopulmonary arrest and the immediate need for cardiopulmonary resuscitation (CPR). The anesthesia care provider must pay particular attention to the patient's neurologic status. Both manual and pharmacologic maneuvers to secure an airway and provide artificial ventilation affect the ability to perform a neurologic examination and to evaluate its results. Therefore, the anesthesia care provider must be cognizant of the patient's baseline neurologic status before performing maneuvers to protect the airway (2). A simple neurologic evaluation tool is the Glasgow coma scale (GCS) (see Table 7.3); a patient's score is based on evaluation of the size and reactivity of the pupils as well as a quick assessment of the motor strength of all four extremities.

Once the anesthesia care provider is sure that the patient is receiving appropriate emergency treatment, the preanesthetic diagnosis continues in an orderly fashion. The history and details of the injury can help focus diagnostic efforts and should be sought from the patient, paramedics, or family.

---

**Figure 6.1.** The anesthesia "cockpit" in an operating room of the R Adams Cowley Shock Trauma Center of the Maryland Institute for Emergency Medical Services Systems. **Plate A.** *A*, Two-channel strip recorder compatible with all monitoring equipment. *B*, Programmable multichannel monitor capable of displaying simultaneous two-lead ECG and four invasive pressures (e.g., arterial, central venous, pulmonary artery, intracranial). *C*, "Slave" unit displays all information processed by *B* and is visible by the surgical team and observers in hallway. *D*, Used needle and hazardous waste receptacle. *E*, Integrated mass spectrometer and infrared capnography. *F*, Pulse oximeter, *G*, Integrated ventilator/anesthesia machine. *H*, Freestanding exchange cart system with crystalloid and colloid volume expanders, as well as antibiotic and nonanesthesia drugs. *I*, Large trash receptacles. *J*, Two identical computer work stations (one for anesthesia care team use, one for operating room nursing personnel) integrated with *K* (telephone). *L*, Anesthesia multidrawer cart system with all necessary anesthetic and emergency drugs drawn up in syringes ready for use; drug label dispenser. **Plate B.** *A*, "Level 1" fluid warmer/power infuser (see Fig. 4.11) (Level 1 Technologies, Marshfield, MA). *B*, "Christmas trees" anesthesia circuit holder with clear face mask. *C*, Respiratory gas warmer/humidifier. *D*, Anesthesia airway management equipment kept ready (e.g., laryngoscope, endotracheal tubes). **Plate C,** *A*, Five-lead ECG ready on operating table. *B*, Noninvasive blood pressure cuff ready on armboard. **Plate D.** Infrared heaters in the operating room ceiling capable of heating the room at a rate of 2°C per minute. (Courtesy of B. G. McAlary M.D. MIEMSS Dept of Anesthesia).

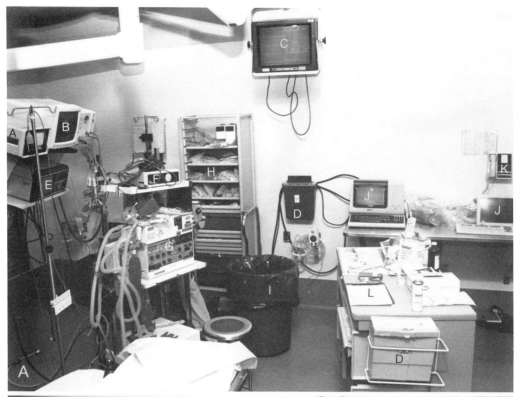

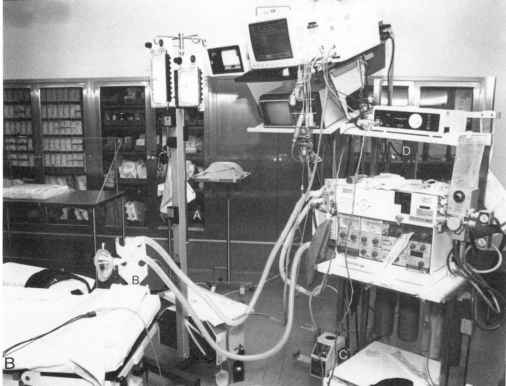

**Figure 6.1.    A** and **B.**

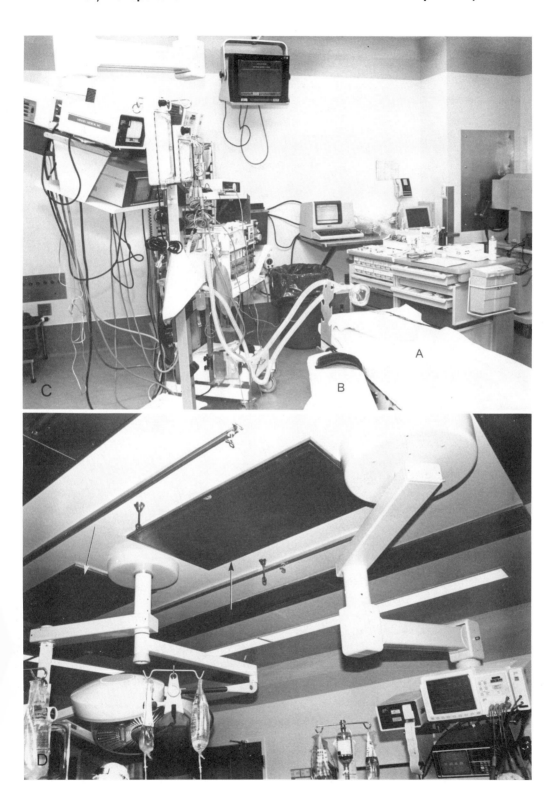

**Figure 6.1.** C and D.

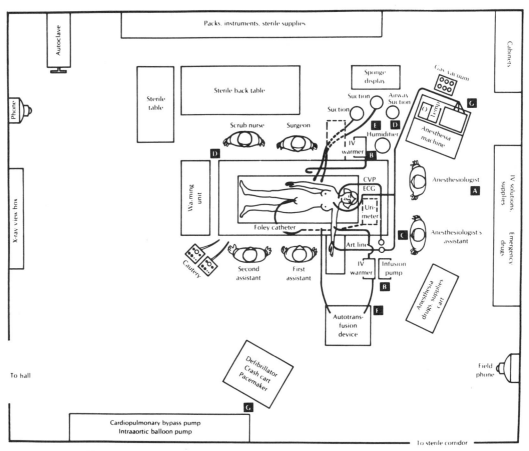

**Figure 6.2.   Floor plan for trauma operating room.** (From Stryler WF: Operating room organization for the trauma patient. In Moore EE, Eiseman B, Van Way CW III (eds): Critical Decisions in Trauma. St. Louis, CV Mosby, 1984, pp 70–73.)

### Mechanisms of Injury: Blunt versus Penetrating Trauma (see also Chapter 2)

Because humans demonstrate a characteristic, reproducible physiologic response to injury, the term "traumatic disease" is justified, even though an almost infinite array of injury mechanisms is possible (6). Knowledge of the specific mechanism of injury is important because it determines the anatomic pattern of injury. This knowledge focuses the treatment priorities for a given patient (see Chapter 2). For example, acute oxygen deprivation from drowning requires immediate attention to restoration of tissue oxygen delivery to prevent massive cellular necrosis (see Chapter 4). Penetrating thoracic trauma often requires the immediate placement of a tube thoracostomy (chest tube) to drain the pleural space of air and blood; such a patient may not require further surgery. Blunt chest trauma, as described below, signals the need for immediate attention to respiratory gas exchange because widespread pulmonary contusion often complicates skeletal instability of the chest wall. In these cases, myocardial contusion and traumatic aneurysm of the thoracic aorta must also immediately be considered and ruled out.

The distinction between blunt and penetrating trauma is important in the primary survey (ATLS) of the trauma patient because the treatment priorities may be different. For example, in penetrating injuries caused by a bladed instrument (e.g., knife, spear) or missile (e.g., bullet, bomb fragment), energy is focused and thus tissues in the penetrating tract are stretched and crushed (7). Such an injury is likely to disrupt a large blood vessel (or the heart), which may cause the patient to exsanguinate rapidly. For penetrating injuries, treatment priorities mandate rapid surgical hemostasis. Thus, it is often advantageous to transfer these patients directly to the OR for treatment and diagnosis, which ultimately rely on surgical intervention.

Blunt trauma, associated with widespread energy transfer to the patient's body, frequently causes massive disruption of the microcirculation. The enormous amounts of energy transferred over wide areas of the body produce anatomic injury wherein the limits of load tolerance are exceeded (8). Thus, blunt trauma may cause multiple fractures and avulsions of extremities, soft tissue disruption, and degloving injury within the same patient. Treatment priorities mandate rapid replacement of blood and intravascular fluid that have been sequestered in injured tissues (see Chapter 4). Unlike the normal handling of penetrating trauma, priorities here must also include stabilization of fractures, support of ventilation, and accurate diagnosis of the various multiple injuries before transfer to the OR for surgical intervention.

### Preanesthetic History

Preanesthetic history includes information generated from the scene of the accident, either from witnesses or the patient's own description. Information as to how the injury occurred will help the anesthesiologist prepare for both surgical and nonsurgical correction of occult injuries. For example, an unrestrained driver who has sustained bilateral femoral fractures in a frontal collision may also have a traumatic aneurysm of the thoracic aorta as a result of sudden chest deceleration on the steering wheel. Clues to such an injury may be provided by knowledge of a bent or broken steering wheel. Traumatic aortic aneurysm, myocardial and/or pulmonary contusion, flail chest, diaphragmatic rupture, cervical spine instability, maxillofacial injuries, and difficulties with airway management may then all be anticipated, in addition to the more obvious orthopaedic trauma of the extremities.

Other important information to be learned from the emergency medical technicians (EMTs) includes the patient's vital signs when the EMTs arrived at the scene, history of loss of consciousness at the scene or during transport, estimates of blood loss, and the patient's response to treatment.

Trauma patients must be treated as though they have "full stomachs," but careful inquiry into the actual time and type of last oral intake should be undertaken. It may reveal a variable potential for quantity and quality of stomach contents (see Chapter 3) (9).

Preoperative information concerning allergies, preexisting diseases and drug therapy, previous operations, and response to anesthetics must be obtained from the trauma patient, just as from any other surgical patient (2, 10). If the patient cannot communicate effectively, medical information may be obtained from relatives. If the patient's name is known, it is important to see if a medical record is on file in a given hospital with the primary care physician. The anesthesiologist also needs information regarding the patient's history of tobacco smoking, alcohol ingestion, marijuana smoking, cocaine intake, and other drug use.

A high index of suspicion is useful for the TA/CCS to prepare for complications of preexisting diseases in a trauma patient who is comatose and thus unable to provide a history. A knowledge of disease prevalence in a given population (e.g., the distribution of ischemic heart disease or diabetes for various age groups) will help the TA/CCS prepare for adverse anesthetic outcomes based on estimations of the patient's age and state of health (11, 12).

Of interest here is the fact that malignant hyperthermia (MH) reactions occur more frequently after surgery for trauma (13) (see Chapter 13). Because many patients with MH react only to their second or subsequent anesthetics, a negative history of MH cannot totally rule out this disease.

A recent study of the effects of preexisting chronic disease on the mortality of trauma patients admitted to hospital concluded that cirrhosis of the liver increased the probability of trauma mortality dramatically (11). Congenital coagulopathies were also associated with a marked increase in the probability of dying from traumatic injury. Surprisingly, ischemic heart disease and chronic obstructive pulmonary disease only moderately increased the probability of traumatic death, whereas diabetes mellitus only slightly increased the overall probability of traumatic death (11). On the other hand, diabetes can present a problem for the anesthesia care provider because many diabetics have treated themselves with long-acting insulin before their injury, which can complicate management (12).

Last, self-medication with psychoactive drugs is a particular problem with trauma patients (14). Careful questioning will frequently reveal a pattern of psychopathologic substance abuse followed by injury, which is especially prevalent in chronic alcoholics (15, 16). Trauma patients frequently are intoxicated with marijuana, cocaine, phencyclidine, and opiates, often in combination with ethanol (17). A history of chronic substance abuse or acute intoxication should alert the anesthesiologist to prepare for unusual responses to anesthetic agents.

**Physical Examination**

A preanesthetic physical examination, including appropriate laboratory testing, must be performed and recorded. This examination will initially concentrate on the respiratory, circulatory, and nervous systems, in accordance with the well-established ABCs (Airway, Breathing, Circulation) of any life-support management system (e.g., Acute Cardiac Life Support [ACLS], ATLS).

The upper airway should be examined in the nonintubated patient to evaluate poten-tial intubation difficulties (see Chapters 3 and 8). Bear in mind that immobilization of the cervical spine may increase the difficulty of performing intubation. Routine evaluation of the airway includes an estimate of tongue size and of the ability to visualize the tonsilar pillars (18). The teeth must be examined carefully, especially in cases of facial trauma, which frequently fractures or loosens the teeth. Loose teeth may be inhaled and obstruct the airway. Direct injury to the airway increases the difficulty and urgency of intubation.

The circulatory system is evaluated for signs of hemorrhagic shock and blood loss (see Chapters 4 and 5). Preexisting blood loss can be quantified according to changes in vital signs as described in Chapter 4 (Table 4.2). To complete the evaluation of the circulatory system, the TA/CCS should examine the chest for signs of pneumothorax, myocardial contusion, and pericardial tamponade.

The trauma patient who presents with hypotension must be presumed to have major fluid loss that should be replaced rapidly, unless it is demonstrated that the patient has a cervical spine injury with no hemorrhagic losses (i.e., spinal shock, see Chapter 4). Although complications of anesthesia are reduced if the TA/CCS replenishes the trauma patient's cardiovascular volume before induction of anesthesia, patients in traumatic (hemorrhagic) shock frequently require induction of anesthesia and initiation of surgery as part of definitive therapy, simultaneously with fluid resuscitation.

As stated above, the status of the central nervous system (CNS) is evaluated with a brief neurologic examination. Level of consciousness, GCS score, pupil size and reactivity, and motor function of each extremity are assessed.

Arterial blood gases, chest and cervical spine roentgenograms, hemoglobin and hematocrit measurements, serum glucose, urea nitrogen, creatinine, and electrolytes, as well as an electrocardiogram (ECG), round out the laboratory analysis (see below).

Once the patient's history and physical examination have been completed, the TA/CCS must assign an American Society of Anesthesiologists (ASA) physical status designation to the patient (Table 6.3). Several rating scores are used exclusively in trauma management. They were developed to quantify the extent of injury, which is useful in anticipating the prognosis of acutely injured patients (19). Prospective physiologic and anatomic scoring systems such as the Trauma Score and the Injury Severity Score (see Chapter 2) are also used to predict outcome and direct patients to appropriate facilities. The ASA physical status system has been demonstrated to predict mortality from blunt trauma, but it is not very useful for discriminating small differences among severely injured patients (20) (see Chapter 1). A patient with a low Trauma Score has sustained serious trauma, which probably equates to an ASA physical status of 4E or 5E. Many of these patients are in frank cardiac arrest or dead on arrival and can be assigned ASA physical status 5E.

Measuring core body temperature on admission is an additional method for evaluating severity of injury. Temperature is negatively correlated with the Injury Severity Score, as illustrated in Figure 6.3. This is a simple measurement that provides information to confirm the TA/CCS's preoperative suspicions of the patient's extent of injury.

**Table 6.3. American Society of Anesthesiologists Physical Status Diagnoses[a]**

| | |
|---|---|
| PS-1 | A normal healthy patient |
| PS-2 | A patient with a mild systemic disease |
| PS-3 | A patient with severe systemic disease |
| PS-4 | A patient with severe systemic disease that is a constant threat to life |
| PS-5 | A moribund patient who is not expected to survive without the operation |
| PS-6 | A declared brain-dead patient whose organs are being removed for donor purposes |
| E | Placed as a suffix to the PS designation for emergency patients |

[a] From the American Society of Anesthesiologists, Chicago, IL.

## Treatment

As stated above, during the immediate preoperative period the TA/CCS is primarily concerned with physiologic management of the respiratory system, circulatory system, and CNS and the pharmacology of anesthesia/analgesia. Airway maintenance and ventilatory support (Chapter 3) are important not only to save the lives of patients who are apneic and/or have ventilatory failure, but also as adjunctive treatments for those in shock and those with head injuries (see Chapters 4 and 7).

Shock, frequently a result of major trauma, separates the trauma patient from other emergency patients. The treatment of hemorrhagic shock is so important to the overall care of trauma patients that the term "golden hour" has been coined to describe the necessity of treating circulatory shock as rapidly as possible to optimize survival of the trauma patient (see Fig. 4.1). Treatment of hemorrhagic shock must begin when the patient arrives and continue throughout the perioperative period. Successful shock therapy requires control of traumatic hemorrhage, as well as appropriate fluid replacement. Shock has many definitions based on changes in blood pressure and other vital signs; however, the basic defect is ultimately regarded as inadequate microcirculatory blood flow and suboptimal cellular oxygen delivery and utilization. Shock treatment is being refined continuously in terms of both diagnostics (e.g., early, aggressive invasive monitoring in the pre/intraoperative phase) and therapeutics (e.g., achieving an optimum cardiovascular profile as early as possible).

Sophisticated, integrated shock resuscitation must address CNS management simultaneously. Because this intervention includes maneuvers to ensure adequate perfusion of the brain with oxygenated blood (Chapter 7), it has been termed "cardiopulmonary cerebral resuscitation" (21). Similarly, the TA/CCS must be especially careful to avoid aggravating a spinal cord injury.

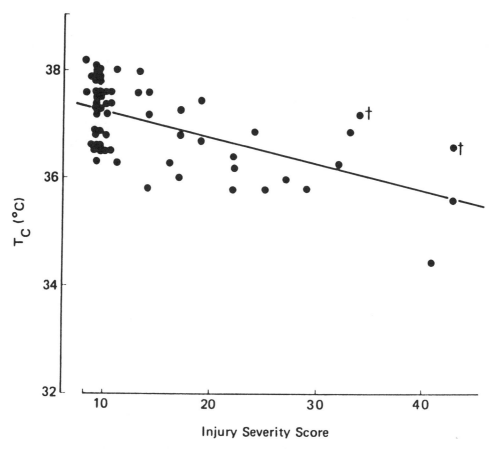

**Figure 6.3.   Increasing severity of injury associated with decreasing body temperature.** This is probably the result of decreased heat production when oxygen delivery and cellular oxygen consumption are impaired by hemorrhagic shock. (From Irving MH, Stoner HB: Metabolism and nutrition in trauma. In Carter DC, Polk HC Jr (eds): Surgery 1 Trauma, London, Butterworths, 1981, pp 302–318.)

## MONITORING

Besides respiratory management, shock resuscitation, and CNS care, the TA/CCS must be concerned about technical details related to the surgical treatment of the injury. Definitive surgical treatment is governed by the trauma patient's injuries. The patient's position on the OR table and the difficulties the TA/CCS will encounter in preparing the patient for surgery are subsequently established. The type of surgical treatment planned and the patient's general condition dictate the type of monitoring required. The trauma surgeon must communicate clearly with the TA/CCS about the proposed operation, anticipated difficulties, and other technical aspects of both anesthetic and surgical management (5). The TA/CCS must verify that the patient has been readied for the appropriate monitoring techniques before surgical preparation and draping. These requirements normally include placement of at least two large-bore intravenous catheters (Chapter 4) and the use of basic and/or advanced monitors.

### Basic Noninvasive Monitoring Techniques

Use of modern medical electronic monitoring products can never adequately replace the attentive and intelligent care of a well-trained anesthesia care provider. The well-trained anesthesia care provider is the most basic element of monitoring and should always be present with the anesthetized patient. Standards published by the ASA for minimum required monitoring of the anesthetized patient recognize the primacy of the well-trained anesthesia care provider by mandating his/her presence with the patient as the first standard (Table 6.4) (22).

The basic *look, listen, and feel* approach to monitoring must not be forgotten in a sophisticated OR of a modern trauma center. It may be all that is available on a battlefield or at a disaster scene, in a primitive hospital, or at an accident site during extrication of a seriously injured patient (23–25). The anesthesia care provider should observe patients closely, looking at the eyes for tearing, at the pupils for size and motion, and at the skin and nail beds for blanching of color and for speed of capillary refill after applying pressure. Palpation of the pulse with the fingers can give approximate systolic blood pressure (BP) (see Table 4.6). The skin is evaluated for temperature and moisture and the arms for muscle tone. Using such techniques, for example, hypercarbia can be suspected without a capnometer when the patient's skin becomes moist, heart rate rapid, and pulse bounding and strong.

Basic noninvasive monitoring utilizing instrumentation includes auscultation of the intensity of heart sounds and breath sounds with a precordial or esophageal stethoscope. The arterial BP is monitored noninvasively with an inflatable *sphygmomanometer* around an arm or leg. Needle oscillations on an aneroid manometer during cuff deflation are used to measure systolic BPs. Auscultation of Korotkoff sounds generated in an artery distal to the cuff provide more specific measurements of systolic and diastolic pressure. Current *noninvasive BP monitors* include electronic devices that oscillometrically measure BP (26). The advantage of using such automated equipment in the trauma patient is that it is accurate to fairly low BPs, it yields reproducible results, and it can be relied upon to measure BP regularly while leaving the clinician free to attend to other tasks during the early, hectic moments of trauma management (26). Other noninvasive monitors, such as *Doppler* probes, can detect systolic and diastolic BP during cuff deflation, can also detect air emboli in the heart, and may be used to enhance cardiovascular monitoring.

The *electrocardiograph (ECG)* is one of the most basic monitors of circulatory system function. The ECG is usually incorporated as part of a comprehensive electronic physiologic monitor. Both a limb lead (e.g., lead II) and a precordial lead (e.g., lead V5)

**Table 6.4.  Basic Monitoring of the Trauma Patient**

| | |
|---|---|
| Personnel | Trained anesthesia care provider continuously with the patient |
| Oxygenation | Pulse oximeter |
| | Oxygen analyzer on anesthesia machine or ventilator to monitor oxygen supply |
| | Mass spectrometer[a] or similar device to monitor inspired and expired oxygen concentrations |
| Ventilation | Tidal volume and respiratory rate monitored by observation of breathing bag or respirator or by auscultation of breath sounds |
| | Impedence pneumograph |
| | Carbon dioxide—inspired and expired gas monitored using a capnograph with waveform display |
| | Airway pressure monitor to signify disconnection from mechanical ventilation |
| Circulation | ECG—to monitor pulse rate and cardiac rhythm |
| | Arterial blood pressure—noninvasive monitor of arterial blood pressure—arm or leg cuff (oscillometric, Doppler, Korotkoff sounds) or digital (Finipress) |
| | Capillary perfusion—inspection of capillary refill or pulse oximeter |
| Temperature | Core temperature should be monitored by thermister in esophagus, rectum, or bladder or on tympanic membrane |

[a] Optional equipment.

should be monitored simultaneously to detect ischemia in the patient with coronary artery disease.

A *pulse oximeter* has become a standard noninvasive monitor of the circulatory system because it monitors heart rate and arterial oxyhemoglobin saturation $(SaO_2)^a$ (27–29). Intact cutaneous microcirculatory blood flow is required for the pulse oximeter to record; therefore, the presence of a pulse signal indicates that the patient has both adequate blood volume and enough cardiac output to perfuse the skin. One of the determinants of $SaO_2$ is pulmonary blood flow, which is adversely affected by traumatic shock. A low $SaO_2$ indicates inadequate pulmonary gas exchange due to impairment of either ventilation or perfusion. Conversely, a high $SaO_2$ suggests adequate pulmonary blood flow and ventilation.

The most basic monitoring of the respiratory system is following both rate and depth of respiration. Pulmonary ventilation is assessed qualitatively by listening for breath sounds with a stethoscope and quantitatively with a respirometer. Many anesthesia machines and ventilators have *respirometers* that give continuous digital displays of respiratory frequency, tidal volume, and minute ventilation. Ventilators also monitor airway pressures and are often equipped with low-pressure (disconnect) and high-pressure alarms and high- and low-volume alarms.

Respiratory gas monitoring may be used to evaluate pulmonary gas exchange, which is determined by both ventilation and perfusion. Either a *capnometer* or a *mass spectrometer* can be used to analyze inspired and expired respiratory gases. A capnometer indicates the concentration of $CO_2$ in exhaled gas and displays respiratory rate (30). A mass spectrometer intermittently or continuously reads out inspiratory and expiratory gases such as $O_2$, $CO_2$, $N_2$, $N_2O$, and

halogenated anesthetic agents. Alternatively, colorimetric semiquantitative devices are now available to monitor breath-by-breath end-tidal $CO_2$ for about 2 hours (31). Impedance pneumography monitors relative tidal changes in thoracic gas volume with respiration (26). The ECG leads on the physiologic monitor can be used to generate both an ECG and the impedence pneumogram (32).

Body temperature should be monitored continuously as part of the basic monitoring of the trauma patient (see Chapter 13). *Thermistors* with relatively rapid response times are designed to record temperature as part of either the esophageal stethoscope or the Foley urinary catheter; they can be used on the skin, on the tympanic membrane, or in the rectum (33). Alternatively, skin temperature can be recorded by *liquid crystal display patches* placed on the forehead. However, core temperature is more closely approximated by a thermistor in the rectum, the bladder, the esophagus, the tympanic membrane, or the esophagus or as part of a pulmonary artery catheter (33). All of these probes can be purchased to connect to the same thermistor amplifier so that the TA/CCS may choose the temperature monitoring route appropriate to the patient's injuries and surgery.

Other techniques that are useful for noninvasive monitoring of cardiopulmonary function during trauma anesthesia management include (*a*) *oxygen saturation finger plethysomographs* that display pulse waves, (*b*) *transesophageal echocardiography*, (*c*) *impedance plethysmography* to measure cardiac output by changes in thoracic blood volume during the cardiac cycle, (*d*) *transcutaneous oxygen and carbon dioxide sensors*, and (*e*) a two-beam, pulsed-Doppler, suprasternal probe to measure cardiac output (28, 34–40).

Noninvasive monitoring of the trauma patient is not complete without neuromuscular transmission monitoring. Transcutaneous stimulation of motor nerves generates muscular activity that is inversely proportional to the degree of blockade of neuro-

---

$^a$ Some authors refer to arterial oxyhemoglobin saturation measured with a pulse oximeter as $SpO_2$. We will use $SaO_2$.

muscular receptors produced by muscle relaxants. Either mechanical or electromyographic activity of the muscle is used to assess neuromuscular transmission and the degree of blockade (41, 42). Percutaneous stimulation of nerves should be as routine as continuous temperature monitoring.

Noninvasive monitoring devices coupled with talented, concerned anesthesia care providers using human senses will most likely remain our most economical and productive monitors, yet modern technology should not be ignored if available. *Computer analysis* can supplement human interpretation of noninvasive monitoring signals (for example, in arrhythmia detection or hemodynamic tracking) (43, 44). Data generated from monitors can be fed into computers for storage, retrieval, and trend analysis. As an example, respiratory data from a mass spectrometer can be used to calculate oxygen consumption, carbon dioxide production, and nutritional needs.

### Minimally Invasive Monitoring Techniques

Use of these monitors (Table 6.5) increases the morbidity associated with monitoring as compared with that associated with purely noninvasive monitoring. The risks, however, are frequently less than the risks of not adequately monitoring the trauma patient. For example, insertion of intraarterial catheters to measure arterial BP continuously may be associated with hematoma formation, thrombosis, infection, vascular insufficiency, discomfort, and even undetected hemorrhage from accidental disconnection (45). Alternatives are available, such as pulse plethysmography for continuous pulse wave monitoring and noninvasive oscillometric BP monitors that provide reasonably accurate and frequent BP readings (26, 28). There must be a medical indication to insert an invasive monitor. For example, the need to analyze arterial blood samples frequently is certainly an acceptable reason for the insertion of a catheter into the radial or ulnar artery.

An *indwelling urinary catheter* (Foley) is a minimally invasive monitor that is indicated (as part of the ATLS protocols) as a means of following urine output in the severely injured patient (3). However, the Foley catheter provides a route for bacteria to enter the urinary tract and thus increases the risk of urinary tract infection if it is left in place for several days. The risk of urinary tract infection is probably greater, however, if the patient cannot void spontaneously and develops bladder distension (46). Furthermore, urinary output is an important

**Table 6.5.   Advanced Monitoring of the Trauma Patient**

| | |
|---|---|
| Depth of anesthesia | Mass spectrometer or anesthesia gas analyzer to monitor end-tidal anesthetic concentrations |
| | Blood concentrations of fixed drugs |
| | EEG and sensory-evoked potentials |
| Oxygenation | Arterial blood gases (in combination with "oxygenation" equipment listed in Table 6.4) |
| Circulation | Arterial catheter for continuous intraarterial pressure monitoring |
| | Central venous catheter for continuous right atrial/superior vena caval pressure monitoring |
| | Pulmonary artery catheter for monitoring central venous pressure, pulmonary artery pressure, and wedge/left atrial pressure |
| | Cardiac output—monitored by thermal dilution using a pulmonary artery catheter, by transthoracic electrical impedance, or by Doppler to monitor pulsatile volume changes in aorta |
| | Indwelling urinary catheter (to monitor urinary output as a function of adequacy of perfusion status) |
| | Transesophageal echocardiography |
| Ventilation | Mass spectrometer to monitor carbon dioxide waveform |
| | Oxygen consumption, carbon dioxide production at the airway (indirect calorimeter) |

endpoint of organ perfusion and effectiveness of fluid resuscitation (see Chapter 4). Direct trauma to the urethra, suggested by blood at the urethral meatus, is an absolute contraindication to the insertion of a Foley catheter (3).

*Instrumentation of the esophagus* provides a minimally invasive route to monitor cardiac performance. Esophageal probes can include a thermistor-containing stethoscope, an esophageal ECG lead, a Doppler probe to measure cardiac output, an ultrasound probe to perform transesophageal echocardiography, and an esophageal balloon to record distal esophageal muscle tone as a correlate of the depth of anesthesia (34). The morbidity of these devices is low if one is careful to avoid insertion in patients with esophageal disease (e.g., varicosities).

Monitoring of CNS function via *electroencephalographic* (EEG) recording of responses to various stimuli is an important component of neurosurgical anesthesia (47) and thus applies to "neurotrauma anesthesia." This method is equally important for monitoring the patient with nonoperative trauma to the CNS, as well as injured patients with impaired cerebral perfusion (47). *Visual, auditory, and somatosensory evoked potentials* are recorded via electrodes placed on the scalp (48). The number and location of electrodes increase the ability to monitor specific areas of CNS function. Changes in EEG waveform, frequency, and intensity from peripherally administered somatosensory input may indicate a change in impulse transmission through the spinal cord (49). This change could indicate a decrease in blood flow to an area in the cord. Increases in EEG "latency" recorded after visual stimulation by strobe light flashes could indicate an increase in intracranial pressure (ICP). These changes in latency are found in patients with elevated ICP and possibly cerebral edema secondary to hypoxia or other intracranial pathological conditions (50). Auditory evoked responses can also be used to monitor brain stem CNS function (48).

Flash visual evoked responses (VERs) can be recorded with a basic evoked potential system using either calibrated LED goggles or a calibrated strobe with acoustic shielding or "white noise" to mask the sound of the strobe as a signal source. Four channels may be the optimal EEG montage for recording cortical VERs. Pattern-reversal VERs are a fairly reliable and consistent test of cortical function (50). Brainstem somatosensory potentials (BSEP) are a reliable and consistent test of the entire somatosensory track, using peripheral nerve, subcortical, and cortical generators (49). Brainstem auditory response (BAER) will test brainstem function (48). Also, delta waves on EEG can be recorded using four channels to follow cortical perfusion (47).

## Laboratory Monitoring

When a patient is admitted, arterial blood gases (ABGs) should be measured to evaluate cardiorespiratory function (see Chapter 4) (51). Measuring the ABGs while the spontaneously breathing patient inhales room air provides a known $FIO_2$ so that the $PaO_2$ can be evaluated as an index of gas exchange. Intubated patients receive oxygen via either a bag-valve-mask apparatus or a ventilator, both of which deliver a precise $FIO_2$ relative to an oxygen mask. Hematologic monitoring of the trauma patient includes hematocrit (HCT), hemoglobin (Hgb), white cell count, platelet count, prothrombin time, partial thromboplastin time, and fibrinogen concentration. The chemistry laboratory measurements should include serum electrolyte concentration (sodium, potassium, chloride, bicarbonate $[CO_2]$), glucose concentration, blood urea nitrogen (BUN) concentration, creatinine concentration, serum osmolarity, and ionized calcium concentration (Table 6.6). It may be useful to monitor serum lactate, magnesium, total calcium, and phosphorus concentrations in critically ill trauma patients being managed in intensive care units. Drug levels (both premorbid illicit drugs and therapeutic drugs) should also be monitored

**Table 6.6.   Laboratory Monitoring of the Trauma Patient**

| | |
|---|---|
| Pulmonary | Frequent arterial blood gases |
| | Occasional mixed venous blood gases and pulmonary shunt determination |
| Hematologic function | Hematocrit/hemoglobin concentration |
| | White blood cell count |
| | Platelet count |
| | Prothrombin time |
| | Partial thromboplastin time |
| | Fibrinogen concentration |
| | Blood type and crossmatch |
| Chemistry laboratory | Sodium concentration (serum) |
| | Potassium concentration (serum) |
| | Chloride concentration (serum) |
| | Carbon dioxide content (serum bicarbonate) |
| | Urea nitrogen concentration (serum) |
| | Creatinine concentration (serum) |
| | Glucose concentration (serum) |
| | Toxicology for prescribed/illicit agents (serum and urine) |
| | Calcium (ionized) concentration (serum) |
| | Phosphorus concentration (serum) |
| | Urinary sodium concentration |
| | Urinary creatinine concentration |
| | Osmolarity (serum/urine) |

when indicated (see preanesthetic history section above).

## Invasive Monitoring Techniques

Indications for pulmonary artery pressure monitoring and calculation of derived indices are listed in Table 6.7. Cardiac profiles can be generated from data gathered from pulmonary artery catheters, arterial catheters, and the clinical laboratory and fed through a computer (44).

The TA/CCS must use clinical judgment to decide when to institute invasive procedures to monitor patients better and thus achieve a greater margin of safety. Hazards associated with the placement and continued use of catheters in central veins and arteries range from vessel thrombosis to bacteremia and sepsis. The TA/CCS should be prepared to defend professionally the use of any invasive monitoring instrument when indicated. Thus, the TA/CCS must understand and appreciate the value of these measurements before placing central vascular lines that may be associated with

**Table 6.7.   Indications for Pulmonary Artery Catheterization in the Trauma Patient**

1. To measure cardiac output
2. To measure oxygen content of mixed venous blood
3. To assess hemodynamic indices:
   mean arterial pressure (MAP)—arterial line
   cardiac index (CI)—pulmonary artery line
   stroke volume (SV)
   stroke volume index (SVI)
   systemic vascular resistance (SVR)
   left ventricular stroke work index (LVSWI)
4. To measure derived indices in conjunction with other monitors such as oxygen consumption ($VO_2$) by the Fick principle (CO × A-$VO_2$)
5. To measure right heart (CVP) and left heart filling pressures (PAWP) for
   a.  Shock
   b.  Expected large volume shifts
   c.  Myocardial dysfunction
6. To continuously monitor mixed venous oxygen saturation ($SvO_2$)

significant morbidity. Additionally, to make appropriate decisions on whether to administer fluid and/or pharmacologic agents (inotropes, vasodilators) or to consider the use of an intraaortic balloon pump or a left ventricular assist device, one must be able to interpret data gathered and derived from pulmonary artery catheters.

Preoperative evidence of hemodynamic instability (for example, decreased myocardial contractility, decreased cardiac preload from ongoing and anticipated hemorrhage, or increased cardiac afterload) mandates invasive monitoring with a pulmonary artery catheter (52) (Table 6.7).

Aggressive perioperative use of invasive hemodynamic monitoring reduces the mortality and reinfarction rate in those surgical patients with a history of myocardial infarction (53). Although the issue has not been studied systematically, hemodynamically unstable trauma patients seem to derive as much benefit from invasive cardiovascular monitoring as elective surgical patients who have had a myocardial infarction.

Continuous measurement of hemoglobin saturation of mixed venous blood with oxygen ($SvO_2$) is a real-time indication of the adequacy of tissue oxygenation. A decrease in $SaO_2$, Hgb, or cardiac output (CO) or an increase in oxygen consumption ($VO_2$) will decrease $SvO_2$. A decrease in $SvO_2$ suggests either a compromise in oxygen delivery relative to $VO_2$, or, less frequently, increased extraction of oxygen from the Hgb at the cellular level. For example, septic patients can have a normal or high $SvO_2$ during the "early" (hyperdynamic) phase of sepsis, as well as a decreased $SvO_2$ in "late" sepsis when oxygen delivery exceeds $VO_2$ (54). Thus, venous saturation should be used as an overall index of the oxygen supply/demand balance.

## PHARMACOLOGY AND CHOICE OF ANESTHETIC DRUGS

Regional anesthesia is most useful for the patient with an isolated limb injury; for example, a brachial plexus block is used for an open reduction of a humeral fracture. Conversely, general anesthesia has several advantages over regional anesthesia (see Chapter 12) for the severely injured trauma patient (2, 55). Mechanical ventilation through an endotracheal tube improves outcome from shock resuscitation (see Chapter 4); therefore, these patients are frequently endotracheally intubated before entering the operating room (56). Hemodynamic changes are more easily compensated during general anesthesia than during regional anesthesia (2, 57, 58). The TA/CCS must carefully choose the agents for the general anesthetic prescription to ensure a safe, efficacious procedure, as well as to avoid aggravating shock (1, 57–60). Additionally, the TA/CCS should consider choosing several different drugs to provide the four components of anesthesia—sleep (hypnosis), amnesia, analgesia, and muscle relaxation—in a "balanced" technique to optimize the patient's physiologic stability (57–61).

Studies of the effects of anesthetic drugs on the outcome of experimental shock in research animals have not produced a consensus of the "best" agents for use (62–69). Various clinical reports on the management of series of trauma patients similarly fail to identify one single "best" anesthetic technique (70–77). However, the principle of preserving mechanisms of lactate clearance will unify these diverse reports (63–67, 69, 72).

Although many studies of anesthetic interaction with shock have concentrated on changes in hemodynamic variables, preservation of visceral blood flow to the liver and kidneys to maintain lactate clearance is very important. Early studies of hemodynamic changes and survival after experimental shock demonstrated that cyclopropane and fluroxene were associated with very high mortality rates (62, 64). Also found were increased catecholamine and lactate concentrations as compared with results produced by anesthetics such as halothane, which caused hypotension but were associated with increased survival. Central-lobular hepatic necrosis was found in animals that died under the influence of the sympathomimetic anesthetics cyclopropane and fluroxene (64). Suprisingly, ketamine, also a sympathomimetic anesthetic, is not associated with a similarly high degree of shock-induced mortality. This may be caused by ketamine's enhancement of $\beta$-adrenergic, not $\alpha$-adrenergic, sympathetic stimulation. This is supported by the fact that $\beta$-adrenergic, but not $\alpha$-adrenergic, blockade causes a poor outcome when administered with ketamine in experimental shock (78).

An increased mortality noted in trauma patients with preexisting cirrhosis of the liver is consistent with the importance of maintaining hepatic perfusion and lactate clearance capabilities. Hemorrhagic shock reduces microcirculatory oxygen delivery to the gut and skeletal muscles (see Chapter 4), which increases their production of lactic acid as the endpoint of the anaerobic metabolism of glucose (79, 80). Both the liver and the kidney clear lactate from the circulation and use it both as an energy source through the Krebs cycle (via pyruvate) and as a gluconeogenic substrate.

A well-oxygenated intracellular state (i.e., high redox potential) is required in the liver and kidney to metabolize lactate (79, 80). Thus, hepatic and renal ischemia will impair lactate clearance because these organs require well-maintained perfusion to deliver both the lactate and the oxygen required for its metabolism.

When the visceral clearance of lactate falls below its production, lactic acidosis develops, defined as a serum lactate concentration of >5 mmol/liter and a pHa of <7.25 (81). Because these high levels of lactate will have a negative inotropic effect on the heart, which is already compromised in the shock state, lactic acidosis will contribute to a downward cycle, eventually ending with irreversible heart failure seen in "terminal shock" (see Chapter 4) (80, 81). The high mortality rate seen in experiments with anesthetics that sacrificially reduce splanchnic blood flow to maintain systemic BP is

consistent with this concept and with the observation that cirrhosis of the liver increases the probability of dying from trauma much more than any other preexisting chronic illness (11). Thus, this hypothesis is that impairment of hepatic lactate clearance allows lethal lactic acidosis to develop during hemorrhagic shock, which promotes further lactic acidosis and eventually "terminal shock." Therefore, we believe that anesthetics used in the management of acute trauma patients must not impair visceral blood flow and/or hepatorenal clearance of lactate. Furthermore, we suggest that future research with respect to the effects of anesthetics in traumatic shock should focus on hepatic lactate clearance, as well as hemodynamic stability.

Bearing these points in mind, the following discussion will briefly focus on the relative merits of selected hypnotics (induction agents), general anesthetics, muscle relaxants, and opioids. Table 6.8 outlines useful anesthetic drugs for acute trauma patients. Table 6.9 outlines useful drugs for "chronic" trauma patients, who are returning to the OR for follow-up surgery with increasing frequency as trauma care continues to improve and who account for a large portion of the operating schedule at major trauma centers.

### Intravenous Hypnotic Agents (see Chapter 3)

Hypnotic drugs are used to induce sleep in the trauma patient; however, the dose of these highly lypophilic drugs must be decreased for the patient presenting with significant hemorrhage (82). The reduced blood volume will cause an increased drug concentration to be delivered to the brain and heart (2, 63). These drugs can also be used to conduct a total intravenous anesthetic, but this is more difficult in the acute trauma patient than in the general patient population presenting for surgery.

#### THIOPENTAL SODIUM

The "granddaddy" of intravenous anesthetics, thiopental, plays an important part

**Table 6.8.  Useful Anesthetic Agents for Emergency Trauma Surgery**

Emergency room
  Hypnotics
    Thiopental++++
    Ketamine+++
    Etomidate++
    Midazolam++/++++[a]
    Propofol+
  Inhalation anesthetics
    Enflurane−
    Halothane−
    Isoflurane−
    $N_2O$ ±[b]
  Muscle relaxants
    Pancuronium++
    Succinylcholine++
    Vecuronium++++
    Atracurium+
  Opioids
    Fentanyl++
    Morphine+
    Nalbuphine+++
    Sufentanil+++
Operating room
  Hypnotics
    Thiopental++++
    Ketamine+++
    Etomidate+
    Midazolam+++[a]
    Propofol+
  Inhalation anesthetics
    Enflurane++
    Halothane++
    Isoflurane++++
    $N_2O$−[b]
  Muscle relaxants
    Pancuronium++
    Succinylcholine++
    Vecuronium++++
    Atracurium++
  Opioids
    Alfentanil++
    Fentanyl+++
    Morphine+
    Nalbuphine++
    Sufentanil++++

− not useful, + minimally useful, ++ somewhat useful, +++ useful, ++++ very useful.

[a] Midazolam during emergency surgery for unstable trauma is somewhat useful as a hypnotic induction agent; it is very useful as an anesthetic, at this point in management. During intraoperative management it becomes less useful as the stabilized trauma patient is able to better tolerate a potent inhalent.

[b] $N_2O$ accumulates in closed air spaces—contraindicated for patients with pneumothorax, pneumocephalus, or ileus.

**Table 6.9.  Useful Anesthetic Agents for Elective (Follow-up) Trauma Surgery**

Hypnotics
  Thiopental ++++
  Ketamine ++
  Etomidate +++
  Midazolam +++
  Propofol +++
Inhalation anesthetics
  Eenflurane +++
  Halothane ++
  Isoflurane ++++
  $N_2O$ +
Muscle relaxants
  Pancuronium ++
  Succinylcholine +++
  Vecuronium ++++
  Atracurium ++++
Opioids
  Alfentanil ++++
  Tentanyl ++++
  Morphine ++
  Sufentanil ++++

− not useful, + minimally useful, ++ somewhat useful, +++ useful, ++++ very useful.

providing anesthesia to a young civilian with a serious gunshot wound in the same issue of *Anesthesiology* in 1944 (73, 74, 83). Animal studies and human case reports support the efficacy of thiopental used carefully as an induction drug for the trauma patient (2, 58, 60, 67, 70, 72). However, to avoid inducing hypotension, one must be sure that dosages are reduced and carefully titrated to effect. In our experience, a "test dose" of 25 to 100 mg intravenously is usually sufficient, depending upon the severity of injury, degree of resuscitation, age, and preexisting diseases.

**KETAMINE HYDROCHLORIDE**

This dissociative anesthetic has been very popular in clinical series of trauma patients because it is widely regarded as capable of increasing heart rate and thus supporting BP (70–72, 75–77, 84). Further, ketamine does not seem to impair hepatic lactate clearance (85). However, the drug is not a panacea for trauma management. Ketamine may cause cardiovascular depression in the setting of a high preinduction sympathetic tone (86).

Also, ketamine has been contraindicated

in the history of trauma anesthesia: it was both damned for causing excess mortality at Pearl Harbor (which almost led to its removal from the market) and praised for in patients with head injury because of its propensity to increase ICP (86, 87). However, a recent animal study demonstrated an increase in cerebral perfusion pressure (CPP) (see Chapter 7) when ketamine was given to animals with both a space-occupying intracerebral lesion and hemorrhagic shock (88). Thus, the use of ketamine may have to be reevaluated for head injury and trauma in general. However, the agent continues to be very useful in field anesthesia situations (e.g., battle, disasters) because of its ease in use, portability, and desirable storage characteristics. Furthermore, ketamine anesthesia induction does not cause the same degree of dependent pulmonary atelectasis and venous admixture caused by other induction agents (89).

## ETOMIDATE

Etomidate is another popular anesthetic induction agent for trauma anesthesia (albeit more so in Europe than in the United States) because of its alleged lack of cardiorespiratory depression (60, 90). However, normal clinical doses of etomidate will decrease blood pressure in the hypovolemic patient. Etomidate does not seem to interfere with hepatic metabolism (90). This agent also suppresses adrenal steroid secretion after an induction or continuous infusion, which may compromise the trauma patient (57). Other drawbacks of etomidate use include elevation of intraocular pressure from myoclonus and its potentiation of nondepolarizing muscle relaxants (90–92).

## MIDAZOLAM

The benzodiazepines, diazepam and midazolam, have been used to induce anesthesia while maintaining cardiovascular stability in patients with cardiovascular disease (58, 59, 87, 90). Midazolam is the more useful of the two drugs because it has increased water solubility, which keeps it dissolved in solution when injected intravenously. Midazolam also is more potent than diazepam. Although midazolam must be given in reduced doses to elderly patients and in patients premedicated with opioids to avoid cardiovascular depression, the young, unpremedicated trauma patient may require a full induction dose (0.3 mg/kg) (90). Midazolam causes a slow anesthetic induction and emergence compared with the other hypnotics described in this section; however, the intravenous administration of a potent opioid (e.g., fentanyl, sufentanil) before midazolam induction will markedly enhance the speed of induction and allow reduction of the induction dose (90). The benzodiazepines do not interfere with hepatic metabolism, but they reduce renal blood flow (90).

The true usefulness of midazolam in the management of acute trauma is its action as an amnestic (93, 94). Because trauma patients usually have a tenuous hemodynamic state during the early stages of care, anesthesia care providers tend to use minimal amounts of or even completely withhold most anesthetic agents. Often, early pharmacologic management is confined to the use of oxygen alone (the "oxygen-and-a-prayer" technique) or in combination with a muscle relaxant. As a result, an inordinately high degree of perioperative recall has been demonstrated in the trauma patient population (95). Besides ethical and moral considerations, medicolegal issues regarding this phenomenon loom on the horizon. Thus, midazolam is very attractive (Table 6.8). Used in small, incremental intravenous doses (1 to 3 mg), this agent seems to satisfy the requirements for amnesia without promoting the detriments of hypotension. Benzodiazepine-induced amnesia is confined to anterograde impairment of memory (93). Verbal memory is preferentially abolished, and painful stimuli require larger doses of benzodiazepines (94). Therefore, midazolam must be started early in the anesthetic to abolish the patient's total recall of the event. Frequent small doses of midazolam must be given because the drug's time of effect is similar to its elimination half-life (94).

## PROPOFOL

The newest hypnotic available in the United States, propofol, is a highly lipophilic drug that must be injected in an oily emulsion (90, 96). Propofol causes cardiopulmonary depression similar to that seen with thiopental use. However, propofol has an extremely rapid emergence, so it can be titrated accurately as a continuous intravenous infusion to sedate the patient whose airway reflexes are stimulated by an endotracheal tube and mechanical ventilation (96). Because there are no reports of impaired hepatic function with propofol, it is unlikely that the agent interferes with hepatic lactate clearance; however, this warrants further investigation (90). Propofol may eventually become a very useful hypnotic for the trauma patient because of its rapid onset and emergence. Total intravenous anesthesia with propofol and an opioid may also become useful for trauma cases (97). The use of propofol has not been well-studied in trauma patient populations; therefore, we recommend caution with its initial use for the hemodynamically unstable trauma patient. On the other hand, for the "chronic" trauma patient returning for elective follow-up surgery, its use should not be significantly different from that for all other surgical patients (Table 6.9).

## Inhalational Anesthetics

Isoflurane, enflurane, and halothane are three widely available, halogenated hydrocarbon, volatile anesthetics. They all reduce blood pressure and cardiac output during experimental hemorrhagic shock but maintain visceral perfusion (62–66, 68). Probably because of this maintenance of hepatic blood flow, excess mortality associated with the use of these agents in experimental hemorrhagic shock has not been documented. Thus, they are extremely useful as a "basal anesthetic" to maintain hypnosis and amnesia in the trauma patient (57, 58). Low concentrations may be used safely in the person with a reduced blood volume, as the depth of anesthesia can be altered rapidly via inhalational concentration changes. This ability becomes important in "touch-and-go" trauma cases wherein the

need to eliminate advance hemodynamic effects rapidly sometimes is crucial. Interestingly, the relationship between hemorrhagic shock and minimum alveolar concentration (MAC) has not been well studied; MAC may be reduced in shock (98).

Although studies of the effects of inhalational anesthesia on hemorrhagic shock have not demonstrated a distinct advantage of any particular agent, theoretically isoflurane is the inhalational anesthetic of choice for trauma management (66, 68). Isoflurane increases ICP in a manner similar to that of halothane and enflurane. However, the ICP increases less with isoflurane, and patients maintain the normal relationship of ICP to $PaCO_2$ during isoflurane anesthesia (99). Furthermore, the epileptiform EEG seen with high-dose enflurane does not occur with deep isoflurane anesthesia even when the cerebral metabolic levels are markedly reduced, providing cerebral protection (99). Hypotensive anesthesia induced with isoflurane is associated with maintenance of cerebral $O_2$ balance (99).

Isoflurane causes less decrease in cardiac output than halothane and enflurane, both of which cause dangerous reductions in cardiac output with increased concentrations. Conversely, arterial BP is decreased similarly by all three anesthetics because systemic vascular resistance is decreased more by isoflurane than by enflurane or halothane. Isoflurane is a strong arterial dilator of coronary, skin, muscle, intestinal, renal, and cerebral vascular beds. Although vasodilation is important to maintain nutrient blood flow, one drawback of isoflurane is a preferential "steal" of coronary blood flow by normal over ischemic vessels (100).

Isoflurane biotransformation is less than that associated with either halothane or enflurane. Both halothane and enflurane release greater amounts of fluoride during metabolism. Enflurane metabolism causes enough fluoride release potentially to damage ischemic kidneys. All three agents decrease renal blood flow and glomerular filtration rate (GFR) and are associated with decreased urine flow (99).

Hepatic blood flow, oxygen consumption, and lactate removal are well maintained by isoflurane (99, 101). Halothane decreases hepatic oxygen demand and hepatic perfusion via both hepatic arterial and portal venous flows (101). Although halothane protects the liver at normal CO and BP, when perfusion pressure is reduced, the liver begins releasing lactate earlier with halothane than with isoflurane (101). Therefore, isoflurane provides better tissue perfusion than the other inhalation anesthetics and is also superior at maintaining hepatic lactate removal.

Nitrous oxide ($N_2O$) has not been studied systematically in hemorrhagic shock. This anesthetic is considered by many to be hemodynamically inert; however $N_2O$ is actually a potent vasoconstrictor, as shown under hyperbaric conditions where concentrations greater than 1 atm can be administered (102). Less-than-hyperbaric concentrations of $N_2O$ may cause undesirable cardiovascular depression, especially when combined with opioids in patients demonstrating cardiovascular instability (103). Furthermore, $N_2O$ may aggravate increased ICP, as do other inhalational anesthetics, because it decreases the cerebral metabolic rate more than the cerebral blood flow (104).

Because of the propensity of $N_2O$ to expand a closed air space, it is contraindicated in the trauma patient with a potential pneumothorax, pneumocephalus, or bowel obstruction. Nitrous oxide should be avoided if laser surgery in the airway is planned because it supports combustion ($N_2O$ is added to high-performance race car fuel to increase power output) and would enhance fires of endotracheal tubes. Furthermore, $N_2O$ is not metabolically inert: it inhibits the methionine synthetase enzyme, causing a functional vitamin $B_{12}$ deficiency (105). Considering the drawbacks to $N_2O$, it should not be used routinely for trauma patients. Thus, all anesthesia machines used for trauma should have compressed air capability.

## Muscle Relaxants

Succinylcholine has long been used to relax muscles and thus facilitate endotracheal intubation of the trauma patient (57–60). Although succinylcholine does not cause cardiovascular depression (except for bradycardia occasionally seen in children, especially with repeated doses), it has been associated with increased intraocular pressure (see Chapter 8); therefore, it has been relatively contraindicated in patients with open eye injuries. Recent experience with succinylcholine in eye injuries indicates that it may be used safely (106). Elevations in plasma potassium concentrations may be exaggerated when succinylcholine is administered to patients with large cutaneous burns (see Chapter 9) and to patients with high spinal cord lesions (107). This effect of succinylcholine, caused by the release of potassium from sensitized muscle cells when depolarized, is clinically important from about 48 hours after injury (but sometimes earlier) until either the burns heal or the muscles denervated by the spinal cord lesion complete their atrophy (usually 3 to 6 months). The sensitization involves an increase in acetylcholine receptors on the muscle membrane, especially outside the neuromuscular junction (107). Treatment of cardiac standstill caused by the inadvertent administration of succinylcholine to a burned patient or one with a high spinal cord lesion requires cardiovascular support with CPR while calcium chloride, insulin, and glucose are given intravenously to lower the serum potassium concentration rapidly.

Vecuronium bromide has become another muscle relaxant of choice for the trauma patient because of its relatively short half-life, its lack of hemodynamic side effects, and its high potency. Additionally, the dose of vecuronium may need to be elevated when used in burned patients (see Chapter 9).

Vecuronium is very useful for intubating the acute trauma patient in shock because of the lack of cardiovascular side effects. As a nondepolarizing muscle relaxant, vecuronium does not have the drawbacks of increased intraocular, intracranial, and intragastric pressure observed with succinylcholine (99). Increasing doses of vecuronium are associated with decreasing time to complete relaxation so that complete relaxation can be achieved in little over a minute with 0.25 mg/kg; higher doses can be given if necessary (108). Pancuronium has also been popular in the past because of its vagolytic and sympathomimetic effects (57, 70–72, 76, 99). However, a case report has described repeated boluses of pancuronium to be associated with tachycardia, hypotension, and histamine release when used in intubating doses (77). Atracurium, another intermediate-acting, nondepolarizing muscle relaxant, is not as useful for acute trauma management because the large doses necessary for rapid intubation are associated with significant degrees of hypotension and histamine release (99–108). However, atracurium becomes very useful for prolonged muscle relaxation in the patient with hepatic and renal impairment because its metabolic clearance is minimally affected by hepatorenal disease (99).

## Opioids

Opioids have been used to provide analgesia as a component of balanced anesthesia, to reduce the requirement for inhalational anesthesia, and to provide total intravenous anesthesia for cardiovascular surgery. The phenylpiperidine opioids—fentanyl, alfentanil, and sufentanil—possess little intrinsic myocardial depression characteristics, although they do cause significant myocardial depression in combination with benzodiazepines and/or $N_2O$ (85, 91). Vasodilatory effects of opioids due to direct action and secondary to histamine release from morphine limit the total dose that can be given to a trauma patient in hemorrhagic shock. We have seen profound hypotension caused by decreased systemic resistance (SVR) when attempting to utilize a "cardiac anesthetic" with high-dose fen-

tanyl for a patient who suffered both an acute myocardial infarction and blunt abdominal trauma. Such hypotension is usually responsive to intravenous fluid administration or naloxone therapy as an extreme measure. However, we advise against attempts to use these potent opioid agonists as the sole intravenous anesthetic in seriously injured individuals.

Sufentanil seems to offer pharmacologic advantages for use as a low-dose continuous intravenous infusion in trauma patients. The extreme potency and specificity of receptor binding by sufentanil, as compared to fentanyl, will allow the desired level of analgesia to be achieved at a much lower serum concentration than would be required to stimulate undesirable (hemodynamic) side effects. This is illustrated by the extremely large margin of safety of sufentanil (lethal dose 50%/effective dose 50%) compared to that of fentanyl demonstrated in animal studies (90).

Furthermore, sufentanil binds more tightly to the active $\mu$-opioid receptors than does fentanyl and thus remains bound much longer. Because the elimination half-life of sufentanil is significantly shorter than that of fentanyl, rate adjustments of a constant infusion will more rapidly change the serum levels of sufentanil. A typically useful dose for sufentanil is a loading dose of 0.5 $\mu$g/kg, followed by an infusion of 0.5 $\mu$g/kg/hr.

Nalbuphine hydrochloride, an opioid agonist/antagonist, increases blood pressure and cardiac output when given in large doses to experimental animals in shock (109). Nalbuphine has strong $\mu$-opioid receptor antagonism, which probably is the cause of its tendency to elevate BP in shock while it maintains analgesia through $\kappa$-opioid receptor agonism. (The opioid receptors are divided into several classes associated with different activities: (a) $\mu/\delta$-opioid receptors cause analgesia, hypotension, and respiratory depression; (b) $\kappa$-opioid receptors provide spinal level analgesia and sedation; and (c) $\sigma$-opioid receptors are associated with psychotomimetic effects

(99).) Normal clinical doses (0.5 to 1.0 mg/kg) required for the use of nalbuphine as a component of balanced anesthesia enhance the hemodynamic stability of the trauma patient (110).

## Pharmacokinetic Considerations

General anesthesia is conducted safely in the patient with multiple injuries by administering agents that minimize cardiovascular depression and intracranial hypertension. As discussed below, small doses of highly lipophilic drugs such as thiopental and sufentanil can be titrated to desired anesthetic effect without causing profound hypotension. Combinations of intravenous drugs as balanced anesthesia are also beneficial to trauma patients by maintaining those pulmonary ventilation-to-perfusion relationships that optimize gas exchange (111). Although pharmacokinetic data during hemorrhagic shock are limited, these patients appear clinically to reach desired drug effects from extremely small intravenous doses (112, 113). A dual effect occurs because of the reduction in blood volume, which probably concentrates the delivered dose at the active site in the brain and reduces hepatic blood flow, which decreases metabolic clearance, thus prolonging drug plasma concentrations. However, normal doses of muscle relaxants should be used to achieve the rapid paralysis necessary for emergency tracheal intubation. The drugs outlined in Table 6.8 for induction and intubation are useful in the OR as well as the emergency room.

Maintenance of cardiovascular homeostasis and adequate cerebral perfusion often has a higher priority than hypnosis or amnesia in the trauma patient. Thus, knowledge of unwarranted drug effects is extremely important for trauma anesthesia (Table 6.10).

Anesthesia machines for use with trauma patients should be equipped to deliver air along with oxygen because air/oxygen mixtures, instead of $N_2O/O_2$, should be used to decrease $FIO_2$. Another gas that is useful to combine with oxygen is helium. Heliox ($He/O_2$) mixtures (up to 80% He, 20% $O_2$) reduce the viscosity of gas so that a patient with profound obstruction of the large airways may be able to generate adequate spontaneous ventilation until the obstruction can be removed surgically.

**Table 6.10.  Contraindications to the Use of Various Anesthetic Agents in Trauma Patients**

Hypnotics
   *Shock*—a relative contraindication: All hypnotics should be carefully titrated to effect (sleep) to avoid aggravating hypotension.
   *Closed head injury*—Ketamine is contraindicated because it potently increases ICP.
Inhalational anesthetics
   *Closed air space* (pneumothorax, pneumocephalus, bowel distension)—$N_2O$ is contraindicated because it will accumulate and place air space under tension.
   *Air embolism*—$N_2O$ is contraindicated (see above).
   *Head injury*—All inhalational anesthetics are relatively contraindicated because cerebral blood volume increases and increases ICP; however, those effects are countered by deliberate hyperventilation and limiting administration to moderate concentrations (see Chapter 7).
   *Malignant hyperthermia*—Halothane, enflurane, and isoflurane are contraindicated.
   *Myocardial depression*—$N_2O$ aggravates myocardial depression.
Muscle relaxants
   *Shock*—All histamine-releasing muscle relaxants (e.g., curare, atracurium) aggravate shock.
   *Malignant hyperthermia*—Succinylcholine is contraindicated.
   *Burns*—For 48 hours after injury, succinylcholine is contraindicated because it exaggerates $K^+$ increase.
   *Spinal cord injury*—Use of succinylcholine between 48 hours and 6 months of injury is contraindicated because it exaggerates $K^+$ increases
Opioids
   *Shock*—relative contraindication: Use caution and titrate to effect to avoid aggravating hypotension.

## POSTOPERATIVE CONSIDERATIONS

### Emergence from Anesthesia

Anesthesia care begins with and should end with oxygen. All monitoring instituted during the preoperative and operative phases should be continued while the patient recovers from anesthesia. Some methods such as pulmonary artery pressure monitoring may be discontinued during transport to the postanesthesia care unit/recovery room (PACU/RR) complex if this is considered safe and appropriate. Small portable ECG, $SaO_2$, heart rate (HR), pulse wave, and pressure (arterial, ICP, venous, etc.) monitors are available for transfer operations (see Chapter 15).

Recovery of neuromuscular transmission must be ensured before a patient can be considered for extubation. Nondepolarizing neuromuscular blockade can be reversed competitively by acetylcholine, serum levels of which increase when an anticholinesterase drug (e.g., neostigmine, pyridostigmine, edrophonium) is administered. However, it is frequently advantageous to allow intermediate-duration neuromuscular blocking drugs (e.g., vecuronium) to clear the system spontaneously without reversal. Neuromuscular transmission is assessed by the nerve stimulators, which are also used in the OR. The ability to sustain head lifts (≥5 seconds) is a good clinical sign that the patient has recovered enough neuromuscular transmission to maintain ventilation and pulmonary toilet (42). "Light levels" of anesthesia, analgesia, amnesia, and sedation should be continued until adequate reversal or recovery of function is demonstrated.

Recovery from inhalation anesthetic agents follows predictable washout curves when the inspired concentration is discontinued and inspired oxygen concentrations are increased to 100% (114). Monitoring the percent concentration of inhalational anesthetics in both inspired and expired gases with a mass spectrometer allows the anesthesia care provider to follow the washout of inhalational anesthetic. Although a pro-

longed, very low level washout of anesthetics from fatty tissues will occur, the patient will be awake once the inhalation anesthetic falls to ≤0.1% end-tidal concentration. In a similar manner, intravenous drugs must be metabolized and/or excreted for the patient to "wake up." Liver and kidney disease will retard the excretion of intravenous agents.

### Extubation

In preparation for removal of a translaryngeal tracheal airway, the anesthesia care provider must ensure that a number of conditions exist (Table 6.11). After sufficient excretion of inhalation anesthetic agents and redistribution and/or excretion of intravenous analgesics and hypnotics, the patient should be observed closely for incontrovertible evidence of return of protective airway reflexes. The demonstrated presence of swallowing and the ability to follow commands should always precede tracheal extubation, except when deliberately precluded (for example, in patients with reactive airway diseases). The stomach should be decompressed via a gastric tube and

**Table 6.11. Criteria for Extubation of Trauma Patients after Prolonged Ventilatory Support**

Prolonged ventilatory support indicated for:
1. Inability to breathe
2. Unstable chest wall
3. Ventilation impairment secondary to abdominal trauma
4. Major fractures with associated hypoxia
5. Excess pulmonary secretions
6. Need for profound analgesia with systemic opioids

Extubation
1. Presence of protective oropharyngeal reflexes
2. Presence of adequate spontaneous ventilation
3. No need for profound systemic analgesia
4. Adequate recovery of CNS from anesthesia (e.g., follows commands)
5. No need for tracheobronchial suctioning of secretions
6. No need to reduce anatomic pulmonary dead space
7. Mechanical ventilatory function
   a. Sustained handgrip/head lift >5 sec
   b. Negative inspiratory pressure <−25 cm $H_2O$
   c. Vital capacity >15 ml/kg

suction before extubation. When possible, the head of the OR table, transport stretcher, or hospital bed should be elevated and the oropharynx suctioned before any tracheal airway is removed. The need for tracheal suctioning before tracheostomy or endotracheal tube removal is based upon the presence or absence of tracheal and/or lower airway secretions. The presence of secretions can be determined easily by auscultation. Negative suctioning pressures should always be $<-150$ cm $H_2O$ for tracheal suctioning. High suction pressures are usually needed to remove thick oropharyngeal and gastric liquid and semiliquid contents.

Before extubation, measured negative inspiratory force should exceed $-20$ cm $H_2O$. Vital capacity should exceed 15 ml/kg in adult patients. However, elderly and/or poorly nourished patients may have difficulty demonstrating the recommended vital capacities and negative inspiratory pressures. A patient with proven adequate spontaneous ventilation, protective oropharyngeal reflexes, and appropriate responses to commands can usually be extubated safely with minimal risk of regurgitation of gastric contents and subsequent aspiration.

## Controlled Recovery from Anesthesia

We do not recommend reversal of opioid drugs with specific antagonists (e.g., naloxone), as this may increase levels of circulating catecholamines. This is an undesirable effect in trauma patients for a number of reasons, such as elevation of ICP and aberrations in microcirculatory hemodynamics. Further, if hypertension and tachycardia are noted, even after administration of sufficient quantities of analgesic medications, antihypertensive drugs may be used to control arterial hypertension. Useful antihypertensive drugs include labetolol, esmolol, propranolol, hydralazine, nitroprusside, nitroglycerine, and trimethophan. Tachycardia is extremely common in the posttrauma "ebb" phase of injury (recovery).

Posttraumatic tachycardia should be treated only when indicated by myocardial ischemia or pathologic tachyarrhythmias. $\beta$-Adrenergic blocking drugs or calcium channel blocking drugs are the indicated agents to treat tachycardia after the TA/CCS has ruled out pain as a cause of tachycardia.

Recovery from anesthesia does not have to be rapid. In fact, a controlled, slow awakening in a PACU/RR may benefit many trauma patients. Patients with coronary artery disease undergoing trauma anesthesia and surgery are not appropriate candidates for testing of their cardiovascular system with the extra stress of fast recoveries from the anesthetized state.

## Critical Care during the Immediate Postoperative Period

A modern, well-equipped PACU/RR is capable of continuing the critical care started in the OR. Management of trauma patients during their recovery from anesthesia, while being weaned from mechanical ventilators and vasoactive drugs, requires a cadre of PACU nurses with critical care nursing skills. TA/CCSs must continue critical care management of their patients in PACU/RR units. For example, if epidural, subarachnoid, or interpleural analgesia or patient-controlled anesthesia (PCA) is to be used postoperatively, the PACU/RR is an appropriate location for this type of pain management program to be initiated. Frequent monitoring of vital signs after the initiation of postoperative pain management is a prerequisite for safe critical care management.

Transfer of a patient back to the critical care unit is a suitable alternative when it is appropriate to bypass the PACU/RR for eduction from anesthesia. Critical care nurses may have less experience in recovering patients from inhalation, intravenous, and conduction anesthesia than do PACU nurses, but they may know "the total patient" better than do PACU/RR nurses. The anesthesia care provider should formally transfer the care of the patient over to the critical care unit physicians (many of whom will be TA/CCSs) by direct communication. The transfer of responsibility must be accepted before the anesthesia care provider leaves the patient (see Chapter 18). Written documentation of the anesthetic must include a record of events that occurred during transportation from the OR to the PACU/RR and/or critical care unit. It is not an acceptable practice for anesthesia care providers to return to the OR to start another case until the patient's postoperative condition has stabilized, the transfer has been accepted, and the responsibility formally transferred.

When to extubate a patient's trachea is a question asked daily in the PACU/RR or critical care unit. When extubating victims of major trauma, it is usually better to be conservative, slow, and safe rather than aggressive, fast, and sorry. Extubation criteria for trauma patients are presented in Table 6.11.

Also included in Table 6.11 are criteria for prolonged ventilatory support. Frequently trauma patients will benefit from prolonged mechanical pulmonary ventilation, and the decision to extubate should be postponed until the patient no longer benefits by ventilatory support. The indications for prolonged mechanical ventilation in the trauma patient include: (a) neuromuscular injury that prevents adequate ventilatory response, (b) chest wall injury that prevents adequate spontaneous ventilation, (c) abdominal injury that prevents adequate spontaneous ventilation, (d) major fracture associated with hypoxia (fat embolism or thromboembolism), (e) excessive pulmonary secretions, and (f) the need for profound analgesia with systemic opioids.

One exception to this slow approach to extubation may be the patient with reactive airway disease and a tracheal tube in place after a follow-up procedure. In this instance, extubation should be done while the patient's reaction to the tube is pharmacologically controlled. Bronchodilators and intravenous analgesics will help prevent cough-induced bronchospasm as a reaction to the tracheal tube. Intravenous lidocaine in doses used to prevent cardiac arrhythmias (approximately 1.5 mg/kg bolus and 1 to 2 mg/min infusion) may also be useful to prevent cough-induced bronchospasm.

The procedure itself should be done only when those capable of reintubating the patient are immediately available (except in cases of war or disaster management, where numbers of trained personnel are lacking). Appropriate equipment and drugs must also be present. Preoxygenation and oropharyngeal suctioning should be done before extubation, and humidified oxygen should be immediately available. If postextubation stridor develops, an aerosol of racemic epinephrine (0.5 ml of racemic epinephrine solution in 2 to 3 ml of saline) should be administered to the vocal cords as soon as possible. Increasing the nebulized humidity is also very helpful to control stridor; a single dose of corticosteroid may be considered as well. Prevention of total upper airway obstruction due to vocal cord edema requires close observation, early recognition of vocal cord swelling, and appropriate treatment. Patients demonstrating excessive head motion with long-term intubation are more likely to develop postextubation stridor because the constant motion of the endotracheal tube against the arytenoid cartilages causes ankylosis of the thyroarytenoid joint. Thus, it is necessary for anesthesia team members to stay in close touch with the critical care staff in case any of these postextubation complications develop.

## Postanesthesia Emergence Delirium and/or Delayed Emergence

The differential diagnosis of a slow emergence from anesthesia in the trauma patient includes an occult head injury that was not obvious preoperatively. The patient may be either depressed or agitated. Illicit drug use just before admission; relative drug overdose in the diagnostic or admitting area, OR, or PACU/RR; as well as unusual reactions to administered medications are also causes of unanticipated delayed recoveries from anesthesia.

## LONG SURGICAL/ANESTHESIA PROCEDURES

Prolonged surgery, which frequently occurs in level I trauma centers, may present additional problems for anesthesia care providers. A change in anesthesia care providers may cause loss of continuity of care and familiarity with the patient's problems and perioperative events. Large doses of drugs may accumulate and delay recovery from anesthesia. Hypothermia may occur secondary to the prolonged poikilothermic state of the anesthetized patient (see Chapter 13) (33).

Prolonged trauma surgery usually is associated with major hemorrhage, which reduces the oxygen-carrying and clotting components of the blood, as well as intravascular volume. Oxygen-carrying capacity must be maintained by ensuring a level of at least 7 gm of hemoglobin per deciliter (Chapter 4). Circulating intravascular volume should be as close to normal as possible to maintain adequate renal blood flow, glomerular filtration, and a urine output of at least 1 ml/kg/hr. An increase in urine output, along with an increase in serum sodium, may indicate the onset of neurogenic or nephrogenic diabetes insipidus. A decrease in urine volume may signal an inadequate circulating blood volume causing renal hypoperfusion or inappropriate secretion of antidiuretic hormone secondary to inadequate release of atrial natriuretic peptides. Laboratory monitoring should proceed as outlined above.

Combined epidural and general anesthesia ("epigeneral") is being used more frequently for long surgical procedures such as acetabular reconstructions. Similarly, combination of an axillary block and general anesthesia is useful in long cases of digit reimplantation. Trauma patients may be operated upon by general, vascular, neurosurgical, orthopedic, or plastic surgical teams simultaneously and/or sequentially during a single anesthetic. With the magnitude of surgery, sequelae that may be associated with prolonged anesthesia need to be considered, ameliorated, or prevented. Translocation of fluids from the intravascular space can decrease cardiac output and oxygen delivery as well as cause edema of organs such as the lung and brain as well as subcutaneous tissues. Third-spacing of fluids out of the intravascular space may become a problem, especially when patients return for repeat operations. Thus, the fluid status must be evaluated appropriately and invasive monitoring implemented as necessary.

## MULTIPLE (FOLLOW-UP) OPERATIONS

After primary surgical repair of damaged organs, many trauma patients return to the operating room for repeat operations. Repeat procedures are frequently done in the acute phase of the initial hospital admission, especially after orthopedic trauma as well as major burns. Frequent multiple operations may be associated with decreased clotting factors, proteins, and oxygen-carrying capacity as well as electrolyte disturbances, ventilation/perfusion mismatching, multisystem organ failure, ARDS, malnutrition (semistarvation), and the need for multiple medications (i.e., many intravenous lines and infusion controllers [pumps]).

A second peak in repeat operations occurs during the rehabilitative phase, when patients return for plastic surgery or orthopedic reconstruction. Orthopedic procedures include the delayed removal of hardware used to fixate fractures, usually 6 to 18 months after injury. Repeat operations on stable patients do not usually present anesthetic problems because their medical problems are known and, theoretically, are now under control. Repeat general anesthetics with halogenated agents and/or regional anesthetic techniques should not increase morbidity and mortality. However, the repeated need for blood products increases the risk of acquiring transfusion-associated diseases, as described in Chapter 5. For this reason, asanguineous fluids such as colloids (hetastarch, albumin) and balanced electrolyte solutions (Ringer's lactate, Plasmalyte) should be used whenever possible rather than component blood therapy. Repeat operations on HIV-positive patients means repeated exposure of anesthesia care providers to the AIDS virus (see Chapter 10). Repeat operations may therefore place stress on patients, the hospital system, and anesthesiology department personnel and equipment.

## THORACOABDOMINAL TRAUMA

Thoracoabdominal injuries are among the classic injuries that anesthesiologists consider when they imagine a trauma patient being rushed from the ambulance to the OR for resuscitative surgery. Furthermore, thoracic injuries are especially worrisome because they affect cardiopulmonary function, the source of most serious anesthetic complications (115).

The concerns of the TA/CCS for patients with thoracic trauma include the need for immediate endotracheal intubation and mechanical ventilation, even if surgery is not needed. Other patients with thoracic injuries will require general anesthesia for emergency surgery to correct life-threatening injuries. Thoracic injuries also initiate injury responses indirectly in other organ systems by affecting pulmonary gas exchange and cardiac output (Table 6.12) (116). Indications for intubation include respiratory arrest, hypoxia, chest wall instability, airway obstruction, shock, and the need to control ventilation during open chest surgery.

### Penetrating Neck Trauma

Penetrating injuries to the neck from gunshot wounds, stab wounds, or penetrating foreign bodies (e.g., construction tools, car parts, bomb fragments) are potentially life-threatening because of the anatomic proximity of cardiovascular, respiratory, and neurologic systems in the neck (117). Initially the TA/CCS will be most interested in airway and vascular injuries that need rapid surgical intervention. Many surgeons recommend exploration of neck wounds

**Table 6.12. Direct and Indirect Effects of Thoracic Injuries**

Direct effects
  Penetrating
    Neck
      Laceration/rupture of any vessel or airway structure
    Lung
      Laceration of parenchyma and/or conducting airway
      Air embolism
    Chest wall
      Open/closed pneumothorax
      Vessel laceration with hemothorax
      Diaphragmatic rupture
      Combined pneumohemothorax
    Heart
      Rupture of any chamber and/or valve
      Coronary artery laceration
      Pericardial tamponade
    Other
      Laceration of aorta or aortic arch vessels
      Laceration of vena cava or great veins
      Laceration of thoracic duct
      Laceration of recurrent laryngeal nerve
  Blunt
    Neck
      Laceration/rupture of any vessel or airway structure
      Cervical spine fractures
      Nerve root traction injuries
    Lung
      Contusion
      Laceration
      Air embolism
    Chest wall
      Contusion
      Rib fractures with vessel lacerations
      Diaphragmatic rupture
    Heart
      Concussion
      Contusion
      Rupture of any chamber and/or valve
      Pericardial tamponade
    Other
      Traumatic aneurysm of aorta or branches
      Avulsion of vena cava or tributaries
      Avulsion of thoracic duct
Indirect effects
  Traumatic asphyxia
  Shock (extends to the microcirculatory level)
  Air embolism
  Hypoxia
  Respiratory acidosis
  Metabolic derangements

that penetrate the platysma muscle; however, recent developments in diagnostic studies have defined a patient population that may be treated by close observation.

Knowledge of potential wound tracts will help predict potential injuries.

Penetrating injury to the larynx or trachea is diagnosed by air bubbling through the penetrating tract, hoarseness, dysphonia, subcutaneous emphysema, and/or loss of laryngeal contours on inspection and palpation of the neck. Distal tracheal injuries may be managed by inserting a cuffed endotracheal tube through the penetrating wound into the trachea, followed by tracheal repair around the tube, which is then left as a tracheostomy tube. Trauma to structures higher in the airway such as laryngeal injuries will require primary repair around a stent with a distal tracheostomy for ventilation.

The surgical anatomy of the neck is defined by three zones: the lower neck from the cephalad border of the clavicle to the cricoid cartilage, the middle neck from the cricoid cartilage to the angle of the mandible, and the upper neck from the angle of the mandible to the base of the skull (118). Penetrating injuries to the lower and upper zones usually require preoperative arteriography to define vascular injury. Exploring middle neck injuries without arteriography is controversial (117).

Trauma surgeons recommend that injuries to the aortic arch vessels and the carotid arteries be repaired unless repair is impossible because of exsanguinating hemorrhage, in which case ligation is the treatment of choice. High lesions of the internal carotids may be inaccessible and require ligation followed by extracranial-to-intracranial anastomosis. Controversy also exists concerning carotid arterial repair or ligation if patients have a serious neurologic deficit. Unilateral lesions to the vertebral artery are treated by ligation above and below the lesion (117).

Cervical venous injuries are almost all treated by ligation, except for accessible internal jugular venous injuries, which are repaired. The TA/CCS must be aware of the potential for venous air embolism through open cervical veins. Thus, the patient should be kept flat or in a slight Trendelenburg position with pressure ventilation to increase venous pressure in the neck (117).

Laryngeal injuries may force the TA/CCS to perform life-saving endotracheal intubation carefully with a small endotracheal tube before tracheostomy (see Chapter 3). Cricothyroidotomies are relatively contraindicated in laryngeal trauma. The laryngotracheal cartilage must be repaired during the initial surgery, with mucosal closure and stent placement for several weeks to prevent stenosis. Early airway management with endotracheal intubation is also recommended to protect patients from airway closure secondary to an expanding hematoma. However, no simple method can be adopted uniformly. For example, anesthetic induction prior to endotracheal intubation is recommended to prevent dislodgement of a hemostatic clot by coughing and straining during intubation (117). Conversely, some anesthesiologists prefer awake intubation for patients with penetrating neck trauma (see Chapters 3 and 8). Blunt trauma to the bony structures of the neck is discussed in Chapter 3.

### Thoracic Trauma

Penetrating and blunt trauma to the chest may injure several structures and thus compromise optimal resuscitation. These structures include the chest wall, the lungs and airways, the heart and pericardium, and the great vessels of the thorax. Injuries to these structures will also compromise anesthesia care by affecting gas exchange and cardiac output.

If the trauma patient is still in shock despite vigorous resuscitative measures, the differential diagnosis of traumatic shock must be reviewed again, other etiologies must be sought aggressively, and specific injuries may need to be treated immediately. This is particularly true in cases of penetrating and/or blunt trauma of the chest and/or abdomen. Some of these etiologies, besides being responsible for continued hemodynamic compromise, may also compromise ventilation, either through direct effects on the lungs and airways or indirectly via pulmonary effects of the cardiovascular pathology. The combination of shock and acute respiratory failure in a trauma patient with chest trauma carries a very high mortality rate (>70%) (119).

Several conditions that interfere with resuscitation can be eliminated quickly and easily (e.g., hypothermia, cardiac arrhythmias, inaccurate monitoring) or sought empirically with little risk to the trauma patient (e.g., hypocalcemia). Proper placement of the endotracheal tube should be ensured, either by directly visualizing the passage of the endotracheal tube through the cords with a laryngoscope or by examining a capnographic trace (see Chapter 3). All the causes of "mediastinal shock" (i.e., tension pneumothorax, pericardial tamponade, myocardial contusion) should be investigated quickly. An upright inspiratory chest x-ray will greatly assist in detecting these injuries; however, chest tube insertion or pericardiocentesis may be required based

solely on clinical signs without a roentgenogram for a patient in extremis.

The extent and nature of a trauma patient's injuries may raise the clinical suspicion of occult hemorrhage or fluid sequestration. For example, in a burn patient, extracellular fluid and plasma may be lost in extremely large quantities. Crush injuries can also sequester large amounts of fluid.

A compartment that can conceal large amounts of fluid is the abdomen (120). It must never be assumed that lack of abdominal distension negates intraabdominal bleeding as a cause of hypotension. The abdomen can be thought of as a cylinder: the effects of internal hemorrhage on its geometry are shown in Figure 6.4. Other areas of the trunk that may contain large amounts of "third space" fluid include (*a*) a retroperitoneal hematoma in the pelvis (up to 2 liters), (*b*) a hemothorax (2–3 liters per hemithorax), (*c*) buttocks, and (*d*) retroperitoneum. Therefore, if the TA/CCS, during the "rapid overview phase" (ATLS, Table

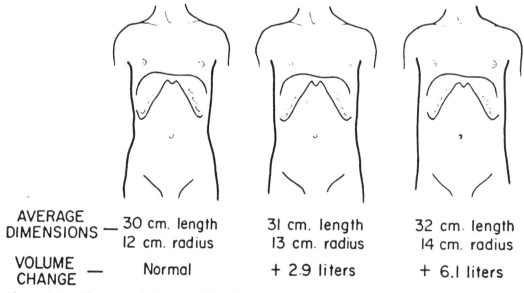

| AVERAGE DIMENSIONS — | 30 cm. length 12 cm. radius | 31 cm. length 13 cm. radius | 32 cm. length 14 cm. radius |
| VOLUME CHANGE — | Normal | + 2.9 liters | + 6.1 liters |

**Figure 6.4. Dimensional changes of the abdomen with increasing hemorrhage.** The abdomen acts as a cylinder in which volume accumulation is accommodated by elevation of the diaphragm, which increases the length of the cylinder with minimal change in radius. Thus, the abdomen can hide significant hemorrhagic volume without obvious distension. (From Trunkey DD, Sheldon GF, Collins JA: The treatment of shock. In Zuidemia GD. Rutherford RB, Ballinger WF (eds): The Management of Trauma, ed 4. Philadelphia, WB Saunders, 1985, pp 105–125.)

6.1), suspects that the trauma patient has sustained an injury to one of these areas, he/she should consider additional volume replacement.

### LIFE-THREATENING CONDITIONS

The conditions discussed in this section (a) are immediately life-threatening, (b) are not always obvious or dramatic (as opposed to the traumatic amputation of an extremity with massive hemorrhage), and (c) require immediate intervention, even before complete diagnosis, because the risk of treating these problems is less than the risk of not treating them.

#### Tension Pneumothorax

A tension pneumothorax (TPT) develops when the pleural cavity (parietal or visceral pleura) is punctured, creating a one-way valve that controls flow of air into this cavity. With each breath, more air becomes trapped in this space, increasing intrapleural pressure to the point that it eventually exceeds all other intrathoracic pressures. The enlarging pleural cavity will then collapse the ipsilateral lung, as well as shift structures of the mediastinum (trachea,

great vessels, heart) into the opposite hemithorax and thereby compress the contralateral lung (Fig. 6.5).

A TPT will compromise pulmonary function because the collapsed lung has little surface area available for gas exchange, causing hypercarbia and hypoxia. A TPT compromises the circulatory system by reducing venous return secondary to vena caval compression. The vena cavae are compressed by both the high pleural pressure and the mediastinal shift that kinks the vena cavae, increasing the resistance to venous return. As the venous return flow is compromised, cardiac output will eventually decrease.

Pleural puncture may occur during chest wall trauma or iatrogenically during the placement of central lines, traumatic intubation attempts, or mechanical ventilation barotrauma. The size of a pneumothorax rapidly increases during positive pressure ventilation (PPV), especially if gases that are more diffusible than nitrogen (e.g., nitrous oxide) are used. For example, a 50/50 mixture of nitrous oxide and oxygen (Nitronox [or Entonox]) is supplied "ready-

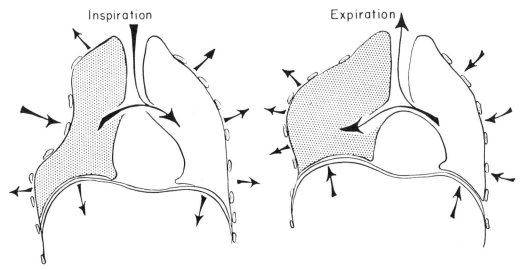

**Figure 6.5. Paradoxic motion of chest wall associated with flail chest.** The volume of the affected side is reduced during inspiration and increased during expiration. (From Wilkins EW: Noncardiovascular thoracic injuries: chest wall, bronchus, lung, esophagus, and diaphragm. In Burke JF, Boyd RJ, McCabe CJ (eds): Trauma Management: Early Management of Visceral, Nervous System, and Musculoskeletal Injuries. Chicago, Year Book, 1988, pp 140–152.)

mixed" in tanks to be used for analgesia in the field and during transport (23). Use of Nitronox in a trauma patient with a pneumothorax will expand the pneumothorax and possibly cause a TPT.

A hypotensive trauma patient with subcutaneous emphysema of the neck or chest, a unilateral decrease in breath sounds (which is difficult to appreciate in a noisy emergency room), diminished chest wall motion, hyperresonance to percussion of one hemithorax, distended neck veins, or tracheal shift should be suspected to have a TPT. If feasible, an upright expirational chest x-ray should be obtained. However, if the trauma patient is unstable, a largebore IV catheter should be inserted into the second intercostal space (ICS) along the midclavicular line (3) (Fig. 6.6). A "hissing" sound may be created by the escaping air under pressure. The catheter can then be attached to an IV extension tubing and placed under "water seal" by submerging it in a liter bottle of sterile water. Care must be taken to keep the water bottle beneath the level of the trauma patient. Otherwise, flow

may be reversed and the water will enter the thorax, thereby causing a hydrothorax.

Alternatives for emergency treatment of a TPT include using a one-way Heimlich valve or a McSwain dart. The McSwain dart is a 16-French polyethylene catheter fitted over a sharp needle stylet. A small skin incision is made over the second ICS in the midclavicular line or the fifth ICS of the anterior axillary line. The dart is inserted, the stylet is withdrawn, and the catheter remains. The end of the catheter has a one-way flutter valve that allows air to exit. This system may also be connected to a pleurevac or a three-bottle suction apparatus (Fig. 6.7). Use of the McSwain dart may prove useful in the field or during transport in cramped spaces (see Chapter 15).

Temporizing devices should be replaced as soon as possible by the more definitive closed-system tube thoracostomy. It is somewhat controversial exactly where to place a thoracostomy tube(s) in the trauma patient (second versus fifth ICS, midclavicular vs. midaxillary line). This choice is probably best guided by review of the chest x-ray, as well as consideration of the following factors: (a) Is this a pneumotho

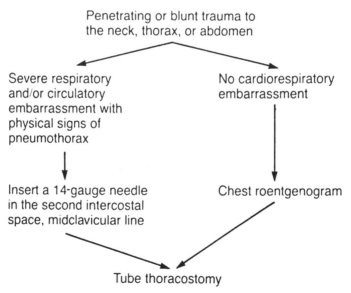

Figure 6.6. **Algorithm for the diagnosis and management of tension pneumothorax.** (From Symbas PN: Cardiothoracic trauma. In Symbas PN (ed): Cardiothoracic Trauma in Trauma. Philadelphia, WB Saunders, 1989, pp 303–343.)

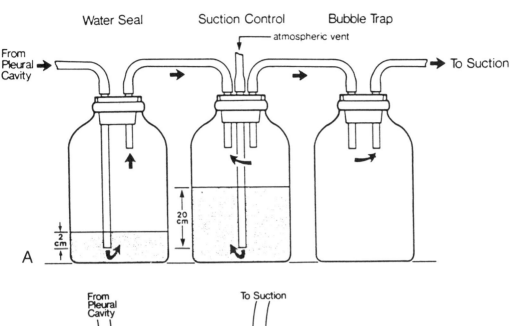

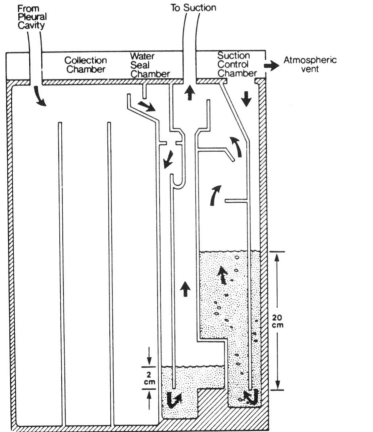

**Figure 6.7.** **A, Three-bottle system for chest tube drainage.** The underwater seal in the bottle placed closest to the patient prevents air from reentering the pleural space during inspiration. The chest tube should not be disconnected from this bottle to prevent a recurrent pneumothorax. **B,** **Underwater seal drainage system** designed to incorporate all functions of the three-bottle system in one compact unit. (From Symbas PN: Cardiothoracic Trauma. Philadelphia, WB Saunders, 1989, pp 3–15.)

rax, hemothorax, or pneumohemothorax? (b) In what position will the patient be maintained and nursed (supine versus head-elevated, supine versus lateral)? The combination of these factors will determine where the thoracostomy will be placed, how many will be placed, and what size chest tube will be used. For example, the trauma patient who has a combined pneumohemothorax with large clots, as well as a severe head injury with an increased ICP, who must be nursed with his head elevated may need two chest tubes. In the head-up position, the air and fluid components of the pneumohemothorax will separate: the air will migrate to the nondependent portion of the hemithorax anterior and cephalad and the blood will migrate to the dependent position of the chest, posterior and caudad. Thus, one chest tube should be placed superiorly to evacuate the air. It is advisable to also place this tube anteriorly (midclavicular line) and direct the tube in a cephalad direction. A second chest tube can be placed in the lower thorax, posteriorly (midaxillary or posterior axillary line), with the tube directed caudally. Because there are larger clots to be evacuated, a chest tube with a larger bore should be chosen to evacuate the hemothorax (121).

Regardless of which insertion site is chosen, the technique is as follows. A surgical prep is applied to the site and an incision 3 cm long is made through to the deep fascia. Anesthesia (generous infiltration with local anesthetics) is administered to conscious trauma patients. A blunt clamp is then inserted into the wound to expose the pleura and puncture it (Fig. 6.8A and B). The incision is enlarged and a gloved finger is inserted to ensure that the pleural space is free without adherent lung parenchyma in the area that may be entered by the chest tube (Fig. 6.8C). The chest tube is then grasped at its tip with a clamp and pushed through the opening until its proximal

fenestration is well inside the chest (Fig. 6.8D). The tube is directed to ensure the predetermined final position as discussed above. A horizontal mattress suture is used to hold the tube in place. This suture will later be used to close the wound. The chest tube is then attached to an evacuation apparatus (three-bottle suction or equivalent) and 15–25 cm $H_2O$ of suction is applied. Occlusive petrolatum gauze is then applied around the tube at the skin, and a secure dressing is placed over this.

In a trauma patient, a chest tube allows continual monitoring of thoracic blood loss, ensures lung expansion (which also arrests hemorrhage from the low-pressure pulmonary vessels due to a tamponade effect), and provides maximal evacuation of nonclotted blood from the pleural space. The overall complication rate of chest tube thoracostomy has been cited as 9.1% (122).

If there is no response to therapeutic chest tube insertion, or if there is persistent large air leak, then tracheobronchial or esophageal rupture must be suspected. This is an indication that bronchoscopy and/or esophagoscopy should be performed. Thoracotomy following intubation with a double-lumen endotracheal tube may be necessary. Also, the trauma patient may have bilateral TPT or a TPT on one side and a massive hemothorax on the opposite side.

### Massive Hemothorax

The mechanisms by which a hemothorax compromises the respiratory and circulatory systems are very similar to those described above for TPT. Additionally, since each hemithorax can accumulate 30–40% of the circulating blood volume, venous return and cardiac output may be more seriously compromised by extreme hemorrhage. Bleeding sources include the heart and great vessels, as well as the vessels of the chest wall and diaphragm. These injuries are

**Figure 6.8. Technique of thoracostomy tube insertion.** (From Symbas PN: Cardiothoracic Trauma. Philadelphia, WB Saunders, 1989, pp 3–15.)

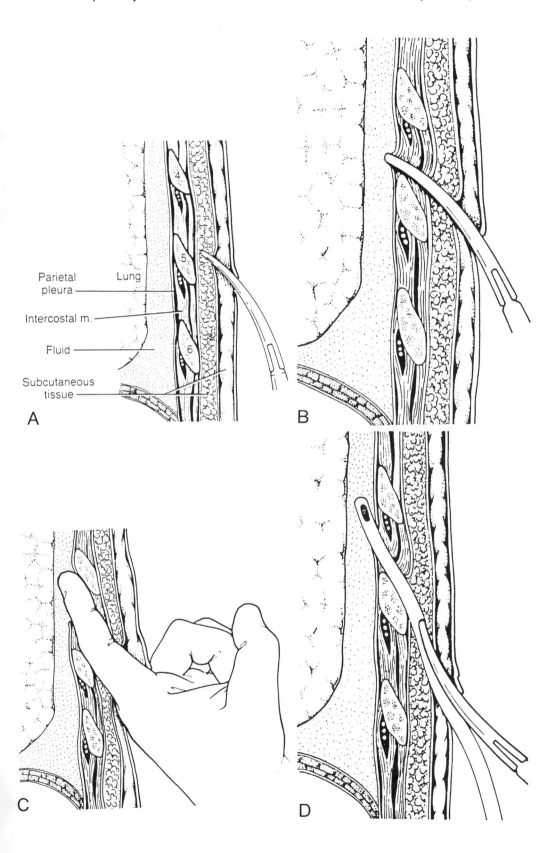

Parietal pleura

Lung

Intercostal m.

Fluid

Subcutaneous tissue

A

B

C

D

associated with a very high mortality rate (119).

The signs of massive hemothorax are similar to those of TPT, except that neck veins will most likely be flat and the involved hemithorax is dull to percussion. Diagnosis is usually made from upright chest x-ray. Confirmation is obtained by the aspiration of blood after insertion of a needle into the eighth intercostal space at the posterior axillary line.

Treatment differs from that of TPT. If the hemithorax is decompressed first, any tamponading effect on the bleeding source will be negated and additional hemorrhage will occur, possibly causing cardiac arrest. Therefore, the first step is rapid intravenous volume replacement. Then tube thoracostomy may be performed (usually more inferiorly and posteriorly than for TPT). Great effort should be made to collect all draining blood and to autotransfuse it; substantial volumes may be recovered (see Chapter 4). Clotted blood left in the pleural space can form fibrinogenolytic and fibrinolytic substances that may cause continued bleeding from the original source. If more than 1500 ml is drained within the first hour, or if more than 200 ml/hr is collected over the next 3 to 4 hours, or if the rate of bleeding increases, thoracotomy is indicated. Placement of a double-lumen endotracheal tube may be necessary. In these cases, a lacerated internal mammary or intercostal artery will most likely be the source of bleeding, because injury to larger vessels usually results in a quick death. The pulmonary vascular system is a low-pressure system (15 mm Hg) and thus would not be expected to contribute excessive bleeding if the lung parenchyma has been reexpanded.

## Pericardial Tamponade (PCT)

Although two types of PCT exist (acute and chronic), the acutely injured trauma patient in the emergency room or OR will usually demonstrate the former. Acute traumatic PCT is caused by the collection of either blood or other fluid (e.g., serous exudate) within an intact pericardial sac. This eventually restricts filling of the cardiac chambers during diastole and produces a fixed low cardiac output (123). Positive pressure ventilation will lower cardiac output even further, as will any cardiac depressant such as many anesthetic agents (124, 125).

Diagnosis of PCT requires a high degree of clinical suspicion. The trauma patient with PCT may occasionally present with the classic Beck's triad: low arterial blood pressure, elevated venous pressure, and distant heart sounds. However, the majority of patients present without the entire triad (3, 126). Other signs are cervical venous distension in the face of systemic hypotension, narrowing of pulse pressure with paradoxic pulse, or equalization of pressures across the heart measured by a pulmonary artery catheter. The chest x-ray may reveal a large globular heart shadow. ECG will be either normal or show nonspecific ischemic changes.

Pericardiocentesis, which is both diagnostic and therapeutic, is performed with an 18-gauge needle placed by subxiphoid puncture. The needle is directed at a 45-degree angle to the horizontal and toward the left shoulder (Fig. 6.9). If this maneuver fails, other less-recommended alternatives include (a) making a subxiphoid puncture but directing the needle toward the *right* shoulder at a 45-degree angle or (b) puncturing the fifth ICS, 1 cm lateral to the sternal edge to a depth of 1.5 to 2.0 cm (127). Accuracy is enhanced by attaching an alligator clip to the needle and observing the V lead on ECG. When the epicardium is contacted, the polarity of the QRS complex will reverse. Aspiration of as little as 10 ml of fluid may provide dramatic improvement.

The conventional wisdom that pericardial blood does not clot because it is defibrinated has been disputed. False-negative pericardial "taps" occur at a rate of approximately 15% (as well as a certain number of false-positives) because of clotting. Therefore, the creation of a subxiphoid

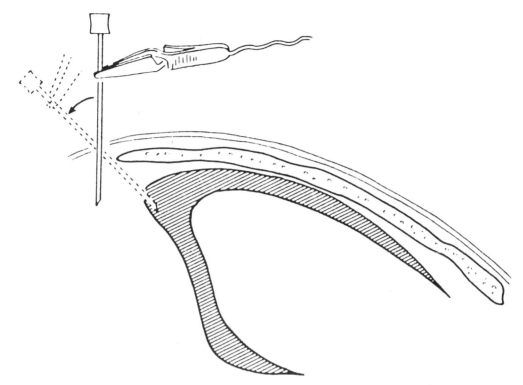

**Figure 6.9.   Pericardiocentesis technique.** The needle is connected to an ECG lead by an alligator clip and directed at a 45° angle downward beneath the sternum and then upward toward the apex of the heart. Lead V of the ECG can be used to identify contact with the myocardium by the appearance of an injury current. (From McSwain NE Jr: Pulmonary chest trauma. In Moylan JA (ed): Trauma Surgery. Philadelphia, JB Lippincott, 1988, pp 77–122.)

pericardial window has been advocated (128). This procedure requires the trauma patient's condition to be stable enough to allow a somewhat time-consuming operation. However, some traumatologists prefer to proceed directly to the pericardial window.

Thoracotomy and pericardiotomy are indicated if a patient has an unstable hemodynamic profile and there is a high degree of clinical suspicion of PCT or if pericardiocentesis has been unsuccessful. If the trauma patient with thoracoabdominal injures is already in the OR for laparotomy when the diagnosis of PCT is suspected, a diagnostic transdiaphragmatic pericardiotomy may be performed. During all of the procedures, volume infusion should be augmented in an effort to raise cardiac

chamber filling pressures and cardiac output (125). The addition of inotropic agents such as isoproterenol may be necessary.

### Cardiac Rupture (without Pericardial Tamponade)

Survival of a trauma patient with cardiac rupture long enough to reach a trauma center is rare, as exsanguination is extremely rapid (126). Penetrating injuries to the shaded areas of Figure 6.10 occur in 57–85% of penetrating chest injuries (129). In one study, it was found that the chamber most likely to be damaged is the right ventricle, owing to its more anterior position (126). The second most likely area to be wounded is the left ventricle. However, in another study, *all* chest wounds were surveyed (Fig. 6.11) and the most common entrance site was the left upper parasternal area (129). These authors concluded that the left ven-

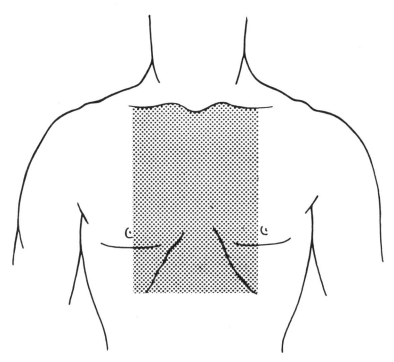

**Figure 6.10. "Danger zone" for central chest penetrating injuries.** Injuries in this zone are associated with a high incidence of cardiac tamponade. (From Harman PK, Trinkle JK: Penetrating cardiac trauma. In Hurst JW (ed): Common Problems in Trauma. Chicago, Year Book, 1987, pp 70–77.)

tricle is the most likely cardiac wound to occur if the thoracic cage is violated. If one examines the studies closely, it can be appreciated that the numerical differences between left and right ventricular wounds are small. Therefore, a more correct statement might be that the most likely chamber to be injured by a penetrating thoracic wound would be *either* the left or the right ventricle.

The mortality rate associated with left ventricular penetrating wounds is highest of all chamber wounds because the pressure generated in that chamber leads to rapid exsanguination into the mediastinal and pleural cavities. However, if the penetrating wound is small enough (i.e., a PCTA catheter puncture) the more muscular left ventricle may have the greatest ability to effectively close the wound.

The degree of cardiac injury sustained during blunt trauma is probably related to the phase of the cardiac cycle at the time of injury and the wounding mechanism. In late diastole or early systole, all chambers are full and the valves are closed. Rapid compression of the heart (as during abrupt decelerations) under these conditions will be more likely to result in rupture of one or more chambers. Structural cardiac injury in blunt trauma is more difficult to categorize than in penetrating trauma, as the wounds vary greatly. The position of the trauma patient when impact occurs during a high-speed motor vehicle accident (MVA) or a fall from a great height will also govern which areas of the heart will be affected (see Chapter 2).

Blunt cardiac trauma is more difficult to diagnose than penetrating injuries, as there is commonly no localized external stigmata to facilitate diagnosis. In fact, associated tramatic injuries may detract attention from the thoracic area. Therefore, a high degree of clinical suspicion must be maintained and inferences from "signpost" injuries such as

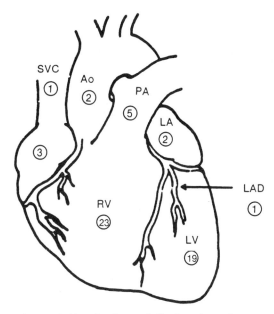

**Figure 6.11.    Regions of the heart most commonly injured in a series of 56 penetrating injuries.** (From Gold JP, Durban L, Krieger KH, Isom OW: Penetrating cardiac trauma. In Callaham ML (ed): Current Therapy for Emergency Medicine, Toronto, BC Decker, 1987, p 131.)

fractured upper ribs and long bone fractures must be utilized. The reported cases of blunt cardiac injuries in the literature are associated with high morbidity. The high morbidity is associated with delayed diagnosis and severe irreparable injury. The trauma patient who does survive transport to a trauma center would be expected to have various combinations of massive hemothorax, TPT, and cardiac structural damage, with underlying severe hypotension due to hypovolemia, pump failure, and other possible complicating factors (secondary to TPT, etc.).

Management of cardiac rupture is the same as that for PCT, except that exsanguination makes emergency thoracotomy more urgent. The techniques for emergency thoracotomy are discussed briefly below.

### Great Vessel Injury: Traumatic Aortic Rupture and Others

Injury to the thoracic aorta has received more attention than injury to any other great vessel of the thorax. In some instances, the aorta may be thoroughly transected, in which case exsanguination occurs rapidly. Alternatively, an intimal tear with formation of a dissecting aneurysm may occur. Causes of aortic injury include (a) penetrating trauma, (b) crush injuries (e.g., from the collapse of buildings), (c) large animal kicks (e.g., horse, cow), (d) falls from great heights, and (e) the most notorious of all, steering wheel impact during a MVA (130). In fact, one study showed that one in six MVA deaths was due to traumatic aortic rupture. The majority of trauma patients with aortic rupture will die "on the spot." Extremely rapid exsanguination is not surprising considering that intraaortic pressures may rise to over 1000 mm Hg upon impact. Survivors of the initial injury will probably have either a small transection with hemorrhage that is controlled or tamponaded by surrounding structures or a dissection in one of the tissue planes (i.e., media, intima) (126).

The most common sites of traumatic aortic rupture are (a) just distal to the origin of the left subclavian artery at the ligamentum arteriosum (80–90%), (b) at the root of the aorta (with possible dissection back to the coronary ostia), (c) avulsion of the innominate artery from the aortic arch, and (d) at the aortic hiatus in the diaphragm, or below the diaphragm (Fig. 6.12) (131). The abrupt intraluminal pressure rise at the time of impact, coincident with the shearing forces of a mobile aorta against these fixed structures, contributes to aortic rupture. With respect to blunt trauma, the horizontal deceleration and shearing forces associated with an MVA will rupture the aorta just distal to the left subclavian artery in 90% of cases (Fig. 6.13) (132). Vertical deceleration associated with falls from great heights causes a greater proportion of aortic rupture at the ascending aorta, as a result of acute lengthening. Multiple aortic tears occur in 20% of MVA's but survival in these cases is very rare (133, 134).

The natural history of penetrating injury to the aorta is different. There is a large difference in survival between intrapericar-

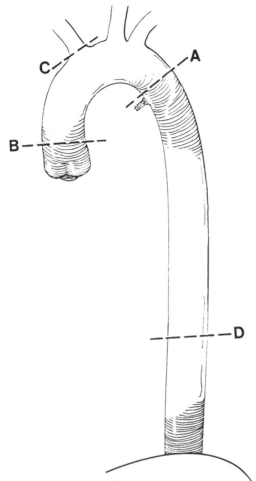

**Figure 6.12.  Sites of traumatic aortic disruption in descending order of frequency.** *A*, Most common site adjacent to the ligamentum arteriosum. *B*, Ascending aorta. *C*, Avulsion of the innominate artery from the aortic arch. *D*, Lower descending aorta. (From Hilgenberg AD: Trauma to the heart and great vessels. In Burke JF, Boyd RJ, McCabe CJ (eds): Trauma Management: Early Management of Visceral, Nervous System, and Musculoskeletal Injuries. Chicago, Year Book, 1988, pp 153–175.)

dial and extrapericardial aortic injuries. The better prognosis of trauma patients with intrapericardial traumatic aortic rupture is dependent upon concurrent PCT. More than 50% of penetrating injuries to the aorta are associated with massive hemorrhage. Concurrent injury of adjacent arterial and venous structures may result in fistulization.

External evidence of trauma is absent in up to one-third of trauma patients; therefore, a high degree of clinical suspicion is required (126). Common symptoms in the conscious trauma patients with TAR include (*a*) retrosternal or interscapular pain that does not vary with respiration, (*b*) ischemic-type extremity pain, (*c*) dysphagia (due to esophageal compression), and (*d*) dyspnea and hoarseness (due to traction of the recurrent laryngeal nerves). Signs of aortic rupture include (*a*) acute onset of upper extremity hypertension with relative hypotension in the lower extremities (pseudocoarctation syndrome), (*b*) a new, harsh systolic murmur over the precordium or posterior interscapular area, (*c*) a pulsatile mass at the base of the neck, (*d*) carotid bruits or decreased carotid pulses, and (*e*) paraplegia.  Associated injuries include steering wheel imprints on the chest wall; rib, sternal, or scapular fractures (see below); massive hemothorax; and TPT (130).

Diagnosis is most often made or confirmed by anteroposterior chest x-ray. Roentgenographic indicators of aortic disruption include the classic, widened upper mediastinum (126). Most trauma patients with ruptured aorta have a widened upper mediastinum, whose presence in a blunt trauma patient is an indication for arteriography of the aorta (126). Aortography may precipitate a potentially lethal aortic rupture in this situation; thus, a cardiothoracic surgical team should be standing by. Digital subtraction angiography offers a less dangerous alternative.

Damage to the major pulmonary vessels or the subclavian or innominate arteries may all be fatal as well. Vena caval injuries are also associated with high mortality rates. As opposed to the thick-walled aorta, bleeding from the thin-walled vena cava is especially lethal, as subsequent surgical exposure and control are more difficult. Because of similar problems with rapid exsanguination, difficulties of exposure and control, and the severity of inevitably associated trauma, rupture of the iliac, femoral, and renal veins many carry an even higher mortality. Thoracotomy to allow cross-clamping of the

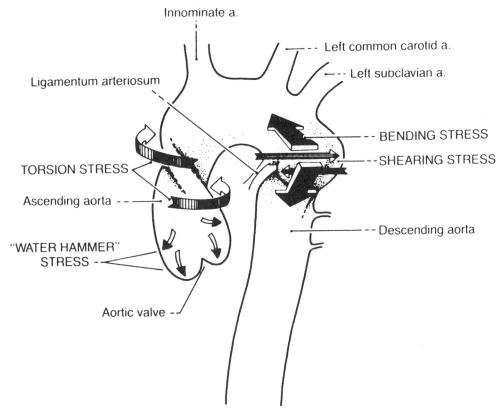

**Figure 6.13.  Mechanisms of injury to different sites of the aorta.** (From Symbas PN: Cardiothoracic Trauma. Philadelphia, WB Saunders, 1989, pp 160–231.)

aorta prior to laparotomy in the trauma patient with suspected injuries of these vessels has been advocated, but the results are questionable (126).

**Air Embolism**

Systemic air embolism, thought to be rare, may occur in approximately 14% of patients with major thoracic injuries. The incidence is three times greater following penetrating injuries than following blunt trauma. Air embolism may occur either on the venous side of the circulation (affecting right heart stroke volume, obstructing pulmonary outflow, or causing pulmonary hypertension) or on the left side of the heart (resulting in coronary artery embolization or cerebrovascular embolization). An air embolism in the left heart is entrained through a bronchopulmonary venous fistula (126, 135). For example, an open pneumothorax may lead to air entrainment through an open pulmonary vein; or positive pressure ventilation may lead to air embolism in a patient with a closed chest, tracheobronchial injury with traumatic bronchopulmonary venous fistula. Air embolism may also occur in a patient with an open skull fracture and exposed diploic veins or iatrogenically during central venous catheterization. Hypovolemia and positive pressure ventilation are predisposing factors.

As with other problems in this section, a high degree of clinical suspicion is necessary for timely diagnosis and treatment. Suggestive scenarios are (*a*) the sudden unexplained deterioration of a trauma patient with severe chest trauma, (*b*) the trauma patient who has no obvious head trauma but who has localized findings on neurologic examination, such as paraplegia or hemiplegia, and (*c*) sudden hemodynamic collapse after endotracheal intubation and initiation of positive-pressure ventilation.

Associated signs include hemoptysis, air visualized in the retinal veins during fundoscopic examination, or froth obtained during aspiration of arterial blood for blood gas analysis.

Overall mortality (immediate and delayed) is extremely high. Treatment of suspected air embolism involves emergency thoracostomy and/or immediate compression in a hyperbaric chamber and subsequent hyperoxygenation.

Hyperbaric therapy is the *only* definitive treatment for air embolism (see Chapter 14). However, when considering treatment, one must be aware of both the secondary problem (air embolism) and the causative (primary) problem which may require definitive treatment to prevent further air embolism. For example, if the primary problem is a pneumothorax, it must be attended to immediately by the placement of a thoracostomy tube. Due to the urgency of treatment of air embolism, hyperbaric compression should be initiated prior to thoracostomy tube insertion if a large hyperbaric chamber is available. In a facility that lacks a large hyperbaric chamber, immediate thoracotomy to obtain control of the site of air entry should be performed followed by thoracostomy tube placement at surgical closure.

If the primary problem was entrainment of air through an intravascular catheter in a central vein with subatmospheric pressure, then right heart air embolism may need corrective treatment. Air collected in the right ventricle, which can obstruct pulmonary arterial outflow, may have to be evacuated by a percutaneous needle puncture or formal thoracotomy. For further discussion see Chapter 14.

## CONDITIONS THAT PREVENT OPTIMAL RESUSCITATION

This category includes problems in trauma management that are not usually as life-threatening as the previously described conditions but that may hinder complete resuscitation and rehabilitation of the trauma patient. If these problems are unrec-

ognized and untreated, they may contribute to the patient's deterioration and ultimate death. These injuries occur as a constellation of injuries to the chest wall and its underlying structures. For example, the ribs may be contused, singly fractured, or multiply fractured. The lung may be concussed, contused, or lacerated. Similarly, the heart may be concussed, contused, or lacerated.

### The Chest Wall
*Simple Rib, Scapular, Clavicular, or Sternal Fractures.*   Rib fracture is the most common injury sustained after blunt chest trauma (126, 134). Not much force is necessary to fracture a rib, especially in geriatric trauma patients. Special attention must be given to fractures of the upper ribs, which are well-protected by the clavicles anteriorly and the scapulae and the heavy musculature of the back posteriorly. Fractures of these ribs may signal that severe trauma has been sustained by the entire body and may be associated with major chest, abdominal, or vascular injuries.

Previously, it had been taught that only first rib fractures were to be regarded as harbingers of serious blunt chest trauma. One classic study found that first rib fracture was associated with major chest injury in 64% of patients, with major abdominal trauma in 33% of patients, and cardiac injuries in 14% of patients. Also noted was a high degree of local injury to the subclavian artery and the brachial plexus (136). Later studies stressed that a high degree of suspicion for associated injuries should not be limited to first rib fractures, but extended to fractures of the first through the third ribs (3, 137–140). Because of this relationship of upper rib fractures with multiple organ system trauma, obtaining an aortogram and a diagnostic peritoneal lavage (DPL) should be strongly considered in the trauma patient with upper rib fractures. Alternatively, fractures of the lower ribs are associated with a high degree of hepatic and/or splenic injury (137).

Although they are simple injuries, rib fractures may cause complications of atelectasis and pneumonia, especially in the elderly or those with underlying pulmonary disease. These problems occur secondary to the associated splinting (poor inspiratory effort) and weak cough. Therefore, a hand-held Wright's spirometer or incentive spirometer should be used to measure tidal volume (VT) and forced vital capacity (FVC). A VT of less than 5 ml/kg or a FVC of less than 10 ml/kg signals severe splinting. Taping the ribs or binding will result in even more splinting and further compromise. Furthermore, the use of systemic analgesics may lead to central respiratory depression. Therefore, the best current therapy consists of intercostal nerve block which can be performed with an indwelling catheter in patients with fractures of three or fewer ribs or with thoracic epidural analgesia if more than three are concerned (138, 141). Intrapleural injection of local anesthetics has recently been promoted for analgesia for chest wall trauma. Preliminary results appear promising in certain cases (142).

Sternal fractures occur in only a few patients with chest injuries, but they are associated with serious intrathoracic injuries (approximately 30% of patients with sternal fractures die) (139). These associated injuries include aortic rupture, myocardial contusion, tracheobronchial rupture, esophageal rupture, and intercostal or internal mammary artery laceration (137). Most sternal fractures are nondisplaced or stable, but a number of them require open reduction (139). Sternal fractures or sternocostal separations contribute to a deterioration in respiratory function similar to that seen with rib fractures (143). A "sternal flail" may occur when there is bilateral disruption of rib attachments.

Scapular fractures occur less frequently than sternal fractures. However, similar to other injuries in this group, scapular fractures can be considered a harbinger of more serious internal injuries, with an associated mortality of approximately 15%. Most deaths are due to pulmonary contusion, clavicular fracture, or injury to the subclavian, brachial, or axillary arteries.

The clavicle may be fractured coinciden-tally with ribs, sternum, or scapulae. Other associated injuries include damage to the brachial plexus and phrenic nerve roots. Trauma to the phrenic nerve may lead to diaphragmatic paralysis, which in turn may cause respiratory embarrassment (139). As an isolated injury, diaphragmatic paralysis may not be significant. However, in conjunction with other thoracic injuries or in the trauma patient with lung disease, diaphragmatic paralysis may cause severe incapacity.

*Flail Chest (FC).* Flail chest (FC) injuries are defined as fractures in more than one place of at least three adjacent ribs. This produces a segment of the chest wall that responds to changes in pleural pressure, as opposed to the muscular action of the chest wall, resulting in a "paradoxic" respiratory pattern (Fig. 6.5). FC may not be apparent upon simple inspection, as chest wall muscular spasm may be able to splint the segment until the muscles become fatigued. Palpation is more likely to be diagnostic of FC than inspection.

FC may cause hypoxia by two mechanisms: (*a*) shunt due to perfusion of the underlying area of poorly ventilated, contused lung, which almost always accompanies FC injuries, and (*b*) atelectasis caused by compromised ventilatory mechanics. A third reason, the pendeluff phenomenon, mentioned only for historical reasons, was once thought to make a significant contribution to hypoxemia, but recently this has been disproven. The pendeluff phenomenon is an increase in dead space ventilation caused by air oscillating from one mainstem bronchus to the other during the ventilatory cycle. This is no longer believed to occur.

A FC can be stabilized immediately in the field by placing a heavy object like a sandbag on the flail segment, but this is of little value for long-term management. An alternative method is to use towel clips and an orthopedic extension set. The disadvantage of this technique is that added stress is placed upon the already compromised respiratory musculature. Definitive therapy of FC has passed through several phases, beginning with *external* stabilization by taping and strapping. External stabilization was later abandoned in favor of *internal* stabilization, which is accomplished by tracheal intubation and PPV. In extreme cases, tracheostomy and mechanical ventilation to the point of alkalotic apnea were continued for 3 to 5 weeks (143). This mode of therapy was not free of morbidity and mortality. The subsequent development of more sophisticated mechanical ventilatory modes such as intermittent mandatory ventilation (IMV) and constant positive airway pressure (CPAP) has minimized such problems. Modern management of flail chest is more selective and depends upon evaluation of the trauma patient's ventilatory mechanics (138, 140, 144). The trauma patient in impending respiratory failure, as demonstrated by physical examination, measurement of arterial blood gases, and/or mechanical ventilatory parameters, is intubated emergently and treated with intermittent mechanical ventilation (IMV), pressure support (PS), or continuous positive airway pressure (CPAP). Borderline cases are given a trial of analgesics, provided by continuous thoracic epidural or intercostal nerve block.

In the near future, intermittent or continuous intrapleural analgesia may be useful to treat FC. Ventilatory mechanical measurements (e.g., VT, FVC) are performed before and after regional anesthesia. Improvement should be demonstrated as a function of pain relief (Fig. 6.14). Incentive spirometry, postural drainage, and chest physiotherapy are then added to the therapeutic regimen. Two to five days of therapy are required before the trauma patient is able to ventilate and cough satisfactorily, without the aid of regional anesthesia. Respiratory parameters are followed regularly; if any deterioration is detected, then additional support is implemented. This may be a CPAP mask (controversial due to concerns of forceful aspiration) or endotracheal intubation with ventilator assistance.

Some authors still advocate the use of internal fixation devices for severe injury to the chest wall involving fractures of eight or more ribs (126). In this case, flat metal plates (Jergusen plates) are contoured to the inner surface of the rib and affixed to the rib segments, across the fractures, by large stainless steel wires. Additionally, operative

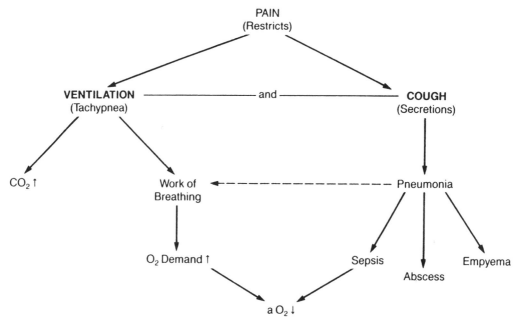

**Figure 6.14.   Pain from chest wall trauma reduces pulmonary reserve and may lead to hypoxia or major infection.** (From Pate JW: Chest wall injuries. Surg Clin North Am 1989;69:59–70.)

stabilization of the flail segments may be chosen if thoracotomy is necessary for another injury.

### The Lung

The most severe types of lung trauma have already been discussed in the previous sections. Others of interest to the TA/CCS are described here.

*Pulmonary Contusion.* Although the most common cause of pulmonary contusion is blast injury, blunt trauma contributes significantly to the development of lung contusion underlying a traumatized chest wall (139, 145). However, the mechanisms causing pulmonary contusion (blast effect or blunt trauma) are the same at the cellular level. A series of high pressure waves combined with instantaneous pressure increases due to thoracic compression rupture the pulmonary capillary membranes, causing extravasation of blood and plasma into the interstitium and alveolae. Blood and plasma are extravasated into the pulmonary extravascular space in an exaggerated manner to that seen with the adult respiratory distress syndrome (ARDS). In fact, the clinical presentation of pulmonary contusion may mimic posttraumatic ARDS. Differentiation may be possible only by consideration of the wounding mechanism. The trauma patient with lung contusion may present with severe dyspnea, tachypnea, and other signs of hypoxia. Arterial blood gases reflect hypoxia in serious cases of contusion, and the chest x-ray usually shows the classic finding of a poorly defined infiltrate, not confined to a segment or lobe, representing combined alveolar and interstitial edema. The timing of the appearance of these findings on chest x-ray is controversial. Some traumatologists believe that radiologic findings will be significant at 1 hour in over 70% of trauma patients with PC. Others feel that useful x-ray results are delayed for 4 to 6 hours or longer. Complete chest film resolution may occur by 72 hours, but in some patients may require up to 3 weeks.

Most authors agree that prevention of fluid overload is of paramount importance in these patients. However, dehydration should also be avoided in the trauma patient whose hemodynamic status is precarious and fluctuating (126). Monitoring cardiac filling pressures with a pulmonary artery catheter will aid the TA/CCS in maintaining a euvolemic state in these patients. Treatment is supportive, and oxygen should be administered to trauma patients with hypoxemia demonstrated by arterial blood gas analysis. Regional anesthesia may obviate the need for controlled ventilation as described above for FC (140, 144). However, intubation and mechanical ventilation may be necessary in the trauma patient unable to meet ventilatory demands because of decreased pulmonary compliance and increased work of breathing produced by severe pulmonary contusion. Pulmonary toilet is also maintained: aseptic technique is mandatory because the most common complication of lung contusion is infection (134). Occasionally, therapeutic bronchoscopy may be necessary. Associated rib trauma should be managed appropriately, as outlined above. Diuretics, steroids, salt-poor albumin, and antibiotics have not been shown to be of definite value unless there is specific indication. However, PEEP can be extremely helpful, especially if instituted early.

*Pulmonary Hematoma.* Pulmonary hematoma, which occurs more commonly with penetrating trauma, is caused by laceration of larger pulmonary vessels that are injured with a contusion. The resultant hemorrhage is usually discreet and localized to a lobe or segment or the bleeding may be contained by the pleura. Clinical presentation is similar to that of lung contusion, but hemoptysis is more common. Chest x-rays may show a *spherical* density due to the compressibility of the surrounding normal elastic tissue. Treatment is conservative and spontaneous. Recovery usually occurs by the third or fourth week (145).

*Pulmonary Laceration.* Pulmonary laceration is a rare form of lung injury, usually caused by the jagged edge of a fractured rib or some form of deep penetrating trauma. There will usually be an associated hemothorax, which will require chest tube thoracostomy. Lung laceration may be associated with a tracheobronchial laceration, which will also cause a TPT and place the patient at risk of an air embolism. Signs and symptoms of pulmonary lacerations are similar to those of pulmonary contusion, but may also include signs of TPT, massive hemothorax, or tracheobronchial laceration. If tracheobronchial laceration is present and the trauma patient is in respiratory distress, mechanical ventilation with a high-frequency technique may be necessary. Thoracotomy may be indicated to control severe hemorrhage or for repair of a significant or persistent air leak (139, 145).

*Tracheobronchial Laceration.* The true incidence of tracheobronchial laceration in the trauma patient is difficult to determine because many patients with this injury die prior to arriving at the trauma center (139). Three theories have been postulated for the mechanism of blunt-trauma-induced tracheobronchial laceration, which attempt to explain why 80% of these injuries occur circumferentially within 2.5 cm of the carina: (*a*) Blunt impact at the time of glottic closure causes pressure buildup in the tracheobronchial tree, which ruptures at its weakest point. (*b*) A mobile carina is sheared away from surrounding mediastinal structures during blunt chest impact. (*c*) Anteroposterior compression of the thoracic cage causes lateral movement of the two lungs in opposite directions, causing tearing at the carina (139, 145).

The clinical presentation of tracheobronchial laceration depends on the degree of violation of pleural space integrity. Symptoms of a small leak are usually confined to a nonproductive cough and are self-limited due to fibrin sealing of the pleura. However, large air leak will result in massive mediastinal and subcutaneous emphysema, hemoptysis, respiratory distress, TPT, and a large amount of air escaping through a chest tube. If the pleural cavity is intact, the laceration may communicate with the me-

diastinum, thus causing only pneumomediastinum.

Diagnosis of tracheobronchial laceration is based on clinical findings and chest x-ray. The chest x-ray might reveal TPT, pneumomediastinum, or subcutaneous emphysema. Bronchoscopy with direct visualization of the tracheobronchial injury is the best diagnostic technique. Treatment requires median sternotomy incision and repair of the laceration.

### Traumatic Diaphragmatic Hernia

Traumatic diaphragmatic hernia may be discovered at the trauma patient's initial evaluation in the trauma center or incidentally at thoracotomy and/or laparotomy performed for other reasons (134, 139, 145). Herniation may occur years after injury and is thought to have a great propensity for incarceration and strangulation, because the defect is usually small and asymptomatic until entrapped viscera become infarcted and/or obstructed.

The incidence of diaphragmatic hernia secondary to both blunt and penetrating trauma is low. These figures would increase if diaphragmatic ruptures found at autopsy on nonsurvivors were included. Diaphragmatic hernia occurs predominantly in males and is more frequent following penetrating trauma than blunt trauma (139, 145).

The majority of diaphragmatic hernias sustained from blunt trauma had been classically thought to occur in the left hemidiaphragm. This was believed because the right hemidiaphragm is relatively protected and buttressed by the liver and the heart. Studies of cadavers support the classic theory by demonstrating congenital weaknesses in the posterior lateral areas of the left hemidiaphragm (146). For penetrating trauma, left-sided injury definitely predominates. This is because most stab wounds are inflicted by right-handed assailants facing their victims.

Diaphragmatic hernia is caused by three factors in blunt trauma: (*a*) The abdominothoracic pressure gradient may exceed the usual maximum value of 100 cm $H_2O$ if the trauma patient gasps against a closed glottis (Meuller maneuver) at the instant that a large external force raises the intraabdominal pressure. (b) Thoracic compression during blunt trauma distorts the anatomy of the diaphragm and tears it with large shearing forces. (c) The trauma patient may have a congenital weakness of the diaphragm (145).

The abdominal organs most likely to herniate transdiaphragmatically are the stomach, omentum, transverse colon, and small bowel. The herniated organs may compress the lung, causing changes in pulmonary compliance and airway resistance, as well as mediastinal shift with resultant circulatory embarrassment. This cardiopulmonary compromise can be further affected by sequelae of trauma such as lung contusion, hypovolemia and TPT.

Diagnosis of diaphragmatic trauma requires a high degree of clinical suspicion by the TA/CCS. Thus injury should be suspected in patients with (a) injuries below the fifth ICS and (b) the injuries associated with high-energy impact, such as fractures of the clavicles, upper ribs, scapulae, sternum, pelvis, or thoracolumbar spine (139, 145).

Clinical symptoms of traumatic diaphragmatic hernia include dizziness, cyanosis, lower chest pain, or upper abdominal discomfort (particularly if referred to the shoulder). Clinical signs that may be noticed are diminished or absent breath sounds, bowel sounds in the chest, tracheal shift, abdominal distension, respiratory distress, or shock. However, these signs and symptoms will prove to be not helpful, unless the TA/CCS suspects a diaphragmatic hernia.

Most preoperative diagnoses of diaphragmatic hernia are made by chest film. The plain chest film may show gas-filled loops of bowel in the chest, a unilaterally elevated hemidiaphragm, or abnormal diaphragmatic contours; if a nasogastric tube (NGT) has been placed, it may be seen coiled in the stomach above the diaphragm. Some surgeons believe that the placement of a NGT prior to x-ray is mandatory in the trauma patient (if there are no contraindica-

tions to its passage), as this also decompresses the stomach. Suspicious findings on a chest radiograph include "plate-like" atelectasis above an indistinct diaphragm, mediastinal shift away from the injured side, gas bubbles or air-fluid levels superior to the diaphragm, unusual shadows above the diaphragm, or pleural effusion. If pleural effusion has been noted, before performing thoracentesis, careful consideration should be given to the possibility of iatrogenically penetrating an entrapped viscera. Thoracoscopy is an alternative.

Radiologic diagnostic pitfalls include (a) a "pseudodiaphragm" formed by the wall of an abdominal viscus mimicking the contour of the diaphragm and (b) an elevated hemidiaphragm caused by phrenic nerve injury. If the radiologic findings are equivocal, further workup includes (a) inspiration and expiration films, which should accentuate visceral herniation, (b) a film done during a positional change (Trendelenburg), (c) the application of external abdominal pressure, (d) fluoroscopy, or (e) contrast studies (except in cases of suspected visceral perforation). Contrast studies may demonstrate contrast-filled viscera above the diaphragm, an abrupt obstruction to flow of contrast media, or a failure of material to progress in serial films. Classic findings include the "amputated fundus sign" showing the fundus of the stomach trapped above the diaphragm. The risk of regurgitation and pulmonary aspiration may be increased by the ingestion of contrast material. Contrast use may also be dangerous in cases of obstruction associated with organ strangulation and necrosis, a condition prone to perforation. These risks may be lessened by use of water-soluble contrast media.

DPL has been used to diagnose traumatic diaphragmatic hernia but it has about a 20% false-negative rate. This may be due to the hemorrhaging portion of the abdominal viscera being entirely isolated above the diaphragm, without contaminating the intraperitoneal space. Diagnostic pneumoperitoneum has also been used with similar results. Air embolism is a risk associated with this procedure; the risk may be reduced by using carbon dioxide as the insufflation gas. Thoracoscopy for the diagnosis of diaphragmatic hernia is under investigation (165). Computed tomography is not useful for diagnosing this condition (146).

Surgical correction of diaphragmatic hernia depends on the time of discovery (preoperatively versus intraoperatively) and associated facilities. Therefore, discussion of whether the procedure of choice is laparotomy, thoracotomy, or a combined thoracoabdominal procedure is beyond the scope of this chapter.

Anesthetic induction or endotracheal intubation for respiratory distress in the trauma patient with diagnosed or occult diaphragmatic hernia must be performed carefully. A lung collapsed by the pressure of abdominal viscera may be prone to reexpansion pulmonary edema.

### The Heart

The more devastating cardiac injuries, such as myocardial rupture, have already been discussed in the previous section. Anesthetic considerations associated with other heart injuries are discussed below.

*Myocardial Concussion.* This form of blunt cardiac trauma is usually very difficult to diagnose. Myocardial concussion is caused by a direct blow to the anterior chest, usually limited to the sternum, which initiates a sudden, transient dysrhythmia (ventricular tachycardia or fibrillation) or complete asystole. Hypotension and unconsciousness will often follow, with death occurring in many cases. Postmortem examination will usually find no demonstrated myocardial histopathology or evidence of damage. A classic example of myocardial concussion is a man wearing a bulletproof vest who sustains a low-velocity "hit" from a handgun to the center of the chest, is "knocked down" and unconscious, and then regains consciousness moments afterward. The bullet did not penetrate the vest, but the force of the impact was transmitted through the sternum to the heart. Other causes of myocardial concussion include punches, kicks, baseballs, and even the "precordial thump." Treatment is supportive until spontaneous cardiac activity returns.

*Myocardial Contusion.* Reported in about 15 to 70% of trauma patients sustaining blunt chest trauma, myocardial contusion is the most common cardiac injury due to nonpenetrating trauma. The contusion is hemorrhagic and well-circumscribed, varying from subendocardial, epicardial, intramural, to transmural, affecting one or more cardiac chambers (Fig. 6.15). It may be associated with pericarditis, pericardial effusion, tamponade (due to either a hemorrhagic or sympathetic reaction) and pulmonary contusion. A force sufficient to cause cardiac rupture will also cause some degree of myocardial contusion (126, 147). Blunt chest trauma is much more commonly associated with myocardial contusion than penetrating chest trauma. In most instances, either the heart is compressed between the sternum and spine, or it is affected by instantaneous increases in intrathoracic pressure (133, 148). Iatrogenetic trauma due to closed-chest massage during CPR may also be responsible for myocardial contusion. The right ventricle is injured more frequently than the left during CPR due to its proximity to the chest wall. However, the valves in the left heart (especially the aortic valve) are more susceptible to injury than those in the right heart. Additionally the coronary arteries may be thrombosed or lacerated or become spasmodic because of direct trauma from the sternum or spine. Consequently, univenticular or biventricular failure may occur. The reduction in cardiac output that occurs from myocardial contusion is proportional to the mass of damaged cardiac muscle (126, 133, 149). If the coronary arteries or valves are affected, sequelae are similar to the clinical response to cardiac rupture (described above). After injury, the damaged myocardium is extremely sensitive and prone to develop arrhythmias (126, 133, 150). Interestingly, the chest wall need not be involved at all in myocardial contusion. The term "hydraulic

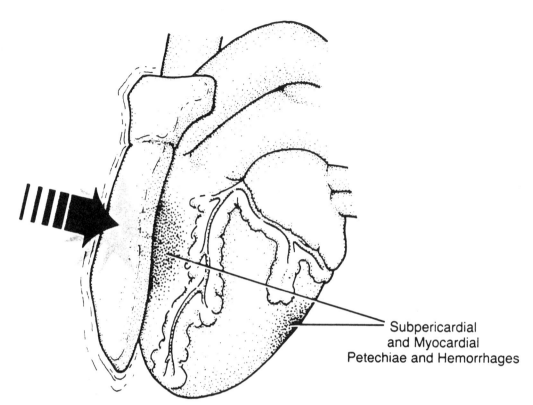

Subpericardial
and Myocardial
Petechiae and Hemorrhages

**Figure 6.15.   Mechanisms of injury for cardiac contusion in blunt chest trauma.** (From Symbas PN: Contusion of the heart. In Symbas PN: Cardiovascular Trauma. Philadelphia, WB Saunders, 1989, pp 55–76.)

ram effect" describes a mechanism whereby abdominal compression as a result of blunt trauma causes a significant increase in transdiaphragmatic pressure to contuse the heart (133).

Symptoms of myocardial contusion may be similar to a myocardial infarction or pericarditis, since anginal chest pain is the most common complaint of patients with myocardial contusion (133). However, contusion pain is *unrelieved* by nitroglycerin (if the trauma patient is able to communicate). Many trauma patients with myocardial contusion report little or no symptoms from their cardiac injury (126, 133, 139, 145, 150).

Ventricular arrhythmias are the most common clinical sign of myocardial contusion (126, 133, 139, 145). Other signs may be injury currents (Q-wave, S-T segments) on the ECG or a pericardial friction rub; there may be no change at all in cardiac

examination. Chemical evidence of myocardial injury can be sought by measuring the myocardial band (MB) fraction of the total serum creatine phosphokinase (CPK-MB). Again, a positive result (greater than 2–5%) is specific only for myocardial cellular injury. The MB fraction will be elevated if the total CPK is extremely high (as in major crush injuries) because skeletal muscle contains a small fraction of the MB isoenzyme of CPK. Although both ECG and CPK-MB results are negative, myocardial contusion cannot be ruled out.

The unreliability of these tests has led to the clinical evaluation of three others: (*a*) the technetium scan (TS), (*b*) a new form of thallium scanning (single-photon emission computerized tomography [SPECT]), and (*c*) echocardiography.

The rationale for TS is calcium uptake by dying myocardial cells. $^{99m}$Technetium pyrophosphate ($^{99m}$Tc PXR) has been found to mimic calcium action at the cell membrane. Currently, the studies performed to evaluate the use of $^{99m}$Tc PXR to detect myocardial contusion in patients with blunt chest trauma have found this test lacking in the sensitivity necessary to confirm the presence of the injury. Furthermore, a large amount of $^{99m}$Tc PXR must be present to provide an acceptable signal-to-noise ratio. Thus, $^{99m}$Tc PXR also requires the presence of a large mass of necrotic myocardium to accurately diagnose myocardial contusion (151).

SPECT is thought to have both the sensitivity and specificity to diagnose myocardial contusion. However, SPECT requires sophisticated and expensive equipment to perform, which limits its utility outside a few sophisticated trauma centers.

Ultrasound can accurately reveal functional and anatomic cardiac chamber abnormalities as well as intracardiac thrombi and shunts. The right ventricle is well-differentiated from the left by ultrasonography (echocardiography). ECG and cardiac isoenzymes must be used as screening tests for the diagnostic sensitivity and specificity of myocardial contusion to remain high. An echocardiographic monitor should be available in the admitting area of a sophisticated trauma center. Personnel expert in interpreting the echocardiographic results should also be available.

Diagnostic pulmonary artery catheterization is useful to monitor patients with myocardial contusion. However, the data generated by a pulmonary artery catheter are not specific for the etiology of cardiac injury, but only for the physiologic dysfunction. Such monitoring may be indicated by the results of diagnostic tests for myocardial contusion. Therapeutic pulmonary artery catheterization is indicated to optimize therapy for the trauma patient with a large contusion, especially for the patient who requires anesthesia and surgery. Patients with small contusions, who exhibit no hemodynamic changes or a few PVCs, do not usually require pulmonary artery monitoring during anesthesia.

The natural history of myocardial contu-

sion depends on the size of the myocardial injury. Large contusions that cause traumatic necrosis of the entire ventricular wall thickness (transmural) including the papillary muscle lead to the rapid development of valvular insufficiency and heart failure. Large transmural contusions can also cause ventricular rupture, which is rapidly fatal. Most contusions are not as devastating and cause a discrete area of interstitial hemorrhage with a modest degree of myocardial cellular necrosis. Although traumatologists tend to treat patients with myocardial contusion as if they had a myocardial infarction, a contusion differs significantly from an infarction because there is no "zone of relative ischemia" surrounding a contusion. Furthermore, the generation of an injury current and/or an irritable focus of ventricular ectopy is much more limited in contusions than in myocardial infarctions. Myocardial contusions tend to heal with a well-vascularized scar that is at less risk for late ventricular rupture, as compared with myocardial infarctions.

Management of myocardial contusion consists of inotropic support, afterload reduction, and dysrhythmia control. If possible, the patient should be maintained in a euvolemic state to minimize secondary pulmonary or renal injury (see Chapter 4). Patients should receive adequate sedation and analgesia to minimize pain and anxiety-induced increases of myocardial oxygen consumption.

A controversial topic is anticoagulating a trauma patient with myocardial contusion and echocardiographically demonstrated mural thrombi. On one hand, anticoagulation can aggravate hemorrhage in a multiple-trauma patient by promoting intramural, myocardial hemorrhage with extension of the area of contusion or increasing the volume of a pericardial effusion. On the other hand, heparinization may prevent embolization. The situation becomes more complicated if an intraaortic balloon pump must be inserted to support the trauma patient hemodynamically because thrombus formation on the balloon can cause also systemic embolization. In some instances, low-molecular-weight dextran has been used for both its antithrombotic effect and its value as a plasma expander.

*Myocardial Infarction.* A myocardial infarction in the trauma patient presents a "chicken and the egg" dilemma. In most cases it is difficult to ascertain if the myocardial infarction occurred first and was responsible for the subsequent traumatic event or if the infarction is a sequela of the traumatic event. Occasionally, the trauma patient's medical history or description of events prior to injury may help, but knowledge of the sequence may not contribute much to the necessary therapy. A myocardial infarction is difficult to differentiate from a myocardial contusion, as described above. A complete discussion of the diagnosis and management of myocardial infarction is beyond the scope of this chapter.

### Abdominal Injuries

Unlike thoracic injuries, which require operative intervention less than 15% of the time, an intraabdominal injury frequently indicates a surgical approach. It is important to define a thoracic injury; however, with abdominal injuries it is most important to decide whether the patient has an abdominal injury and therefore needs an operation rather than to define the exact injury. This section of this chapter will discuss the diagnosis of an intraabdominal injury and the anesthetic implications of celiotomy.

Injuries to the three abdominal regions—the retroperitoneal space, the abdominal cavity, and the pelvis—cause characteristic specific organ injuries that affect the trauma patient's management.

### ANATOMY

The three anatomic regions of the abdomen of concern to the traumatologist are (*a*) the peritoneal cavity, (*b*) the retroperitoneal space, and (*c*) the pelvis.

The peritoneal cavity is further divided into the intrathoracic and abdominal sections. The intrathoracic aobdomen is contained by the rib cage and can rise to the fourth intercostal space when the diaphragm ascends with full expiration. The diaphragm, spleen, stomach, liver, and transverse colon reside in the intrathoracic abdomen. Therefore, penetrating trauma to the lower chest or fractures of the lower ribs

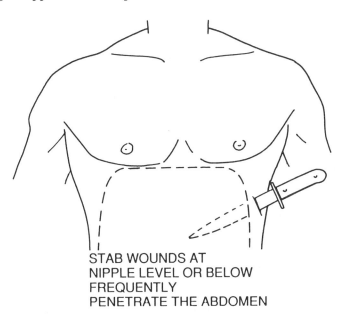

STAB WOUNDS AT
NIPPLE LEVEL OR BELOW
FREQUENTLY
PENETRATE THE ABDOMEN

**Figure 6.16. Stab wounds of the lower rib cage can injure intraabdominal structures.** (From Campbell JE: BTLS: Basic Prehospital Trauma Care. Englewood Cliffs, NJ, Prentice Hall, 1988, p 20.)

may be associated with intraabdominal injuries (Fig. 6.16).

The aorta, vena cava, pancreas, kidneys, ureters, and portions of the colon and duodenum are retroperitoneal structures. Diagnosis of retroperitoneal injuries is difficult but important because life-threatening hemorrhage can occur within this space.

The pelvis contains the rectum, bladder, iliac vessels, and female internal genitalia. The anatomic location of pelvic structures hides them from diagnostic efforts similar to retroperitoneal structures.

### MECHANISMS OF INJURY

Blunt trauma must be distinguished from penetrating trauma because the indications for exploratory celiotomy are different (Table 6.13). Blunt trauma is associated with injuries to solid organs (liver, spleen, and kidneys), which cause significant hemorrhage (3). Improperly applied seat belts will cause rupture of entrapped bowel loops and lumbar spine injuries (152).

Penetrating injuries involve direct effects of the weapon as well as indirect effects of blast injury and temporary cavitation with high-powered gunshot wounds (see Chapter 2). The patterns of injury correspond to the proximity of the abdominal organs to the entrance site and their relative size (3). Common injury patterns involve the liver, small bowel, colon, and stomach. Peritoneal contamination and peritonitis occur commonly with penetrating abdominal injuries.

Wound tracks for bullets may not line up between the entrance and exit wounds in the position the patient assumed when struck. Additionally, the patient's position on the examining table frequently distorts the wound track, making careful exploration mandatory (126).

All penetrating wounds to the lower torso should be explored operatively unless they can be demonstrated to not penetrate the superficial fascia (126).

Significant degrees of bleeding can occur from rupture of solid organs. The abdomen can conceal huge amounts of hemorrhage before becoming distended (Fig. 6.4).

### RETROPERITONEUM

The retroperitoneum contains the abdominal aorta and inferior vena cava as well as the kidneys, ureters, pancreas, and duodenum. Penetrating injuries to the flanks frequently disrupt these organs; blunt trauma may cause injury less often.

#### Major Blood Vessels

Hematoma in the upper central retroperitoneal space should be explored because it is likely to be caused by aortic or vena caval laceration. Blunt trauma usually leads to arterial occlusion from intimal flaps or hemorrhage from venous avulsions. Aortic injuries are explored by mobilizing the mesenteric structures and reflecting them to the right. Arterial injuries are repaired or grafted after proximal and distal control is

---

**Table 6.13.  Management Protocols in Abdominal Injuries**

Penetrating trauma[a]
  Knife (puncture wounds)
    Penetrated abdominal wall, requires exploration
    Peritoneum intact, local exploration only
  Gunshot wounds
    Potential for extensive unpredictable damage should be explored (usually by emergency celiotomy)
Blunt trauma
  Free peritoneal blood—criteria for exploratory celiotomy
    1. Peritoneal lavage—>100,000 RBCs/ml$^3$
    2. CT scan—free air or blood in peritoneal space, retroperitoneal hematoma in cephalad third of abdomen, or expanding hematoma in middle third of abdomen
  Amylase detected in peritoneal lavage—explore
  Elevated WBC count in peritoneal fluid—explore
  Contrast-enhanced CT scan—define injuries to bowel, retroperitoneum—explore

[a] At a certain point, penetrating injuries with sufficient energy begin to exhibit a component of blunt trauma.

achieved. Certain visceral arterial branches of the aorta may be ligated with a very low probability of severe ischemia (126). For example, the common hepatic or left gastric artery can be ligated without causing severe ischemia, but there is a 95% probability of severe ischemia following ligation of the superior mesenteric artery.

Venous injuries are approached by mobilizing and reflecting the intraabdominal organs to the left. Repair of the venous injuries, which hemorrhage as much as arterial injuries, requires initial proximal and distal control by digital pressure (vascular clamps tend to damage the thin-walled veins). Similar to the arterial side, occlusion of some venous branches is tolerated better than others. For example, ligation of the superior mesenteric vein is associated with intestinal edema and a 30% risk of infarction while ligation of the splenic or inferior mesenteric veins is well tolerated.

### Pancreatoduodenal Injuries

Injury to the duodenum and head of the pancreas occurs more frequently from penetrating than blunt trauma. Blunt trauma is associated with injury to the body and tail of the pancreas when the organ is fractured over the vertebral column. Diagnostically pancreatoduodenal injuries are in a silent area. Pancreatic injuries rarely hemorrhage enough to be detected by DPL and contrast enhanced CT may demonstrate duodenal injuries but miss pancreatic injuries. An increased serum amylase concentration is associated with pancreatic injuries. Celiotomy is the most sensitive technique to diagnose pancreatoduodenal injuries. If the mechanism of injury is correct for an injury to the pancreas or duodenum, abdominal examination and amylase determinations should be repeated even if the CT scan is negative. Any suggestion of pancreatic injury should trigger a celiotomy because the injured pancreas is not protected from autodigestion by its own secretions.

Repair of isolated duodenal injuries is feasible, but complex lesions require closure of the pyloris and diversion of the gastric flow through a gastrojejunostomy Roux-en-Y. Injuries to the head of the pancreas and duodenum are treated with Whipple's procedure to resect the gland. The pancreatic duct from the tail of the pancreas and the bilary tree are drained through anastomosis to the jejunum (Roux-en-Y) (126).

### Kidneys/Ureters

The kidneys may be injured directly by penetrating wounds to the retroperitoneum or by blunt trauma which causes avulsion of the renal vascular pedicle or fracture of the parenchyma. Renal injury is diagnosed by the appearance of a nonfilling kidney or dye extravasation during an intravenous pyelogram (IVP). Alternatively an abdominal CT scan will outline an injured kidney or urinary tract.

If a nonpulsatile midabdominal retroperitoneal hematoma is noted at celiotomy and an IVP fails to reveal urine extravasation, the injured kidney should be managed by observation alone. However, an expanding or pulsatile retroperitoneal hematoma demands exploration. Vascular injuries should be repaired if possible. Crush injuries of the parenchyma, confined to an upper or lower pole, may be debrided and the remaining kidney closed. Major crush injuries or total vascular avulsion are best treated with nephrectomy as long as the other kidney is functioning well. If the contralateral kidney does not function properly, efforts should be made to preserve renal function. In the extreme situation, the kidney may be removed and autotransplanted into the iliac fossa.

Injuries to the renal pelvis, ureters, or bladder are repaired. An ureteral stent may be necessary to prevent stricture of the ureter at the repair site. If both ends of a lacerated ureter are not readily available, nephrostomy urinary diversion may be necessary. If the distal ureter is injured, it may be reimplanted into the bladder. Bladder injuries are repaired by primary closure, with bladder drainage via a urinary catheter. Membranous urethral injuries diagnosed by blood at the urethral meatus, a high riding prostate, or extravasation of urine into the scrotum are treated by cystostomy, urinary drainage, and delayed repair 3 to 6 months later. If an injury to the membranous urethra or bladder neck is diagnosed as above or by urethrograms, no attempt should be made to catheterize the urethra. Injuries to the anterior urethra are treated by primary repair. Injuries to the female urethra are very rare.

## INTRAPERITONEAL INJURIES

### Spleen

The spleen, which lies in the intrathoracic abdomen, can be injured by blunt or penetrating trauma to the left lower rib cage. Celiotomy is indicated for suspected or confirmed splenic lacerations. Treatment involves splenorrhaphy to salvage if possible. The decision to salvage the spleen and thus preserve its immunologic function is based on the patient's stability and degree of blood loss. With less than 500 ml of hemorrhage, the spleen is packed off while the abdomen is explored. If no further bleeding occurs, the abdomen is closed. If the spleen continues to hold, it is repaired. Following 500 to 1000 ml of hemorrhage, the spleen is debrided of all devitalized tissue and sutured closed. Following more than 1000 ml of hemorrhage, splenorrhaphy is reserved for isolated splenic injuries. With this amount of hemorrhage, splenectomy is indicated in the unstable multiple injured patient.

### Liver

Celiotomy is indicated to evaluate suspected hepatic injuries as well as those injuries diagnosed by CT scan. Nonbleeding liver injuries in a stable patient with less than 500 ml of hemorrhage are treated by removal of intraperitoneal blood clots and observation. If the liver rebleeds or is bleeding during celiotomy, the Pringle maneuver—digital compression of the portal triad—is used to gain control of hemorrhage while lacerations are sutured closed.

Massive hemorrhage from a liver injury is treated by suturing with the Pringle maneuver used to control hemorrhage. Packing the injury with pressure to tamponade the hemorrhage followed by reoperation (second look) 4 to 48 hours later to evaluate and remove the packs may be successful with large liver lacerations. Continued hemorrhage following the above procedure suggests inferior vena caval or hepatic venous injury. Vascular isolation of the liver by shunting the vena caval flow past the hepatic veins and occluding the portal venous and hepatic arterial inflow with the Pringle maneuver can control hemorrhage to allow identification of the injury site. Hepatic venous injury will require resection of the liver lobe drained by its respective hepatic vein. It has been noted frequently that liver injuries involving the hepatic veins and/or inferior vena cava cause the patient to deteriorate with anesthesia induction. Anesthesia is associated with a loss of abdominal muscle tone and positive pressure ventilation, which elevates the inferior vena caval pressure. Both of these effects of anesthesia induction will increase hemorrhage from hepatic venous injuries.

The bilary tract may be injured by penetrating trauma; blunt injury is rare. Small lacerations are closed with primary repair. Larger or irregular lacerations are treated by anastomosis to the jejunum.

### Stomach, Small Bowel, Colon, Rectum

When hollow organs are injured, usually by penetrating trauma, the peritoneal space can be contaminated by their contents. A seat belt worn over the abdomen may cause perforation of an entrapped loop of bowel during impact (152). Diagnosis is made by identifying free air on an abdominal CT scan, an increased white cell count in peritoneal lavage fluid, signs of peritoneal irritation on repeat physical examination, or exploratory celiotomy. In the very unstable patient, a shunt is required and definitive treatment is performed at a later operation. The stomach may be treated with simple closure similar to resection and closure of small bowel wounds. Colon lesions may be treated either by resection or colostomy and mucous fistula with later closure. The treatment decision depends on the degree of colonic injury and the patient's physical condition. Rectal injuries, usually associated with pelvic fracture or gunshot wounds to the buttocks, are treated by diversion of the stool by colostomy, irrigation of the mucous fistula to clear, and perirectal drains.

## DIAGNOSIS

As many as 20% of patients with significant hemoperitoneum initially present with a normal abdominal examination (3). Diagnosis of intraabdominal injury is based on an index of suspicion aroused by the mechanisms of injury and the patient's cardiovascular stability. Suspected abdominal injuries are confirmed by serial physical examination of the abdomen and hematocrit measurement, diagnostic peritoneal lavage, CT scan with contrast enhancement, and/or exploratory celiotomy (Fig. 6.17).

Observation, repeat physical examination of the abdomen and monitoring of the hematocrit are used to diagnose intraabdominal injuries in the majority of trauma patients. Blunt trauma patients who are cardiovascularly stable and available for repeat abdominal examination are excellent candidates for observation and repeat physical examination. Delayed presentation of peritonitis in these patients who have no other reason for peritoneal signs signifies the need for celiotomy and repair of injuries. Similarly, a progressive decrease in hematocrit and slow change in abdominal examination also are indications for celiotomy (126).

Diagnostic peritoneal lavage (DPL) can be used to screen patients for hemoperitoneum. DPL is especially useful in mass casualty situations where large numbers of patients can be screened rapidly for hemoperitoneum. A positive DPL is an indication for immediate celiotomy. The sensitivity of DPL for hemoperitoneum is 96% and its specificity is 99% compared to celiotomy (153).

If DPL is performed, the lavage fluid is examined for red blood cells (RBC), white blood cells, amylase, bile, and gram stain. Although most centers use an absolute value of greater than 100,000 RBC/mm$^3$ as a positive result, the presence of 50,000,

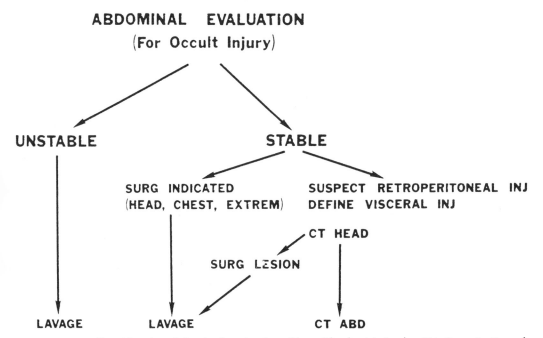

Figure 6.17. Algorithm for abdominal evaluation. (From Rhodes M, Brader AH: Organization of a trauma resuscitation system. Adv Trauma 1989;4:19–41.)

10,000, or even as few as 1,000 RBC/mm$^3$ may be considered an indication for operation depending upon the trauma center and the surgeon's overall evaluation of the situation (i.e., an elevated index of suspicion for a particular case).

Although a DPL can be performed easily, safely, and correctly by either TA/CCSs or emergency medical physicians, they should probably perform this procedure only if patient transfer depends on the results. On one hand, a negative result suggests that the peritoneal cavity has not been contaminated by either blood or bowel contents. False-negative results are possible due to retroperitoneal bleeding or inadequate lavage of the peritoneal cavity. On the other hand, a positive result indicates that a surgical consult is imperative. Unfortunately, DPL alters the examination of the abdomen by introducing both intraabdominal fluid and free intraperitoneal air. Also the DPL can be painful and cause abdominal tenderness. Thus, the consulting surgeon will be forced to accept the reports of the patient's signs and symptoms and DPL results or repeat the DPL because the signs and symptoms of injury will be altered.

An attractive alternative to DPL is a double contrast enhanced CT scan of the abdomen. The CT scan enhanced with 100 ml of intravenous contrast agent and 400 ml of intragastric contrast agent has a good sensitivity for intraabdominal hematoma, solid organ injuries, free intraperitoneal fluid, and free intraperitoneal pain. This procedure does not interfere with the abdominal physical exam and may be repeated frequently (126, 153). Although the CT scan defines the diaphragm poorly, it is superior to the DPL for defining retroperitoneal injury (125, 154). The CT scan is preferable to DPL for patients who have multiple blunt injuries that will preclude frequent examination of the abdomen (e.g., closed head injury, orthopedic injuries requiring prolonged surgery).

Exploratomy celiotomy is indicated for penetrating wounds to the lower rib cage, abdomen, and/or fluids (126, 155). Celiot-

omy allows evaluation of injuries to the diaphragm, solid organs, bowel, and retroperitoneal space. Furthermore, definitive repair of the injuries requires celiotomy. Limited celiotomy incision for exploration of blunt trauma victims has been recommended for patients with serious injuries that have a high probability of causing multiorgan failure (126).

## ANESTHETIC CONCERNS

Anesthetic problems with abdominal trauma include (a) hemorrhage, (b) hypothermia, (c) sepsis, and (d) interference with ventilation. Major hemorrhage is associated with fractures of solid organs, liver, spleen, and kidney as well as vascular injuries and pelvic fractures. The TA/CCS must prepare the patient with at least two large-bore intravenous cannulae prior to draping for surgery. Serious consideration should be given to monitoring unstable patients with abdominal trauma with an intraarterial catheter. The arterial line will allow close monitoring of blood pressure as well as provide a route for sampling blood for blood gases, hematology, and chemistry.

Hypothermia is a frequent complication of abdominal trauma surgery because of both increased heat loss through the open mesentery and reduced heat production as a consequence of shock and anesthesia (see Chapter 13).

## PRIORITIES IN MULTITRAUMA

Blunt trauma that causes transection of the thoracic aortic is often associated with intraabdominal injuries. This raises the therapeutic dilemma of whether to perform angiography, laparotomy, or thoracotomy first (3, 126). Those who stress repair of the aortic injury first point to the high mortality rate among patients with aortic transection who do survive the initial insult, but succumb within the first few hours. However, it is not clear if their deaths are due to aortic rupture and exsanguination or to associated injuries. Therefore, others have concluded that without aortic rupture or large external blood losses, the most likely cause of persistent shock is an intraabdominal injury (126). Successful laparotomies have been performed on patients with traumatic aortic aneurysms without rupture. Recommendations are for performance of angiography in the stable postresuscitation trauma patient followed sequentially by laparotomy and thoracotomy. However, if the trauma patient is unstable, the recommendation is that laparotomy precede the other two procedures. Simultaneous operations on the thoracic and abdominal injuries are possible, but optimal positioning of the patient at surgery is a problem.

## OTHER CONSIDERATIONS

The common major injuries that may prevent an optimal patient response to appropriate resuscitation have been discussed in the preceding two sections. If these injuries are ruled out in the trauma patient who does not respond to resuscitation, the following must be considered.

### Spinal Shock

The trauma patient may have suffered a high spinal cord injury, which has caused maximal vasodilation in the face of a low blood volume. Spinal shock can be differentiated from traumatic shock (see Chapter 4).

### Coincident (Preexisting) Disease

Similar to a myocardial infarction, associated diseases are often responsible for precipitating the traumatic event and complicate resuscitation (11). Adrenal apoplexy is another example. Either the trauma patient had this condition pretraumatically or it resulted from bilateral injury or hemorrhage into the adrenal glands. Adrenal insufficiency, either chronic or acute, will aggravate hemorrhagic shock.

### Effect of Drugs

The trauma patient may be a drug abuser, with one or more illicit substances "on board" at admission. Or a medication may have been given for therapeutic reasons and is interacting with a prescribed medication already in the trauma patient's system. An example is the interaction between meperi-

dine and monoamine oxidase inhibitors (MAOI).

### Effect of Transport

Physiologic stress due to the rigors of transport may interfere with adequate shock resuscitation (see Chapter 15) (156, 157).

## Emergency Thoracotomy

Currently there is a debate between surgeons and nonsurgeons regarding emergency thoracotomy. The debate focuses on who is *allowed* to perform this procedure, not who *can* or *should* perform this procedure, emphasizing the nonmedical facets of this argument. Currently, there are institutional variations in answer to this question, depending on the medical staff organizations. It seems logical that a responsible, licensed physician with special interests and advanced training in traumatology, should be permitted to perform a *life-saving* procedure on *appropriate* patients.

Once the chest has been opened, the aorta has been cross-clamped, open chest cardiac massage has been performed successfully, and the trauma patient stabilized, an additional 30 minutes of time has been "bought" without significant additional morbidity (126). Thus efforts should be directed toward optimizing the selection, training, qualification, and utilization of physicians who can contribute to the care of the *appropriate* trauma patient who would acutely benefit from emergency thoracotomy, instead of wasting time and effort on nonproductive medicopolitical arguments.

Four major points need to be considered before engaging in an emergency thoracotomy. (*a*) Indications for the procedure include control and repair of cardiac wounds with or without tamponade, control and repair of great vessel rupture, internal cardiac compression in hypovolemic arrest (in cases of inadequate closed chest cardiac massage), in air embolism performance of open cardiac massage and cross-clamping of the pulmonary hilum, and cross-clamping of the descending aorta to control distal hemorrhage and maximize cardiocerebral perfusion. (*b*) *Contraindications* to emergency thoracotomy include prolonged cardiac arrest with no electrical activity of the heart and signs of neurologic death. (*c*) The proposed operator must be qualified to perform emergency thoracotomy and the necessary equipment for the procedure must be available. (*d*) The institution must have the equipment and personnel to provide postresuscitative critical care.

The techniques for actually performing emergency thoracotomy can be found elsewhere. Sources include most comprehensive surgical or emergency medicine texts (3).

## ORTHOPAEDIC INJURIES

### Incidence

Although orthopaedic injuries are not immediately life-threatening and are considered in the secondary survey (ATLS) of the trauma patient, they should be of extreme interest to the TA/CCS (60). Orthopaedic injuries occur frequently in blunt trauma patients. High-energy blunt trauma such as motor vehicle accidents cause complex, highly comminuted fractures with extensive overlying soft tissue destruction (158). Urgent surgical repair of these fractures is necessary to reduce long-term disability. Appropriate rehabilitation of the trauma patient with high-energy fractures will require multiple operative procedures. Patients with highly comminuted fractures

will require prolonged surgical repair, as well as multiple procedures to repair the injury. Major hemorrhage associated with fractures will require massive intraoperative fluid resuscitation, although rapid exsanguination from major fractures is unlikely. Finally, orthopaedic trauma is associated with far-reaching systemic physiologic derangements such as shock, fat emboli, thromboemboli, and hypoxic respiratory failure (e.g., ARDS) (1, 158, 159).

Therefore, the TA/CCS will be anesthetizing patients for orthopaedic procedures more frequently than for any other operative procedures. This involvement and appropriate intervention will affect long-term morbidity and mortality.

The MIEMSS Shock Trauma Center experience has been that approximately 50% of trauma patients require the services of an orthopaedic surgeon for initial resuscitative surgery. Further, the majority of follow-up cases are orthopaedic surgery. Many of the patients with Grade III open fractures of the tibia (Table 6.14) (i.e., with extensive soft tissue loss, see below) require multiple operations over 1 to 2 years. One MIEMSS Shock Trauma Center patient was anesthetized more than 20 times for serial procedures.

Consistent patterns of fractures occur with different injury patterns (Fig. 6.18). Penetrating trauma from high-velocity missiles causes massive bone destruction if the bullet strikes a limb. Low-velocity bullets

**Table 6.14.   Fracture Description**

Location—diaphyseal, metaphyseal, juxta articular, or intraarticular
Closed/open—skin condition: any laceration over fracture site is considered an open fracture
  a. grade I, wound <1 cm long
  b. grade II, wound <5 cm long without contamination or crush
  c. grade III, large laceration with associated crushing and contamination (includes traumatic amputation)
Comminution—has many pieces
  a. simple fracture, 2 pieces
  b. comminuted fracture <2 pieces
Displacement—length, alignment or angulation
   a. reference point of distal in relation to proximal fragments
  rotation
  opposition of fragments
Neurovascular status
  distal pulses
  neurologic function

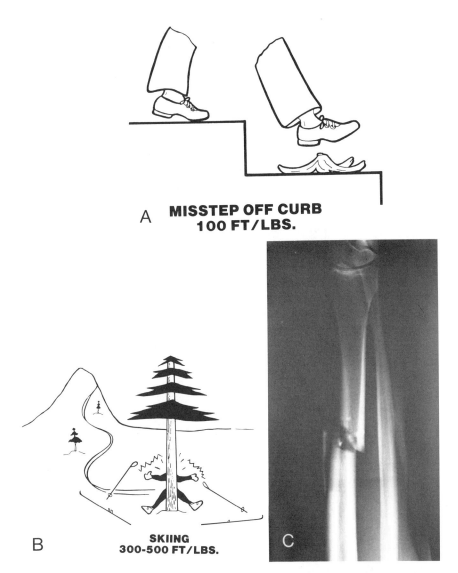

**Figure 6.18.  Approximate energy associated with four mechanisms of fracture.** The greater the energy transfer, the more extensive the bone and soft tissue destruction. **A,** Misstep off curb leads to simple ankle fracture. **B,** Ski injury. **C,** X-ray illustrates typical ski injury, a moderate energy fracture. Note fractured tibia with minimal comminution; the fibular remains intact. **D,** Gunshot. **E,** X-ray shows fractures of femur caused by low-velocity handgun, typical of inner city violence as opposed to military (high-velocity) wounds. Note bullet fragments and minimal displacement. **F,** High-energy bumper injury. **G,** X-ray shows periarticular long-bone fracture surrounding the knee. Note severe comminution and significant displacement. These wounds are often accompanied by significant soft tissue destruction. (Cartoons and x-rays courtesy of Andrew Burgess, M.D. Director of Orthopaedic Surgery, MIEMSS.)

cause less extensive bone destruction but will fracture bones that are crossed by the permanent cavity. Blunt trauma from low-energy falls—skiing, falls at home, or sports injuries—causes relatively simple fractures. High-energy blunt trauma—falls from a great height, pedestrian struck by an automobile, or high-speed motor vehicle injuries—causes complex, highly comminuted fractures with extensive soft tissue loss.

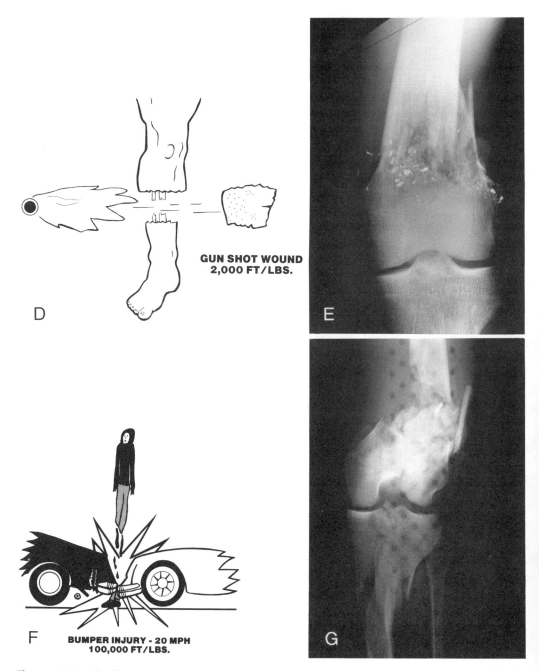

**Figure 6.18.  D–G.**

## Associated Injuries

Fractures, especially high-energy fractures, are associated with a number of interesting clinical problems: (*a*) neurovascular injuries, (*b*) shock, (*c*) compartment syndrome, and (*d*) fat emboli (1, 159). The TA/CCS will work in concert with the orthopaedic specialist to address these problems, as well as provide the proper perioperative conditions for surgical repair of these fractures. The presence of one or more of these problems will affect the type of resuscitative care and of anesthetic care required by these patients.

Associated secondary neuromuscular trauma results from the edges of a fractured bone being driven into nerves and blood vessels in proximity to the fracture site (160). Pelvic fractures are notorious for mechanically damaging nerves and blood vessels that exit via the pelvis to the perineum and lower extremities (158, 159). This displacement of pelvic fragments, which disrupts nerves, arteries, and veins, can cause major hemorrhage into the retroperitoneal space (161). Continued hemorrhage from constant movement of these unstable fragments will shear away hemostatic elements that have formed in these ruptured blood vessels. This is a major cause of mortality and morbidity from pelvic fractures. Prompt stabilization of the unstable pelvic elements will minimize this risk and also is the best method to control massive hemorrhage from this injury. Early emergent placement of an external fixator (Hoffman device) is frequently the only appropriate technique to stabilize firmly an inherently unstable fracture of the pelvic ring (158, 162). Stabilization of the fragments of a pelvic fracture will allow angiographic embolization of arterial bleeding to proceed more successfully than if the fracture is allowed to remain mobile.

Similarly, the neurovascular bundle that crosses an unstable joint injury is also likely to be injured with a fracture of the bones that support the joint (163–165) (Table 6.15). The vascular injuries range from complete obstruction with distal ischemia to vascular wall damage that leads to late aneurysm formation. Brachial plexus injuries with upper extremity trauma and popliteal artery injuries after fractures around the knee are frequent examples of such neurovascular injuries (166). Long-term morbidity requiring difficult rehabilitation is caused by these types of peripheral nerve injuries. Severe trauma may cause permanent loss of nerve function and thus may lead to amputation of the extremity. A working prosthetic limb is considered to be more functional than a native limb without nerve function (165).

Increased pressure in the myofascial compartments is a third cause of neurovascular injury in a traumatized limb (159, 161). The tissue pressure in these compartments is normally lower than both capillary and venous intravascular pressure and can rise high enough to prevent microcirculatory blood flow after injury. Edema or hematoma formation that increases the volume contained within the relatively noncompliant fascial compartment causes the pressure to rise quickly as soon as the volume limit of the compartment is exceeded ("closed box" phenomenon). Edema formation may be secondary to direct tissue damage or to ischemic increases in microvascular permeability. Pain is the most frequent symptom associated with increased compartment pressure (158). During the secondary survey (ATLS) of the trauma patient with fractures, the peripheral pulses and the sensory and motor nerve function must be evaluated in all extremities (3). Decreased pulses distal to fracture sites should be a warning of either vascular injury or compartment syndrome. Although full neurologic evaluation is rarely possible in the severely traumatized limb,

**Table 6.15.   Vascular Injuries Associated with Fractures**[a]

| Bone Injury | Artery Involved |
| --- | --- |
| Fractures and dislocations around the shoulder and clavicle | Axillary artery |
| Supracondylar fractures: humerus | Brachial artery |
| Supracondylar fractures: femur | Popliteal artery |
| Pelvic fractures | Iliac artery |
| Femoral shaft fractures | Femoral artery |
| Knee dislocation | Popliteal artery |
| Proximal tibial fractures | Posterior tibial artery |
| Fracture of the forefoot | Dorsalis pedis artery |

[a] From Gurd AR: The repair of bone and fracture healing. In Odling-Smee W, Crockard A (eds): Trauma Care. London, Academic Press, 1981, pp 339–377.

the presence of sensation and motor activity distal to a fracture site suggests that peripheral nerve damage, if any, is not complete. Compartment pressures should be measured in all closed myofascial compartments in the vicinity of a fracture (158). Compartment pressures should also be measured in nonfractured limbs eliciting complaints of extreme pain or in which the mechanism of injury suggests prolonged ischemia ("crush injury"). The most reliable diagnostic method is to measure the compartment pressure with a properly placed needle connected to a fluid-filled transducer (i.e., "wick pressure"). If increased compartment pressure is not relieved by a fasciotomy, severe muscle necrosis or peripheral nerve damage can be caused by elevated compartment pressures resulting in severe postinjury disability.

Significant fractures are associated with major hemorrhage from rupture of intraosseous blood vessels and laceration of blood vessels close to the fracture (159, 160).

Frequently, large volumes of blood are collected in a perifracture hematoma without major changes in the external dimensions of the limb (120). Although hemorrhage from a fracture accumulates relatively slowly, the patient can eventually lose enough blood to cause shock and death (see Chapter 4) if not given adequate intravenous therapy (Fig. 6.19). Traumatic hypovolemic shock is a major complication of fractures, especially long bone fractures. The TA/CCS must be aware of the potential hidden blood loss associated with various fractures and must closely monitor and replace ongoing intraoperative blood loss (covered in detail in Chapter 4). Table 6.16 outlines expected hemorrhagic volumes from different fracture sites.

Fractures disturb oxygenation to some degree in most patients with orthopaedic trauma (159, 161, 167). Fractures of the long bones of the lower extremities lead to a severe impairment of oxygenation that has been called "fat embolism" (168–171). Frac-

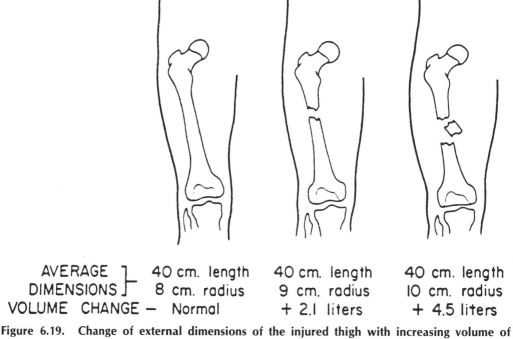

AVERAGE     40 cm. length     40 cm. length     40 cm. length
DIMENSIONS   8 cm. radius      9 cm. radius     10 cm. radius
VOLUME CHANGE — Normal         + 2.1 liters      + 4.5 liters

Figure 6.19.   Change of external dimensions of the injured thigh with increasing volume of hematoma. (From Trunkey DD, Sheldon GF, Collins JA: The treatment of shock. In Zuidema GD, Rutherford RB, Ballinger WF (eds): The Management of Trauma. Philadelphia, WB Saunders, 1985, pp 105–125.)

**Table 6.16.  Hemorrhagic Volumes from Various Fracture Sites**[a]

Potential blood loss from closed fractures
Expect up to 500 ml blood loss from:
  Forearm fractures of radius and/or ulna
Expect up to 750 ml blood loss from:
  Elbow fracture
  Tibial fracture
  Ankle fracture
Expect up to 1000 ml blood loss from:
  Humerus fracture
  Femoral shaft fracture
Expect up to 1250 ml blood loss from: Hip fracture
Expect greater than 1500 ml blood loss from pelvic
  fracture

[a] Adapted from Shumaile GM: Extremity trauma. In Baxt WG (ed): Trauma: The First Hour. East Norwalk, CT, Appleton-Century-Crofts, 1985, pp 221–237.

tures of long bones release fragments of various types of bone tissue into the venous circulation. Many of these mobilized products are fat globules from the marrow compartment. Because all venous blood flow eventually collects in the pulmonary circulation, the pulmonary capillary bed traps much of the fracture-derived debris. Ultimately, respiratory gas exchange is impaired by the presence of fracture debris in the pulmonary capillary bed. In severe cases, pulmonary damages associated with fractures are similar to ARDS (see Chapter 4) and may be followed by a systemic response, termed the fat emboli syndrome, consisting of respiratory failure, focal neurologic defects, and widespread petechiae (167–169). Prevention of the fat emboli syndrome requires early fracture fixation to prevent ongoing showers of marrow fragments into the circulation, in combination with aggressive respiratory critical care, which includes intubation and mechanical ventilation with large tidal volumes to prevent pulmonary atelectasis and venous admixture (1, 158, 159, 161, 169, 171, 172).

Arterial blood gases should be evaluated for adequacy of oxygenation in all patients with musculoskeletal trauma. Oxygenation defects can be diagnosed by comparing the arterial oxygen partial pressure ($PaO_2$) to the alveolar oxygen partial pressure ($PAO_2$) (173) (see also Chapter 3). The ratio of the

two oxygen partial pressures ($PaO_2/PAO_2$) is not influenced by carbon dioxide partial pressure ($PaCO_2$) or inspired oxygen fraction ($FIO_2$). However, the $FIO_2$ must be known for calculatation of $PAO_2$. It is impossible to define the $FIO_2$ precisely if the patient is wearing an oxygen mask. Thus, blood gases should be evaluated while the spontaneously breathing patient, with a natural airway, is breathing room air. However, the $FIO_2$ can be measured precisely for a patient with an artificial airway (i.e., endotracheal tube, tracheostomy tube). Endotracheal intubation and mechanical ventilation should be initiated immediately on all patients demonstrating impaired oxygenation—$PaO_2/PAO_2 < 0.6$. In patients who require a pulmonary artery catheter for hemodynamic monitoring, mixed venous blood gases should be measured, as should ABGs. Pulmonary shunt fraction ($Qs/Qt$) can be monitored directly in the patient with a pulmonary artery catheter. Indices of oxygenation such as $(Pa/PA)O_2$ should be followed when a pulmonary artery catheter is not available (1).

## Anesthetic Management

Orthopaedic injuries may be difficult anesthetic challenges to the TA/CCS because many of these patients require prolonged operation for complex fracture reconstruction. The proposed length of the operation will often determine the use of general and/or regional anesthesia.

Regional anesthesia has the advantages of limiting the anesthesia effects to the location of the operation and minimizing the systemic effects of anesthesia (55, 174). Patients can also remain awake and alert with full command of their faculties during operation under regional anesthesia. More specifically, the trauma patient with a mild head injury can be questioned continuously to follow trends in the effects of the head trauma. Similarly, the patient can be queried to evaluate symptoms of occult injuries. Furthermore, the trauma patient with a full stomach can maintain control of protective airway reflexes during regional anesthesia. Postoperative analgesia is another advantage of regional anesthesia if performed with a continuous catheter technique. Because of these considerations, regional anesthesia is used for patients with isolated limb injuries (who have been properly resuscitated) or for prolonged posttraumatic analgesia in the ICU.

Intravenous regional anesthesia is advocated by some authors as ideal for simple fractures of the forearm, wrist, or hand (175–179). Also, intravenous regional anesthesia does not produce prolonged analgesia; therefore, it is not indicated if prolonged operation is contemplated or prolonged postoperative analgesia is needed. The rapid onset of analgesia and the simple equipment needed are definite advantages of intravenous regional anesthesia for emergency room use for reducing closed fractures.

The disadvantages of regional anesthesia become most apparent in the multitrauma patient (2, 58). Patients with multiple injuries tend not to tolerate long periods of enforced stillness on the operating table during the repair of complex fractures. General anesthesia with endotracheal intubation to protect the airway is safer for these trauma patients than sedation alone. In addition, many patients with multiple injuries and/or shock will require endotracheal intubation and mechanical ventilation as a vital component of their medical management (1, 56, 158, 159, 161) (see Chapters 3 and 4). Positive-pressure ventilation reduces the pulmonary damage associated with long bone fractures—fat emboli (1, 159, 161, 169–171, 180). These patients should be monitored as described above for efficacy of pulmonary oxygen exchange. Extubation should be delayed until the patient demonstrates adequate oxygen exchange.

Because the ideal time to fix open fractures operatively is within the first few hours after injury, all patients brought to the operating room for emergency surgical repair of fractures must be considered to have "full stomachs" and are anesthetized using techniques aimed at minimizing the risk of aspiration (181). It is impractical to wait for the stomach to empty so that mask anesthesia may be used. Gastric emptying time is quite variable, especially after trauma (see Chapter 3). The priorities of providing timely fracture fixation to reduce infectious complications and malalignment and instituting mechanical ventilation to improve oxygen exchange must take precedence over theoretic concerns about stomach contents. The incidence of significant gastric acid aspiration is relatively small (182). A smooth, well-conducted anesthetic induction with properly applied cricoid pressure will further reduce the risk of aspiration pneumonia to much less than the risk of fracture complications that may arise from prolonged delays in definitively treating the fracture.

Hypoxic respiratory failure is extremely common after long bone fractures (1, 159, 161, 168, 183). All patients with major fractures, especially of the lower extremities and pelvis, should receive frequent monitoring of ABGs. Endotracheal intubation and mechanical ventilation with large tidal volumes are recommended to treat fracture-induced hypoxia and prevent further lung damage (1, 159, 161, 164, 180, 183, 184).

Operative reduction and fixation of complex, highly comminuted fractures and multiple fractures frequently results in very long procedures. However, the benefits of aggressively correcting all injuries are great enough to outweigh the risks of prolonged operation.

Very little is written concerning the effects of long operation on a patient's outcome. The improvement in respiratory management in the critical care unit as a result of immobilizing fractures as opposed to immobilizing the patient is considerable (1, 158, 159, 161, 181). Fat embolism syndrome notwithstanding, the immobilized patient is also at risk for hypostatic pneumonia, deep venous thrombosis, and pulmonary embolism. Immobilization of the fracture will allow the patient to be moved frequently in bed. The mortality rate from femur fractures is significantly reduced by early operative fixation instead of balanced skeletal traction (181).

Thus, the task of providing optimal intraoperative care must be expertly undertaken. The TA/CCS must carefully monitor and maintain the patient by providing a true critical care environment in the OR. Frequent measurement of ABGs and respiratory minute volume will allow the TA/CCS to adjust the ventilator to the patient's requirements. Fluid administration must be carefully titrated to the patient's needs. Serum electrolytes should be analyzed frequently enough to guide administration of appropriate replacements. Similarly, blood replacement must be guided by assessment of losses and hemoglobin and hematocrit levels. The coagulation status also must be monitored frequently by asking the surgeon about abnormal bleeding in the surgical field and measuring prothrombin times, activated partial thromboplastin times, and platelet counts (see Chapter 5). The patient's temperature should be controlled by warming all fluids, humidifying inspired gases, and maintaining a euthermic operating temperature (see Chapter 13).

Surgery should not be discontinued before all fracture sites are repaired on unfounded theoretic grounds such as "the patient has had too much surgery." The decision to postpone surgery before all multiple injuries are repaired should be based on objective signs of physiologic instability. Refractory hypothermia or refractory shock are indicators that the patient should be transferred to the critical care unit as soon as all life-threatening injuries have been treated.

## SUMMARY

In this chapter the reader has been exposed to the multitude of issues that arise in the perioperative anesthetic management of the trauma patient. These include philosophical, basic scientific, and clinical issues. One of the philosophical issues is the role of the anesthesiologist in trauma management. When considering mechanisms of injuries,

one bridges the gap between philosophical and basic scientific issues. Other basic science subjects necessary for optimal care of the trauma patient include pharmacology of anesthetic drugs in the shock model and purely technical issues such as monitoring techniques. Clinical science issues include preoperative, intraoperative, and postoperative anesthetics performed in the context of organ system injuries. The organ system injuries discussed in this chapter included thoracoabdominal and orthopaedic injuries. An understanding of thoracoabdominal injuries is crucial for the trauma anesthesiologist to perform optimally because these injuries are often immediately life-threatening. Orthopaedic injuries often provide the largest volume of cases for a trauma operating room but also may be limb-threatening if not treated appropriately. In addition, because of subtle, far-reaching implications that are only beginning to be understood, orthopaedic injuries may actually be life-threatening in terms of long-term recovery.

## References

1. Bone L, Bucholz R. The management of fractures in the patient with multiple trauma. J Bone Joint Surg (Am) 1986;68A:945–949.
2. Stene JK. Anesthesia for the critically ill trauma patient. In Siegel JH (ed): Trauma: Emergency Surgery and Critical Care. New York, Churchill Livingstone, 1987, pp 843–862.
3. American College of Surgeons, Committee on Trauma: The Advanced Trauma Life Support Program. Instructors Manual. Chicago, American College of Surgeons, 1989.
4. American College of Surgeons, Committee on Trauma: Resources for Optimal Care of the Injured Patient. Chicago, American College of Surgeons, 1990.
5. Grande CM, Stene JK, Barton CR. The trauma anesthesiologist. Md Med J 1988;37:531–536.
6. Committee on Trauma Research. Injury in America: A Continuing Public Health Problem. Washington, DC, National Academy Press, 1985.
7. Fackler ML. Physics of missile injuries. In McSwain NE Jr, Kerstein MD (eds): Evaluation and Management of Trauma. East Norwalk, CT, Appleton-Century-Crofts, 1987, pp 25–41.
8. McSwain NE Jr. Mechanisms of injuries in blunt

trauma. In McSwain NE Jr, Kerstein MD (eds): Evaluation and Management of Trauma. East Norwalk, CT, Appleton-Century-Crofts, 1987, pp 1–24.

9. Hardy JF. Large volume gastroesophageal reflex: a rationale for risk reduction in the perioperative period. Can J Anaesth 1988;35:162–173.

10. Grande CM, Tissot M, Bhatt V, et al. Preexisting compromising conditions. In Capan LM, Miller S, Turndorf H (eds): Trauma: Anesthesia and Intensive Care. Philadelphia, JB Lippincott (in press).

11. Morris JA, MacKenzie EJ, Edelstein SL. The effect of preexisting conditions on mortality in trauma patients. JAMA 1990;263:1942–1946.

12. Rembert FC. State of health at time of injury. In Giesecke AH Jr (ed): Anesthesia for the Surgery of Trauma. Philadelphia, FA Davis, 1976, pp 17–24.

13. Britt BA. Malignant hyperthermia. Can Anaesth Soc J 1985;32:666–677.

14. Caldwell TB III. Anesthesia for patients with behavioral and environmental disorders. In Katz J, Benumof J, Kadis LB (eds): Anesthesia and Uncommon Diseases, ed 2. Philadelphia, WB Saunders, 1981, pp 672–777.

15. Whetsell LA, Patterson CM, Young DH, Schiller WR. Preinjury psychopathology in trauma patients. J Trauma 1989;29:1158–1162.

16. Soderstrom CA, DuPriest RW Jr, Benner C, Maekawa K, Cowley RA. Alcohol and roadway trauma: problems of diagnosis and management. Am Surg 1979;45:129–136.

17. Marzuk PM, Tardiff K, Leon AC, Stajic M, Morgan EB, Mann JJ. Prevalence of recent cocaine use among motor vehicle fatalities in New York city. JAMA 1990;263:250–256.

18. McIntyre JWR. The difficult tracheal intubation. Can J Anaesth 1987;34:204–213.

19. Trunkey DD, Siegel J, Baker SP, Gennarelli TA. Panel: current status of trauma severity indices. J Trauma 1983;23:185–201.

20. Koch JP, McClelland BA, Wortzman D, Berton SG, Szalai JP. Is the ASA physical status classification adequate in predicting mortality in blunt trauma? Anesthesiology 1987;67:A482.

21. Safar P, Bircher NG. Cardiopulmonary Cerebral Resuscitation, ed 3. London, WB Saunders, 1988.

22. House of Delegates. Standards for Basic Intraoperative Monitoring. Chicago, American Society of Anesthesiologists, Directory of Members, 1988, p 590.

23. Baskett PJF. The trauma anesthesia/critical care specialist in the field. Crit Care Clin 1990; 6:13–24.

24. Donchin Y, Wiener M, Grande CM, Cotev S. Military medicine: trauma anesthesia and critical care on the battlefield. Crit Care Clin 1990; 6:185–202.

25. Grande CM, Baskett PJF, Donchin Y, Bernhard WN. Trauma anesthesia for disasters: anything, anywhere, anytime. Crit Care Clin (in press).

26. Finnie KJC, Watts DG, Armstrong PW. Biases in the measurement of arterial pressure. Crit Care Med 1984;12:965–968.

27. Yelderman M, New NJ. Evaluation of pulse oximetry. Anesthesiology 1983;59:349–352.

28. Anonymous. Pulse oximeters. Health Devices 1989;18:185–230.

29. Severinghaus JW, Naifeh KH. Accuracy of response of six pulse oximeters to profound hypoxia. Anesthesiology 1987;67:551–558.

30. Gravensteon JS, Paulus DA, Hayes TS. Capnography in Clinical Practice. Boston, Butterworths, 1989.

31. Goldberg JS, Rawle PR, Zehnder JL, Sladen RN. Colorimetric end-tidal carbon dioxide monitoring for tracheal intubation. Anesth Analg 1990; 70:191–194.

32. Anonymous. Apnea monitoring by impedence pneumography. Health Devices 1987;16:80–81.

33. Imrie MM, Hall GM. Body temperature and anaesthesia. Br J Anaesth 1990;64:346–354.

34. Urbanowicz JH, Shaaban MJ, Cohen NH, Cahalan MK, Bolvinick EH, Chatterjee K, Schiller NB, Dae MW, Matthay MA. Comparison of transesophageal echocardiographic and scintigraphic estimates of left ventricular end-diastolic volume index and ejection fraction in patients following coronary artery bypass grafting. Anesthesiology 1990;72:607–612.

35. Spinale FG, Smith AC, Crawford FA. Relationship of bioimpedence to thermodilution and echocardiographic measurements of cardiac function. Crit Care Med 1990;18:414–418.

36. Huch R, Lubbers DW, Huch LA. The transcutaneous measurement of oxygen and carbon dioxide tensions for the determination of arterial blood-gas values with control of local perfusion and peripheral perfusion pressure. In Payne JP, Hill DW (eds): Oxygen Measurements in Biology and Medicine. London, Butterworths, 1975, pp 121–137.

37. Niclou R, Teague SM, Lee R. Clinical evaluation of a diameter sensing Doppler cardiac output meter. Crit Care Med 1990;18:428–432.

38. Wong DH, Mahutte CK. Two-beam pulsed Doppler cardiac output measurement: reproducibility and agreement with thermodilution. Crit Care Med 1990;18:433–437.

39. Wong DH, Tremper KK, Stemmer EA, O'Connor D, Wilbur S, Zaccari J, Reeves C, Weidoff P, Trujillo RJ. Noninvasive cardiac output: simultaneous comparison of two different methods with thermodilution. Anesthesiology 1990;72:784–792.

40. Clements FM, Harpole DH, Quill T, Jones RH, McCann RL. Estimation of left ventricular volume and ejection fraction by two-dimensional transoesophageal echocardiography: compari-

son of short axis imaging and simultaneous radionuclide angiography. Br J Anaesth 1990; 64:331–336.

41. Ali HH, Miller RD. Monitoring of neuromuscular function. In Miller RD (ed): Anesthesia, ed 2. New York, Churchill Livingstone, 1986, pp 871–887.

42. Sharpe MD, Lam AM, Nicholas JF, Chung DC, Merchant R, Alyafi W, Beauchamp R. Correlation between integrated evoked EMG and respiratory function following atracurium administration in unanaesthetized humans. Can J Anaesth 1990;37:307–312.

43. Sramek BB. The impact on diagnosis and therapy of computerized integration, processing and display of noninvasive hemodynamic and cardiodynamic parameters. Intensive Care World 1989;6:205–210.

44. Stene JK, Long JF. Hemodynamic monitoring with use of a bedside computer terminal. CVP 1982;10(1):66–71.

45. Soderstrom CA, Wasserman DH, Dunham CM, Caplan ES, Cowley RA. Superiority of the femoral artery for monitoring: a prospective study. Am J Surg 1982;144:309–312.

46. Michelson JD, Lotke PA, Steinberg ME. Urinary-bladder management after total joint-replacement surgery. N Engl J Med 1988;319:321–326.

47. Anonymous. EEG monitors. Health Devices 1986;15:71–95.

48. Grundy BL. Intraoperative monitoring of sensory-evoked potentials. Anesthesiology 1983; 58:72–87.

49. Judson J, Cant BR, Shaw NA. Early prediction of outcomes from cerebral trauma by somatosensory evoked potentials. Crit Care Med 1990; 18:363–368.

50. York D, Legan M, Benner S, Watts C. Further studies with a noninvasive method of intracranial pressure estimation. Neurosurgery 1984;14: 456–461.

51. McLaughlin JS, Suddhimondala C, Mech K Jr, Llacer RL, Houston J, Blide R, Attar S, Cowley RA. Pulmonary gas exchange in shock in humans. Ann Surg 1969;169:42–56.

52. Sprung CL. The Pulmonary Artery Catheter: Methodology and Clinical Applications. Baltimore, University Park Press, 1983.

53. Rao TLK, Jacobs HK, El-Etr AA. Reinfarction following anesthesia in patients with myocardial infarction. Anesthesiology 1983;59:499–505.

54. Siegel JH, Vary TC. Sepsis, abnormal metabolic control, and the multiple organ failure syndrome. In Siegel JH (ed): Trauma: Emergency Surgery and Critical Care. New York, Churchill Livingstone, 1987, pp 411–501.

55. Desai SM, Bernhard WN, McAlary B. Regional anesthesia: management considerations in the trauma patient. Crit Care Clin 1990;6:85–101.

56. Peters RM. Fluid resuscitation and oxygen exchange in hypovolemia. In Siegel JH (ed): Trauma: Emergency Surgery and Critical Care. New York, Churchill Livingstone, 1987, pp 157–179.

57. Brown DL. Anesthetic agents in trauma surgery: are there differences? Int Anesthesiol Clin 1987; 25(1):75–90.

58. Stene JK, Grande CM. General anesthesia: management considerations in the trauma patient. Crit Care Clin 1990;6:73–84.

59. Graves CL. Management of general anesthesia during hemorrhage. Int Anesthesiol Clin 1974; 12(1):1–49.

60. Nicholls BJ, Cullen BF. Anesthesia for trauma. J Clin Anesth 1988;1:115–129.

61. Clarke RSJ, Carson IW. Anaesthesia for trauma and shock. In Nunn JF, Utting JE, Brown BR (eds): General Anaesthesia, ed 5. London, Butterworths, 1989, pp 686–695.

62. Smith DP, Fabian LW, Carnes MA. Comparative evaluation of Fluothane & cyclopropane anesthesia during hemorrhagic hypovolemia: changing concepts in the management of anesthesia. Anesth Analg 1961;40:137–147.

63. Theye RA, Perry LB, Brzica SM Jr. Influence of anesthetic agent response to hemorrhagic hypotension. Anesthesiology 1974;40:32–40.

64. Longnecker DE, Sturggill BC. Influence of anesthetic agent on survival following hemorrhage. Anesthesiology 1976;45:516–521.

65. Bavister PH, Longnecker DE. Influence of anaesthetic agents on the survival of rats following acute ischemia of the bowel. Br J Anaesth 1979;51:921–925.

66. Weiskopf RB, Townsley MI, Riordan KK, Chadwick K, Baysinger M, Mahoney E. Comparison of cardiopulmonary responses to graded hemorrhage during enflurane, halothane, isoflurane, and ketamine anesthesia. Anesth Analg 1981; 60:481–491.

67. Weiskopf RB, Bogetz MS, Roizen MF, Reid IA. Cardiovascular and metabolic sequelae of inducing anesthesia with ketamine or thiopental in hypovolemic swine. Anesthesiology 1984;60: 214–219.

68. Bogetz MS, Weiskopf RB. Cardiovascular effects of the volatile anesthetics during hypovolemia. Anesthesiology 1984;61:A51.

69. Shibata K, Yamamoto Y, Murakami S. Effects of epidural anesthesia on cardiovascular response and survival in experimental hemorrhagic shock in dogs. Anesthesiology 1989;71:953–959.

70. Jowitt MD, Knight RJ. Anaesthesia during the Falklands campaign. Anaesthesia 1983;38: 776–783.

71. Lenz G, Stehle R. Anesthesia under field conditions: a review of 945 cases. Acta Anaesthesiol Scand 1984;28:351–356.

72. McGown RG. A technique of anaesthesia in

haemorrhagic shock. Anaesthesia 1975;30:616–623.

73. Halford FJ. A critique of intravenous anesthesia in war surgery. Anesthesiology 1943;4:67–69.

74. Anonymous. The question of intravenous anesthesia in war surgery. Anesthesiology 1943;4:74–77.

75. Kuznetsova Olu, Marusanov VE, Biderman FM, Danilevich Ela. Anesteziia ketalarom na dogospital 'nom etape u postradavshikh s tiazheloi travmoi i tramaticheskim shokom. (Ketalar anesthesia in the first-aid stage with the victims of severe injury and traumatic shock.) Vestnik Khirurgii Imeni I Grekova 1984;132(7):88–91. (Vestn-Khir)

76. Chasapakis G, Kekis N, Sakkalis C, Kolios D. Use of ketamine and pancuronium for patients in hemorrhagic shock. Anesth Analg 1973; 52:282–287.

77. Christian CM, Naraghi M, Adriani J. Adverse effects of pancuronium in patients with hemorrhagic shock. South Med J 1979;72:1113–1115.

78. Kaukinen S. Effects of antihypertensive medication on the cardiovascular response to ketamine in rats. Acta Anaesthesiol Scand 1978; 22:437–446.

79. Haljamäe H. Lactate metabolism. Intensive Care World 1987;4:118–120.

80. Kruse JA. Blood lactate and oxygen transport. Intensive Care World 1987;4:120–125.

81. Bersin RM, Arieff AI. Recent advances in therapy of lactic acidosis. Intensive Care World 1987; 4:128–133.

82. Fragen RJ, Avram MJ. Comparative pharmacology of drugs used for the induction of anesthesia. In Stoelting RK, Barash PG, Gallagher TJ (eds): Advances in Anesthesia, vol 3. Chicago, Year Book, 1986, pp 103–132.

83. Adams RC, Gray HK. Intravenous anesthesia with pentothal sodium in the case of gunshot wound associated with severe traumatic shock and loss of blood: report of a case. Anesthesiology 1943;4:70–73.

84. Yamamura T, Harada K, Okamura A, Kemmotsu O. Is the site of action of ketamine anesthesia the n-methyl-d-aspartate receptor? Anesthesiology 1990;72:704–710.

85. Lacoumenta S, Walsh ES, Waterman AE, Ward I, Paterson JL, Hall GM. Effects of ketamine anaesthesia on the metabolic response to pelvic surgery. Br J Anaesth 1984;56:493–497.

86. White PF, Way WL, Travor AJ. Ketamine: its pharmacology and therapeutic uses. Anesthesiology 1982;56:119–136.

87. Corssen G, Reves JG, Stanley TH. Intravenous Anesthesia and Analgesia. Philadelphia, Lea & Febiger, 1988, pp 99–173.

88. Klase R, Hartung HJ, Kotsch R, Walz T. Experimentalle Untersuchungen zur intracaniellen Drucksteigerung durch ketamine beim hamorrhagischen Shock. Anaesthesist 1982;31:33–38.

89. Hedenstierna G. Gas exchange during anaesthesia. Br J Anaesth 1990;64:507–514.

90. Dundee JW, Wyant GM. Intravenous Anaesthesia. Edinburgh, Churchill Livingstone, 1988.

91. Berry JM, Merin RG. Etomidate myoclonus and the open globe. Anesth Analg 1989;69:256–259.

92. Booij LHDJ, Crul JF. The comparative influence of gamma-hydroxy butyric acid, Althesin and etomidate on the neuromuscular blocking potency of pancuronium in man. Acta Anesthesiol Belg 1979;30:219–223.

93. Lister RG. The amnesic action of benzodiazepines in man. Neurosci Biobehav Rev 1985; 9:87–94.

94. Ghoneim MM, Mewaldt SP. Benzodiazepines and human memory: a review. Anesthesiology 1990;72:926–938.

95. Bogetz MS, Katz JA. Recall of surgery for major trauma. Anesthesiology 1984;61:6–9.

96. Sebel PS, Lowdon JD. Propofol: a new intravenous anesthetic. Anesthesiology 1989;71:260–277.

97. Leeuwen LV, Zwirmond WWA, Deen L, Helmes HJHJ. Total intravenous anesthesia with propofol, alfentanil and oxygen-air: three different dosage schemes. Can J Anaesth 1990;37:282–286.

98. Eger EI II, Saidman LJ, Brandstater B. Minimum alveolar anesthetic concentration: a standard of anesthetic potency. Anesthesiology 1965;26: 756–763.

99. Wood M, Wood AJJ. Drugs and Anesthesia: Pharmacology for Anesthesiologists, ed 2. Baltimore, Williams & Wilkins, 1990.

100. Mangano DT. Perioperative cardiac morbidity. Anesthesiology 1990;72:153–184.

101. Nagano K, Gelman S, Parks DA, Bradley EL. Hepatic oxygen-supply-uptake relationship and metabolism during anesthesia in miniature pigs. Anesthesiology 1990;72:902–910.

102. Russell GB, Snider MT, Richard RB, Loomis JL. Hyperbaric nitrous oxide as a sole anesthetic agent in humans. Anesth Analg 1990;70: 289–295.

103. Eisele JH. Cardiovascular effects of nitrous oxide. In Eger EI II (ed): Nitrous Oxide/N₂O. New York, Elsevier, 1985, pp 125–156.

104. Frost EAM. Central nervous system effects of nitrous oxide. In Eger EI II (ed): Nitrous Oxide/N₂O. New York, Elsevier, 1985, pp 157–176.

105. Nunn JF, Chanarin I. Nitrous oxide inactivates methionine synthetase. In Eger EI II (ed): Nitrous Oxide/N₂O. New York, Elsevier, 1985, pp 211–233.

106. Libonati MM, Leahy JJ, Ellison N. The use of succinylcholine in open eye surgery. Anesthesiology 1985;62:637–640.

107. Gronert GA, Theye RA. Pathophysiology of

hyperkalemia induced by succinycholine. Anesthesiology 1975;43:89–99.

108. Lennon RL, Olson RA, Gronert GA. Atracurium or vecuronium for rapid sequence endotracheal intubation. Anesthesiology 1986;64:510–513.

109. Hunt LB, Guril NJ, Reynolds DG. Dose-dependent effects of nalbuphine in canine hemorrhagic shock. Circ Shock 1984;13:307–318.

110. McGruder MR, Cristofforette R, Difazio CA. Balanced anesthesia with nalbuphine hydrochloride. Anesthesiol Rev 1980;7:25–29.

111. Anjow-Lindskog E, Broman L, Broman M, Holmgren A, Settergren G, Öhqvist G. Effects of intravenous anesthesia on VA/Q̇ distributions. Anesthesiology 1985;62:485–492.

112. Wilkinson GR. Pharmacokinetics in disease states modifying body perfusion. In Benet LZ (ed): The Effects of Disease States on Drug Pharmacokinetics. Washington, DC, American Pharmaceutical Association, 1976, pp 13–32.

113. Hug CC Jr. Pharmacokinetics of drugs administered intravenously. Anesth Analg 1978;57:704–723.

114. Eger EI II. Anesthesia Uptake and Action. Baltimore, Williams & Wilkins, 1974.

115. Caplan RA, Posner KL, Ward RJ, Cheney FW. Adverse respiratory events in anesthesia: a closed claims analysis. Anesthesiology 1990;72:828–833.

116. Craven KD, Oppenheimer L, Wood LDH. Effects of contusion and flail chest on pulmonary perfusion and oxygen exchange. J Appl Physiol 1979;47:729–737.

117. Gens DR. Cervical soft tissue injuries. In Cowley RA, Conn A, Dunham CM (eds): Trauma Care, Volume 1, Surgical Management. Philadelphia, JB Lippincott, 1987, pp 88–105.

118. Roon AJ, Christensen N. Evaluation and treatment of penetrating cervical injuries. J Trauma 1979;19:391–397.

119. Wilson RF, Gibson DB, Antonenko D. Shock and acute respiratory failure after chest trauma. J Trauma 1977;17:697–705.

120. Trunkey DD, Sheldon GF, Collins JA. The treatment of shock. In Zuidema GD, Rutherford RB, Ballinger WF (eds): The Management of Trauma, ed 4. Philadelphia, WB Saunders, 1985, pp 105–125.

121. Hood RM. Techniques in General Thoracic Surgery. Philadelphia, WB Saunders, 1985, p 172.

122. Symbas PN. Cardiothoracic Trauma. Philadelphia, WB Saunders, 1989, pp 3–15.

123. Casson WR. Delayed cardiac tamponade. Anaesthesia 1985;40:48–50.

124. Stanley TH, Weidauer HE. Anesthesia for the patient with cardiac tamponade. Anesth Analg 1973;52:110–114.

125. Lake CL. Anesthesia and pericardiac disease. Anesth Analg 1983;62:431–443.

126. Holcroft JW, Blaisdell FW. Trauma to the torso. In Wilmore DW, Brennan MF, Harken AH, Holcroft JW, Meakins JL (eds): American College of Surgeons: Care of the Surgical Patient. New York, Scientific American, 1989, sect IV, ch 1, pp 1–56.

127. McSwain NE Jr. Pulmonary chest trauma. In Moylan JA (ed): Trauma Surgery. Philadelphia, JB Lippincott, 1988, pp 77–122.

128. Koster JK, Saunders JH Jr. Thoracic injuries. In May HL (ed): Emergency Medicine. New York, John Wiley & Sons, 1984, pp 365–377.

129. Harman PK, Trinkle JK. Penetrating cardiac trauma. In Hurst JM (ed): Common Problems in Trauma. Chicago, Year Book, 1987, pp 160–168.

130. Newman RJ, Jones IS. A prospective study of 413 consecutive car occupants with chest injuries. J Trauma 1984;24:129–135.

131. Hilgenberg AD. Trauma to the heart and great vessels. In Burke JF, Boyd RJ, McCabe CJ (eds): Trauma Management: Early Management of Visceral, Nervous System, and Musculoskeletal Injuries. Chicago, Year Book, 1988, pp 153–175.

132. Symbas PN. Trauma to the great vessels. In Symbas PN (ed): Cardiothoracic Trauma. Philadelphia, WB Saunders, 1989, pp 160–231.

133. Cohn PF, Braunwald E. Traumatic heart disease. In Braunwald E (ed): Heart Disease: A Textbook of Cardiovascular Medicine, ed 2. Philadelphia, WB Saunders, 1984, pp 1528–1539.

134. Lewis FR. Thoracic trauma. Surg Clin North Am 1982;62:97–104.

135. Graham JM, Beall AC Jr, Mattox KL, Vaughn GD. Systemic air embolism following penetrating trauma to the lungs. Chest 1977;72:449–454.

136. Richardson JD, McElvein RB, Trinkle JK. First rib fracture: a hallmark of severe trauma. Ann Surg 1975;181:251–254.

137. Besson A, Seageesser F. Color Atlas of Chest Trauma and Associated Injuries. Oradell, NJ, Medical Economics Books, 1983, pp 153–198.

138. Worthly LIG. Thoracic epidural in the management of chest trauma. Intensive Care Med 1985;11:312–315.

139. Jones KW. Thoracic trauma. Surg Clin North Am 1980;60:957–981.

140. Kwa BH. Experiences in the management of chest injuries and a review of current management. Ann Acad Med Singapore 1983;12:474–478.

141. Graziotta PJ, Smith GB. Multiple rib fractures and head injury: an indication for intercostal catheterization and infusion of local anesthetics. Anaesthesia 1988;43:964–966.

142. Reiestad F, Stromskag KE, Holmqvist E. Intrapleural administration of bupivicaine in postoperative management of pain. Anesthesiology 1986;65:A204.

143. Avery EE, Morch ET, Benson DW. Critically crushed chests: a new method of treatment with

continuous mechanical hyperventilation to produce alkalotic apnea and internal pneumatic stabilization. J Thorac Surg 1956;32:291–311.

144. Robinson JS. Respiratory care after injury. Injury 1978;10:46–48.

145. Mulder DS, Shennib H, Angood P. Thoracic injuries. In Maull KI, Cleveland HC, Strauch GO, Wolferth CC (eds): Advances in Trauma. Chicago, Year Book, 1986, vol 1, pp 193–216.

146. Rehm CG, Sherman R, Hinz TW. The role of CT scan in evaluation for laparotomy in patients with stab wounds of the abdomen. J Trauma 1989;29:446–450.

147. Getz BS, Davies E, Steinberg SM, Beaver BL, Koenig FA. Blunt cardiac trauma resulting in right atrial rupture. JAMA 1986;255:761–763.

148. Doty DB, Anderson AE, Rose EF, Go RT, Chiu CL, Ehrenhaft JL. Cardiac trauma: clinical and experimental correlations of myocardial contusion. Ann Surg 1974;180:452–460.

149. Sutherland GR, Calvin JE, Driedger AA, Holliday RL, Sibbold WJ. Anatomic and cardiopulmonary responses to trauma with associated blunt chest injury. J Trauma 1981;21:1–12.

150. Saunders CR, Doty DB. Myocardial contusion. Surg Gynecol Obstet 1977;144:595–603.

151. Brantigan CO, Burdick D, Hopeman AR, Eiseman B. Evaluation of technetium scanning for myocardial contusion. J Trauma 1978;18:460–463.

152. Williams JS, Lies BA Jr, Hale HW. The automotive safety belt: in saving a life may produce intra-abdominal injuries. J Trauma 1966;6:303–315.

153. Meyer DM, Thal ER, Weigelt JA, Redman HC. Evaluation of computed tomography and diagnostic peritoneal lavage in blunt abdominal trauma. J Trauma 1989;29:1168–1172.

154. Hauters P, de Canniere, Michell A. Pneumoperitoine diagnostique uniquement au CT scan. Acta Chir Belg 1989;89:325–328.

155. Buck GC III, Dalton ML, Neely WA. Diagnostic laparotomy for abdominal trauma: a university hospital experience. Am Surg 1986;52:41–43.

156. Gentleman D, Jennett B. Audit of transfer of unconscious head-injured patients to a neurosurgical unit. Lancet 1990;335:330–334.

157. Andrews PJD, Piper IR, Dearden NM, Miller JD. Secondary insults during intrahospital transport of head-injured patients. Lancet 1990;335:327–334.

158. Burgess AR, Brumback RJ. Early fracture stabilization. In Cowley RA, Conn A, Dunham CM (eds): Trauma Care, Volume 1, Surgical Management. Philadelphia, JB Lippincott, 1987, pp 182–203.

159. Bolhofer BR, Spiegel PG. Prevention of medical complications in orthopedic trauma. Clin Orthop 1987;222:105–113.

160. Coleman SS. Early care of the patient with multiple fractures. Am J Surg 1959;97:43–48.

161. Burgess AR, Mandlebaum BR. Acute orthopedic injuries. In Siegel JH (ed): Trauma: Emergency Surgery & Critical Care. New York, Churchill Livingstone, 1987, pp 1049–1074.

162. Rubash HE, Mears DC. External fixation of the pelvis. Instr Course Lect 1983;32:329–348.

163. Arnold WD. Principles of fracture management. In Shires GT (ed): Principles of Trauma Care, ed 3. New York, McGraw-Hill, 1985, pp 370–384.

164. Briggs SE, Seligson D. Management of extremity trauma. In Richardson JD, Polk HC, Flint LM (eds): Trauma: Clinical Care and Pathophysiology. Chicago, Year Book Medical Publishers, 1987, pp 535–562.

165. Alden PA, Shaw WW. The evolution of the surgical management of severe lower extremity trauma. Clin Plast Surg 1986;13:549–569.

166. Berg E, Kimbrough EE. Trauma to the pelvis and the extremities. In McSwain NE Jr, Kerstein MD (eds): Evaluation and Management of Trauma. East Norwalk, CT, Appleton-Century-Crofts, 1987, pp 167–193.

167. Sheikh MA. Respiratory changes after fractures and surgical skeletal injury. Injury 1982;13:489–494.

168. Collins JA. The causes of progressive pulmonary insufficiency in surgical patients. J Surg Res 1969;9:685–704.

169. Gossling HR, Pellegrini VD. Fat embolism syndrome. Clin Orthop 1982;165:68–78.

170. Riska EB, Myllynen P. Fat embolism in patients with multiple injuries. J Trauma 1982;22:891–894.

171. Lavarde G. L'embolic graisseuse post-traumatique: a propos de 272 cas francais. J Chir (Paris) 1975;109:221–252.

172. Riska EB, vonBonsdorff H, Hakkinen S, Jaroma H, Kiviluoto O, Paavilainen T. Prevention of fat embolism by early internal fixation of fractures in patients with multiple injuries. Injury 1977;8:110–116.

173. Gilbert R, Keighley JF. The arterial alveolar oxygen tension ratio, an index of gas exchange applicable to varying inspired oxygen concentrations. Am Rev Respir Dis 1974;109:142–145.

175. Zauder HL. Intravenous regional anesthesia. In Zauder HL (ed): Anesthesia for Orthopaedic Surgery. Philadelphia, FA Davis, 1980, pp 119–125.

176. Goodwin DRA, Rubenstein N, Otremski I. Intravenous anaesthesia in the upper limb: a review of 225 cases. Int-Orthop 1984;8:51–54.

177. Turner RL, Batten JB, Hjorth D, Ross RS, Eyres RL, Cole WG. Intravenous regional anaesthesia for the treatment of upper limb injuries in childhood. Aust NZ J Surg 1986;56:153–155.

178. Olney BW, Lugg PC, Turner PL, Eyres RL, Eyres RL, Cole WG. Outpatient treatment of upper

extremity injuries in childhood using intravenous regional anaesthesia. J Pediatr Orthop 1958; 8:576–579.

179. Maletis GB, Watson RC, Scott S. Compartment syndrome: a complication of intravenous regional anesthesia in the reduction of lower leg shaft fractures. Orthopedics 1989;12:841–846.

180. Holmstrom FMG. Respiratory support in the orthopaedic patient. In Zauder HL (ed): Anesthesia for Orthopaedic Surgery. Philadelphia, FA Davis, 1980, pp 181–197.

181. Keever JE, Rockwood CA Jr. Early mobilization of the severely injured patient. In Zauder HL (ed): Anesthesia for Orthopedic Surgery. Philadelphia, FA Davis, 1980, pp 21–28.

182. Olsson GL, Hallen B, Hambraes-Jonzon K. Aspiration during anaesthesia: a computer-aided study of 185, 358 anaesthetics. Acta Anaesthesiol Scand 1986;30:84–92.

183. Modig J. Posttraumatic pulmonary insufficiency caused by the microembolism syndrome. Acta Chir Scand 1980;Suppl. 499:57–65.

184. Modig J, Busch C, Olerud S, Saldeen T. Pulmonary microembolism during intramedullary orthopaedic trauma. Acta Anaesth Scand 1974; 18:133–143.

# Perioperative Anesthetic Management of Central Nervous System Trauma

*Elizabeth A. M. Frost*

Central nervous system (CNS) trauma is not only a major medical emergency but also a serious socioeconomic problem because of the generally young age of the victims. The trauma anesthesiologist, as part of the "trauma team," is important in providing initial resuscitation, stabilization during neurodiagnostic testing, and selection of appropriate anesthetic management and intensive care.

## HEAD INJURY

Head injury constitutes a dynamic process and has a variable course, depending both on the initial injury and on secondary brain damage. The initial brain damage resulting from the impact is not amenable to treatment. Therefore, the goals of management are to prevent secondary brain damage resulting from the development of intracranial or extracranial complications and to provide the brain with the optimal physiologic environment to maximize the potential for recovery.

After the initial injury, subsequent neurologic deterioration and systemic complications leading to a poor outcome or death should be preventable (1). This is exemplified in a group of patients known to have talked before dying from head injury (2). The most common extracranial causes of death were hypoxia and shock and the most frequent intracranial complications were misdiagnosis or delays in diagnosis of intracranial hematomas due usually to transfer of the patient from the initial hospital to the tertiary care center.

### Emergency Care

The anesthesiologist contributes to the emergency care of the head-injured victim in several areas: establishment and maintenance of the airway, normalization of cardiovascular status, and control of intracranial pressure (ICP) (3, 4).

#### RESPIRATORY CARE

That an ischemic injury can be aggravated by hypoxia has been shown in a fluid percussion model (5). Seventy per cent of rats sustained a deficit or died in the presence of hypoxia, whereas only 20% had injury if normoxia persisted. Therefore, the emergency room management should be directed toward establishing an optimal level of cerebral oxygenation and perfusion and a prompt recognition of intracranial hematomas (6).

The oxygen requirement of the injured brain is higher than that of the normal brain. Borderline hypoxia tolerated by healthy cerebral tissue can produce hypoxic insult after acute injury. Respiratory abnormalities occur almost immediately after severe head injury (7). Blood gas values obtained at the scene of the accident and on admission to the hospital after craniocerebral trauma indicate that hypercapnia correlates with the severity of head injury (8). Glasgow coma scores below 9 have been associated with arterial $CO_2$ tension ($PaCO_2$) levels over 50 mm Hg. Also, patients who have sustained a prehospital hypoxic event have significantly poorer outcomes (9).

Transient respiratory arrest at the time of injury is not uncommon and may cause diffuse microatelectasis and hypercarbia. Time to intubation is critical. In a study of almost 2000 patients over a 28-month period, the adjusted mortality rate was 22.5% in those intubated within 1 hour of injury and 38.4% if intubation was delayed for more than 1 hour ($P < 0.01$) (10).

Indications for ventilatory assistance include oxygen saturation (as measured by pulse oximetry) below 94%, arterial oxygen partial pressure ($PaO_2$) of less than 70 mm Hg on room air, $PaCO_2$ above 45 mm Hg, respiratory rate below 10 or above 30, and any abnormality of respiratory patterns.

How the airway is secured is very important. Attempting to intubate the trachea of an otherwise healthy, young, muscular, semicomatose male may precipitate extreme struggling and enormous rises in ICP, with risk of tentorial herniation. The preferred technique is to perform intubation after supplemental oxygen administration (hyperventilation if possible) and the intravenous administration of thiopental and/or lidocaine and a short-acting muscle relaxant (see also Chapter 3). Cricoid pressure should

be used. Diazepam and midazolam have long half-lives and, at the doses required to allow atraumatic intubation, may significantly interfere with neurologic examination for hours. Nasal intubation is not indicated because of the risk of hemorrhage and contamination if the patient has a basal skull fracture. These principles also apply if a cervical injury is suspected or has not been ruled out. Before intubation, which must be done as atraumatically as possible, the cervical vertebrae should be distracted by applying manual in-line axial traction or by simply pulling on the hair and stabilizing the neck in as neutral a position as possible. It is not advisable to administer muscle relaxants or benzodiazepine derivatives before stabilization of the neck because the unstable bony fragments may be maintained in their position only by muscular spasm. Cervical fractures are rare, however, especially in young children, as compared with the frequent occurrence of hypoxia in patients with head injury (11). Therefore, the need for establishing an airway should take precedence over the concern for potential cervical instability. If the operator is skilled in fiberoptic techniques and there is no blood in the mouth, oral intubation by this method is recommended. Again, nasotracheal instrumentation is not recommended (12).

## CARDIOVASCULAR SUPPORT

Hypotension in adults after head trauma usually indicates other injuries (e.g., ruptured spleen or liver) because intracranial hematomas do not become large enough to cause hypovolemic shock. Thus, sustained hypotension after severe head injury is usually due to brainstem failure and is a terminal event (13). In infants, however, intracranial hemorrhage, especially if it is due to subgaleal hemorrhage, may be sufficient to cause hypovolemia.

High spinal cord injury concomitant with head injury may also cause shock due to loss of sympathetic innervation. Elevating the legs, using antishock trousers (MAST suit), or administering atropine are the therapies of choice.

By far the commonest cardiovascular response to head injury is hypertension and tachycardia, due primarily to the combination of activation of the autonomic nervous system and hypoxia (14). Heart rates over 120 beats/min have been reported in over 45% and systolic blood pressures over 160 mm Hg in 25% of head-injured patients admitted to a hospital (15).

Autoregulation is no longer homogeneous after cerebral injury (16). At both ends of the autoregulatory curve, penumbral areas are very sensitive to hypotension. Hypotension increases cerebral blood flow (CBF), especially in the parietal cortex, which may worsen edema (17). All attempts should be made to maintain normal cerebral perfusion pressure (CPP = mean arterial blood pressure − ICP).

β-Blockade has been effective in improving CPP. Propranolol may be infused at a rate of 1 mg/15 min until the systolic blood pressure is less than 160 mm Hg and the diastolic pressure is below 90 mm Hg (15). Comparison between propranolol and tetratolol to control the hyperdynamic state of head injury has indicated that the latter drug preserves renal perfusion better (17). Sodium nitroprusside and hydralazine all increase CBF by a cerebral vasodilatory action and should not be used in the head-injured patient before the skull is opened (18, 19).

Many electrocardiographic (ECG) abnormalities have been described after head injury, again usually due to increased sympathetic tone. The most common include tachycardia, prolonged Q–$T_c$ interval, large U waves, and T and ST wave changes (20). Peaked P waves, long P–R intervals, prolonged Q–$T_c$ intervals, and U waves indicate a poor prognosis (21). Although major ventricular extrasystoles and heart blocks are rare, fatal dysrhythmias have been reported in young patients with no preexisting heart disease (22). Therapy includes correction of hypoxia and excess vagal tone, sympathetic pharmacologic blockade as in-

dicated, and reduction of intracranial hypertension.

## INTRACRANIAL PRESSURE

ICP refers to cerebrospinal pressure within the cranial cavity. Biomechanically, the intracranial vault consists of three compartments: the brain (84%), the cerebrospinal fluid (CSF) (12%), and blood (4%). An increase in one results in a decrease in the others, as stated by the Monro-Kellie doctrine, to maintain stable ICP. Normal ICP ranges between 5 and 15 mm Hg. Greater than 40 mm Hg is considered severely increased ICP. The adult CSF volume is 150 ml; it is replaced three times daily (18 ml/hour) and is not affected by variations in ICP. Elevations in ICP result from changes in CSF absorption and cerebral circulation and from intracranial abnormalities. The deleterious effect of increased ICP is based on the reduction in perfusion pressure and CBF below the critical level (60 mm Hg), resulting in brain ischemia. Once a critical compensatory point is reached, rapid elevation in ICP occurs with minimal provocation (Fig. 7.1).

Using a ventricular cannula, one can ascertain intracranial dynamics by calculation of the pressure-volume index (PVI). The PVI is defined as the volume (milliliters) necessary to raise the CSF pressure by a factor of 10, as shown in the following formula (23).

$$PVI = \frac{V}{\log_{10}\frac{P_p}{P_0}}$$

where $V$ is volume injected into the lateral ventricle, $P_0$ is initial ICP, and $P_p$ is peak ICP.

Clinically, the PVI is derived by adding or withdrawing fluid from the ventricular system and noting pressure changes. Calculation of this number allows approximation of the pressure-volume curve to a straight line. A high number indicates good compliance, whereas a low number suggests a "tight" compartment.

Several methods to measure ICP are

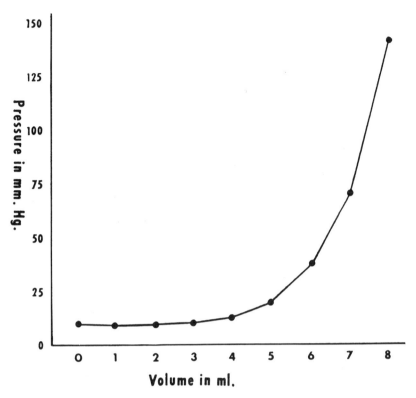

**Figure 7.1.   Pressure/volume compliance curve.**

currently available (Table 7.1). Measurement of ICP by ventriculostomy, although an old technique, remains the most reliable method for ICP assessment. Cerebral compliance, CSF production rate, and outflow resistance can be determined, in addition to permitting rapid reduction in ICP by CSF extraction when indicated. Alternatives to ventriculostomy, when cannulation of ventricles proves difficult, include epidural and subdural ICP monitoring techniques. Although the risk of infection or bleeding may be less with these alternatives, correlation with ventricular pressures can be spurious and extraction of CSF is not possible. Epidural pressure sensor implantation directly on the dura mater yields higher values than actual ICPs, and maintenance of meticulous calibration is problematic. Subdural bolt pressure monitoring, although lacking correlation, can be used to estimate intracranial compliance. Frequent clogging and inaccessibility for CSF drainage are other disadvantages of subdural pressure monitoring. High-resolution computed axial tomographic (CT) scanning provides a static but accurate indication of ICPs. If CT scanning reveals a marked shift of the

**Table 7.1   Methods of Measuring ICP**

| Method | Advantages | Disadvantages |
|---|---|---|
| Subarachnoid | Simple | Cannot drain CSF<br>Compliance measurement difficult |
| Intraventricular catheter | CSF drainage possible<br>Compliance measurements more<br>   accurate | Difficult if edema present |
| Implanted epidural transducer | Infection unlikely<br>Simple | Cannot drain CSF<br>Calibration more difficult to maintain |
| CT scan | Simple, noninvasive | One-time measurement only |

ventricles, then subdural monitoring is preferred.

Increased ICP may be treated by pharmacologic means (barbiturates, diuretics), by decreasing $PaCO_2$ (hyperventilation), or mechanically (releasing hematoma, drainage of CSF, head-up position) (Table 7.2).

Although "brain edema" and "brain swelling" are terms that are often used interchangeably to indicate a cause for raised ICP, these terms can be more precisely applied to two distinct and temporal processes that occur after head injury. The pathophysiologic distinction between cerebral edema and swelling after head injury has led to a logical approach to their management. Brain swelling is defined as an increase in the cerebral blood volume. It is postulated to result from cerebral vasoparalysis with resulting hyperemia and may last several hours to several days. Prolonged hyperemia of the brain may lead to vasogenic edema and possibly to increased ICP with brain herniation. The CT scan characteristic of cerebral hyperemia shows slightly increased brain density and compressed ventricles. This increased density can be enhanced further by use of intravenous contrast infusion. Appropriate therapy includes hyperventilation or other means to increase vasoconstriction (e.g., barbiturates)

Brain edema, on the other hand, is defined as increased water content of the extravascular spaces of the brain. The white matter density of edematous brain is less than that of normal brain on CT scanning. Water content, which can be quantitatively determined by tissue density, is higher in edematous than in normal brain. Diuretic

**Table 7.2.   Reduction of Intracranial Hypertension**[a]

| Pharmacologic Reduction | Mechanical Reduction |
| --- | --- |
| Diuretics | Release of hematoma |
| Barbiturates | Drainage of CSF |
| | Craniectomy |
| | Hyperventilation |
| | Head-up position |

[a] Maintenance of adequate CPP is essential in head-injured patients.

therapy is indicated. Brain edema, usually focal or unilateral, does not develop shortly after trauma, while hyperemia occurs early.

Although steroids continue to be used in many neurosurgical centers, the use of high-dose dexamethasone in 130 patients with severe head injury showed no advantageous effect on clinical outcome. Moreover, a study of the effects of steroid administration in children indicated a detrimental effect by potentiation of posttraumatic catabolic response and increased protein breakdown (24).

Both mannitol and furosemide decrease ICP. Although a bolus of mannitol may initially aggravate intracranial hypertension, the time of elevation of ICP is short and there are apparently no ill effects (25, 26). Nevertheless, in infants or in elderly patients with cardiac disease, the hyperosmolar effect of mannitol may precipitate cardiac failure.

Mannitol has also been shown to decrease blood viscosity, thus increasing oxygen delivery to the brain and causing reflex vasoconstriction (27). Furosemide lowers ICP and brain water content alone and in combination with mannitol. It does not seem to increase ICP or blood volume and may be advantageous in patients with cardiac or renal disease (28, 29). Less disturbance of electrolyte balance is recorded (28). In large doses, furosemide reduces CSF formation and may reduce water and ion penetration across the blood-brain barrier (29). Furosemide prolongs the effectiveness of mannitol (30). Reductions in ICP are greater in duration by combination of the two agents. Administration of mannitol, 0.5 g/kg, followed after 15 minutes by furosemide, 0.5 mg/kg, is most effective in causing prompt and adequate brain shrinkage. However, fluid and electrolyte losses are consistently increased. The peak loss of sodium is increased five times. Water excretion of up to 42 ml/min has been reported with the use of both drugs, as compared to 17 ml/min with mannitol alone (31). Moreover, the duration of diuresis is prolonged.

A complication of diuretic therapy is

hyponatremia, which has also been associated with increased ICP, altered mental status, and pulmonary edema (32). Close monitoring and appropriate correction of electrolyte balance are indicated. The danger of rapid sodium replacement in increasing neurologic abnormalities has been emphasized (33). Correction of hyponatremia must be slower than 0.55 mmol/liter/hr to avoid further complications.

Both thiopental and propofol reduce ICP. However, CPP is reduced more by propofol, which has marked cardiovascular effects (34). Its use in the patient with severe head injury, while still being investigated, is probably limited.

In the most acute phase after injury, adult comatose patients have a reduced cerebral metabolic rate of oxygen consumption ($CMRO_2$). However, CBF is not as predictable and may be increased, decreased, or normal. A concomitant reduction of CBF when the $CMRO_2$ is decreased reflects preservation of metabolic flow matching. Conversely, normal or increased CBF in the face of decreased $CMRO_2$ reflects a relative or absolute cerebral hypermia and a degree of metabolism flow mismatch.

The feasibility of monitoring arteriovenous oxygen saturation differences across the brain as an indicator of critical cerebral oxygen delivery, CBF, and therapy of intracranial hypertension has been studied (35, 36). Hyperventilation may be titrated against oxygen content differences ($AJDO_2$) by measuring systemic arterial oxygen content and jugular venous bulb (JVB) oxygen content and equating this value to the relationship between metabolism and flow:

$$AJDO_2 = CMRO_2/CBF$$

If normal arterial oxygen saturation and hemoglobin concentration exist, JVB oxygen tension may be used alone. Mechanical passive hyperventilation should be adjusted to levels of JVB oxygen tension of 28 to 30 mm Hg. Also $AJDO_2$ less than 10 indicates that CBF is probably adequate and that intracranial hypertension can be treated by hyperventilation, as is commonly the case in children. Increased oxygen extraction indicates reduced flow, and diuretic therapy is indicated. This situation is more frequently encountered in adults after blunt trauma.

$AJDO_2$ has also been used as a bedside monitor to detect changes in cerebral oxygen delivery. Brief periods of arterial desaturation perhaps related to sporadic increases in ICP are common during the first 72 hours after head injury and respond to increased oxygen delivery.

The best position in which to nurse head-injured patients has been disputed. The controversy is partly resolved by taking account of both mean arterial blood pressure (MABP) and ICP. Increasing head-up tilt in 10° increments from the horizontal results in a progressive fall in CPP because any benefit from the associated fall in ICP is offset by a greater fall in MABP (37). Consideration of the combined effect of MABP and ICP is important because controlling the ICP is of limited value if the MABP is ignored.

Both intracranial hypertension and hypoxia are worsened by status epilepticus, a serious complication that occurs in approximately 7% of posttraumatic patients. Midazolam at an infusion of 7 to 12 mg/hr after a loading dose of 10 mg provides effective control (38). Rapid attenuation of $\alpha$-rhythm occurs. Advantages of midazolam over other benzodiazepines include water solubility, shorter half-life, and lower incidence of cardiorespiratory depression.

## NEURODIAGNOSTIC TESTING

Although not strictly part of immediate resuscitation, the anesthesiologist is called frequently to assist in the diagnostic evaluation of the head-injured patient. Increased ICP, hypoxia, and hypercapnia cause patients to become restless, agitated, or belligerent, often making these studies difficult or the results equivocal. Cooperation is especially difficult to obtain from young children. Patients should be sedated only after the cause of the restlessness has been established and appropriate therapy initiated. Administration of narcotics or barbiturates to a hypoxic patient breathing spontaneously may convert a life-threatening situation to one that is fatal. If there is any doubt as to the adequacy of the airway in restless patients, they must be managed with a general endotracheal anesthetic technique for the duration of the study. Reduction of $PaCO_2$ levels may, by decreasing CBF, allow better angiographic studies. Introduction of CT scanning has greatly facilitated neuroradiologic diagnosis. Although the technique is essentially noninvasive, the patient must be kept motionless for the duration of the study. A recent review emphasized that general endotracheal anesthesia is not only acceptable for the head-injured patient, but also may constitute essential management (39). Magnetic resonance imaging is of particular value in assessing spinal injuries. In restless, hypoxic patients with head injury requiring sedation and ventilation, the need to provide non-ferrous containing apparatus may speak against its use. Although anesthetic machines have been designed for use in magnetic resonance units, they are not yet generally available.

## Anesthetic Management

Only about 20% of head-injured patients have lesions amenable to surgical intervention. In the operative management of head-injured victims, the key aims are establishment and maintenance of an impeccable airway, cardiovascular stability, and optimal intracranial dynamics.

### CHOICE OF ANESTHETIC AGENTS

Controversy continues over what constitutes the preferred anesthetic technique in head-injured victims. Routine administration of preoperative medication is not indicated. Pain is rarely a major complaint and therefore the use of narcotics, which depress respiration, is not justified. Barbiturates and tranquilizers obscure changing neurologic status, and tachycardia caused by belladonna alkaloids may mask excessive blood loss. Phenytoin is the initial drug of choice for seizure control as it causes less

sedation. Side effects (hypotension, cardiac dysrhythmias, and CNS depression) are minimized if the drug is given at an intravenous rate no faster than 50 mg/min.

A primate study compared the cerebral protective effects of isoflurane and barbiturates during focal ischemia and found better neurologic outcome with thiopental (40). When the study was repeated, no difference in outcome was found between the two groups when variables were minimized.

In other studies the safety of isoflurane in maintaining autoregulation at 1.4% end-tidal concentration has been demonstrated (41). Autoregulation is lost at 2.8% end-tidal concentration. An interesting study in a rat model indicated that isoflurane alone improves neurologic outcome compared with nitrous oxide alone (42). However, the addition of nitrous oxide to the inhalation agent did not worsen outcome. In a review of outcome of head-injured patients in our institution, we found significantly better outcome in less severely injured patients when inhalation agents were used. As the pathology of head injury is often one of decreased flow, maintenance of excess flow in relation to metabolic demands may provide better conditions for recovery (i.e., the uncoupling of flow and metabolism provided by isoflurane). Administration of nitrous oxide alone (i.e., 70% with muscle relaxation) yielded uniformly poor results (43). With injuries characterized by diffuse vasodilation (immediately after gunshot wounds and in small children), outcome was slightly better after barbiturate anesthesia. Moreover, the addition of nitrous oxide decreases the amount of inspired oxygen and increases the chances of tension situations developing if pneumothorax or pneumocephalus exist.

Other studies have shown that, although satisfactory control of otherwise refractory intracranial hypertension may be achieved in 25% of patients by barbiturate infusion, outcome is not improved (44). Moreover, considerable patient variability exists in clearance of pentobarbital after head injury and daily monitoring of barbiturate levels is indicated (45).

Succinylcholine is often incorporated in rapid sequence intubation. At least one case of hyperkalemia has been reported after the use of this muscle relaxant given to a nonparetic, comatose patient (46). Other studies have suggested that succinylcholine increases ICP by central and peripheral actions. Whether or not this is the case, the availability of other agents suggests that succinylcholine should not be used in patients with cerebral damage. Vecuronium, while generally effective, may be required in very high doses in patients who have been maintained on antiseizure medications such as phenytoin or phenobarbital for extended periods because of rapid breakdown by microenzymes induced in the liver (47). The breakdown product of atracurium, laudanosine, has been implicated as a seizure-provoking agent in animals, but the dose of atracurium necessary to produce such toxic levels is greatly in excess of that required in neurosurgical procedures (48). Also, if the dose of atracurium is limited to 0.5 mg/kg, problems with histamine-induced hypotension are more theoretical than actual. Until an ultra-short-acting, nondepolarizing agent becomes available, either atracurium or vecuronium can be used to aid intubation in the head-injured victim.

## MONITORING

Appropriate intraoperative monitoring includes continuous electrocardiography with the capability of strip recording and temperature recording. Pulse oximetry and capnography are invaluable, and mass spectrometry of infrared analyses is highly desirable. Arterial cannulation is essential to provide a port for frequent blood gas and serum electrolyte analyses and continuous systemic arterial blood pressure monitoring. Trend recordings with availability of a final hard copy of all parameters provide indications of continued adequate cerebral perfusion during the administration of anesthesia.

Urinary output and fluid balance must be monitored both to balance the enormous fluid shifts caused by blood loss and diuresis and as an early warning of the development of diabetes insipidus.

If the operation is performed with the patient in a head-up position or if the injury involved a venous sinus, Doppler monitoring and prior placement of a right atrial catheter are recommended. However, as pertains also to the insertion of a pulmonary artery catheter, the patient should not be placed in a Trendelenburg position for this maneuver. Also, a subclavian approach causes less interference with cerebral drainage than the internal jugular approach.

In patients with acute arterial epidural hematomas, probably one of the most emergent of all neurosurgical cases because of the potential for complete survival if the clot is released promptly, preanesthetic time should not be devoted to cannulation of vessels other than a peripheral vein. Rather, as soon as possible the patient should be anesthetized and the trachea intubated. After the operation has commenced, an arterial route can be established. During the interim period, continuous assessment of blood pressure may be obtained by use of finger plethysmography, and pulse oximetry can monitor the adequacy of arterial flow (49).

To compare initial findings with those on subsequent examinations, the neurologic examination must be succinct and reproducible. Assessment and monitoring of level of consciousness, eye examination, and brainstem function are of special importance. The Glasgow coma scale (GCS), first described as a prognostic indicator of outcome in head injury, is also used as an indicator of progress (50, 51) (Table 7.3). Motor response is the most sensitive component and correlates best with extent and outcome of severe injury indicated by a motor score of 4 or less. Such patients commonly score only 2 additional points and obtain a total GCS score of 6 or below.

For GCS scores greater than 6, other circumstances may confound the score. For example, patients who are in shock, hy-

**Table 7.3.　The Glasgow Coma Scale**

| | |
|---|---|
| Best verbal response | |
| None | 1 |
| Incomprehensible sound | 2 |
| Inappropriate words | 3 |
| Confused | 4 |
| Oriented | 5 |
| Eyes open | |
| None | 1 |
| To pain | 2 |
| To speech | 3 |
| Spontaneously | 4 |
| Best motor response | |
| None | 1 |
| Abnormal extensor | 2 |
| Abnormal flexion | 3 |
| Withdraws | 4 |
| Localizes | 5 |
| Obeys | 6 |
| Total coma scale | 15–3 |

poxic, intoxicated, or postictal may have a GCS score that does not accurately reflect the degree of brain damage. In addition, associated injuries, such as bilateral orbital trauma or cervical cord damage, may interfere with reliable interpretation of the scale. In the agitated, uncooperative, dysphasic, or intubated patient, accurate scoring may be impossible (52). The GCS cannot be applied to preverbal children. Furthermore, because the motor score is obtained from the side with the best response, it fails to reflect unilateral deterioration. For example, the coma score in a patient who can localize the stimulus bilaterally and then becomes unilaterally decerebrate remains the same. This misrepresentation can be avoided by recording the motor response of both sides. Hence, the GCS must be regarded as a crude quantitative measure of consciousness and not as a substitute for a detailed neurologic assessment.

## Fluid Management

The blood-brain barrier (BBB), which is based on tight junctions between the endothelial cells of the cerebral capillary walls, is often disrupted after head trauma. Thus, substances of high molecular weight such as albumin (MW 69,000), which would normally be excluded, pass into the brain and remain after the plasma levels decrease, thus considerably increasing cerebral edema (53). Although hydrostatic forces are not an important determinant of water flow into the brain when the BBB is intact, with disruption a relatively high intraluminal pressure forces fluid out of the capillaries and into the surrounding brain; this outflow increases proportionally with intraluminal pressure. There is often concomitant dysfunction of local cerebrovascular autoregulation, which normally maintains intraluminal pressure and velocity of blood flow within narrow ranges. Dysautoregulation permits a higher intracapillary pressure and, therefore, enhances the formation of cerebral edema. In patients with an area of dysautoregulation, elevation of blood pressure, therapeutic or otherwise, worsens the situation regionally, although adequate perfusion of other areas of the brain endangered by a rising ICP may be achieved.

Despite its low molecular weight, sodium passage across the BBB requires 2 to 4 hours to reach equilibrium. Rapid infusion of isotonic saline increases ICP transiently, probably because of an acute increase in total blood volume (54). If the BBB is disrupted, there is no impediment to the influx of sodium into the brain. Thus, brain sodium levels equilibrate much more rapidly.

Catecholamine excretion after head injury is common, causing hypertension that may mask an iatrogenically induced hypovolemia that may first be realized during induction of anesthesia. Rapid infusion of fluids may help to correct hypotension but may be deleterious to the brain. Thus, the type of fluids and the rate of administration are critical choices in the treatment of patients with CNS trauma.

Based on the supposition that head-injured patients should be maintained "dry" to decrease cerebral edema, tradition has demanded the establishment of a negative fluid balance. However, such treatment may prove detrimental in these patients for the following reasons:

1. Despite complete fluid restriction in animals,

cerebral water content decreases minimally or not at all (55).

2. Hypovolemia may cause hypotension, which increases hypoxia.

3. Hypovolemia decreases oxygen transport, which causes vasodilation and intracranial hypertension.

4. An unstable anesthetic course is frequently due to preoperative hypovolemia.

Treatment of preoperative hypovolemia, hypokalemia, or hyperosmosis should be started whenever possible before operative intervention. Central venous pressure monitoring is a useful guide in fluid replacement if time permits placement of the catheter. After decompression of the brain, blood loss from vascular injuries may be considerable and replacement should be available. A time-honored tradition has been to administer glucose intraoperatively to prevent hypoglycemia, provide energy, conserve protein, and prevent ketosis. However, studies have shown that hyperglycemia existing before an ischemic or hypoxic event enhances ischemic damage (56). This effect is probably due to the failure of oxidative metabolism of glucose in the presence of ischemia or hypoxia. Hence, glycolysis, with lactate as an end product, increases. Withholding glucose or giving it in moderation to maintain blood glucose levels below 150 mg/dl is recommended whenever brain ischemia may occur (56).

Spurred by the observation in the neurosurgical unit that patients with cerebral edema deteriorated significantly after infusions of crystalloid solutions, Tranmer and colleagues studied the effects of different intravenous fluids on ICP in dogs with cerebral lesions. In animals receiving sodium chloride, ICP increased 90%; in the dextrose group, the increase was 141%, but no increase was seen when 6% Hetastarch was used. The authors suggest that fluid resuscitation for patients with cerebral edema may be safer with colloid agents than with crystalloids.

Mild isovolemic hemodilution may enhance cortical blood flow to ischemic regions of brain. Experimentally, hemodilu-

tion with normal saline increases CBF significantly and is associated with a moderate increase in ICP. Hypertonic lactated Ringer's solution also elevates CBF but may decrease ICP (57). Rapid fluid replacement should be avoided as sudden volume expansion may elevate ICP.

Maintenance of a hematocrit at 28 to 32% does not decrease oxygen delivery and does decrease viscosity, permitting improved rheologic conditions (58).

Thus, after head injury, it would seem appropriate to avoid sugar-containing solutions and perhaps all crystalloids and to maintain systemic pressure with colloid infusions at a rate adjusted according to central pressures.

## COMPLICATIONS OF FLUID BALANCE

Several complications of fluid balance occur in neurosurgical patients and may lead to postoperative coma or seizure activity. Damage to the hypothalamus either directly or associated with increased ICP may manifest itself, even intraoperatively, as diabetes insipidus. Urinary output increases to as much as 1 liter/hour, urinary osmolality decreases, and hypernatremia develops. Large amounts of fluid replacement and frequent serum electrolyte determination are required. Muscle irritability, seizures, and loss of consciousness occur at serum sodium levels of 160 mEq/liter. Urinary output should be replaced hourly with hypotonic solutions such as 0.25 to 0.5% sodium chloride with additional potassium chloride. If the polyuria exceeds 150 ml/hour, pitressin tannate in oil, 5 units subcutaneously, should be given. In cooperative patients, control can be obtained in minutes by nasal insufflation of 1-desamino-8-D-arginine vasopressin (DDAVP). This drug is also available as a subcutaneous preparation. Parenteral pitressin should be given slowly and the electrocardiogram monitored carefully as dysrhythmias may occur. The syndrome usually resolves spontaneously in 72 hours. If it has been diagnosed after severe hypernatremia has developed, too rapid correction of the hyperosmolar state may cause fatal cerebral edema or brain damage. Half of the calculated free water deficit should be replaced within the first 24 hours and the rest over the next 1 to 3 days (in addition to the normal daily requirements). The decreased total body water is estimated as follows:

$$\text{Actual body water} = \frac{\text{Desired serum Na}^+}{\text{actual serum Na}^+}$$
$$\times \text{ normal total body water}$$
$$(60\% \text{ of body weight in kg})$$

Replacement with sugar-containing solutions should be avoided to prevent the development of nonketotic, hyperglycemic coma (59). This syndrome is characterized by loss of consciousness, seizures, and even respiratory arrest. Laboratory values show serum sodium of 145 to 155 mEq/liter, serum osmolality of 350 to 380 mOsm/kg, and serum glucose around 1000 mg/dl. Therapy includes administration of pitressin, withdrawal of sugar solutions, and small doses of regular insulin (60).

Other complications of fluid therapy can often be avoided by careful monitoring and prompt appropriate revision of fluid administration. In the desire to prevent dehydration, excessive fluids may be given, especially if more than one vein has been cannulated. Generally, if the fluid balance exceeds 1 liter, some degree of overhydration exists. Delayed return to consciousness and dilutional hyponatremia may result.

Water retention secondary to antidiuretic hormone secretion or excess water administration may cause hyponatremia. The syndrome of inappropriate secretion of antidiuretic hormone (SIADH) has been found in 9 to 15% of neurosurgical patients (61, 62). The time course of development of hyponatremia dictates the neurologic signs observed. Therefore, the more rapidly it develops, the more water will move into the relatively hyperosmolar brain, causing edema and disturbed consciousness. If hyponatremia occurs more gradually, mental status changes may not be observed until serum sodium levels are reduced to about 130 mEq/liter, as there will be more time for

equilibration to occur. As the serum sodium concentration falls below 120 mEq/liter, confusion and delirium develop and the clinical picture progresses to seizures, tremors, aphasia, hypo- or hyperreflexia, hemiparesis, rigidity, and coma. An acute decrease of serum sodium below 125 mEq/liter can cause irreversible brain damage within 12 hours.

The amount of sodium necessary to correct the deficit can be estimated:

$$(\text{Desired Na}^+ \text{ concentration}$$
$$- \text{ initial Na}^+ \text{ concentration})$$
$$\times 0.5 \text{ (body weight in kg)}$$
$$= \text{mEq Na}^+ \text{ required}$$

The treatment of hyponatremia is with isotonic or hypertonic saline (3–5%) depending on the time course and severity of the sodium deficit. Hypertonic saline should be used circumspectly because of the risk of fluid overloading. Furosemide, 20 mg intravenously, can be given initially to promote negative fluid balance. To avoid neurologic complications, correction of severe hyponatremia must be done slowly (63).

Acute hypokalemia is not uncommon after the combined administration of mannitol and furosemide. Complications include potentiation of neuromuscular blockade, cardiac dysrhythmias, and even respiratory arrest (64). Mineralocorticoids, glycosuria, and metabolic alkalosis enhance renal potassium excretion. Careful monitoring and addition of potassium to the infusion as necessary are required.

## Postanesthetic Care

The postanesthetic care of the head-injured patient requires careful monitoring, exquisite attention to maintenance of cardiorespiratory stability, and frequent neurologic assessment. With release of an intracranial mass lesion, many patients regain consciousness promptly. As soon as the patient is able to follow commands and the respiratory status is stable, early extubation can decrease the likelihood of pneumonic complications and improve the ability to cough. Patients in whom considerable cerebral edema was demonstrated preoperatively must be carefully observed for the development of hypercapnia, alteration in the sensorium, and further increase in ICP. Should any of these conditions occur, reintubation and assisted ventilation must begin immediately.

Multimodality evoked potential and electroencephalographic monitoring may reliably be used during the postoperative period or in the intensive care unit to follow the course of head-injured patients (65). Evoked potential techniques allow differentiation between patients with drug-induced electroencephalographic changes and those with brain injury and evaluation of functional state and prognosis. Patients with raised ICP undergo characteristic alterations in flash- and brainstem evoked potentials.

It is critical to evaluate coagulation factors pre- and postoperatively. An indicator of developing complications after head injury is activation of the complement system by enzymes that cleave clotting factors (66). Disseminated intravascular coagulopathy and adult respiratory distress syndrome may result. Early diagnosis by measurement of total hemolytic serum complement activity, prothrombin time, and partial thromboplastin time can be made, and therapy with fresh frozen plasma or other appropriate blood products can be commenced.

Much recent work has suggested that brain injury may be diminished and recovery accelerated by early parenteral hyperalimentation (67).

## SPINAL CORD INJURY

The level of the spinal column at which the injury has occurred determines the complications that may develop. Patients with high cervical traumatic spinal cord injuries (SCIs) are prone to many complications, including respiratory, cardiovascular, and thermoregulatory dysfunction (Table 7.4). Although the move now is away from early surgical intervention, deteriorating neurologic function may necessitate emergency operation to release a hematoma or stabilize a fracture.

After complete transection of the cord at C5, intercostal muscle activity is lost. The patient depends on diaphragmatic respiration and auxiliary means of chest expansion, such as contraction of the sternocleidomastoid muscle. If the vital capacity is less than 1 liter preoperatively, a means of assisted ventilation must be used postoperatively to prevent respiratory failure. Occasionally, a patient may have marginal respiratory embarrassment preoperatively. During anterior cervical spine fusion, sufficient spasm and edema occur in the auxiliary muscles to precipitate ventilatory failure. Continuous positive airway pressure (CPAP) must be used cautiously; its increase of the functional residual capacity hampers diaphragmatic action and decreases vital capacity.

Hypoxemia, due mostly to neuromuscular deficit, is found in about 50% of patients with high SCI. Tracheal suctioning or mechanical irritation of tracheal vagal sensory receptors during intubation may cause reflex bradycardia or even cardiac arrest due to vasovagal reflex in sympathectomized patients.

The spinal cord-injured patient presenting with hypotension may have hemorrhagic shock from concurrent multiple trauma. However, the presence of an abnormal heart rate is not reliable in differentiat-

**Table 7.4.  Complications of High SCIs**

Respiratory
  Marginal embarrassment
  Apnea
  Ondine's syndrome
Cardiovascular
  Bradycardia
  Hypotension
Hypothermia
Urinary retention
Gastric distension
Sensory loss
  Pressure necrosis
  Hallucinations
Autonomic hyperreflexia
Malnutrition
  Negative nitrogen balance

ing the cause of hypotension. Although tachycardia usually accompanies hemorrhagic shock, bradycardia may indicates neurogenic etiology and volume depletion.

ECG changes consistent with subendocardial ischemia have been demonstrated in clinical and experimental cord transections at C5–C6 (68). Other ECG changes include sinus pauses, shifting sinus pacemaker, atrial fibrillation, multifocal premature ventricular contractions, ventricular tachycardia, and ST–T wave changes (69).

Systolic blood pressure commonly stabilizes at 90 to 100 mm Hg, which is considered adequate for cord perfusion in the supine position. However, loss of sympathetic tone and the compensatory mechanism for postural changes may jeopardize cord perfusion during repositioning and periods of operative blood loss. Spinal cord perfusion pressure should be adequately maintained with judicious volume loading using crystalloid or colloid solutions or blood replacement. Atropine, 0.4 mg, may be given to correct bradycardia. If hypotension persists despite reasonable fluid administration, the judicious use of vasopressors to replace the loss of neurogenic vasoconstriction will usually promptly restore the blood pressure to normal. Patients in the acute phase of injury have a marginal capacity to respond to volume stress and may develop pulmonary edema. Placement of a central venous catheter is essential for optimal volume resuscitation before surgery. In patients with high cord transection, an adequate guide to appropriate fluid management may only be achieved by trend recordings from a pulmonary artery catheter. Urine output should also be used as a guide to volume administration and should be optimally maintained at 0.5 to 1.0 ml/kg/hr. Blood loss must be adequately replaced to achieve a preoperative hematocrit close to 30%.

Two interesting and apparently conflicting studies concern anesthesia and acute SCI. High doses of naloxone or methylprednisolone afforded improved quality of survival after experimental cord injury in cats (70). Combination of the drugs increased mortality. The use of a narcotic antagonist might suggest that narcotic anesthesia would not be indicated. After experimental injury in a rat, the greatest degree of spinal cord protection was demonstrated in animals anesthetized with fentanyl, 57 μg/kg, and 65% nitrous oxide (71). Clearly, more work must be done in this area.

The onset of the intermediate phase of recovery from SCI develops approximately 1 month after injury. It is characterized by the resolution of spinal shock and the appearance of autonomic hyperreflexia. In this condition, afferent somatic sensory and visceral impulses arising from below the level of the lesion enter the isolated spinal cord and elicit a massive sympathetic response from the adrenal medulla and sympathetic nervous system, which is no longer modulated by the normal inhibitory impulses arising from the brainstem and hypothalamus. Autonomic hyperreflexia occurs in 85% of patients with spinal cord transections above the T5 level in whom splanchnic outflow remains intact. Afferent impulses originating from bladder or bowel distension, childbirth, manipulations of the urinary tract, or surgical stimulation are transmitted along the pelvic, pudendal, or hypogastric nerves to the isolated spinal cord. Vasoconstriction occurs below the lesion; reflex activity of carotid and aortic baroreceptors produces vasodilation above the lesion, which is often accompanied by bradycardia, ventricular dysrhythmias, and even heart block. The anesthesiologist must be aware that the potential for this complication arising during operation is maximal 4 weeks after injury. Although it gradually subsides, autonomic hyperreflexia may recur after many years (72).

In the chronic phase of SCI, renal function may deteriorate because of repeated infections and stone formation secondary to hypercalciuria. Ascending pyelonephritis and chronic renal failure result in loss of serum protein, sodium, and potassium. In addition, serum blood urea nitrogen (BUN) and creatinine become elevated.

Preoperative evaluation of electrolytes, protein, BUN, and creatinine is essential. Efforts must be made to restore these values to within normal limits before any elective surgery is undertaken. Urinary tract infections should be resolved with appropriate antibiotic therapy.

Compounding protein and electrolyte abnormalities is the negative nitrogen balance into which the spinal-cord-injured patient enters almost immediately after injury. In addition to skeletal muscle wasting, visceral wasting may also ensue, secondary to inactivity or denervation. Wasting of the diaphragm is potentially dangerous to a patient who may rely entirely on diaphragmatic activity for breathing. As patients enter the chronic stage of SCI, they become more susceptible to limb fracture during periods of movement and positioning for surgery. When spinal shock resolves, muscle spasm and contractures are seen because of the development of unmodified reflex circuits below the level of the injury. Spasm and contracture may cause technical difficulties in locating intravenous sites and during positioning for regional anesthesia and surgery.

## SUMMARY

Appropriate anesthetic management for the patient with CNS trauma is critical to outcome. Establishment of the airway, maintenance of stable intracranial dynamics, appropriate choice of anesthetic agents, and careful postoperative monitoring can all help to ensure maximal neuronal survival.

## References

1. Reilly PL, Adams JH, Graham DJ, Jennett B. Patients with head injury who talk and die. Lancet 1975;2:375–380.
2. Rose J, Valtonen S, Jennett B. Avoidable factors contributing to death after head injury. Br Med J 1977;2:615–618.
3. Singbartl G, Cunitz G. Pathophysiology, emergency care and anesthesia in patients with severe head injury. Anaesthesist 1987;36:321–332.
4. Landolt H, Gratzl O. Craniocerebral trauma—

bases, immediate risks and management. Ther Umsch 1987;44:553–558.
5. Ishige N, Pitts LH, Hashimoto T, Nishimura MC, Barkowski HM. Effect of hypoxia on traumatic brain injury in rats: part 1. Changes in neurological function, electroencephalograms and histopathology. Neurology 1987;20:848–853.
6. Andrews BT, Chiles BW, Olsen WL, Pitts LH. The significance of intracerebral hematoma location on clinical outcome and the risk of tentorial herniation. In Proceedings of the Annual Meeting of the American Society of Neurological Surgeons, Toronto, Ontario, April 1988, paper 40.
7. Frost EAM, Domurat MF. Cardiopulmonary changes after head injury. In Miner MM, Wagner KA (eds): Neurotrauma. Boston, Butterworth, 1986, pp 29–40.
8. Pfenninger E, Ahnefeld FW, Kilian J, Dell U. Blood gases at the scene of the accident and on admission to hospital following craniocerebral trauma. Anaesthesist 1987;36:570–576.
9. Eisenberg HM, Cayard O, Papanicolaou AC. The effects of 3 potentially preventable complications on outcome after severe closed head injury. In ICP V. Tokyo, Springer-Verlag, 1983, pp 549–553.
10. Gildenberg PL, Makela ME. The effect of intubation and ventilation on outcome following head trauma. In Symposium of Neural Trauma, Charlottesville, VA. New York, Raven Press, 1982.
11. Bayless P, Ray VG. Incidence of cervical spine injuries in association with blunt head trauma. Am J Emerg Med 1989;7(2):139–142.
12. Grande CM, Barton CR, Stene JK. Appropriate techniques for airway management of emergency patients with suspected spinal cord injury. Anesth Analg 1988;67:714–715.
13. Clifton GL, McCormick WF, Grossman RG. Neuropathology of early and late deaths after head injury. Neurosurgery 1981;8:309–314.
14. Brown RS, Mohr PA, Corey JS. Cardiovascular changes after cranial cerebral injury and increased intracranial pressure. Surg Gynecol Obstet 1967;125:1205–1211.
15. Miner ME, Allen SJ. Cardiovascular effects of severe head injury. In Frost E (ed): Clinical Anesthesia in Neurosurgery, ed 2. Boston, Butterworth, 1990.
16. Mendelow AD. Head injuries. Current Opinions Neurosurg Neurol 1988;1(1):37–45.
17. Leeman M, Naeje R, Degaute JP, et al. Acute central and renal hemodynamic responses to tetratolol and propranolol in patients with arterial hypertension following head injury. J Hypertens 1984;4:581–588.
18. Cottrell J, Patel K, Ransohoff J, et al. Intracranial pressure changes induced by sodium nitroprusside in patients with intracranial mass lesions. J Neurosurg 1978;48:329–331.
19. Overgaard J, Skinhoj E. A paradoxical hemody-

namic effect of hydrolazine. Stroke 1975; 6:402–404.

20. Boddin M, Van Bogaert A, Dierick W. Catacholamines in blood and myocardial tissue in experimental subarachnoidal hemorrhage. Cardiology 1973;58:229–237.

21. Cruickshank JM, Neil-Dwyer G, Brice J. Electrocardiographic changes, their prognostic significance in subarachnoid hemorrhage. J Neurol Neurosurg Psychiatry 1974;37:755–759.

22. Hersch C. Electrocardiographic changes in head injuries. Circulation 1961;23:853–860.

23. Dearden NM, Gibson JS, McDowall DG, Gibson RM, Cameron MM. Effect on high dose dexamethasone and outcome from severe head injury. J Neurosurg 1986;64:81–88.

24. Ford EG, Jennings LM, Andrassy RJ. Steroid administration potentiates urinary nitrogen losses in head injured children. J Trauma 1987;27:1074–1078.

25. Ravussin P, Archer DP, Meyer E, Abou-Madi M, Yamamoto L, Trop D. The effects of rapid infusions of saline and mannitol on cerebral blood volume and intracranial pressure in dogs. Can Anaesth Soc J 1985;32:506–515.

26. Abou-Madi M, Trop D, Abou-Madi N, Ravussin P. Does a bolus of mannitol initially aggravate intracranial hypertension? A study at various $PaCO_2$ tensions in dogs. Br J Anaesth 1987; 59:630–639.

27. Nelson PB, Kapoor W, Rinaldo G, Robinson AG, Fu F. Hyponatremia associated with increased intracranial pressure, altered mental status and pulmonary edema following a marathon run. In Proceedings of the Annual Meeting of the American Society of Neurological Surgeons, Toronto, Ontario, April 1988 (paper 49).

28. Muiselaar JP, Lutz HA, Becker DP. Effects of mannitol on ICP and CBF correlation with pressure autoregulation in severely head-injured patients. J Neurosurg 1984;61:700–706.

29. Pollay M, Fullenwider C, Roberts PA, et al. Effect of mannitol and furosemide on blood-brain osmotic gradient and intracranial pressure. J Neurosurg 1983;59:945–950.

30. Roberts PA, Pollay M, Engles C, Stevens FA. Effect on intracranial pressure of furosemide combined with varying doses and administration rates of mannitol. J Neurosurg 1987;66:440–446.

31. Schetinni A, Stakurski B, Young HF. Osmotic and osmotic loop diuresis in brain surgery: effects on plasma and CSF electrolytes and ion excretion. J Neurosurg 1982;56:680–684.

32. Sterna RH: Severe symptomatic hyponatremia. treatment and outcome. Ann Intern Med 1987; 107:656–664.

33. Weissman JD, Weissman BM. Routine myelinolysis and delayed encephalopathy following the rapid correction of acute hyponatremia. Acta Neurol Scand 1989;46:926–927.

34. Hartung HT. Intracranial pressure after propofol and thiopental administration in patients with severe head trauma. Anaesthesist 1987; 36:285–287.

35. Raphaely RC. Central nervous system trauma in children. In Rogers M (ed): Current Practice in Anaesthesiology. Toronto, BC Decker, 1988, pp 268–272.

36. Allen SJ, Cruz J, Abouleish BA, Miner ME. Immediate detection of critical transient hypoxic episodes in acute head injuries. Anesth Analg 1987;66:S2, (abstract).

37. Rosner MJ, Coley IB. Cerebral perfusion pressure, intracranial pressure, and head elevation. J Neurosurg 1986;65:636–641.

38. Anson JA, Sundberg S, Stone JL. Treatment of status epilepticus with continuous midazolam infusion. In Proceedings of the Annual Meeting of the American Society of Neurological Surgeons, Toronto, Ontario, April 1988 (paper 146).

39. Walters FJM. Anaesthesia for neuroradiology. Br J Hosp Med 1987;38(suppl 4):351–357.

40. Nehls DG, Todd MM, Spetzler RF, Drummond JC, Thompson RA, Johnson PC. A comparison of the cerebral protective effects of isoflurane and barbiturates during temporary focal ischemia in primates. Anesthesiology 1987;66:453–464.

41. McPherson RW, Traystman RJ. Effects of isoflurane on cerebral autoregulation. Anesthesiology 1987;67(suppl 3A):A576.

42. Baughman VL, Hoffman WE, Albrecht RF, Miletich DJ. The interaction of $N_2O$ and isoflurane on regional cerebral ischemia in the rat. Anesthesiology 1987;67(suppl 3A):A578.

43. Frost EAM, Kim B, Thiagarajah S. Anaesthesia and outcome in severe head injury. Br J Anaesth 1981;53:310–311.

44. Gokaslan ZL, Robertson CS, Narayan RK, Pahwa R. The effect of barbiturates on cerebral blood flow and metabolism. In Proceedings of the Annual Meeting of the American Society of Neurological Surgeons, Toronto, Ontario, April 1988 (paper 288).

45. Wermeling DP, Blouin RA, Porter WH, Rapp RP, Tibbs PA. Pentobarbital in patients with severe head injury. Drug Intell Clin Pharm 1987;21:459–463.

46. Frankville DD, Drummond JC. Hyperkalemia after succinylcholine administration in a patient with closed head injury without paresis. Anesthesiology 1987;67:264–266.

47. Ornstein E, Matteo RS, Schwartz AE, Silverberg PA, Young WL, Diaz J. The effect of phenytoin on the magnitude and duration of neuromuscular block following atracurium or vecuronium. Anesthesiology 1987;67:191–196.

48. Chapple DJ, Miller AA, Ward JB, Wheatley PL. Cardiovascular and neurological effects of laudanosine. Br J Anaesth 1987;59:218–225.

49. Friesen RH. Pulse oximetry during pulmonary artery surgery. Anesth Analg 1985;64:376.
50. Teardale G, Jennett B. Assessment of coma and impaired consciousness: a practical scale. Lancet 1974;2:81–84.
51. Overgaard J, Hrid-Hansen O, Land A, Pedersen KK, Christensen S, Haase J, Hein O, Tweed WA. Prognosis after head injury based on early clinical examination. Lancet 1973;2:631–635.
52. Bouzarth WF. Coma scale. J Neurosurg 1978; 49:477–478.
53. Gazendam J, Gwan Go K, Van Zanten AK. Composition of isolated edema fluid in cold-induced edema. J Neurosurg 1979;51:70–77.
54. Weed LH, McKibben PS. Pressure changes in the cerebrospinal fluid following intravenous injection of solution of various concentrations. Am J Physiol 1919;48:512 530.
55. Jelsma LF, McQueen JD. Effect of experimental water restriction on brain water. J Neurosurg 1967;26:35–40.
56. Sieber FE, Smith DS, Traystman RJ, Wollman H. Glucose: a re-evaluation of its intraoperative use. Anesthesiology 1987;67:72–81.
57. Todd MM, Tommasino C, Moore S. Cerebral effects of isovolemic hemodilution with a hypertonic saline solution. J Neurosurg 1985; 63:944–948.
58. Wood JH, Simeone FA. Failure of intravascular volume expansion without hemodilution to elevate cortical blood flow in regions of experimental focal ischemia. J Neurosurg 1982;56:80–91.
59. Park BE, Meacham WF, Netsky MG. Nonketotic hyperglycemic hyperosmolar coma. J Neurosurg 1976;44:409–417.
60. Shucart WA, Jackson I. Management of diabetes insipidus in neurosurgical patients. J Neurosurg 1976;44:65–70.
61. Fox JL, Falik JL, Shalhoub RJ. Neurosurgical hypernatremia. The role of inappropriate diuresis. J Neurosurg 1971;34:506–514.
62. Doczi T, Bende J, Huszka E, et al. Syndrome of inappropriate secretion of antidiuretic hormone after subarachnoid hemorrhage. Neurosurgery 1981;9:394–397.
63. Sterns RH: Severe symptomatic hyponatremia. treatment and outcome. Ann Intern Med 1987; 107:656–664.
64. Dorin RI, Crapo LM. Hypokalemic, respiratory arrest in diabetic ketoacidosis. JAMA 1987;257: 1517–1518.
65. Nau HE, Rimpel J. Multimodality evoked potentials and electroencephalography in severe coma cases—clinical experiences in a neurosurgical intensive care unit. Intensive Care Med 1987; 13:249–255.
66. Becker P, Zieger S, Rother U, Lutz H, Osswald PM. Complement activation following severe head injury. Anaesthesist 1987;36:301–305.
67. Rapp RP, Young B, Twyman D, Bivans BA, Haack D, Tibbs PA, Bean JR. The favorable effect of early parenteral feeding on survival in head injured patients. J Neurosurg 1983;58:906–912.
68. Greenhoot JH, Reichenbach D. Cardiac injury and subarachnoid hemorrhage: clinical pathologic correlation. J Neurosurg 1969;30:521–531.
69. Kopaniky DR, Frost EAM. Management of spinal cord trauma. In Frost E (ed): Clinical Anesthesia in Neurosurgery. Boston, Butterworth, 1984, pp 375–395.
70. Young W, Decrescito V, Flamm ES, Blight AR, Gruner JA. Pharmacological therapy of acute spinal cord injury: studies of high dose methylprednisolone and naloxone. Clin Neurosurg 1988; 34:675–697.
71. Cole DJ, Shapiro HM, Drummond JC, Zivin JA. Anesthesia protects against spinal cord injury in the rat. Anesthesiology 1987;67(suppl 3A):A585.
72. Cottrell JE, Newfield P, Giffin JP, Shwiry B. Spinal cord injury. In Cottrell JE, Newfield P (eds): Handbook of Neuroanesthesia: Clinical and Physiologic Essentials. Boston, Little, Brown & Co, 1983, pp 339–351.

# 8

# Perioperative Anesthetic Management of Maxillofacial and Ocular Trauma: Injuries of the Craniocervicofacial Complex

*Christopher M. Grande, Chet I. Wyman,*
*and William N. Bernhard*

## MAXILLOFACIAL INJURIES

Because of the proximity of the airway, which begins at the oronasopharynx, to the face, there is probably no area in trauma management in which the anesthesiologist will have more input than in maxillofacial injury. From a general standpoint, there is probably no area that is more important to the patient's well-being than proper management of trauma of the craniocervicofacial complex (CCFC). Because of the relationship of the face to the remainder of the head and to the neck, a triad of injuries to these regions is often found (1, 2). The face itself is of paramount importance to the individual because of all of its functions: sensory reception (i.e., sight, smell, hearing), eating, breathing, speaking, and nonverbal communication via facial expression. Also,

facial trauma is associated with significant social ramifications (1, 2).

Maxillofacial trauma is certainly one of the most visually impressive injuries to present to the trauma anesthesiologist; its appearance can intimidate the unprepared physician (Figs. 8.1 and 8.2). However, facial injuries, which may present with bleeding, massive swelling, and appalling deformity, rarely represent an immediate threat to life unless accompanied by compromise of the airway or associated massive vascular injury. In fact, airway obstruction is the leading cause of death in patients with maxillofacial injuries (1). Because maxillofacial injuries are frequently dramatic, they can easily divert attention away from other less obvious and often potentially fatal injuries. Thus, it must be remembered that other injuries, both obvious and occult, can greatly affect both patient outcome and anesthetic management. The trauma anesthesiologist must be prepared to deal with these life-threatening injuries and must keep a high index of suspicion for associated injuries during the anesthetic care of the trauma patient with injuries of the CCFC (3, 4).

Perioperative management of injuries to the maxillofacial area can usually be divided into several discrete steps, which may overlap and sometimes must be addressed simultaneously: initial assessment, airway management, hemorrhage control, resuscitation, damage assessment, preoperative planning and preparation, intraoperative management, and a realm of postoperative events (recovery, critical care, and subsequent reconstructive operations). In this chapter, some of these areas are examined

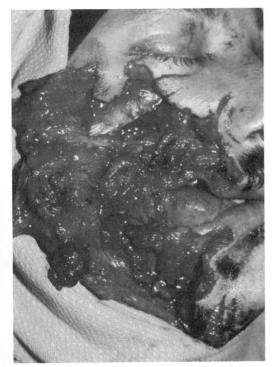

**Figure 8.1.    Shotgun wound to the lower face.** Note avulsed soft tissue (including parotid gland and buccal mucosa), extensive edema (including the tongue), and fractures of the maxilla and mandible. The patient underwent tracheostomy. (Courtesy of Paul N. Manson, M.D.)

individually; the remainder are discussed in other sections of the book.

### Scope of the Problem

The CCFC, like any other portion of the body, may be subject to any of the major mechanisms of injury (i.e., blunt, penetrating, thermal; see Chapter 2). Depending upon the circumstances, the factors responsible for trauma will vary. These differences can basically be broken down into those that occur in the military and those that occur in the civilian sphere. In war situations, most maxillofacial injuries are caused by penetrating trauma. In civil situations, blunt trauma (usually from motor vehicle and motorcycle accidents) claims the major responsibility (5, 6).

However, even within one epidemiologic group of injuries, the pattern of the various contributors will change. In the Viet Nam War, fragmentation weapons (e.g., artillery, rockets, mortars, and grenades) caused the majority of penetrating injuries (7). In World War I, which consisted primarily of trench warfare, there were many injuries to the upper face as result of soldiers being shot as they attempted to look over the lip of a trench (1).

Once again, one will appreciate a difference in the patterns that emerge in the distribution of injuries as they apply to the facial bones themselves. For example, in the Viet Nam War the bone most commonly fractured was the mandible, followed by the maxilla, zygoma, and nose, in order of decreasing frequency (7). In the civilian sphere, the nasal bones are most often injured, followed by the zygoma, mandible, orbital floor, and then the maxilla (6, 8).

The severity of injuries to the CCFC will depend primarily on the amount of energy imparted to its structures. Therefore, the higher the change of velocity in a blunt trauma episode (see Chapter 2), the greater the likelihood of damage. In the case of penetrating missile trauma, the higher the velocity of a bullet or fragment, the greater the damage. Damage from secondary mis-

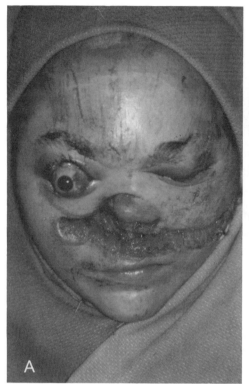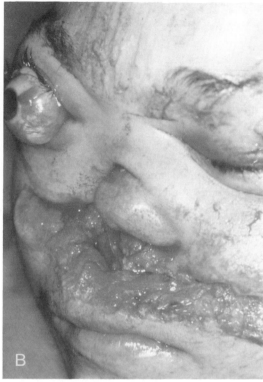

**Figure 8.2.    Mixed mechanical trauma secondary to motor vehicle accident.** There are panfacial fractures and retrusion of the midface, multiple deep lacerations, an extruded globe (as a result of optic nerve severance), and massive facial edema. (Courtesy of Paul N. Manson, M.D.)

siles (e.g., bone fragments, teeth) is also more likely, as these objects are accelerated by the energy transferred from the missile to the tissues (7, 9).

The use of certain devices will modify the pattern of injury. For example, the use of a three-point restraint in a car (lap/shoulder belt combination) will markedly decrease the amount of upper and midfacial injuries but, because of the dynamics of body motion upon impact, will not significantly alter the amount of lower facial (mandibular) injuries (5).

Also, since the late 1960s general improvements have been made in automobile windshields. Before that time, the head and neck of a victim who was not wearing a restraining device would travel through the windshield and be injured by that impact. A second avulsing-type injury was incurred from the jagged windshield as the motion reversed and those parts of the body reentered the passenger compartment (6, 10). Now the safety glass used in windshields should fragment and prevent these types of injuries.

As pertains to the CCFC itself, one should appreciate that the number of related injuries is indeed significant: of patients with a maxillofacial injury, 20% will have a concurrent cervical spine injury and 50 to 70% will have associated closed head trauma (11–13). There need not be any external evidence of head injury; mechanisms such as whiplash and contrecoup can be responsible for intracranial trauma. Because of the dynamics of these types of injury, injuries of the upper face (e.g., the frontal bone) may be associated with hyperextension injuries of the cervical spine (11). Associated cervical spine injuries will be more common with blunt trauma than with penetrating trauma (especially low-energy stab wounds). Concurrent head injury will be less likely if the cause of blunt facial trauma was interpersonal violence (e.g., a fist fight) rather than a motor vehicle accident, as sufficient energy probably would not be present (4).

### Initial Evaluation and Resuscitation

The importance of preanesthetic evaluation cannot be overemphasized in any patient, particularly someone with facial trauma. The trauma anesthesiologist will be intimately involved in initial evaluation, resuscitation, and stabilization. As with any trauma patient, initial priorities are to establish airway control, ensure ventilation, control bleeding, and treat shock. The facial injuries themselves may take a lower priority than other life-threatening injuries; although not currently desirable, treatment of facial injuries usually can be delayed for several days, often with still excellent results (2, 6). Shock is rarely caused by blood loss from maxillofacial injury alone (unless there are extensive lacerations of the scalp, which is very vascular, especially in children) (2, 9, 14). A diligent search for occult bleeding must be initiated and maintained during the initial resuscitation of the patient. The chest, abdomen, and pelvis must be evaluated as possible sources of shock-producing hemorrhage (see Chapter 6) (14). Bleeding from injuries to the head and neck usually can be controlled with direct pressure (2).

### Airway Management: Concepts

Trauma patients initially are managed according to the standard "ABCs," which always must be followed specifically: **A**irway, **B**reathing, and **C**irculation. Airway management is of utmost importance and receives immediate attention.

Airway obstruction in the trauma patient can be divided into three main categories: (a) The first group comprises patients with complete or nearly complete airway obstruction who present with frank hypoxia, hypercarbia, agitation, and confusion if they are not unconscious (15). (b) The second group of patients with airway compromise are those with progressive obstruction. They may initially present with stridor, labored breathing, intercostal retractions, tracheal tugging, and agitation (15). They may be alert and cooperative and thus may lull the naive anesthesiologist into a false sense of security. These patients may quickly fatigue or progress to complete obstruction (e.g., the burn patient with thermal trauma of the upper airway). Though the situation may allow for planned airway management, this group also deserves immediate attention (see below). (c) The final group consists of those patients with insidious airway obstruction (15). They may have occult injuries that slowly and progressively compromise the airway if not sought out aggressively. The signs are subtle and require diligent evaluation. Throughout the entire resuscitation, the airway should be continually reassessed if it has not been secured or protected adequately.

Probably no other case will be more provocative and lead to greater stimulation of opinions among a group of anesthesiologists than the topic of airway management of a trauma patient with maxillofacial injuries. Issues that will be discussed include the "full stomach," the route and techniques of intubation and any devices to assist in its completion (e.g., fiberoptic bronchoscope), the use of pharmacologic adjuncts, and consideration of associated injuries and preexisting medical conditions.

Initial ventilation with a bag-valve-mask apparatus may be almost impossible because of difficulty in achieving a satisfactory seal secondary to facial damage (16). One may attempt to improve the situation by applying damp pieces of gauze around the mouth and nose to "fill in" the defects (17). In the patient with a pathologic communication between the oronasopharynx and the subdural space (e.g., fractured cribriform plate), the possibility of meningitis secondary to positive-pressure mask ventilation exists (3, 18).

Facial swelling or upper airway edema may severely impair access to the oropharynx. The mouth may have limited opening secondary to pain, muscle spasm, or fractures of the mandible (3, 4). A fracture of the zygoma may be displaced medially and impinge upon the coronoid process of the mandible, making oral intubation difficult, if not impossible. (Formal tracheostomy under local anesthesia may be another alternative for airway control in the elective situation.)

Blood, saliva, and teeth or dentures may collect in the pharynx and impair ventilation. If dentures are found, they should be kept safely, as they will be indispensable in establishing various measurements and skeletal relationships during reconstructive surgery (9). Suction is essential. The tongue, or remnants of the tongue, and soft tissue may severely impair the airway, especially when mandibular fractures are present. An initial "chin-lift" or "jaw-thrust" maneuver may easily clear an obstructed airway. Again, care must be taken not to hyperextend the neck and compromise the cervical spinal cord (see Chapter 3). If these basic maneuvers are ineffective, the tongue and other soft tissues may be displaced with a surgical clamp or a strong suture, thus opening the airway (1). This may be all that is required to secure what may have appeared to be a very severely compromised airway on initial inspection.

Positioning of the patient with extensive oropharyngeal bleeding is also very important. The patient should be placed in the position that optimizes drainage of blood and secretions away from the airway (19). In awake patients who are breathing spontaneously, the sitting (or prone) position usually is best. We have found that, with the patient in the left lateral decubitus position, gravity works with us during the intubation. A stable patient with fairly active pharyngeal bleeding should be placed in the lateral position with the head in a downward tilt.

Throughout the literature it is easy to find many prescribed "cookbook" methods for managing the airway of injured patients. Similarly, algorithms that direct the user through several "yes/no" decision points abound. However, neither the cookbook

approaches nor the algorithms should be regarded highly (although they may be useful as learning tools) because exceptions are frequent in trauma patients. Further, if one were to consider all possible variables that could be present in a given situation (e.g., presence/absence of head injuries or cervical pathology, consciousness or unconsciousness, stable or unstable hemodynamics), by binary permutation there would be thousands of possibilities; it is impossible to make any "blanket" recommendations of techniques to cover all of them. Therefore, the authors suggest that the practitioner strive for a thorough conceptual knowledge that can be applied as the situation demands. General concepts (Table 8.1) that must be considered when managing any victim of maxillofacial trauma include those listed here.

*No single method of airway control can be uniformly adopted for all injuries of the CCFC.* This is the most basic concept and is heavily dependent on all of the concepts that follow.

*Determine the absolute urgency of the situation.* Does the situation demand action *now*, or is there some amount of time available during which alternatives can be examined, precautions taken, and a plan developed that provides for "safeties" (secondary plans of action should the primary plan fail)? Two factors of most importance in making this determination are the status of the respiratory system (airway and breathing) and hemodynamic status (Table 8.2).

**Table 8.1.  General Concepts of Airway Management in the Patient with Maxillofacial Trauma**

No single method of airway control can be uniformly adopted for all injuries of the CCFC.
Determine the absolute urgency of the situation.
When possible, always proceed with a backup plan.
Consider the possibility of concomitant head injury.
Consider the possibility of concomitant cervical injuries.
Consider the possibility of concomitant ocular injuries.
Remember the need to visualize.
Remember "full stomach" considerations.
Suspect airway obstruction by foreign bodies.

**Table 8.2.  Items of Potential Concern in Airway Management of the Patient with Maxillofacial Trauma**

Obstruction to mouth opening
  Cervical collar
  Bimandibular fracture
  Condylar fracture
  Postoperative jaw wiring
  Trismus
  Pain
Obstruction of upper and lower airway
  Blood
  Secretions
  Teeth
  Bone fragments
  Foreign body (e.g., coin)
Associated injuries
  Intracranial
  Cervical
  Other (e.g., thoracoabdominal, orthopedic)
Associated conditions
  Hypoxia
  Shock
  Other (e.g., respiratory: tension pneumothorax)

*When possible, always proceed with a backup plan.* No matter what the primary choice is for achieving airway control, it is usually prudent to have devised at least one plan of action to fall back on if the former fails. This planning includes having all of the necessary equipment and personnel ready.

*Consider the possibility of concomitant head injury.* Establishing the likelihood or definite presence of head injury will affect most strongly the adjunctive use of pharmacologic agents to control changes in intracranial pressure (ICP) and in the other hemodynamic determinants of brain perfusion and oxygenation (see Chapter 7). Here a delicate balance must be maintained: if the chosen drugs are not used properly, then either ICP will rise and cause further ischemic damage (or, at the far end of the spectrum, tentorial herniation) or systemic blood pressure will collapse, also resulting in a diminished level of brain perfusion secondary to hypotension or general circulatory shock (with cardiac arrest at the far end of this side of the spectrum).

Clues regarding head injury will be received from four sources: (*a*) information from the field care providers, which details the mechanisms of injury (see Chapter 2); (*b*) the initial neurologic examination performed as part of the Advanced Trauma Life Support protocols (i.e., the Glasgow coma scale and the examinations performed during the primary and secondary surveys [see Chapter 7]); (*c*) diagnostic studies, which time may or may not permit to be performed (skull roentgenography, computed tomographic [CT] scanning, magnetic resonance imaging [MRI]); and (*d*) consultation with the other members of the trauma team, in this case, primarily the neurosurgeon. Input from these four sources will be melded and tempered by the trauma anesthesiologist's experience with these types of cases.

*Consider the possibility of concomitant cervical injuries.* For the purpose of this discussion, cervical injuries may be divided into three categories: those directly affecting the airway (i.e., pharynx, hypopharynx, larynx, trachea, and bronchi), those directly affecting the cervical spine, and those affecting the vasculature and other soft tissue structures. These types of injuries may be present alone or in combination. Proper management, from an anesthesia standpoint, of these injuries as regards damage to both the airway and the cervical spine is discussed in depth in Chapter 3.

*Consider the possibility of concomitant ocular injuries.* As described below in a separate section, the crux of the matter here is the management of open (penetrating) eye injuries, because of concerns of elevating intraocular pressure (IOP), which secondarily may result in extrusion of some vitreous humor. Control of IOP is within the anesthesiologist's abilities but requires meticulous timing and the use of appropriate pharmacologic agents. Again, a delicate balance must be maintained, which encompasses airway management, systemic hemodynamics, and the eye injury. In certain cases, decisions that prioritize the value of life, limbs, and eyesight will have to be made.

*Remember the need to visualize.* The anesthesiologist must be concerned about occult injury to three regions when managing the airway of the patient with injury to the CCFC: (*a*) the cribriform plate and nasopharynx, (*b*) the oropharynx and hypopharynx, and (*c*) subglottic structures.

In trauma of the CCFC, fractures of the *cribriform plate* may occur (3). Although this defect is usually seen in conjunction with high-energy midfacial damage (e.g., one of the LeFort fractures, fractures of the anterior table of the frontal sinus [see below]), it is possible with any type of CCFC injury (15, 20). Classically, rhinorrhea of cerebrospinal fluid (CSF) has been described as pathognomonic for this injury. This may be true, but it is extremely difficult to rely solely upon the presence or absence of CSF coming from the nostrils, because it may be absent (e.g., because of its flow back into the nasopharynx if the patient is supine, as most severe trauma patients are) or obscured by epistaxis or efflux of mucus from the nostrils (although the "ring test" may be applied and useful, it also cannot be depended upon). Therefore, relying solely upon this sign as to whether to proceed with a nasal intubation, especially considering the dire consequences if one is in error, may be ill-advised (15).

Besides the possibility of damage to the cribriform plate, the possibility also exists for altered anatomy of other structures of the *nasopharynx* (e.g., conchae, septum). Passage of any type of device (nasogastric or nasotracheal tubes) through these areas without definite knowledge of the situation may lead to iatrogenic damage (15, 21). Additionally, in view of these possibilities, delayed infectious complications (e.g., meningitis, sepsis) are concerns (22, 23). Also, placement of a nasotracheal tube will often interfere with the surgical management of midfacial fractures. Thus, in the majority of patients with severe trauma to the CCFC, nasal intubation is best avoided in the acute situation unless time is available to "scout" the area (e.g., with a fiberoptic bronchoscope), although this route might be quite useful and, in fact, is often preferred in elective follow-up surgery after the area has been evaluated thoroughly.

If one considers the most commonly encountered mechanisms of injury (i.e., blunt, penetrating, thermal) and their effects on the CCFC, it is not difficult to imagine the ways in which occult injuries to the *oropharynx* and *hypopharynx* might occur. For example, in blunt trauma of the CCFC, bony shards from a fractured mandible or teeth may cause lacerations to these areas (7, 9). Similarly, the high-velocity missiles involved in gunshot wounds of the face or neck may impart energy to these "secondary missiles" (see Chapter 2). The path of a bullet is often difficult to predict, even if an entrance and exit wound can be identified (i.e., the course of a missile is not always linear) (9). Possible injuries in the hypopharynx include laceration of the piriform fossae or the anterior commissure and fracture of the epiglottic cartilage. Alternatively, the burn patient may have severe edema of the epiglottis and glottic aperture, which necessitates the use of a very small caliber endotracheal tube (see Chapter 3). Because of these possibilities, the "need to visualize" is again stressed, and oral laryngoscopy becomes the "gold standard." However, even here the reader is cautioned that careful introduction of the laryngoscope blade is warranted to avoid its passage into damaged areas. For the above reasons, other "blind" techniques (e.g., nasotracheal), including both oral and nasal "digital" (tactile) intubation (with or without transillumination), and the "retrograde" method are also probably best avoided, unless no other alternatives exist (e.g., a field situation without a functioning laryngoscope).

Because of the high energy associated with motor vehicle accidents and some gunshot wounds, occult injuries may affect the integrity of *subglottic structures* (larynx, trachea, and bronchi) without obvious external signs. Once again, the trauma anesthesiologist's experience and understanding of mechanisms of injury will raise his/her level of suspicion and sensitivity to these possibilities. The first clue might be the cervical emphysema that appears after the institution of positive-pressure ventilation with a bag-valve-mask apparatus due to a ruptured trachea. As discussed in Chapter 3, these injuries have a high mortality rate. For patients with these injuries who reach a hospital alive, the diagnosis and management are difficult and may require the use of special devices (such as the extracorporeal membrane oxygenator). Good results are often tied to good fortune. Visualization of the injury is difficult under any circumstances but, at minimum, requires the use of a flexible or rigid bronchoscope.

*Remember "full stomach" considerations.* As in any trauma patient, the concept of the "full stomach" (see Chapter 3) raises concerns related to "protecting" the airway against aspiration of regurgitated gastric contents. Cricoid pressure (cricoesophageal compression, Sellick's maneuver) is the mainstay here, as well as avoiding abolition of protective airway reflexes by inappropriate use of local anesthetics on airway structures or pharmacologic induction of unconsciousness. Although controversial, "acceptable" procedures include topical application of anesthetizing agents to the mucosa of the pharynx and hypopharynx, as well as direct blockade of the superior laryngeal nerves bilaterally (24). "Unacceptable" maneuvers include the transtracheal application of local anesthetic, as this will suppress protective lower airway reflexes (25).

*Suspect airway obstruction by foreign bodies.* Because of the high likelihood of obstruction of either the upper or lower airway by any number of foreign bodies (e.g., bone fragments, teeth, avulsed soft tissues), one should always maintain a high degree of clinical suspicion for this possibility. Obstructions of the upper airway normally are easy to clear by using gravity (i.e., a head-down position), a "sweeping" device (e.g., a finger or a Yankauer suction tip), or a set of forceps. Obstructions of the lower airway are more problematic and may require the use of a rigid bronchoscope to facilitate removal of the object, high frequency jet ventilation via a percutaneous needle (26), a flexible bronchoscope to attempt to bypass the object and then jet ventilation via the suction port, or a technique that ventilates without use of the lungs (15).

## Damage Assessment: Facial Injuries

The face, consisting of soft tissue and bone, is easily damaged when force is applied to its relatively unprotected structures. In facial trauma, mild bleeding is usually the result of muscle and mucosal tears. Vessels in the face capable of producing significant hemorrhage are the anterior and posterior ethmoidal arteries, the greater palatine artery, the temporal artery, and the internal maxillary artery (6, 8). However, facial bleeding usually can be controlled with digital pressure or packing and rarely requires ligation. Blind probing with clamps in the presence of important cranial nerves must be avoided (2, 8). Although the skin and subcutaneous tissues have a generous blood and lymphatic supply, it is unlikely that lacerations of these vessels will cause shock (except in some patients with scalp lacerations) (2, 9, 14).

Beneath the layers of skin, subcutaneous tissue, and mimetic muscles is the facial skeleton. This complex array of alternating areas of thin and thick bone forms a series of arches and buttresses that reinforce the facial architecture with a system of horizontal and vertical structural supports (2, 3).

In civilian situations, the most commonly fractured portion of the facial skeleton is the nose (6, 8). Clinical signs include nasal deformity with or without obstruction to air passage, epistaxis, abrasion, laceration or hematoma of the nasal dorsum, and crepitation of the dorsum on palpation. Airway obstruction may result from a nasal fracture that causes dislocation of the nasal septum from the maxillary crest.

The second most common fracture of the facial skeleton is that of the mandible. The mandible is a circular or tubular structure when considered in relation to the skull. Because of its tubular structure, it tends to redistribute applied forces so that they very rarely will extend to cause fractures of the skull. Being a tubular bone, the mandible derives its strength from its cortex and is thus weakest where the cortex is thinnest. Thus, fractures are usually oblique and occur most commonly in the subcondylar angle and parasymphyseal areas (2). The most important presenting sign of a mandibular fracture is malocclusion (2). The anesthesiologist can usually ask the patient whether the teeth meet correctly (3).

On the other hand, the maxilla will redistribute the force from a blow so that the fracture may extend into the base of the skull (2). This membranous bone is very vascular and can account for a great deal of blood loss in both the prehospital and the intraoperative settings (27, 28).

Rene LeFort, in 1901, using cadaver experiments, demonstrated that there is little relationship between external signs of facial trauma and fractures of the facial skeleton. He described the three classic patterns of fractures of the facial skeleton which now bear his name (Fig. 8.3) (29).

A LeFort I fracture involves a dentoalveolar horizontal fracture and separates the entire maxillary alveolus as a unit from the remainder of the midface (2, 3). A LeFort II is a pyramidal or triangularly shaped fracture of the nasomaxillary segment from the adjacent zygomas and upper portions of the facial skeleton, essentially separating the maxilla from the zygoma (2, 3). The fracture line traverses the infraorbital foramen or travels near it and progresses across the infraorbital rim, traveling in the thin portion of the orbital floor, and then superiorly to the medial portion of the orbit to separate a portion of the nose from the nasal process of the frontal bone. Thus, a central fragment involving the maxillary alveolus, portions of the medial orbit, and the nose is separated: hence, the term *pyramidal fracture*. The LeFort III fracture is a complete disjunction of the facial bones from the cranial skeleton, the facial bones being separated through the upper orbits (2, 3).

In reality, most LeFort fractures are a complex combination of the above three: LeFort III fractures rarely exist as isolated fractures but as comminuted combinations of the other two LeFort fracture complexes. In the LeFort II and III groups, a fracture of the plate of the ethmoid bone can, as mentioned before, extend into the cribriform plate, resulting in a CSF leak (2, 3).

Presenting signs of a LeFort fracture include malocclusion due to downward displacement of the maxilla, massive facial swelling, ecchymosis, step-off deformities at

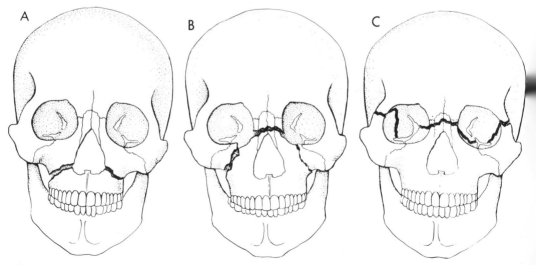

**Figure 8.3.** LeFort fractures. **A**, LeFort I; **B**, LeFort II, **C**, LeFort III. (From Krizek TJ: Management of maxillofacial trauma. In Maull KI (ed): *Advances in Trauma*. Chicago, Year Book, 1987, vol 2, pp 131–161.)

the fracture site, and mobility of the midface (1, 2). With LeFort III fractures periorbital swelling is the clue.

Fracture of the zygoma, also known as a "tripod fracture," is actually a fracture/dislocation of the malar bone. The zygomatic arch, which is also actually fractured, may be displaced medially and impinge upon the coronoid process of the mandible, making orotracheal intubation extremely difficult (3).

Generally, there are two patterns of facial injury. In one, associated with low-energy mechanisms, isolated fractures limited to one anatomic area (e.g., zygoma) are the norm. For the second, associated with high-energy mechanisms, "panfacial fractures" occur. These usually include combinations of LeFort fractures, fractures of the nasoorbitoethmoid complex, or fractures of the frontal bone (anterior table) (2).

## Perioperative Planning and Preparation: Multisystem Evaluation

Once the airway is secure, the patient's associated injuries must be evaluated. The coexisting injuries and diseases will dictate the monitoring and anesthetic management rather than the presence of facial injuries. As stated above, most trauma patients with extensive facial injuries present with coexisting neurotrauma, either open or closed. The anesthesiologist should perform a brief neurologic examination to document the level of consciousness, spinal cord injury, or other gross neurologic impairment before administering an anesthetic. Two exams are in common use for evaluating the trauma patient in the acute setting. The first is the "A,V,P,U" exam for describing the level of consciousness. This refers to the patient being Alert, responding only to Voice or Pain, or being Unresponsive. The second assessment is the Glasgow coma scale (see Table 7.3). It is based on adding the sum of scores from three different areas: spontaneous eye opening, best verbal response, and best motor response. The maximal score a patient can receive is 15, and the minimum is 3. Any patient with a Glasgow coma scale score of 8 or less is classified as being in a state of coma and has a high likelihood of an intracranial injury with increased ICP. This will usually require a method of monitoring ICP, normally initiated after further investigation with either CT scanning or MRI, and evaluation by a neurosurgeon. In this situation one should measure ICP directly (see Table 7.1) rather than use central vascular pressures as a reflection of ICPs. At the Shock Trauma Center of the Maryland Institute for Emergency Medical Services Systems (MIEMSS), patients with facial injuries who will undergo long procedures in the operating room may receive an intracranial monitor before the administration of a general anesthetic as a means of following developments intraoperatively.

The patient's respiratory function also requires thorough evaluation. A great many patients present not only with massive hemopneumothoraces but also with massive underlying pulmonary contusions. It is not uncommon for our patients to present with large alveolar-to-arterial oxygen gradients of over 500 mm Hg, many requiring mechanical ventilation with equipment that is capable of generating the high inspiratory pressures necessary to support adequate ventilation (e.g., a Seimens Servo-Ventilator).

Cardiac function tends not to be a problem in our young patient population, but these parameters need to be evaluated carefully in many patients presenting with facial trauma, especially the elderly. Again, monitoring should be individualized by the particular patient's needs. For example, in the event of a severe myocardial contusion, a pulmonary arterial catheter may be inserted as a guide for management of intravenous fluids and inotropic cardiac support.

Last, plans may need to be made for reestablishing an airway to permit better surgical management. For example, an oral or nasal endotracheal tube may have to be exchanged for a tracheostomy. This should be done under controlled elective conditions.

## Intraoperative Anesthetic Management

The immediate goals for anesthesia personnel dealing with maxillofacial trauma are to provide a safe and effective anesthetic for the patient's associated injuries and a secure uninterrupted airway both intraoperatively and in the recovery period, while also providing a relatively unobstructed field for the surgeon. At the same time, the anesthesia provider should have a clear view of the operative field and as much access to the patient's airway as possible. Good communication between the surgeon and the anesthesia team is essential in this situation.

A great many procedures can and should be carried out under local infiltration and nerve block if the patient's condition permits (30). Regional anesthesia is normally preferable to "field" blocks as the possibility of swelling and contamination is minimized (31). The supraorbital, infraorbital, nasal, maxillary, and mandibular nerves may all be blocked (32). For some larger procedures, sequential nerve blocks can provide anesthesia to entire regions (see Chapter 12). However, local anesthetic infiltration with epinephrine added to the solution will provide not only a painless field but also reasonable hemostasis. A minimal amount of epinephrine should be used as its vasoconstrictor effects may lead to tissue necrosis and wound dehiscence in poorly vascularized, traumatized areas (31). Cocaine hydrochloride, if used properly, may also provide a relatively pain-free and bloodless field.

For more extensive and longer procedures or in the patient with multisystem injury, a general anesthetic will usually be required (20). Again, the anesthetic techniques, as well as the monitoring, will be dictated more by the associated injuries than by the maxillofacial trauma itself (see Chapter 6). As most of the procedures are quite long, the anesthetist will have to maintain a constant vigil and a high index of suspicion for ongoing neurologic, respiratory, and renal injury. Many procedures involving the head, face, and neck will involve large venous structures, with the field being relatively higher than the heart. This introduces the possibility of a venous air embolus. At the MIEMSS Shock Trauma Center, mass spectrometers are available in every operating room; by monitoring exhaled gases, clinicians can detect venous air embolism by the appearance of a "nitrogen spike." For those operating rooms without these capabilities, one may use a precordial Doppler stethoscope in addition to a central venous or pulmonary arterial catheter.

For induction of anesthesia, ketamine should be avoided because of problems with raising ICP. Any of the benzodiazepines, thiopental, etomidate, or a potent narcotic can be used as long as the agent is titrated carefully against the patient's hemodynamic status. All of these agents decrease cerebral blood flow and thus would also decrease ICP. Thiopental and etomidate also decrease cerebral metabolic oxygen consumption, have better cardiovascular stability in the hypovolemic patient, and thus have some advantages. Narcotics and benzodiazepines can be used as long as respiratory depression is controlled to prevent a rise in arterial $CO_2$, which would increase ICP. For induction, the synthetic narcotics fentanyl and sufentanil work well as part of a balanced technique for longer plastic reconstructive procedures.

General anesthesia can be maintained by inhalational agents, by a balanced narcotic-muscle relaxant technique, or by a combination of both. Again, the choice is dictated by the coexisting injuries.

Nitrous oxide probably should be avoided; for an amnestic effect supplemental midazolam or a low-dose inhalational agent can be used instead. Nitrous oxide has been shown to have several deleterious effects, including promotion of tension pneumocephalus, myocardial depression, and increasing cerebral metabolism and limitation of the amount of oxygen that can be delivered to the patient (33, 34). In most severe trauma patients, an undiagnosed pneumothorax should always be suspected. Nitrous oxide can quickly convert a small pneumothorax into a tension pneumothorax. As mentioned earlier, many of these patients will have underlying pulmonary contusions and thus will need maximal oxygenation.

At the MIEMSS Shock Trauma Center, isoflurane tends to be the most widely used inhalation agent for supplementation of narcotic techniques. It provides good amnesia in low dosage, is the least metabolized of all inhalational anesthetics, decreases cerebral metabolic rate, and does not increase ICP if hyperventilation is instituted (35, 36). This anesthetic agent is used in combination with oxygen or an air-oxygen mixture. (Nitrous oxide is usually avoided, as noted above.) With this technique, a high concentration of agent may be required to provide a total anesthetic, and this may compromise hemodynamic stability in some patients. However, using an inhalational technique early during intraoperative management is useful because it can be discontinued quickly if the patient suddenly becomes unstable. An example is the patient who becomes profoundly hypotensive once a fluid-filled abdomen is opened, thereby negating any tamponade effect. Once stability is achieved and most "unknowns" become known, it may be of benefit to begin converting to a balanced technique.

Narcotic infusions work very well as part of a balanced technique for these procedures. At the MIEMSS Shock Trauma Center, these procedures can take in excess of 12 hours and patients usually are not extubated at the end of the operation. Fentanyl or sufentanil infusions can provide excellent analgesia with minimal hemodynamic compromise. The dosage rates may vary depending upon the amount of supplementation with an inhalation agent.

Muscle paralysis can be achieved by any of the nondepolarizing neuromuscular blocking agents. Hemodynamic side effects are perhaps one theoretic limitation to be considered for each agent; there are effects on various pressures (e.g., ICP, IOP). Vecuronium has the fewest cardiovascular side effects, but giving repeat bolus doses during long procedures should be accompanied by monitoring of neuromuscular blockade. A continuous infusion, with monitoring of neuromuscular transmission with a peripheral nerve stimulator, provides excellent control of depth of paralysis, as well as convenience. Pancuronium will also provide excellent paralysis. Of course, the possibility of producing tachycardia and hypertension must be kept in mind for patients with these relative contraindications. On the other hand, these may be desirable effects in the early management of a young hypotensive patient. Curare and atracurium should be used with caution because their hemodynamic effects tend to be unpredictable, especially in the hypovolemic patient, because of histamine release.

Head and neck surgery is by no means bloodless. Positioning of the patient tends to be very important during surgical repair of facial trauma. One alternative is to utilize a hypotensive technique, but this may be contraindicated by the patient's other injuries. Alternatively, the surgical field can be positioned higher than the level of the heart to decrease blood loss and allow the surgeon a clearer field in which to work. Again, the anesthesia provider must be ever alert to the possibility of a venous air embolus.

Of course, crystalloid and then colloid solutions are used early to replace intravascular volume (see Chapter 4). Transfusion of blood products will be governed by serial hematocrit measurements, coagulation studies, and the patient's general medical condition (see Chapter 5).

A Foley catheter will usually have been inserted in these patients during the initial resuscitation. If not, one should be inserted to measure urinary output as a guide to fluid requirements and as a measure of renal perfusion. The length of these procedures usually mandates the use of a urinary catheter.

## Complications

Probably the most significant complication during facial reconstruction or repair involves loss of the airway. This is perhaps the most devastating and yet preventable of all complications. Because most surgeons will desire access to the entire area around the head intraoperatively, many surgeons will elect to perform a tracheostomy before beginning the main operative procedure. This does not guarantee complete airway control, however. One may consider armored or metal endotracheal tubes that can be sutured into the tracheostomy site. Again, this does not ensure airway protection. The best method of ensuring adequate protection of the airway during surgery is maintenance of good communication between the anesthesia and surgical teams (e.g., notifying the anesthesiologist before moving the patient's head) and unwavering vigilance on the part of the anesthesia team. It may also be wise to use sutures to secure even oral or nasal tubes because sutures are more reliable than tape and because tape can distort or contaminate the tissues (6).

Another complication seen in these patients is intraoperative hyperthermia. Although malignant hyperthermia will usually present with hypertension, tachycardia, and profound respiratory and metabolic acidosis (see Chapter 13), the fever associated with surgery for facial injury is a gradual steady increase in temperature unassociated with any cardiovascular or acid/base changes. The most likely cause of benign intraoperative fever is bacteremia from traumatized perinasal sinuses. Also, heavy draping will interfere with heat loss during long surgical procedures.

Aspiration of blood and secretions is another complication of injuries of the CCFC. Many of these patients have aspirated before arrival at the trauma center and before control of the airway was gained. Intraoperatively, aspiration may present as fever, hypoxia, and hemodynamic instability. With severe tracheobronchial injury, patients may have high airway pressures with very low pulmonary compliance. These patients may require high inspiratory pressures, large amounts of positive expiratory-end pressure (PEEP), and judicious use of bronchodilators.

Other complications include pneumomediastinum, pneumopericardium, and subcutaneous emphysema, which may result from dissecting air. Again, avoidance of nitrous oxide will tend to minimize the development of these problems.

Many patients with facial trauma will present for multiple reoperations for reconstruction during ensuing months and years. Some of them may develop tracheal stenosis as a complication of multiple and prolonged intubations or tracheostomy without meticulous control of intracuff pressures (37). This possibility should be evaluated thoroughly before induction of a general anesthetic. If tracheal stenosis is documented or suspected, precautions should be taken (e.g., having smaller endotracheal tubes ready).

### Recovery Period

The recovery period can be one of the most challenging and difficult periods in the management of these patients. One must decide when to extubate patients who have not had a tracheostomy as part of the operative procedure. Because most of these procedures tend to be very long, many will opt to keep these patients intubated overnight to ensure adequate ventilatory function and eduction from anesthesia. For those who choose to extubate, very strict criteria should be followed to judge whether the patient can protect the airway. Many of these patients will have intermaxillary fixation, making an emergent laryngoscopy nearly impossible or at least not expedient (wire cutters should be kept readily available at the bedside). The patient should be awake and oriented, being able to display some cognitive function and not just follow simple commands. All muscle relaxants should be fully reversed, and the patient should demonstrate a 5-second head lift, if not contraindicated by the surgical procedure or initial injury. As with any patient recovering from anesthesia, a good tidal volume (10–15 ml/kg) and negative inspiratory force (of at least −20 mm Hg) should be demonstrated. In some instances laryngeal incompetence secondary to facial trauma may present. The cause is multifactorial, but the anesthesiologist should be aware of this possibility (38).

If possible, an orogastric or nasogastric tube should be placed before or during operation. Through this tube, the stomach should be evacuated before extubation. The pharynx should also be suctioned as thoroughly as possible before extubation.

Again, the anesthesia team and recovery personnel should be alert for signs of occult respiratory obstruction. These patients need constant vigilance throughout the recovery period.

## OCULAR INJURIES

Despite the fact that many articles have addressed the issue of intubating and anesthetizing the patient with ocular trauma, much of the information is conflicting. Thus, at present it is very difficult to make recommendations regarding the anesthetic management of patients with this type of injury. In this section, however, several pertinent issues are reviewed and relevant information is presented.

### Increased Intraocular Pressure

When discussing the subject of perioperative anesthetic management of the patient with ocular trauma, the main concern is additional extrusion of vitreous humor from an open globe secondary to a raised IOP (Fig. 8.4). IOP, as far as the anesthesia care provider is concerned, is elevated by at least three separate but interrelated issues: (a) extraocular muscle fasciculation caused by the administration of a depolarizing neuromuscular blocking agent (NMBA); (b) adrenergic stimulation caused by manipulation of the airway in an inadequately anesthetized patient, for example, during intubation; and (c) secondary effects of abnormal blood gas tensions (hypercarbia and/or hypoxia) (39–42). All of these subjects are tied to the initial management of the trauma patient, which most importantly focuses on airway management. In-

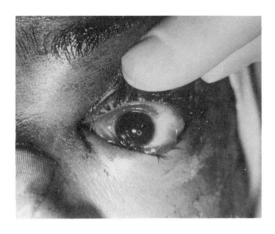

**Figure 8.4.** Ruptured globe secondary to blunt trauma. (Courtesy of Paul N. Manson, M.D.)

tubation is facilitated by the use of NMBAs and anesthetic agents; if intubation and/or ventilation is unsuccessful, $PCO_2$ levels will rise acutely. In the patient with an open globe injury, concerns common to all trauma patients influence the ability of the anesthesiologist to manage effectively those factors that affect IOP. For example, "full stomach" considerations will affect choices of techniques for airway management as well as the pharmacologic adjuncts used. Hypovolemic shock will limit the amount of anesthetic agents that can be used. Prioritization of other injuries in the multiple trauma patient may also enter into consideration (i.e., "loss of life" versus "loss of eyesight").

### Muscle Relaxants

A review of extraocular muscle fasciculation must begin with an examination of the effects of the mainstay of NMBAs, succinylcholine, and then proceed to the other agents currently in use. The majority of the literature shows that succinylcholine uniformly increases IOP by at least 6 to 12 mm Hg. The increases are rapid in onset, peak within 1 to 2 minutes, and dissipate by 2 to 6 minutes (39, 40, 43). Thus, during operation on the intact globe succinylcholine can be used without concern, as these effects would be gone by the time the globe is incised. However, in the case of the open globe, this is not true.

Once the globe has been opened either by the ophthalmologist or as a result of trauma, the IOP equals atmospheric pressure. However, administration of a depolarizing NMBA such as succinycholine will cause fasciculation of the extraocular muscles, which may literally squeeze the contents of the eye out through the opening (39, 40, 42). A similar additive effect is postulated on the basis of succinylcholine's action upon the vascular system of the eye (42).

The extraocular muscles have been described as "resistant" to the effects of succinylcholine; at least one team of investigators has demonstrated a dose-related difference in effect (39). A number of studies have examined the possibility of modifying this effect by prior administration of a nondepolarizing NMBA ("precurarization") (44–47). Although the administration of such agents has been demonstrated to be effective, the result is not to be depended upon in each and every case because of variable effects. Administration of "taming" doses of succinylcholine before the main bolus has also been suggested but is controversial (48, 49).

Succinylcholine's measured effect of increasing IOP may be confounded by simultaneous increases in systemic blood pressure when these measurements are performed in subjects who have not been given (adequate) anesthesia (50). The IOP-depressing effects of most anesthetic agents (see below) can be used to balance the opposite effects created by succinylcholine. This is a matter of timing. In one study, succinylcholine, 1 mg/kg, administered 2 minutes after thiopental, 3 mg/kg intravenously, produced no appreciable difference in IOP (51). Although the exact results vary, similar relationships have been shown by others (52).

Other investigators have examined the effects of administration of acetazolamide before injection of succinycholine. One study showed that acetazolamide (500 mg intravenously) was effective in this regard, but the reasons are not clear (53). The use of

mannitol has also been successful in preventing increases in IOP subsequent to the use of succinylcholine (41).

As an alternative to the use of succinylcholine, the sole use of nondepolarizing NMBAs has been examined (54–65). This practice has been made more attractive by the introduction of the "priming principle," in which a fraction of the total intubating dose is given several minutes before the remainder, resulting in a quicker onset of effect and an overall reduced dose (66). Still, some might disagree with using this technique in the patient with a "full stomach," as it does not permit a "rapid sequence" induction. An answer to this problem would be using a "modified rapid sequence" technique, which includes the continued application of cricoid pressure and mask ventilation with oxygen after the NMBA is administered and which would probably be more appropriate in the multitrauma patient who may have a good cause for oxygen desaturation (see Chapter 3). This would also avoid the possibility of raising intragastric pressure that is associated with succinylcholine. Additionally, whether there is a significant difference at all between using succinylcholine for "crash induction" and using a slower-acting nondepolarizing NMBA has been questioned (67, 68).

Another choice besides using the priming principle is using nondepolarizing NMBAs (which do not cause fasciculation) in a "high-dose" mode, with its associated quicker onset (69). One must then, however, suffer the consequences of a prolonged duration of action. This factor would not usually be of major importance in the multitrauma patient in whom perioperative management (including controlled ventilation) would normally be extensive anyway (see Chapter 3).

Another suggestion is the use of "inhalation induction" (39). Thus, a NMBA may be avoided completely or it may be administered after the inhalation agent has reduced the IOP (see below). The combination of succinylcholine with an inhalation agent would probably result in no net change in IOP or at least in blunting of the increases in IOP.

### Systemic Blood Pressures

The second cause of elevation of IOP is mediated by the relationship of this pressure with systemic vascular pressures (39, 42). Changes in central venous pressure have a greater effect on IOP than those in arterial pressure (42). These effects occur via changes in the blood volume of the choroid plexus of the eye. Laryngoscopy, coughing, "bucking" on an endotracheal tube, and the Valsalva maneuver will increase central venous pressure, which in turn increases the choroidal blood volume and hence IOP (by as much as 40 mm Hg) (39, 50). Similarly, decreases in the systemic pressures will result in decreases in IOP.

Except in the most obtunded trauma patients, introduction of a laryngoscope blade or an endotracheal tube (via the mouth or nose) will activate airway reflexes, stimulate the adrenergic system, and reflexly elevate blood pressure to varying degrees, often in excess of the rise in IOP caused by succinylcholine and tracheal intubation. To quote one source, this increase "in both IOP and ICP is of such magnitude as to render the succinylcholine effect almost inconsequential" (65). However, with sufficient skill and means, these effects are preventable.

The most prudent means available to the anesthesiologist to blunt airway reflexes acutely and control systemic blood pressures is the use of anesthetic induction agents. With the exception of ketamine (and possibly trichloroethylene), all of the other agents, whether inhalational or intravenous, will reduce blood pressure and thus IOP (70–76). This IOP-increasing effect of ketamine may be attenuated by intramuscular administration or by preceding it with other agents such as a diazepam-meperidine combination (77, 78). The issue then becomes one of balancing the effects of the appropriate anesthetic agents (which will decrease

IOP but also may decrease system blood pressures, especially in the hypovolemic trauma patient.) If time and circumstances permit, the use of a topical anesthetic in the pharynx and hypopharynx may attenuate the degree to which the airway is stimulated, with negligible effects on systemic blood pressure. Other approaches that have been suggested include proceeding with tracheal intubation with the patient in a 10° to 15° head-up tilt and avoiding positive-pressure breathing (39, 40).

### Blood Gases

Hypercarbia and/or hypoxia also leads to increases in IOP; therefore, it is important to maintain adequate oxygenation and ventilation (39, 40, 79). This may also mean that premedication with respiratory depressants should be avoided. Postoperative respiratory status must also be followed closely.

### Other Management Considerations

Any time surgery is performed on or near the eye, the anesthesiologist should be aware that the oculocardiac reflex may be activated (39, 41, 80). This reflex may arise when traction is applied to the extraocular muscles. The afferent signal travels via the ciliary branch of the ophthalmic division of the trigeminal nerve to the gasserian ganglion. The reflex is effected by the vagus nerve terminating at the heart, resulting in bradycardia. It can be interrupted by retrobulbar blockade (controversial) or vagal blockade with an anticholinergic agent such as atropine (41, 80).

During emergence from anesthesia, the same considerations regarding IOP must also apply. In elective situations, "deep extubation" (extubation of the trachea during a deep level of anesthesia) has been suggested (39). In the emergent trauma patient with a full stomach, this solution is not applicable, although during anesthesia every attempt should be made to evacuate the stomach contents via a gastric tube. Gastric emptying should also be promoted with metaclopromide, and an antiemetic should be administered (41).

Local or regional anesthesia (combined with retrobulbar and facial nerve blocks) of the ocular area is frequently used in the elective situation, providing many advantages (e.g., minimal intervention). However, in the emergent trauma patient, probably neither would be the method of choice (41). Manipulation of the needle when performing a retrobulbar block and deposition of local anesthetic may extrude eye contents. These techniques carry their own set of risks even in the elective situation (e.g., retrobulbar hematoma, proptosis, globe perforation) (41, 81–83). In cases where a retinal detachment has occurred as well, some ophthalmologists may attempt to use gravity to assist in retinal reattachment, requiring that the patient be placed in positions such as the steep head-up or head-down or the face-down position, which would not be tolerated well except with general anesthesia (41). In the multitrauma patient with ocular injury, ventilatory control via endotracheal intubation promotes the choice of a general anesthetic.

## Recommendation of Technique

In view of the above, it should be clear that there is no panacea. However, in an attempt to address all concerns, one may consider the following technique.

1. Administration of intravenous metaclopromide to reduce the volume of gastric contents (Additional preinduction aspiration pneumonia prophylaxis such as gastric acid neutralization may be preferred.) (84)
2. Preoxygentation with 100% $O_2$
3. Application of topical anesthetic to the mucosa of the pharynx and hypopharynx with small doses of barbiturate, benzodiazepine, and/or narcotic (with all anesthetics titrated to blood pressure and continued respiratory support)
4. Gentle application of cricoid pressure (If applied incorrectly or too vigorously, this pressure may impede venous drainage of the eye and raise IOP.)
5. Continued mask ventilation with 100% $O_2$

with cricoid pressure (with attention to airway pressure)
6. Incremental intravenous sedation (Whether to perform a superior laryngeal nerve block and/or a transtracheal block is a personal choice.)
7. Introduction of minimal amounts of inhalation agent and then gradually increasing levels
8. Administration of a priming dose of the nondepolarizing NMBA of choice or a high dose of the nondepolarizing NMBA of choice
9. Continuation of respiratory support (mask ventilation, cricoid pressure), inhalation induction, and monitoring of the level of neuromuscular blockade with peripheral nerve stimulator
10. Administration of "main bolus" of NMBA if priming dose is used
11. Continuation of respiratory support (as in point 9)
12. Laryngoscopy and intubation when appropriate according to peripheral nerve stimulator monitoring

We realize that this suggestion is not ideal. Besides *theoretically* exposing the patient to an increased risk of aspiration, it is dependent upon achieving a good mask seal. In some patients with associated maxillofacial trauma, this may not be possible. Additionally, the positioning necessary for a good mask seal may interfere with the ocular injury or may raise IOP itself. Perhaps the optimal means of achieving intubation of a patient with an open globe injury will emerge in the near future when new rapid-onset/short-acting vecuronium analogs are available for use.

## SUMMARY

In this chapter we have tried to present basic information that should be appreciated by any anesthesiologist involved in the management of victims of trauma to the CCFC. Management is complex and entails consideration of various factors, including intracranial injury, cervical injury, ocular injury, and possibilities of injuries to the airway throughout its course. Successful management, of course, cannot be guaranteed but can be maximized by internalizing a conceptual understanding of the issues and by keeping a "cool head" as critical experience is gained. Last, the practitioner is reminded that a "good" technique is one that works for the individual.

## References

1. Krizeck TJ. Management of maxillofacial trauma. In Maull KI (ed): Advances in Trauma. Chicago, Year Book, 1987, vol 2, pp 131–162.
2. Manson PN. Maxillofacial injuries. In Siegel JH (ed): Trauma: Emergency Surgery and Critical Care. New York, Churchill Livingstone, 1987, pp 983–1046.
3. Gotta AW. Maxillofacial trauma: anesthetic consideration. In ASA Refresher Courses. Park Ridge, IL, American Society of Anesthesiologists, Inc, 1987, vol 15, pp 39–50.
4. Capan LM. Perioperative management of maxillofacial, neurologic and cervical injuries. Presented at the First Annual Trauma Anesthesia and Critical Care Symposium, Washington, DC, May 1988.
5. Reath DB, Kirby J, Lynch M, Maull KI. Patterns of maxillofacial injuries in restrained and unrestrained motor vehicle crash victims. J Trauma 1989;29:806–810.
6. Hoehn RJ. Facial injuries. Surg Clin North Am 1973;53:1479–1508.
7. Phillips RM. Early management of maxillofacial war injuries. J Oral Surg 1970;28:808–813.
8. Martinez SA. Maxillofacial injury/airway obstruction. In Hurst JM (ed): Common Problems in Trauma. Chicago, Year Book, 1987, pp 3–9.
9. Manson PN, Kelly KJ. Evaluation and management of the patient with facial trauma. Emerg Med Services 1989;18:22–30.
10. Seaton JR. Soft tissue facial injuries related to vehicular accidents. Clin Plast Surg 1975;2:79–92.
11. Manson PN, Saunders JR. Anesthesia in head and neck surgery: head and neck surgery and maxillofacial trauma. Clin Plast Surg 1985;12:115–122.
12. Braunstein PW. Medical aspects of automotive crash injury research. JAMA 1957;163:249.
13. Lewis VL, Manson PN, Morgan RF, Cervillo LJ, Meyer PR. Facial injuries associated with cervical fractures: recognition, patterns and management. J Trauma 1985;25:90–93.
14. Spira M, Hardy SB. Maxims in maxillofacial management. South Med J 1972;65:1136–1137.
15. Brown AC, Sataloff RT. Special anesthetic techniques in head and neck surgery. Otolaryngol Clin North Am 1981;14:587–614.
16. Johnson RP. Anesthesia for maxillofacial injuries. J Am Assoc Nurse Anesth 1971;29:50–52.
17. Marshall M. Anaesthesia for major oral and maxillofacial surgery. Br J Anaesth 1968;40:479.
18. Kitahata LM, Collins WF. Meningitis as a complication of anesthesia in a patient with a basal skull fracture. Anesthesiology 1970;32:282–283.
19. Davies RM, Scott SG. Anesthesia for major oral and maxillofacial surgery. Br J Anaesth 1968;40:202–208.
20. Stene JK. Anesthesia for patients with facial trauma. In Manson PN (ed): Facial trauma. Baltimore, Williams & Wilkins (in press).
21. Seebucher J, Rozik D, Mathiew A. Intracranial introduction of a nasogastric tube, a complication of severe maxillofacial trauma. Anesthesiology 1975;42:100–102.
22. Grande CM, Barton CR, Stene JK. Appropriate techniques for airway management of emergency patients with suspected spinal cord injury. Anesth Analg 1988;67:714–715.
23. Grande CM, Stene JK, Bernhard WN. Airway management: considerations in the trauma patient. Crit Care Clin 1990;6:37–59.
24. Gotta AW, Sullivan CA. Anesthesia of the upper airway using topical anesthetics and superior laryngeal nerve block. Br J Anaesth 1981;53:1055–1058.
25. Gotta AW, Sullivan CA. Superior laryngeal nerve block: an aid to intubating the patient with fractured mandible. J Trauma 1984;24:83–85.
26. Miller J, Iovino W, Fire J, Klain M. High frequency jet ventilation in oral and maxillofacial surgery. J Oral Maxillofac Surg 1982;40:790–793.
27. Everett G, Meyer R, Allen GD. Blood volume changes associated with surgical treatment of fractures of the mandible. J Oral Surg 1969;27:637–639.
28. Myer RA. Blood volume considerations in oral surgery. J Oral Surg 1971;29:617–621.
29. Le Fort R. Etude experimentale sur les fractures de la machoire superieure. Rev Chir 1901;23:208–227, 360–379, 479–507.
30. Small EW. Inside-out and bottom-up: the management of maxillofacial trauma. Milit Med 1971;136:553–557.
31. Kays CR. Local infiltration versus regional anesthesia of the face: case report and review. J SC Med Assoc 1988;84:494–486.
32. Stromberg B. Regional anesthesia in head and neck surgery. Clin Plast Surg 1985;12:123–136.
33. Kitahata LM, Katz JD. Tension pneumocephalus after posterior fossa craniotomy, a complication of the sitting position. Anesthesiology 1976;44:448–450.
34. Pelligrino DA, Miletich DJ, Hoffman WE, Albrecht RF. Nitrous oxide markedly increases cerebral metabolic rate and blood flow in the goat. Anesthesiology 1984;60:405–412.
35. Madsen JB, Gold GM, Hansen ES, Bardrum B. The effect of isoflurane on cerebral blood flow and metabolism in humans during craniotomy for small supratentorial cerebral tumors. Anesthesiology 1987;65:332–336.

36. Messik JM, Casement B, Sharbrough FW, Milde L, Michenfelder J, Sundt TM. Correlation of regional cerebral blood flow with EEG changes during isoflurane anesthesia for carotid endarterectomy. Anesthesiology 1987;66:334–349.

37. Bernhard WN, Yost L, Joynes D, Cothalis S, Turndorf H. Intracuff pressures in endotracheal and tracheostomy tubes: related cuff physical characteristics. Chest 1985;87:720–725.

38. Zachariales N. Laryngeal incompetence following facial trauma. J Oral Maxillofac Surg 1985;43:638–639.

39. Holloway KB. Control of the eye during general anesthesia for intraocular surgery. Br J Anaesth 1980;52:671–679.

40. Cunningham AJ, Barry P. Intraocular pressure—physiology and implications for anesthetic management. Can Anaesth Soc J 1986;33:195–208.

41. Adams AK, Jones RM. Anaesthesia for eye surgery: general considerations. Br J Anaesth 1980;52:663–669.

42. Adams AK, Barnett KC. Anaesthesia and intraocular pressure. Anaesthesia 1966;21:202–210.

43. Pandey K, Badola RP, Kumar S. Time course of intraocular pressure hypertension produced by suxamethonium. Br J Anaesth 1972;44:191–195.

44. Bowen DJ, McGrand JC, Hamilton A. Intraocular pressure after suxamethonium and endotracheal intubation: the effect of pretreatment with tubo-curarine or gallamine. Anaesthesia 1978;33:518–522.

45. Bowen DJ, McGrand JC, Palmer RJ. Intraocular pressures after suxamethonium and intubation in patients pretreated with pancuronium. Br J Anaesth 1976;48:1201–1205.

46. Miller RD, Way WL, Hickey RF. Inhibition of succinylcholine-induced intraocular pressure by nondepolarizing muscle relaxants. Anesthesiology 1968;29:123–126.

47. Meyers EF, Krupin T, Johnson M, Zink H. Failure of nondepolarizing neuromuscular blockers to inhibit succinylcholine-induced increased intraocular pressures: a controlled study. Anesthesiology 1978;48:149–151.

48. Verma RS. "Self-taming" of succinylcholine-induced fasciculations and intraocular pressure. Anesthesiology 1979;50:245–247.

49. Myers EF, Singer P, Otto A. A controlled study of the effect of succinylcholine self-taming on intraocular pressure. Anesthesiology 1980;53:72–74.

50. Libonati MM, Leahy JJ, Ellison N. The use of succinylcholine in open eye surgery. Anesthesiology 1985;62:637–640.

51. Joshi C, Bruce DL. Thiopental and succinylcholine: action on intraocular pressure. Anesth Analg 1975;54:471–475.

52. Cook JH. The effect of suxamethonium on intraocular pressure. Anaesthesia 1981;36:359–365.

53. Carballo AS. Succinylcholine and acetazolamide (Diamox) in anaesthesia for ocular surgery. Can Anaesth Soc J 1965;12:486–498.

54. Balamoutsos NG, Tsakona H, Kanakoudes PS, Iliadelis E, Georgiades G. Alcuronium and intraocular pressure. Anesth Analg 1983;62:521–523.

55. Rich AL, Witherspoon CD, Morris RE, Feist RM. Use of nondepolarizing anesthetic agents in penetrating ocular injuries. Anesthesiology 1986;65:108–109 (letter).

56. Warner DO. Atracurium for open eye injuries. Anesthesiology 1987;66:579–580 (letter).

57. Maharaj RJ, Humphrey D, Kaplan H, Blignaut P, Brocke-Utne JG, Welsh N. Effects of atracurium on intraocular pressure. Br J Anaesth 1984;56:459–463.

58. Schneider MJ, Stirt JA, Einholt DA. Atracurium, vecuronium, and intraocular pressure in humans. Anesth Analg 1986;65:877–882.

59. Tattersall MP, Manus NJ, Jackson DM. The effect of atracurium or fazadinium on intraocular pressure: comparative study during induction of general anesthesia. Anaesthesia 1985;40:805–807.

60. Weiner MJ, Olk RJ, Meyers EF. Anesthesia for open eye surgery. Anesthesiology 1986;65:109–110 (letter).

61. George R, Nursingh A, Downing JW, Welsh NH. Nondepolarizing neuromuscular blockers and the eye: study of intraocular pressure. Br J Anaesth 1979;51:789–792.

62. Lavery GG, McGalliard JN, Mirakhur RK, Shepherd WFI. The effects of atracurium on intraocular pressure during steady state anaesthesia and rapid sequence induction: a comparison with succinylcholine. Can Anaesth Soc J 1986;33:437–442.

63. Bourke DL. Open eye injuries. Anesthesiology 1985;63:727 (letter).

64. Weiner MJ, Olk RJ, Meyers EF. Anesthesia for open eye surgery. Anesthesiology 1986;65:109–110 (letter).

65. Murphy DF, Davis NJ. Succinylcholine use in emergency eye operations. Can J Anaesth 1987;34:101–102 (letter).

66. Foldes F. Rapid tracheal intubation with non-depolarizing neuromuscular blocking drugs: the priming principle. Br J Anaesth 1984;56:663.

67. Barr AM, Thornley BA. Thiopentone and suxamethonium crash induction. Anaesthesia 1976;31:23–29.

68. Barr AM, Thornley BA. Thiopentone and pancuronium crash induction. Anaesthesia 1976;33:25–31.

69. Abbott MA, Samuel JR. The control of intraocular pressure during the induction of anaesthesia for emergency eye surgery: high-dose vecuronium technique. Anaesthesia 1987;42:1008–1012.

70. Magora F, Collins VJ. The influence of general

anesthetic agents on intraocular pressure in man. Arch Ophthalmol 1961;66:806–811.

71. Couch JA, Eltringham RJ, Magauran D. The effect of thiopental and fazadinium on intraocular pressure. Anaesthesia 1976;34:586–590.

72. Runcimann JC, Bowen-Wright RM, Welsh NH, Downing JW. Intraocular pressure changes during halothane and enflurane anaesthesia. Br J Anaesth 1978;50:371–374.

73. Oji EO, Holdcroft E. The ocular effects of etomidate. Anaesthesia 1975;34:245–249.

74. Morton NJ, Hamilton WF. Alfentanil in anaesthetic technique for penetrating eye injuries. Anaesthesia 1986;41:1148–1151.

75. Shroeder M, Linssen GH. Intraocular pressure and anaesthesia. Anaesthesia 1972;27:165–170.

76. Yoshikawa K, Murai Y. The effect of ketamine on intraocular pressure in children. Anesth Analg 1971;50:199–202.

77. Peuler M, Glass DD, Arens JF. Ketamine and intraocular pressure. Anesthesiology 1975;43: 575–578.

78. Ausinch B, Rayborn RC, Munsen ES, Levy NS. Ketamine and intraocular pressure in children. Anesth Analg 1976;55:773–775.

79. Samuel JR, Beaugie A. Effect of carbon dioxide on the intraocular pressure in man during general anaesthesia. Br J Ophthalmol 1974;58:62–67.

80. Arthur DS, Dewan KM. Anaesthesia for surgery in children. Br J Anaesth 1980;52:681–688.

81. Zaturansky B, Hyams S. Perforation of the globe during the injection of local anesthesia. Ophthalmic Surg 1987;18:585–588.

82. Ramsay RC, Knobloch WA. Ocular perforation following retrobulbar anesthesia for retinal detachment surgery. Am J Ophthalmol 1978;86: 61–64.

83. Kimble JA, Morris RE, Witherspoon CD, Feist RM. Globe perforation from peribulbar injection. Arch Ophthalmol 1987;1105:749.

84. Palazzu MGA, Stunin L. Anaesthesia and emesis: II. Prevention and management. Can Anaesth Soc J 1984;31:407–415.

# Burn Anesthesia

*William R. Furman and Judith L. Stiff*

A person who sustains a major burn suddenly is placed in a life-threatening condition that may last for many months. For the physician, the technical and physiologic problems in the care of such patients demand meticulous attention to every detail; a multidisciplinary approach is crucial to the management of burned patients.

Burns of any kind, whether due to heat, chemicals, radiation, or electricity, are characterized according to their depth and extent. The depth of destruction of skin and underlying structures is characterized as first, second, or third degree (superficial, partial-thickness, and full-thickness, respectively). In terms of prognosis, however, it is more useful to make the distinction between *first or superficial second degree* and *deep second or third degree* burns and to observe the presence or absence of associated inhalational injury. Deep second degree and all third degree burns do not heal spontaneously or do so with poor cosmetic and functional result and therefore must be surgically covered. The term fourth degree is sometimes applied when structures beneath the skin such as muscle and fascia are burned (1, 2).

Mortality from burns is greatest in infants and in the elderly and increases with increasing depth and extent of the burn.

Associated inhalational injury appears to add 30 to 40% to the level of morality associated with a burn of any size (Table 9.1) and in any age group (Table 9.2) (3, 4). However, with modern pulmonary care, smoke inhalation unassociated with burns rarely causes death if the victim is conscious on arrival at the emergency department (5). The mortality from high-voltage electrical burns is high relative to the percentage of surface burned.

The care of burned patients may be divided into three phases: the immediate resuscitative phase, the subsequent debridement and grafting phase, and the reconstructive phase (6). In each phase, the anesthesia team, as part of the entire burn care team, must address specific consider-

**Table 9.1. Burn Mortality in Relation to Burn Size and Inhalational Injury**

| % BSA Burned | Mortality (%) | |
|---|---|---|
| | Without Inhalational Injury | With Inhalational Injury |
| ≤20% | 1 | 36 |
| 21–40% | 2 | 38 |
| 41–60% | 18 | 50 |
| 61–80% | 24 | 67 |
| >80% | 47 | 83 |
| Overall | 4 | 56 |

**Table 9.2. Burn Mortality in Relation to Age and Inhalational Injury**

| Age | Mortality (%) | |
| --- | --- | --- |
| | Without Inhalational Injury | With Inhalational Injury |
| ≤4 | 2 | 44 |
| 5–14 | 1 | 38 |
| 15–44 | 5 | 54 |
| 45–59 | 15 | 58 |
| >59 | 24 | 92 |
| Overall | 4 | 56 |

ations in formulating their part of the care plan. The contribution to the team by the trauma anesthesiologist and critical care specialist (TA/CCS) varies among centers. In addition to the usual areas of airway management, safe transport to and from the operating room, and operative anesthesia, it may include fluid resuscitation and monitoring of fluid status, ventilator management and weaning, cardiovascular resuscitation, and overall intensive care. In each instance, communication with the other members of the burn care team is essential.

## IMMEDIATE RESUSCITATIVE PHASE

Three nonsurgical considerations that are of great concern in the care of the acutely burned patient are fluid administration and its monitoring (see also Chapter 4), airway management (see also Chapter 3), and evaluation of associated nonburn injuries (see also Chapter 6). Before any necessary surgical procedures can be contemplated, these three issues must usually be addressed.

### Fluids

All burn victims require large volumes of sodium-containing fluid because of tissue edema, which results from an increase in capillary permeability in the burned area (7). There are several effective formulas for estimating this need (8). In general, these are based upon a requirement for 2 to 4 ml of crystalloid per kg per 1% of body surface area burned over the first 24 hours. Each

formula provides an initial guideline from which care must be individualized based on the patient's clinical response to therapy. Victims at the extremes of age, those with larger burns (>30% total body surface area), and those with electrical burns may require fluids greatly in excess of these calculated needs (9).

Hypoproteinemia often occurs during the first 24 to 48 hours, resulting in edema of all tissues. It remains unresolved whether this hypoproteinemia is due solely to an increase in capillary permeability in the burned tissue or is due to protein leakage in the lungs and nonburned tissues as well (10). Although apparently safe and effective in this setting, the use, timing, and type of colloid remain controversial and vary among the different approaches. Early administration of colloid does not correlate with survival (7, 8, 11, 12); however, the Brooke, Parkland, and Massachusetts General Hospital formulas all prescribe 0.5 ml of colloid per 1% burn per kg during the first 48 hours of resuscitation (Table 9.3).

Secure venous access is required at first to administer the large amounts of fluid required during resuscitation and later for nutritional support and intraoperative management. The requirement for long-term venous access in patients with large burns is often best met by inserting a multilumen catheter into a large vein when the patient is first admitted.

Once initiated, it is necessary to determine the adequacy of resuscitation by observing the weight, vital signs, urine output, skin turgor, and mental status of the patient. If the urine output remains low despite the administration of what seems to be a large amount of fluids, central venous or pulmonary artery pressure monitoring is indicated. This may be particularly necessary in the elderly because, in addition to the problems imposed by preexisting cardiac disease, myocardial depression may occur, presumably as a consequence of mediators released in patients with large burns (8). Nonburned areas are preferred for the insertion of all lines because of problems

**Table 9.3   Fluid Resuscitation Formulas for Burn Patients[a]**

| Formula | First 24 hr | Second 24 hr |
|---|---|---|
| Brooke | | |
| Crystalloid | 2 ml LR/% burn/kg | $D_5W$ maintenance |
| | ½ in 1st 8 hr | |
| | ½ in next 16 hr | |
| Colloid | None | 0.5 ml/% burn/kg |
| Parkland | | |
| Crystalloid | 4 ml LR/% burn/kg | $D_5W$ maintenance |
| | ½ in 1st 8 hr | |
| | ½ in next 16 hr | |
| Colloid | None | 0.5 ml/% burn/kg |
| MGH | | |
| Crystalloid | 1.5 ml LR/% burn/kg | Not specified |
| | ½ in 1st 8 hr | |
| | ½ in next 16 hr | |
| Colloid | 0.5 ml/% burn/kg | Not specified |
| | None in 1st 4 hr | |
| | ½ in 2nd 4 hr | |
| | ½ in next 16 hr | |

[a] Abbreviations: LR, lactated Ringer's solution; $D_5W$, 5% dextrose in water; MGH, Massachusetts General Hospital.

with bacterial contamination; cutdowns also have a high rate of infection (11).

## Airway Management

Endotracheal intubation may be required to treat the four causes of early respiratory dysfunction in burned patients (see Chapter 3). These are carbon monoxide poisoning, upper airway edema, subglottic thermal and chemical burns, and chest wall restriction.

Carbon monoxide (CO) poisoning is an important cause of early mortality in victims of burns. It causes tissue hypoxia because it binds to hemoglobin 200 times more readily than does oxygen, thus greatly decreasing the oxygen carrying capacity of blood. It also increases the stability of the oxyhemoglobin molecule, decreasing release of oxygen to the tissues (13, 14).

Carbon monoxide poisoning should be suspected in all victims of fires, especially fires in confined spaces, such as buildings and automobiles. Such patients appear hypoxic; complain of headache, shortness of breath, nausea, or angina pectoris; and may be tachypneic, irritable, or delirious but are not cyanosed. The diagnosis cannot be made by routine arterial blood gase analysis as the $PO_2$ will be normal and the $PCO_2$ will be reduced by hyperventilation. Likewise, standard pulse oximetry (which measures

light absorbance at two wavelengths) cannot distinguish oxyhemoglobin from carboxyhemoglobin. Newer three-wavelength devices that can report CO saturation are being developed (15).

The diagnosis and quantification of the degree of poisoning can be made by measuring the carboxyhemoglobin level, which is expressed as a percentage of saturation of hemoglobin. Saturation of more than 15% of hemoglobin by CO is usually toxic, and over 50% is almost always lethal. CO poisoning requires the administration of 100% $O_2$, usually through an endotracheal tube, especially in a confused or comatose patient. Oxygen will displace the carbon monoxide and shorten the half-time of its elimination from about 4 hours (breathing room air) to 40 minutes (6, 16). Delayed neurologic symptoms may appear after a lucid interval of days to weeks. This is more common in older patients and those with more severe CO poisoning (17).

The upper airway is compromised within 24 hours of an inhalational injury or a burn of the face and neck. All supraglottic tissues may be affected and, if intubation is not accomplished early, edema may make it impossible later (Fig. 9.1). Upper airway injury should be suspected if the patient was burned in a closed-space fire, is hoarse, or

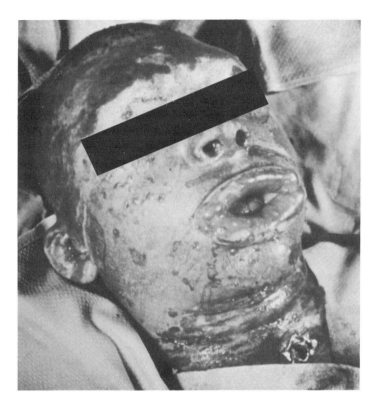

**Figure 9.1.    A patient with severe facial and upper airway burns.** Early intubation was essential in this case. Later, an elective tracheostomy was performed to facilitate management of the facial burns.

has facial burns, an injected tongue, or soot in the nasal or oral secretions. In cases where, on oral examination, the burn does not appear to involve the pharynx, fiberoptic nasopharyngoscopy may be performed to exclude the need to intubate. In mild cases, flow-volume loops may be followed as evidence of improvement or worsening, but they are no substitute for direct examination. In the presence of burned or edematous mucosa, securing the airway early is the treatment of choice (13, 16).

Tracheobronchial (subglottic) thermal injury is rare and occurs only if live steam or explosive gases are inhaled (6). However, many chemicals and products of combustion that are toxic to the tracheobronchial tree can be inhaled. These damage the lower airways during the first 48 hours and may cause bronchospasm, edema of the airways, decreased pulmonary compliance, and poor mucociliary clearance. Airway plugging,

atelectasis, and infection, leading to acute respiratory failure, often result. In particular, victims of fires in homes or buildings containing plastic and synthetic materials often have lung damage due to fumes of hydrogen chloride, a combustion product of polyvinyl chloride. Before the development of pulmonary toxicity, hydrogen chloride can cause myocardial irritation and potentiate CO toxicity (18).

In addition, the fluid, electrolyte, and protein shifts that occur during the early postburn period may exacerbate antecedent pulmonary problems and lead to pulmonary edema. Severe inhalational injuries require early intubation and mechanical ventilation, often with positive end-expiratory pressure. Corticosteroids and prophylactic antibiotics have not proven beneficial; antibiotics are used only to treat documented infections (6, 7, 16).

Circumferential chest wall burns can

compound the dysfunction caused by inhalational injury by producing massive chest wall edema, usually within 24 hours. The pulmonary restriction that results may require early escharotomy (surgical incision of the skin and subcutaneous tissues) (Fig. 9.2).

## Associated Injuries

Victims of fires must be evaluated for the existence of associated traumatic injuries. Bones are often broken when jumping out of burning houses, and blunt or penetrating trauma may occur in motor vehicle accidents that are complicated by fires. Life-threatening injuries occasionally require operative treatment during the initial resuscitation. More commonly, fixation of fractured bones takes place concurrently with the debridement and grafting of burned skin. In an effort to prevent permanent osseous deformities, reduction and fixation of severely comminuted fractures is generally undertaken as early as possible, despite the potential risks of infection.

## Surgical Procedures

In addition to the problems of fluid and airway management discussed above, there are two other major anesthetic considerations when surgery is required during the immediate postburn period. These involve the altered responses of burned patients to muscle relaxants and the problems that arise when it becomes necessary to provide anesthesia in areas outside the operating room, such as the burn unit.

Succinylcholine may provoke a massive release of potassium from muscle if administered to a burned patient, especially if the burn exceeds 10% of the body surface area (19–22). It is speculated that an increase in acetylcholine receptors occurs in the muscle of burned patients and that this is responsible for the sensitivity to succinylcholine, but this has not been confirmed (22). This response is most likely to occur between 5 days and 3 months postburn, with a peak effect between 20 and 60 days. Succinylcholine is therefore considered safe to use

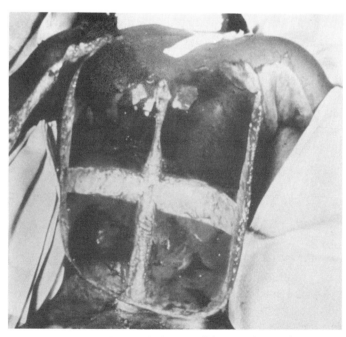

**Figure 9.2.   A patient with circumferential chest wall burns after escharotomy.** The 2- to 3-inch gaps between the cut edges of the incised skin show how tightly restricted the chest had been before the procedure.

during the first 8 to 12 hours but then is not recommended until all of the burned areas have been surgically covered with healed grafts.

Often it is necessary to provide anesthetic care for surgical procedures outside the operating room (in a burn unit). Debridements and early faciotomies or escharotomies may be required when access to the operating room is limited by the existing caseload. In such situations, a preestablished protocol for safely anesthetizing such patients is of great value. Such a protocol should provide for monitoring and resuscitative equipment at the level of current standards of care and should treat the patient in every way as if the procedure were being performed in the operating room.

The degree of pain involved in these procedures can be considerable, and adequate anesthesia with intravenous narcotics, benzodiazepines, butyrophenones, or inhalational agents often produces hypotension in this setting. An anesthetic that is easy to use in such situations is ketamine, which has been used extensively and shown to be efficacious in burn debridements. It usually provides good hemodynamic support and postoperative analgesia and requires neither an anesthesia machine nor scavenging from the environment. In patients who do not require intubation for the management of airway injury or a full stomach, protective reflexes may be preserved, even in the presence of profound analgesia, and prolonged pain relief may facilitate transfer back to the patient's bed. Although hallucinations are a potential undesirable side effect of this agent, they can be greatly minimized by the use of small doses of benzodiazepines or droperidol (19, 23–25).

## DEBRIDEMENT PHASE

After initial hemodynamic and pulmonary stabilization, the task of grafting to cover burned areas begins. Often, burn victims must undergo several operations over a period of weeks to months before all burned areas are successfully covered. As a result, a number of anesthetic problems must be solved once and their solutions applied many times. A valuable tool in such cases is a notebook kept in the department of anesthesiology for the recording of details of how monitoring and support were accomplished, how the airway was managed, and any pharmacologic or other observations that would be of help to teams providing subsequent anesthetic care (Fig. 9.3).

### Monitoring and Support

Simple tasks such as monitoring blood pressure, electrocardiogram (ECG), and oxygen saturation become more complicated when the burn involves the limbs or chest. When an arm or the lower part of a leg has been spared injury, blood pressure can be measured there by auscultation or palpation or with a Doppler device. If no limb is free of injury, a femoral arterial line is usually placed for monitoring during the resuscitation phase and is used in the operating room. An axillary arterial line is an alternative.

ECG electrode placement can be complicated by burns of the trunk and arms. Nonstandard lead placements result, making interpretation of the shape of the QRS complex and diagnosis of the nature of arrhythmias difficult. In nearly total burns, it may be necessary to use needle electrodes to achieve electrical contact. If, however, the upper arms are not part of the operative field, the ECG electrodes may be held in place with a gauze wrap; most of the topical ointments applied to burn wounds are good electrical conductors.

Pulse oximetry has become widely used in operative anesthesia as a noninvasive means of monitoring oxygen saturation in arterial blood. This technology requires that a probe be applied to a part of the body that has a pulse, such as a finger, a toe, an ear, or the nose. In many severely burned patients, successful application of such a probe is not feasible, precluding its use in situations where it would be very helpful. All potential

The
**Francis Scott Key**
Medical Center

4940 Eastern Avenue / Baltimore, MD 21224
(301) 955-0100          **Department of Anesthesiology**
                              Burn Case Record

Name _____ Victim, Burn _____  Date of Burn _____ 3/9/88 _____

History # _ 99-99-99 _____  % Deep 2° & 3° _____ 72 _____ %

Ht 68" Wt 105 kg Age 21 yr Areas Burned Face, chest, hands, back

Medical History Heavy alcohol and cocaine abuse _____

 Heavy smoke inhalation in house fire _____

Meds Morphine, Valium, Oxacillin _____

_____ Allergies None _____

Date 3/12/88 _____  IV's L SC 3-lumen ___  BP Cuff R Calf _____

Pre-op HCT _ 46% ___  Oximeter R 3rd toe   A-Line L Femoral _____

Other Labs BUN 44  ETT 8.5 _____  Other _____

Creat 2.3  K+ 4.5  Ventilator Settings 1200x18 100% O2 5cm PEEP

_____ Operative Management

Operative Site Chest, L arm _____ % BSA ___ 15% _____

Position Supine ____ EBL 3000 ml Fluids 7500 ml Blood 4 u _____

Airway Management Difficult? Already intubated. Face edematous ___

Agents Used Morphine 30 mg, Isoflurane, O2, Pancuronium _____

Date 3/16/88 _____  IV's L SC 3-lumen ___  BP Cuff R Calf _____

Pre-op HCT _ 31% ___  Oximeter R 3rd toe   A-Line L Femoral _____

Other Labs BUN 22  ETT 8.5 _____  Other _____

Creat 1.7  K+ 4.0  Ventilator Settings 1200x18 50% O2 5cm PEEP

_____ Operative Management

Operative Site Back _____ % BSA ___ 10% _____

Position Prone _____ EBL 1800 ml Fluids 3500 ml Blood 4 u _____

Airway Management Difficult? Already intubated. Face edematous ___

Agents Used Morphine 30 mg, Isoflurane, N2O/O2, Pancuronium

**Figure 9.3.** A sample page from the burn case book used at the Francis Scott Key Medical Center (Baltimore Regional Burn Center). Identifying information and a report of the first two anesthetics are entered on the front of the page, with room for three more reports on the reverse side.

monitoring sites must be tried before the technique is abandoned.

Auscultation of breath sounds and heart tones by means of an esophageal stethoscope is not limited by burns. Because of the difficulties inherent in blood pressure, ECG, and oxygen saturation monitoring, this form of monitoring is especially valuable. Temperature must also be monitored either in the esophagus or by a rectal probe.

Vascular access in patients with large burns of the arms and legs usually requires the placement of femoral, central venous, or right atrial catheters (26). Because of the need for administration of intravenous alimentation, fluids, medications, and blood products, large multiport devices containing two to four lumens are very useful. These are usually inserted via a subclavian vein, but internal jugular and femoral sites may also be used. It is not unusual for a patient with a large burn (>40%) to have no other intravascular access than one multiport subclavian venous line and a femoral arterial line. When bacterial infection complicates the course of treatment, difficult decisions are faced regarding whether to change the catheters and whether to do so before, during, or after operative debride-

ment and grafting of burn wounds. This type of situation requires a team approach to weigh the various risks and benefits of each possible course of action and cannot be dogmatically summarized. It is, however, safe to say that continuous intravenous access and ability to measure blood pressure are mandatory, especially in the operating room.

Intraoperative blood loss during excision and grafting of burn wounds can be substantial. As a rule, larger debridements result in greater blood loss, but the relationship between size of debridement and magnitude of blood loss is extremely variable. Figure 9.4 is a scattergram of the relationship between the extent of the procedure (percentage of the body surface area [BSA] excised and grafted) and the

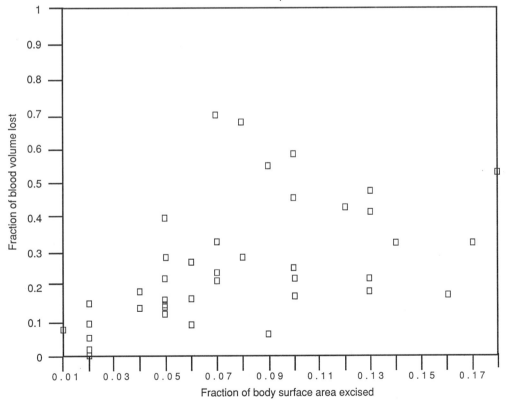

**Figure 9.4.  A scattergram of the relationship between blood loss and excision size in 40 procedures on 23 patients.** The line of best fit by least squares is $y = 0.09 + 2.12\ x$ (correlation coefficient = 0.52).

percentage of the blood volume lost during 40 consecutive debridements performed on 23 patients at the Baltimore Regional Burn Center. The line of best fit (least squares analysis) has a slope of 2.12, indicating that, for each 1% of the BSA excised and grafted, about 2% of the blood volume may be lost during operation. The graph reveals that, despite considerable variation, increasing the extent of the excision results in greater blood loss (correlation coefficient ;eq 0.52) and includes 1 patient who lost as much as 10% of the blood volume for each 1% debrided and grafted. Two previously published studies reported higher average losses, predicting that, for each 1% of the BSA to be excised and grafted, 3 to 6% of the blood volume may be lost during surgery (27, 28). Collectively, these data suggest that the only safe prediction about blood loss during burn surgery is that blood loss will be significant except when very small injuries are treated. Visual estimates of blood loss are often inaccurate; therefore, monitoring of hemodynamics, urine output, and hematocrit is necessary to prevent under- or overtransfusion of these patients.

Using the above data, it can be predicted that, for a 70-kg male patient (blood volume approximately 5250 ml), debridement of 8% of the BSA may require 3 to 4 units of blood over a period of about 60 minutes. Because of this, the importance of secure venous access and sufficient quantities of crossmatched blood available in the operating suite before the operation is begun cannot be overemphasized. In many cases, it is prudent to begin to transfuse packed red blood cells at the beginning of surgery, and it is often necessary to infuse them at a high speed to maintain an adequate intravascular volume during debridement.

Local control of blood loss after debridement (and before grafting) is often attempted by the surgeon via the application of gauze pads soaked in a vasoconstrictor, such as epinephrine. Although the amount absorbed by the patient is not known, it is possible to calculate that each pad may contain 1 to 2 mg of the drug, based on a content of between 100 and 200 ml of a 10-µg/ml solution of epinephrine in saline (10 ml of 1:1000 epinephrine in 1000 ml of 0.9% NaCl solution). In some instances, this may be beneficial, as it will support the blood pressure during a period of rapid blood loss; however, excessive levels of epinephrine can cause ventricular arrhythmias. Infants and children may be most susceptible to this complication because of their high ratio of surface area to volume. In such cases, phenylephrine is a nonarrhythmogenic alternative. Systemic absorption of part of the 1 to 2 mg of a 10-µg/ml solution per gauze pad (1 ml of 1% phenylephrine in 1000 ml of 0.9% NaCl solution) would not be expected to cause arrhythmias.

Loss of heat is a major intraoperative problem. The burned patient is hypermetabolic, a problem exacerbated in a cold environment (29). Because uncovered tissue suffers evaporative and radiant heat loss, exposure to the cold, dry ambient conditions of the operating room can rapidly lower the body temperature (see also Chapter 13). Every method of thermal conservation available should be used in burned patients, especially children. These include warming antiseptic and intravenous solutions, heating the environment above 25°C (77°F) if possible, using a heating pad on the operating table and heat lamps, insulating the patient by covering the head and limbs if not part of the operative field, and covering any part of the field that is not actively being debrided or grafted. Ventilating with heated, humidified gases or at low fresh gas flows may be especially helpful in reducing evaporative heat loss via the respiratory tract.

## Airway Management

Induction of anesthesia and intubation of the airway of a burn patient who has not sustained an inhalational injury are straightforward (Chapter 3), apart from altered muscle relaxant pharmacology (discussed below). A potential exception to this is the patient with facial and neck burns. Topical antibiotic creams applied to the face can make airtight application of an anesthesia mask difficult, and contracture of the skin of the neck and around the lips may limit exposure of even a normal larynx (Fig. 9.5). Depending upon the severity of these problems, gas induction by mask to assure the ability to control the airway or awake intubation, either orally or nasally, may be necessary. A fiberoptic bronchoscope is a very useful adjunct for intubation in this setting.

### Pharmacology

The potency of agents used to induce anesthesia is not altered in burned patients (19). The choice of agent is therefore based, as for any patient, on the cardiovascular status before induction. Thiobarbiturates can be used safely; ketamine and etomidate are preferred in the presence of hypovolemia.

Depolarizing muscle relaxants are known to cause hyperkalemia, especially 20 to 60 days postburn. Although it has not been proven dangerous to use them during the first few days, it is recommended to avoid them after 8 to 12 hours postburn. Likewise, although they are not proven to be unsafe after 90 days, some authors suggest, based on indirect evidence, that they be avoided longer than that (6 to 24 months). This recommendation is based on the theory that the etiology of sensitivity to depolarizing muscle relaxants is related to an increase in acetylcholine receptors. Such an increase is seen after experimental denervation injury (another situation where depolarizing muscle relaxants cause hyperkalemia) and is postulated to occur in burned patients. This increase (in the denervated muscle model) begins after 2 days, is greatest between 1 and 3 weeks, and may persist for as long as 2 years (19–22).

If succinylcholine is administered inadvertently and ECG abnormalities develop, the patient should be treated for presumed hyperkalemia. Calcium, sodium bicarbonate, hyperventilation, and/or glucose and insulin may be required.

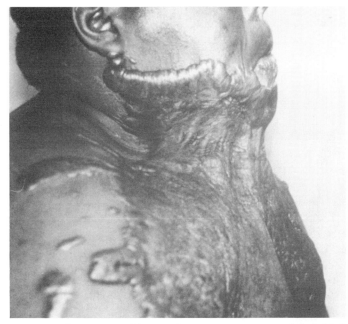

**Figure 9.5.   A 450-pound patient with scarring, contracture, and keloid formation after a chemical burn of the neck.** During both the debridement period and part of the reconstructive period (until excision of these scars was completed), intubations were performed nasally with a fiberoptic bronchoscope because it was not possible to extend the neck during laryngoscopy.

Burned patients are resistant to the nondepolarizing muscle relaxants (NDMRs) in current clinical use, especially if the burned area exceeds 40% of the BSA. Below 10% BSA, this effect is seldom seen. Both the dose and serum concentration level may need to be increased to two to five times what would usually be required to achieve relaxation in a patient of the same age and size. In the case of d-tubocurarine, alterations in protein binding and pharmacokinetics do not seem to explain this abnormality fully (30). Studies fully characterizing the pharmacokinetics of the other NDMRs have not been reported, but it appears that, despite requirements for large doses of these agents, neither their elimination nor the ability to antagonize their effects is significantly altered (19, 22, 30–34). The classic explanation of NDMR resistance in burn victims has been that burn injury leads to an increase in the number of acetylcholine receptors (35). More recently, this theory has been disputed (36), and evidence suggests that the plasma of burn victims has an anticurare effect (37).

Benzodiazepines are often used in anesthetic care to achieve preoperative sedation and intraoperative amnesia. In the burned patient, diazepam and chlordiazepoxide have been shown to have shortened periods of therapeutic efficacy. This is believed to be due to rapid redistribution of the drug from the brain to other tissues caused by the hypermetabolic condition of burn victims. With repeated doses, however, active metabolites of these drugs accumulate (with prolonged half-lives because of impaired hepatic clearance), leading to prolonged sedation (19, 38). The concomitant administration of cimetidine, often used to reduce the risk of stress ulcers, further reduces diazepam clearance. The new $H_2$-blocker, ranitidine, does not seem to affect diazepam metabolism but does increase the soporific effects of the newer benzodiazepine, midazolam (39).

Narcotic analgesics are required by most if not all burn victims, particularly for control of the pain of first and second degree burns (third degree burns include nerve damage and are usually painless). Although narcotics are widely used and suspicions are widely held that burn patients are resistant to their effects, this has not been borne out by research. One pharmacokinetic study indicated that eight burn patients (of whom seven had major burns) were not different from normal controls with regard to plasma concentration-time profiles after the intravenous administration of morphine and that the degrees of pain relief achieved at each plasma level were comparable in the two groups (40). Studies of the pharmacokinetic properties of the other narcotic analgesics have yet to be published; however, they all seem safe to use in operative anesthesia. The common wisdom, however, dictates that narcotics be administered cautiously during excision and grafting of burned areas, at least until the blood loss associated with the procedure is complete and replenished. Once this is done, postoperative pain must be expected to be considerable. No instances of iatrogenic narcotic addiction have been reported in burned patients receiving large doses of narcotics for control of severe pain, even over long periods (19, 40).

Inhalational agents have been used safely for years, and the most experience has been with halothane. Repeated administration of halothane has not been associated with an increased risk of hepatitis. Potential theoretical advantages of isoflurane over halothane and enflurane (least production of metabolic products, least cardiovascular depression) remain to be proven (19). In clinical use, inhalational agents are favored by many because they offer the potential advantage of being easy to eliminate from the patient in the event of severe hypotension resulting from unexpectly rapid blood loss, an advantage not shared by narcotics and other intravenous agents.

## Burn Wound Sepsis

Burn patients suffer immunosuppression, which may lead to septic complications (41). Bacterial infection and septic shock are ever-present concerns and, as aggressive surgical debridement and coverage with allograft are viewed as important measures in the control of infection, it is often necessary to proceed with anesthesia despite hemodynamic instability (12). Maintaining the blood pressure in the face of surgical blood loss in a septic patient can be particularly difficult. It requires an anesthetic technique designed to minimize cardiac depression and vasodilation as sepsis is usually characterized by a low systemic arterial resistance, resulting in hypotension despite a normal or high cardiac output (Chapter 4). The standard management of this problem in intensive care settings is to provide hemodynamic support with dopamine in an effort to restore the systolic blood pressure to normal. When dopamine fails, an agent with greater vasoconstrictive properties, such as norepinephrine or phenylephrine, is often used. The same management is recommended in operative settings, although no studies have shown that outcomes are favorably altered by raising blood pressure toward normal in septic shock, where the cardiac output is high (42).

## Other Considerations

Burn injury may affect major organ systems, and victims who have preexisting disease may have a worsening of their condition (Chapter 6). Often it is necessary to anesthetize a compromised patient, it being neither practical nor advantageous to await the resolution of major organ system dysfunction or failure.

Renal failure (Chapter 4) occurs in up to 30% of burn patients. Causes include toxic effects of chemicals associated with burns such as sodium bichromate, toxic effects of antibiotics, prerenal azotemia due to inadequate fluid resuscitation, acute tubular necrosis due to hemoglobinuria or myoglobinuria, or, most commonly, a form of polyuric renal failure characterized by a low fractional excretion of sodium (43). This last form of acute renal failure usually has its onset 2 to 3 weeks postburn and may be so severe as to require dialysis.

Myoglobinemia and myoglobinuria are often observed after high-voltage electrical and lightning injuries and can also be found in victims of thermal burns (9, 44, 45). Although the mechanism of toxicity of these pigments has not been clearly defined, the current treatment is to induce diuresis with mannitol and to alkalinize the urine (46, 47). In deep muscle damage, such as that occurring in electrical burns, adequate debridement and often amputation are necessary to stop the excretion of myoglobin.

For the anesthesiologist, renal failure from any cause has two important implications. Excretion of agents dependent upon renal clearance will be reduced, resulting in longer half-lives of these drugs. Second, electrolyte and free water clearance will be limited, resulting in a greater sensitivity to the composition of fluids administered intravenously. Excess potassium in fluids or plasma protein may cause hyperkalemia, excess chlorides may cause metabolic acidosis, and inadequate volume may worsen whatever degree of renal failure is present.

When a patient with cardiac disease sustains a burn, a number of insults must be borne by an already damaged heart in addition to myocardial depression caused by mediators released during the immediate postburn period (8). Hypoxia during exposure to carbon monoxide, massive alterations in preload during resuscitation, and major increases in afterload from endogenous catecholamine release during periods of stress from intubation, surgery, or pain from simply moving about can all contribute directly or indirectly to myocardial ischemia and pump failure. Electrically injured patients may sustain cardiac muscle injury, resulting in myocardial damage and arrhythmias.

Such patients are usually continuously monitored in the burn unit with an ECG and pulmonary artery and arterial catheters and are often treated with vasoactive agents. The anesthesiologist needs to understand the management plan initiated in the burn unit and to continue it successfully during transport to the operating room, surgery, and transport back to the burn unit. In addition to safeguarding the integrity of the many monitoring lines and infusion devices in use, adjustment of the rate of delivery of vasoactive agents may be required to offset the effects of changes in blood volume or in depth of anesthesia and surgical stimulation.

Selection of ventilator settings during anesthesia for patients with respiratory failure is relatively straightforward. The settings (rate, depth, inspired oxygen tension, and level of positive end-expiratory pressure, if any) that were successful in the burn unit are selected, and pulse oximetry, end-tidal $CO_2$, and arterial blood gas measurements are used to confirm or modify them. In all burn patients, including those without respiratory problems, the minute ventilation is elevated because both oxygen consumption and carbon dioxide production increase with increasing burn size (48). Additionally, if inhalation injury has occurred, there may be an increased ratio of dead space to tidal volume. At the end of the procedure, mechanical ventilatory support is continued (Chapter 6). Subsequent weaning from mechanical support and eventual extubation are based on the same principles as in any other intensive care setting. Weaning should be deferred in the presence of cardiovascular instability, hypothermia, significant metabolic derangement, sepsis, or signs of worsening pulmonary status (infection, pulmonary edema, compliance, airway resistance, or secretions). Extubation should be delayed if the patient is not alert enough to protect the upper airway from obstruction and aspiration (49).

Often extensive excision and grafting in a patient with a major burn is considered a derangement significant enough to warrant postoperative intubation and ventilatory support for several hours. Even in the absence of other indicators of the need to ventilate, this means of assuring oxygen-ation and ventilation may be indicated during what is viewed as a period of potential risk. Another situation where a patient who has airway mechanics suitable for extubation might need to remain intubated after operation is when the grafts are applied to the patient's back and the postoperative plan calls for the patient to remain prone after surgery. Reintubation in the event of decompensation would compromise the grafts; hence, when in doubt, it may be best to delay extubation.

## RECONSTRUCTIVE PHASE

For months to years after hospital discharge, victims of major burns return for reconstructive procedures to remove or reduce scar tissue, with the aim of improving both cosmetic and functional outcomes. As a rule, these patients can be treated as other plastic surgery patients, although some authors recommend avoidance of depolarizing neuromuscular blocking agents until 2 years after the initial injury (22). The major ongoing problems in this patient group are the physical effects of contractures and the psychologic effects of undergoing repeated procedures over a long period (especially in children) (Chapter 11). Where the contractures affect the face and neck, intubation may continue to be difficult. Limb contractures may require special care in surgical positioning to avoid stretch or pressure on peripheral nerves which might result in a postoperative peripheral neuropathy.

## SUMMARY

The anesthetic management of burn patients is a challenging problem where all aspects of physiology and pharmacology must be considered. Anesthesia care providers function as part of a team where communication and cooperation among all members is essential. It can be most rewarding to participate over the course of months to years in the progressive recovery of these patients from their devastating injuries.

# References

1. Munster AM. Burn wound. In Cameron JL (ed): Current Surgical Therapy. St Louis, CV Mosby, 1986, pp 460–461.
2. Robson MC, Kucan JO. The burn wound. In Wachtel TL, Kahn V, Frank HA (eds): Current Topics in Burn Care. Rockville, MD, Aspen Systems, 1983, pp 55–57.
3. Herndon DN, Thompson PB, Linares HA, Traber DL. Postgraduate course: respiratory injury, part I. J Burn Care Rehabil 1986;7:184–191.
4. Zikria BA, Weston AB, Chodoff M, Ferrer JM. Smoke and carbon monoxide poisoning in fire victims. J Trauma 1972;12:641–645.
5. Heimbach DM. Smoke inhalation: current concepts. In Wachtel TL, Kahn V, Frank HA (eds): Current Topics in Burn Care. Rockville, MD, Aspen Systems, 1983, pp 31–39.
6. Welch GW. Anesthesia for the thermally injured patient. In Artz CP, Moncrief JA, Pruitt BA (eds): Burns: a Team Approach. Philadelphia, WB Saunders, 1979, pp 299–306.
7. Demling RH. Burns. N Engl J Med 1985;313:1389–1398.
8. Moncrief JA. Replacement therapy. In Artz CP, Moncrief JA, Pruitt BA (eds): Burns: A Team Approach. Philadelphia, WB Saunders, 1979, pp 169–192.
9. Luce EA, Gottlieb SE. "True" high-tension electric injuries. Ann Plast Surg 1984;12:321–326.
10. Demling RH, Kramer G, Harms B. Role of thermal injury-induced hypoproteinemia on fluid flux and protein permeability in burned and nonburned tissue. Surgery 1984;95:136–144.
11. Tompkins RG, Burke JF. Fluid and nutritional management of the burn patient. In Cameron JL (ed): Current Surgical Therapy. St Louis, CV Mosby, 1986, pp 466–469.
12. Munster AM. Burn Care for the House Officer. Baltimore, Williams & Wilkins, 1980.
13. Lamb JD. Anaesthetic considerations for major thermal injury. Can Anaesth Soc J 1985;32:84–92.
14. Dreisbach RH. Handbook of Poisoning: Diagnosis & Treatment. Los Altos, CA, Lange Medical Publications, 1974, pp 228–232.
15. Barker SJ, Tremper KK, Hufstedler S, Hyatt J, Zaccari J. The effects of carbon monoxide inhalation on noninvasive oxygen monitoring. Anesth Analg 1986;65:S12 (abstract).
16. Demling RH. Postgraduate course: respiratory injury, part III. J Burn Care Rehabil 1986;7:277–284.
17. Choi IS. Delayed neurologic sequelae in carbon monoxide intoxication. Arch Neurol 1983;40:433–435.
18. Dyer RF, Esch VH. Polyvinyl chloride toxicity in fires. JAMA 1976;235:393–397.
19. Martyn J. Clinical pharmacology and drug therapy in the burned patient. Anesthesiology 1986;65:67–75.
20. Gronert GA, Theye RA. Pathophysiology of hyperkalemia induced by succinylcholine. Anesthesiology 1975;43:89–99.
21. Schaner PJ, Brown RL, Kirksey TD, Gunther RC, Ritchey CR, Gronert GA: Succinylcholine hyperkalemia in burned patients. Anesth Analg 1969;48:764–769.
22. Martyn JAJ, Goldhill DR, Goudsouzian NG. Clinical pharmacology of muscle relaxants in burned patients. J Clin Pharmacol 1986;26:680–685.
23. White PF, Way WL, Trevor AJ. Ketamine—its pharmacology and therapeutic uses. Anesthesiology 1982;56:119–136.
24. Martinez S, Achauer B, de Rios MD. Ketamine use in a burn center: hallucinogen or debridement facilitator?. J Psychoactive Drugs 1985;17:45–49.
25. Demling RH, Ellerbe S, Jarrett F. Ketamine anesthesia for tangential excision of burn eschar: a burn unit procedure. J Trauma 1978;18:269–270.
26. Smith RC, Hartemink RJ, Duggan D. Prolonged multipurpose venous access in burned patients: three years' experience with Hickman right atrial catheters. J Trauma 1985;25:634–638.
27. Snelling CFT, Shaw K. Quantitative evaluation of blood loss during debridement and grafting of burns. Can J Surg 1982;25:416–417.
28. Canizaro PC, Sawyer RB, Switzer WE. Blood loss during excision of third-degree burns. Arch Surg 1964;88:800–802.
29. Wilmore DW, Mason AD, Johnson DW, Pruitt BA. Effect of ambient temperature on heat production and heat loss in burn patients. J Appl Physiol 1975;38:593–597.
30. Martyn JAJ, Matteo RS, Greenblatt DJ, Lebowitz PW, Savarese JJ. Pharmacokinetics of d-tubocurarine in patients with thermal injury. Anesth Analg 1982;61:241–246.
31. Dwersteg JF, Pavlin EG, Heimbach DM: Patients with burns are resistant to atracurium. Anesthesiology 1986;65:517–520.
32. Hagen J, Martyn JAJ, Szyfelbein SK, Goudsouzian NG: Cardiovascular and neuromuscular responses to high-dose pancuronium-metocurine in pediatric burned and reconstructive patients. Anesth Analg 1986;65:1340–1344.
33. Martyn JAJ, Goudsouzian NG, Matteo RS, Liu LMP, Szyfelbein SK, Kaplan RF: Metocurine requirements and plasma concentrations in burned paediatric patients. Br J Anaesth 1983;55:263–268.
34. Mills A, Martyn JAJ: Evaluation of vecuronium neuromuscular blockade in pediatric patients with thermal injury. Anesth Analg 1987;66:S119.
35. Kim C, Fuke N, Martyn JAJ. Burn injury to rat increases nicotinic acetylcholine receptors. Anesthesiology 1988;68:401–406.

36. Marathe PH, Haschke RH, Slattery JT, Zucker JR, Pavlin EG Acetylcholine receptor density and acetylcholinesterase activity in skeletal muscle of rats following thermal injury. Anesthesiology 1989;70:654–659.

37. Storella RJ, Martyn JAJ, Bierkamper GG. Anti-curare effect of plasma from patients with thermal injury. Life Sci 1988;43:35–40.

38. Martyn JAJ, Greenblatt DJ, Quinby WC: Diazepam kinetics in patients with severe burns. Anesth Analg 1983;62:293–297.

39. Kirch W, Hoensch H, Janisch HD: Interactions and non-interactions with ranitidine. Clin Pharmacokinet 1984;9:493–510.

40. Perry S, Inturrisi CE: Analgesia and morphine disposition in burn patients. J Burn Care Rehabil 1983;4:276–279.

41. Munster AM, Winchurch RA, Thupari JN, Ernst CB: Reversal of postburn immunosuppression with low-dose polymixin B. J Trauma 1986; 26:995–998.

42. Breslow MJ, Miller CF, Parker SD, Walman AT, Traystman RJ: Effect of vasopressors on organ blood flow during endotoxin shock in pigs. Am J Physiol 252 (Heart Circ Physiol 21) 1987;H291–H300.

43. Planas M, Wachtel T, Frank H, Henderson LW: Characterization of acute renal failure in the burned patient. Arch Intern Med 1982;142: 2087–2091.

44. Haberal M: Electrical burns: a five-year experience. J Trauma 1986;26:103–109.

45. Walsh MB, Miller SL, Kagen LJ: Myoglobinemia in severely burned patients: correlations with severity and survival. J Trauma 1982;22:6–10.

46. Eneas JF, Schoenfeld PY, Humphreys MH: The effect of infusion of mannitol-sodium bicarbonate on the clinical course of myoglobinuria. Arch Intern Med 1979;139:801–805.

47. Ron D, Taitelman U, Michaelson M, Gad B, Bursztein S, Better OS: Prevention of acute renal failure in traumatic rhabdomyolysis. Arch Intern Med 1984;144:277–280.

48. Saffle JR, Medina E, Raymond J, Westenskow D, Kravitz M, Warden GD. Use of indirect calorimetry in the nutritional management of burned patients. J Trauma 1985;25:32–39.

49. Wallfisch HK. Postgraduate course: respiratory injury, part IV. J Burn Care Rehabil 1986; 7:285–293.

# 10

# The Pregnant Trauma Patient

*Andrew P. Harris, Charles R. Barton,*
*and C. Russell Baker*

Overall, trauma ranks as the third leading cause of death in the United States. Among individuals under the age of 40 years, however, trauma is the leading cause of death. Since pregnancy occurs predominantly in this age group, it is understandable that trauma during pregnancy is not uncommon; in fact, in a recent series, 2.5% of patients admitted to the Maryland Institute for Emergency Medical Services Systems were pregnant (1). Anesthesia providers who practice in similar settings are, therefore, occasionally faced with the challenge of providing resuscitative and anesthetic care to pregnant patients who sustain a variety of injuries, ranging from relatively minor to life-threatening. Once pregnancy is suspected or diagnosed in a trauma patient, a rational plan for anesthetic management can be made by incorporating the principles of fetal and maternal physiology into the usual clinical algorithms for trauma patients.

## ESTABLISHING THE DIAGNOSIS OF PREGNANCY

The possibility of pregnancy should be considered in any injured female of childbearing age, and an attempt to ascertain the diagnosis of pregnancy should be undertaken concurrently with preliminary management. In many situations, the diagnosis of pregnancy can be made simply by observation or manual palpation of a pregnant uterus through the abdominal wall or, if the patient is conscious, by obtaining a menstrual history. When the patient is unable to render an accurate history, family members should be questioned regarding the possibility of pregnancy.

Further testing should be performed when the question of pregnancy remains unanswered after the history and initial physical examination. The uterus can be examined sonographically or radiographically for the presence of a fetus. Sonographic studies are useful as early as 5 weeks of gestation, but specialized pulse-echo sonographic equipment must be used (2). Radiographic detection of pregnancy (by skeletal calcification) can be done as early as 16 weeks, although only one-half of 24-week pregnancies can be positively diagnosed this way (3). The detection of fetal heart tones using a Doppler fetal heart tone monitor can also document pregnancy and is consistently useful as early as 12 weeks of gestation (3). Even in the absence of fetal heart tones, the patient may nonetheless be pregnant because the pregnancy may still be too early to detect or fetal death in utero may have occurred. A large, gravid uterus, especially if injured, presents further risks to the mother even if fetal death has occurred. These risks include vena caval obstruction and coagulopathy (see below).

The most common in vitro test for pregnancy is the detection of human chorionic gonadotropin (hCG) in the blood or urine. Urine latex fixation immunoassay hCG tests may be inaccurate in trauma patients because a false-positive or equivocal result may be obtained in the presence of proteinuria or hematuria (4). The definitive in vitro test of pregnancy is a determination of serum $\beta$-hCG level by either radioimmunoassay (RIA) or radioreceptor assay. The serum RIA can be accurate as early as the 1st week of pregnancy.

Usual trauma protocols can be followed if pregnancy is ruled out. However, whenever pregnancy has not been ruled out or has indeed been confirmed, subsequent care should be modified by giving consideration to the principles outlined in this chapter.

## MATERNAL PHYSIOLOGIC CHANGE DURING PREGNANCY

### Respiratory System

Physical changes of the respiratory system occur during pregnancy and affect anesthetic care (Table 10.1). Capillary engorgement of the respiratory mucosa results in swelling of the membranes lining the pharynx, larynx, and trachea. For this

**Table 10.1.  Respiratory Changes of Pregnancy**

| |
|---|
| Respiratory mucosal engorgement |
| È PaCO$_2$ |
| À PaO$_2$ |
| s1. È Total lung capacity |
| È Functional residual capacity (FRC) |
| È FRC−CV |
| Subjective dyspnea |
| Slight tachypnea |

reason, manipulation and instrumentation of the airway may be more hazardous than in nonpregnant patients; bleeding from traumatic instrumentation occurs more readily, and upper airway obstruction may occur more easily when the patient is rendered unconscious. Smaller endotracheal tubes than usual (e.g., 6.0 to 7.0 mm I.D.) are used routinely, as are smaller nasopharyngeal airways.

Arterial blood gases at term pregnancy differ from nonpregnant values. After the first trimester, hyperventilation and relative hypocapnia are present for the remainder of the pregnancy. PaCO$_2$ is normally 28 to 32 torr at term. Despite hypocapnia, arterial pH is unchanged because of a compensatory decrease in serum bicarbonate resulting in a metabolically compensated respiratory alkalosis. The decrease in PaCO$_2$ does result in a higher alveolar (and therefore arterial) PO$_2$ than normal: PaO$_2$ frequently increases to 100 to 105 torr. These arterial blood gas changes should be taken into consideration whenever arterial blood gases are being evaluated in a pregnant patient because, for instance, a PaCO$_2$ considered within the range of normal in a nonpregnant patient may represent CO$_2$ retention or pulmonary insufficiency at term pregnancy.

Other pulmonary functions also change with pregnancy. Although the enlarging uterus mechanically results in a 4-cm cephalad elevation of the maternal diaphragm, full diaphragmatic excursion is maintained during pregnancy. The anteroposterior and transverse diameters of the thoracic cage increase by approximately 2 cm, with the net effect being changes in the parturient's lung volumes and capacities. Although total lung capacity is either unchanged or decreased by 5% at most, functional residual capacity (FRC) decreases by approximately 20%. This decrease results from concurrent decreases in both expiratory reserve volume and residual volume. When this change in functional residual capacity is combined with increasing oxygen demands of the mother and fetus as pregnancy progresses, it becomes clear (a) why pregnant patients who hypoventilate or become apneic desaturate so rapidly and (b) why protection of the airway, maintenance of normal ventilation, and the use of supplemental oxygen therapy are so important in parturients.

These pulmonary changes have other ramifications as well. As pregnancy progresses, abdominal breathing decreases in favor of thoracic breathing. A pregnant patient with a thoracic injury may thus be unable to maintain normocarbia if the injury impairs her ability to use the chest wall during breathing. The above-mentioned decrease in functional residual capacity also leads to a narrowing of the difference between functional residual capacity and closing volume (FRC−CV). Because FRC further decreases in the supine position, one-third to one-half of pregnant patients near term will actually develop airway closure during normal tidal ventilation when they lie supine (5); this may further contribute to impaired oxygenation.

Normal respiratory changes of pregnancy can confound diagnosis in the traumatized patient. Some women develop subjective dyspnea during normal pregnancy, and this can be confused with dyspnea as a sign of blunt chest injury. Minute ventilation increases approximately 50% during pregnancy, and the accompanying increase in respiratory rate can confuse the diagnosis of respiratory distress secondary to traumatic injury. Finally, even moderate hypoventilation, for reasons mentioned above, results in marked and rapidly occurring hypoxemia, which may seem disproportionate to the extent of the traumatic injury.

## Cardiovascular System

A summary of the changes in the cardiovascular system is given in Table 10.2. Total blood volume, plasma volume, and red blood cell volume increase linearly from the beginning of gestation through the end of the 8th month of pregnancy (6). By term, total blood volume has increased by 40%, plasma volume by 50%, and red blood cell mass by 30%. Cardiac output increases 50% by the 28th week of gestation, with increases in both heart rate and stroke volume (7) paralleling the increase in blood volume.

Several normal cardiovascular changes of pregnancy confound the accurate diagnosis of hypovolemia and hypotension by affecting normally useful clinical and laboratory criteria (see Chapter 4). Heart rate increases during pregnancy, and slight tachycardia may therefore not be reflective of hypovolemia. Mean arterial pressure tends to decrease over the course of pregnancy, and thus diagnosing hypovolemia may be difficult in some cases. Finally, because plasma volume increases during gestation to a much greater extent than red blood cell volume, a "physiologic anemia of pregnancy" results. Although the hematocrit is lower by the end of gestation, total blood cell mass is actually increased. This should be kept in mind when estimating blood loss by conventional laboratory methods and when planning blood replacement.

The pattern of venous return is markedly changed during the second half of pregnancy. As the enlarging uterus grows out of the pelvis, it begins to impair blood flow returning to the heart through the inferior vena cava. Collateral routes develop, including the azygous and epidural venous systems. Despite these collaterals, venous return to the heart from the lower extremi-

**Table 10.2.   Cardiovascular Changes**

| |
|---|
| À Total blood volume |
| À Plasma volume |
| À Red blood cell mass |
| À Heart rate |
| À Cardiac output |

ties can be diminished acutely if the uterus further impinges upon the inferior vena cava, a condition occurring when the pregnant patient lies supine. In the supine position, the baroreceptor reflexes usually are capable of responding to the drop in blood pressure that occurs as a result of decreased venous return to the heart. Tachycardia and vasoconstriction occur; in fact, blood pressure usually normalizes and the heart rate increases in response to vena caval occlusion. Approximately 2 to 10% of pregnant patients are incapable of such compensatory baroreceptor-mediated responses and become hypotensive and bradycardic when they lie supine (the "supine hypotensive syndrome") (8). Because a generalized vasoconstriction is necessary to implement the normal baroreceptor response to supine positioning, this homeostatic capability may be easily overwhelmed in any hypovolemic pregnant patient who cannot further vasoconstrict, and massive hypotension can result. Even if blood pressure could be maintained, this would be accomplished at the expense of vasoconstriction of various vascular beds, including the uterus, and fetal distress might ensue. For all of these reasons, whenever evaluating or treating any pregnant patient past the midpoint of gestation, left uterine displacement should be always utilized and the supine position avoided. Of course, any maternal spinal injuries that may also be present should be taken into consideration.

The electrocardiogram changes during pregnancy as well. Slight left axis deviation is expected, as well as T wave flattening in lead III. The heart is physically displaced by the elevated diaphragm, and the point of maximal impulse is more superior and lateral than would otherwise be expected.

## Coagulation System

As gestation progresses, pregnant women become hypercoagulable. This hypercoagulable state may function to avoid excessive uterine blood loss immediately after delivery. A summary of the changes in coagula-

tion factors and inhibitors during normal pregnancy is given in Table 10.3. With the exception of factors XI and XIII, the levels of the blood coagulation factors listed are either normal or elevated. The level of antithrombin III (also known as heparin cofactor), one of the protease inhibitors that inactivate circulating blood coagulation factors, decreases.

Amniotic fluid has thromboplastin-like activity, and the uterus can be a source of plasminogen activator. Because both uterine and amniotic fluid have procoagulant activity, uterine and placental injuries resulting in hematomas or amniotic fluid emboli may produce a consumptive coagulopathy that progresses to a disseminated intravascular coagulation (DIC). When fetal death occurs in utero, DIC can likewise ensue. In patients with possible traumatic injury to the uterus or in whom fetal death has occurred in utero, the presence of coagulopathy should be ruled out using appropriate clinical or laboratory evaluation.

## Gastrointestinal System

Several changes in the gastrointestinal system occur during pregnancy. The gravid uterus alters the functional anatomy of the stomach and surrounding structures, which results in (a) the gastroesophageal junction becoming relatively incompetent, allowing gastric reflux; and (b) the pylorus being displaced as well, slowing gastric emptying. Hormonal changes associated with pregnancy (e.g., increased progesterone, decreased motilin) produce further delay in gastric emptying and diminished tone of the lower esophageal sphincter. The growing uterus physically increases intraabdominal pressure (and, therefore, intragastric pressure), and this increase may be augmented by the presence of blood in the abdomen of

**Table 10.3.  Coagulation Changes**

À Fibrinogen, factor VIII, factor XII
È Factor XI, factor XIII
À Fibrinopeptide A
À Fibrin monomer complexes

a traumatized patient. The net effect of all of these alterations is a larger volume of gastric contents, with no change in acidity; these contents are more likely to exit the stomach through the esophagus than through the pylorus. For this reason, all parturients are considered at increased risk for aspiration during periods of unconsciousness or heavy sedation. In fact, aspiration of gastric contents is the leading cause of maternal death associated with anesthesia. Two steps are taken to attenuate this risk: (*a*) chemoprophylaxis (e.g., 0.3 M sodium citrate, 30 ml per os) is used, whenever possible, to reduce the acidity and/or volume of gastric contents before the induction of anesthesia, and (*b*) protection of a questionable airway is given paramount consideration.

## Kidney

Renal blood flow increases during pregnancy, as does creatinine clearance. Serum creatinine and urea nitrogen during pregnancy are $0.5 \pm 0.1$ and $9 \pm 1$ mg/dl, respectively (9), and higher values may indicate renal dysfunction in pregnant patients.

The increased filtration rate of solute overwhelms the renal tubules' absorption capabilities, resulting in glucosuria and aminoaciduria. Therefore, the presence of small amounts of glucose in the urine may be insignificant during pregnancy. The normal limits of urinary protein excretion during gestation are also increased, so that slight proteinuria may not be indicative of renal disease.

## Central Nervous System

The minimal alveolar concentration (MAC) of anesthetic agents necessary to produce anesthesia is decreased during pregnancy (10). This change is believed to be due to changes in hormone and endogenous opiate levels during pregnancy. Regardless of the etiology, less anesthetic agent may be necessary when anesthetizing pregnant patients, and overdosing should be avoided. An additional consideration is that

induction of anesthesia using inhalation agents may be more rapid during pregnancy because of the decreased functional residual capacity; however, the normal increase in cardiac output may or may not offset this effect, depending upon the individual clinical situation.

For spinal or epidural anesthesia, the amount of local anesthetic necessary is also decreased during pregnancy. This need for less local anesthetic may be due to increased sensitivity of neuronal tissue to the effect of local anesthetics or decreased volume of the subarachnoid and non-blood vessel epidural space. Usually, the dose is approximately two-thirds the volume or mass of drug used for the nonpregnant patient of the same age. For regional anesthesia outside the spinal/epidural space (e.g., brachial plexus block), the same mass/volume is usually used.

## Liver

Elevations in serum glutamic-oxaloacetic transaminase (SGOT), lactate dehydrogenase (LDH), alkaline phosphatase, and cholesterol normally occur during pregnancy and do not necessarily indicate hepatic disease. Serum bilirubin is unchanged. Total serum protein and the albumin/globulin ratio decrease. Serum pseudocholinesterase activity also decreases but, despite lower mean levels of activity, the resulting prolongation of duration of action of succinylcholine is unpredictable, and normal doses are used when succinylcholine is indicated.

## FETAL PHYSIOLOGY

The fetus depends upon normal placental (and therefore, ultimately, maternal) function to both provide oxygen and remove metabolic waste products, such as $CO_2$ and lactic acid. In general, when oxygen delivery to the fetus is adequate, placental function will allow sufficient metabolic waste excretion from fetus to mother as well. This is true because (*a*) $CO_2$ diffuses across the placenta more readily than $O_2$ and, (*b*) when $O_2$

supply is adequate, the production of harmful metabolic products (i.e., lactic acid) is minimized.

The adequacy of oxygen transfer from mother to fetus is consequent upon normal functioning of several maternal physiologic systems. Alveolar oxygen needs to enter the maternal bloodstream via pulmonary capillaries. Under normal conditions, this depends upon the presence of a normal diffusion barrier and proper ventilation-perfusion matching in the lung. Abnormalities of either will produce hypoxemia of the mother and ultimately the infant. Maternal lung disease or injury, therefore, affects the fetus. Maternal cardiac function must also be sufficient both to perfuse the lungs (allowing oxygenation of maternal blood) and to provide adequate perfusion pressure to the uterine artery.

Assuming adequate oxygenation of maternal arterial blood, oxygen delivery to the placenta becomes dependent on uterine blood flow. Uterine blood flow tends to be proportional to mean arterial pressure and inversely proportional to the resistance of the uterine vasculature. The uterine vasculature is highly innervated with $\alpha$-adrenergic receptors, and significant uterine vasoconstriction probably most often occurs secondary to stimulation of these receptors. In the presence of uterine artery vasoconstriction, maternal mean arterial pressure may be normal and yet uterine perfusion may be compromised. Any stress or pharmacologic manipulation that results in increased $\alpha$-adrenergic tone may, therefore, compromise uterine blood flow, even if blood pressure is "normal." The normal physiologic stress response to trauma or shock (see Chapter 4) may, indeed, be extremely hazardous to fetal well-being, even though that same response will be lifesaving for the mother. With this in mind, one goal of treatment of the pregnant trauma patient should be to reduce the "stress response" as much as possible. Some ways to do this include maintaining intravascular volume, minimizing psychologic stress by communicating extensively and

reassuringly with the patient, avoiding "light" anesthesia, and relieving pain.

The placenta itself, especially the intervillous space, must be maintained intact so that oxygen can be transferred from the maternal blood in the intervillous space to the fetal capillary system within the villi. If the placenta is traumatized (i.e., placental abruption), inadequate oxygen transfer to the fetus may result, and any pregnant patient with an abdominal injury should be monitored for fetal well-being (see below).

Finally, flow through the umbilical cord cannot be compromised if fetal oxygenation is to be optimized. Although there is no evidence of physiologically significant umbilical arterial vasoconstriction in response to endogenous fetal vasoconstrictors (even during severe fetal stress), the umbilical artery certainly can be compressed mechanically. Such compression may be the result of cord entrapment between the uterine wall and the fetus, which is especially likely to occur in the setting of decreased amniotic fluid volume (e.g., after traumatic rupture of the amniotic membranes). Umbilical artery compression can also occur with prolapse of the cord into the birth canal (after rupture of the membranes) or into the abdominal cavity (after uterine rupture).

By whatever means it occurs, impaired fetal oxygenation can frequently be diagnosed by observing the secondary effects of brainstem or myocardial hypoxia on the fetal heart rate. Fetal heart rate patterns indicative of fetal distress include fetal tachycardia, fetal bradycardia, fetal periodic decelerations, and decreased fetal heart rate variability. Fetal tachycardia resulting from fetal distress should be differentiated from fetal tachycardia secondary to infection or maternal fever. Persistent fetal bradycardia (especially with heart rates below 100) is associated with fetal distress and indicates the need to consider immediate surgical intervention to deliver a viable infant. Periodic fetal heart rate decelerations, especially after uterine contractions (i.e., "late" decelerations) may also be indicative of fetal distress. Finally, because fetal heart rate variability is indicative of normal homeo-static autonomic control of heart rate by the brainstem, decreased heart rate variability may be an indicator of fetal brainstem hypoxia and requires further evaluation.

## RESUSCITATION AND PREOPERATIVE PREPARATION

Once a trauma patient is diagnosed to be potentially or definitively pregnant, the goal of preoperative preparation is primarily to optimize the maternal condition to the greatest extent possible, thereby optimizing the fetal condition. Steps must be undertaken to stabilize the cardiovascular and respiratory systems of the mother, diagnose the extent of trauma, evaluate fetal well-being, and formulate a plan to proceed further.

The cornerstone of maternal hemodynamic stabilization is the maintenance of adequate intravascular volume so that endogenous or exogenous vasoconstriction becomes unnecessary to maintain blood pressure. Replacement of lost blood with transfused red cells will also provide the additional benefit of increasing oxygen delivery to the uterus by increasing the oxygen content of uterine arterial blood (see Chapters 4 and 5). When maintenance of blood pressure or volume becomes problematic, direct arterial, central venous, or pulmonary artery monitoring can be used (see Chapter 6). Military antishock trouser (MAST) suits may also be useful in obtaining hemodynamic stability. For most circumstances, only the leg portion, not the abdominal portion, should be utilized in pregnant women with significant uterine enlargement. As always, if the suit has been inflated at a different altitude (e.g., in a helicopter), the suit pressure may need to be adjusted during initial evaluation in the trauma center.

Aggressive maintenance of adequate maternal ventilation and oxygenation is impor-tant. If necessary, invasive monitoring or measurement of arterial oxygenation should be undertaken, but simple, rapid, noninvasive techniques such as pulse oximetry should not be overlooked. Supplemental oxygen therapy should be used whenever the adequacy of oxygen delivery to the fetus is in question because increases in uterine arterial $PO_2$ result in linear increases in fetal umbilical venous $PO_2$ (11). Maternal acidosis should not be treated with bicarbonate administration. Bicarbonate ion may not cross the human placenta readily to buffer fetal acids, but the $CO_2$ produced in the mother does cross readily. The possible result is additional fetal respiratory acidosis, which may be fatal if combined with already-present fetal metabolic acidosis.

Invasive or radiographic evaluation of the traumatized parturient should rarely, if ever, be delayed or modified because of fetal concerns, unless fetal distress is present. For example, potential theoretical radiation exposure risks to the fetus incurred during maternal radiographic evaluation would be far outweighed by potential fetal benefits to be gained by ensuring maternal well-being.

Fetal well-being and fetal gestational age should be evaluated as soon as possible. Fetal gestational age can be determined from the date of the last menstrual period (when a good history can be taken) or by a sonographic evaluation and comparison to published nomograms. The finding of a gestational age consistent with fetal viability (i.e., ≥25 weeks) requires that a decision be made regarding the timing of delivery: whether to attempt resuscitation and treatment of the mother with the fetus in utero or to deliver the fetus by cesarean section before further maternal care. If fetal distress is diagnosed, immediate delivery by cesarean section must be considered. Fetal distress under these circumstances is usually diagnosed by inspection of the fetal heart rate trace; therefore, the fetal heart rate should be monitored continuously during maternal resuscitation whenever a viable fetus is present and delivery is an option.

## ANESTHETIC MANAGEMENT

### The Patient for Immediate Cesarean Section

When a trauma patient is to undergo cesarean section before further operative treatment, the principles that apply to anesthesia for emergent cesarean section in the usual setting apply here as well. The airway must be secured rapidly during induction of general anesthesia, usually by awake intubation or rapid sequence intravenous induction. Agents used during induction in these circumstances may be thiopental (in a hemodynamically stable patient) or ketamine (in an unstable patient) (see Chapter 6). The induction dose of thiopental is limited to 4 mg/kg (to avoid neonatal respiratory depression) and the induction dose of ketamine is limited to 1 mg/kg (because a larger dose causes greatly increased neuromuscular tone in the newborn). Succinylcholine remains the neuromuscular blocker of choice in these circumstances, although recent work indicates that high doses of vecuronium may be useful as an alternative when succinylcholine is absolutely contraindicated (12). Nitrous oxide is not used in such cases, both because it is avoided in polytrauma patients in general (since it tends to expand a pneumothorax or pneumocephalus) and because the omission of nitrous oxide allows the use of high concentrations of inspired oxygen, which generally results in higher fetal $PaO_2$. Narcotics are avoided before the birth of the infant, and a low concentration of a potent inhalation anesthetic is used instead. Once the infant is born, the anesthetic can be modified to include narcotics and the inhalation agent is discontinued because halothane, enflurane, and isoflurane are all myometrial relaxants. High-dose inhalation techniques should be avoided to prevent excessive uterine blood loss.

To minimize the risk of maternal aspiration during the induction of general anesthesia, regional anesthesia may be preferable to general anesthesia for cesarean section if operative requirements will permit and hemodynamic stabilization has been determined. If the cesarean section is to be undertaken before a peripheral operative procedure, then spinal or epidural anesthesia is a reasonable alternative for the cesarean section. If a concurrent abdominal or thoracic procedure is to be done, then general anesthesia is best instituted for both procedures.

### Anesthesia Management When Cesarean Section Is Not Performed

When the fetus is viable and a cesarean section is not to be performed during initial surgery, the anesthetic management of the mother is undertaken with an eye toward minimizing pharmacologic effects of anesthesia, operation, and anesthetic agents on the fetus. Such potential effects include teratogenesis, asphyxia, and preterm labor.

In general, teratogenesis is a concern only during the first trimester of pregnancy, when major organogenesis occurs. During the first trimester, benzodiazepines and phenothiazines are generally avoided as part of the anesthetic management because their use has been suggested in some studies to result in cleft lip/palate and cardiopulmonary anomalies, respectively (13). Although general anesthetic agents commonly used have never been shown convincingly to increase teratogenic risk when administered during pregnancy, there are other drugs that may be used intraoperatively which may be potential teratogens: phenytoin, valproic acid, tetracyclines, streptomycin, and kanamycin.

Several steps are taken to avoid fetal asphyxia intraoperatively. To optimize oxygenation of the fetus, nitrous oxide is avoided to maximize $FIO_2$. Maternal cardiac output should be maintained so that uterine blood flow is not compromised. The maintenance of normal blood volume will minimize autonomic reflexes that may be harmful to the infant, as mentioned previously. Maintaining the hemoglobin concentration at 10 to 11 g/dl will also help ensure efficient oxygen delivery to the intervillous space. Nalbuphine in a dose of 0.1 to 0.5 mg/kg can be used to provide analgesia while maintaining cardiovascular stability (14).

Preterm labor has never been shown to be caused by anesthetic agents, with the exception that ketamine results in a dose-related increase in intrauterine pressure (15). Potent inhalation agents may, indeed, prove to be useful adjuncts during operation because they decrease uterine contractility and thereby decrease the risk of intraoperative labor. Isoflurane is the preferred potent anesthetic agent because (*a*) it lacks both the central nervous system excitatory effects and potential high fluoride levels of enflurane, as well as the arrhythmogenicity of halothane, and (*b*) it may also produce the least myocardial depression of these agents. Surgery itself, regardless of the anesthetic used, roughly doubles the risk of preterm delivery (16).

During operation, the fetal heart rate of viable infants should be monitored, assuming that the diagnosis of fetal distress would result in a change of therapy (e.g., immediate delivery of the infant, altered pharmacologic management). Fetal heart rate monitoring can be accomplished intraoperatively by the use of sterilized probes (if the surgical site includes the abdomen) or by external monitoring (if peripheral operation is being performed). Uterine activity is simultaneously monitored so that preterm labor can be properly diagnosed and treated as indicated. Several classes of drugs, including

inhalation anesthetics, magnesium, and $\beta_2$-adrenergic agonists may be useful acute tocolytics in the event that preterm labor must be treated during the immediate perioperative period (Table 10.4).

When peripheral surgery only is planned, regional anesthesia should be considered for the reasons given above. Fetal well-being should be monitored.

## SPECIAL CIRCUMSTANCES

### Postmortem Cesarean Section

If cardiac arrest has occurred, evacuation of a large, term uterus is essential before effective cardiac resuscitation can be undertaken (17). In this case, the airway should be secured and cesarean section performed. If death has already occurred, cesarean section should be undertaken to deliver any potentially viable infant. Extensive neonatal resuscitation may be necessary in such cases.

### Burns

Pregnant burn patients must be treated aggressively because hypoxemia and hypovolemia are frequent sequelae of serious burns. Hypoxemia may be more easily precipitated in pregnant patients, given their predisposition to arterial oxygen desaturation. Noninvasive oxygen monitoring is more difficult because real-time pulse oximetry monitoring may be rendered clinically useless by the presence of high concentrations of carboxyhemoglobin. Fluid therapy should be initiated promptly to avoid sym-

**Table 10.4.    Tocolytic Drugs**

| Drug | Route of Administration | Comment |
|---|---|---|
| Magnesium | i.m. or i.v. bolus followed by i.v. infusion | Serum level of 5–8 mEq/liter desired |
| Ritodrine | i.v. infusion | Side effects include angina, pulmonary edema, hypokalemia, hyperglycemia, dilutional anemia |
| Inhalational anesthetic agents | Inhaled | Sub-MAC doses are efficacious but impractical |
| Alcohol | i.v. | Infrequently used |
| Indomethacin | p.o. | Used for chronic tocolysis, may cause fetal ductus arteriosus closure in late third trimester |

pathetic-mediated reflexes that may impair uterine blood flow. Finally, if circumferential deep thoracic or abdominal burns are present, escharotomies should be considered early to avoid respiratory or circulatory insufficiency due to the exacerbation of ventilatory and circulatory impairment normally present during pregnancy (see Chapter 9).

## Maintenance of Utero Pregnancy after Maternal Brain Death

When in utero maintenance of pregnancy is undertaken after maternal brain death, appropriate life support measures should be instituted so that maternal cardiac output is maintained and maternal blood remains oxygenated. Maternal dialysis may be necessary if maternal renal failure has occurred. As soon as gestational age compatible with ex utero viability has been reached (i.e., 25 weeks of gestation), periodic tests of fetal well-being such as oxytocin challenge tests can be performed to assure fetal well-being until the time of planned delivery. Consultation with the neonatologist should be undertaken to select an appropriate gestational age for cesarean section delivery.

## Neonatal Resuscitation

Anesthesiologists will occasionally be called upon to render newborn resuscitation in emergency settings and should therefore be familiar with the basic principles involved. Similar to other resuscitations, securing the airway, establishing ventilation, and promoting circulation are the goals. "Neonatal Advanced Life Support" (18), included in the "Standards for CPR and ECC" published by the American Heart Association, outlines the procedures for neonatal resuscitation and should be used as a model for protocols. Several important differences between neonatal and adult resuscitation make familiarity with specific neonatal protocols important (see Chapter 11).

The proper resuscitative environment is essential for neonates. Equipment and med-

ication should be readily available. Additionally, the importance of a warm environment cannot be overstated, especially for infants who have suffered asphyxial damage and as a result do not have intact thermal regulation.

The assessment of the need for resuscitation in neonates is predominantly based on both signs of neurologic activity and the infant's heart rate. As asphyxia develops, the central nervous system begins to dysfunction, resulting in lack of respiration, loss of muscle tone, and loss of reflex response to noxious stimulation. All of these factors are taken into consideration in Apgar scoring, which is the most commonly used indicator for the need for resuscitation. The heart rate is, perhaps, the most important component of this scoring system because hypoxia or asphyxia in the infant results in bradycardia.

When resuscitation begins, the airway should be cleared and maintained. Special mention should be made of the procedures required when meconium aspiration is suspected. When thick meconium is present or if the infant has not begun vigorous respiratory efforts, the trachea is intubated and meconium evacuation is attempted. Suctioning should be repeated until the trachea is clear of meconium, the infant begins to breath spontaneously, or 2 minutes has elapsed.

If positive-pressure ventilation is required during resuscitation, it is performed via either mask or endotracheal tube. Endotracheal intubation is slightly different in neonates: the tongue is larger, the larynx is more anterior, and the cricoid ring (not the vocal cords) is the narrowest part of the airway (see Chapter 11).

Prompt and effective ventilation and oxygenation do not always result in rapid resuscitation of the infant, and chest compressions may be necessary. Chest compressions should be performed at a rate of approximately 120/minute with 40 to 60 breaths/minute of 100% oxygen (see Chapter 11).

As far as medications are concerned, atropine and calcium are no longer recommended as part of neonatal resuscitation. Epinephrine at a dose of 0.01 to 0.03 mg/kg should be used when necessary, and volume expansion with balanced salt solution, 10 ml/kg, or 5% albumin is the most useful pharmacologic therapy. These can be administered via the umbilical vein, peripheral vein, or umbilical artery. If venous access is not available, epinephrine can be administered through the endotracheal tube.

## SUMMARY

Many physiologic changes during pregnancy will potentially affect management of the pregnant trauma patient. These include respiratory, cardiovascular, hematologic, gastrointestinal, renal, and central nervous system changes. Fetal and placental physiology are additional factors to consider. Prompt attention to both fetal and maternal problems will define appropriate management options.

## References

1. Esposito TJ. Pitfalls in resuscitation and early management of the pregnant trauma patient. Trauma Q, 1988;5:1–22.
2. Pritchard JA, MacDonald PC, Gant NF. Williams Obstetrics, ed 17. East Norwalk, CT, Appleton-Century-Crofts, 1985, pp 210–212.
3. Bartholomew RA, Sale BE, Calloway JT. Diagnosis of pregnancy by the roentgen ray. JAMA 1921; 76:912–916.
4. Pauerstein CJ. Diagnosis of pregnancy. In Pauerstein CJ (ed). Clinical Obstetrics. New York, John Wiley & Sons, 1987, p 111.
5. Bevan DR, Holdcroft A, Loh L, MacGregor WG, O'Sullivan JC. Closing volume and pregnancy. Br Med J 1974;1:13–15.
6. Pritchard JA. Changes in blood volume during pregnancy and delivery. Anesthesiology 1965; 26:393–399.
7. Ueland K, Novy MJ, Peterson EN. Maternal cardiovascular dynamics: IV. The influence of gestational age on the maternal cardiovascular response to posture and exercise. Am J Obstet Gynecol 1969;104:856–864.
8. Howard BK, Goodson JH, Mengert WF. Supine hypotension syndrome in late pregnancy. Obstet Gynecol 1953;1:371–377.
9. Ferris TF. Renal diseases. In Burrow GN, Ferris TF (eds): Medical Complications during Pregnancy. Philadelphia, WB Saunders, 1982, p 237.
10. Palahniuk RJ, Shnider SM, Eger EL II. Pregnancy decreases the requirements for inhaled anesthetic agents. Anesthesiology 1974;41:82–83.
11. Rankin JHG, Meschia G, Makowski EL, Battaglia FC. Relationship between uterine and umbilical pO$_2$ in sheep. Am J Physiol 1971;220:1688–1692.
12. Tessem JH, Johnson TD. The evaluation of vecuronium for rapid sequence induction in patients undergoing cesarean section. Anesthesiology 1987;67:A452, (abstract).
13. Wright RG, Shnider SM. Fetal and neonatal effects of maternally administered drugs. In Shnider SM, Levinson G (eds): Anesthesia for Obstetrics. Baltimore, Williams & Wilkins, 1987, p 541.
14. Barton CR, Cunningham P, Smith JD. More unique applications for nalbuphine. AANA J 1986;54:217–218.
15. Galloon S. Ketamine for obstetric delivery. Anesthesiology 1976;44:522–524.
16. Duncan PG, Pope WDB, Cohen MM, Greer N. Fetal risk of anesthesia and surgery during pregnancy. Anesthesiology 1986;64:790–794.
17. Marx GF. Cardiopulmonary resuscitation of late-pregnant women. Anesthesiology 1982;56:156.
18. American Heart Association. Neonatal advanced life support. JAMA 1986;255:2969–2973.

# Anesthesia for Pediatric Trauma

*Randall C. Wetzel*

The leading cause of death in infants and children in the United States is trauma. Thirty thousand children die from trauma each year. Trauma accounts for more than 50% of all childhood deaths. In the first few months of life, birth-related fatalities outnumber those related to motor vehicle accidents, but motor vehicle accidents still account for a higher incidence of death (approximately 18/100,000 infants) in this age group than in any other age group (1, 2). These statistics are appalling enough, but an additional 100,000 children are left permanently disabled each year (3). Clearly, the problem is enormous, and anesthesiologists are frequently involved in the care of acutely traumatized children. In childhood, the overwhelming majority of injuries and fatalities are caused by motor vehicle accidents, with children being involved as passengers, pedestrians, or cyclists; however, this is not the sole cause of death and injury. Additionally, because of the child's anatomy and the lack of suitable passenger restraints, motor vehicle accidents in children have a higher incidence of facial, airway, and intracranial trauma than do such accidents in adults. Penetrating, high-velocity injuries account for only 10% of

pediatric injuries, with approximately 80% resulting from blunt trauma (2).

Apart from motor vehicle accidents, infants and small children are prone to injuries in their frequently chaotic environments. Child abuse continues to play a large role in injuries to children of all ages (4). This can appear as isolated severe head injury superimposed upon a background of chronic injury with multiple fractures, bruises, and cutaneous manifestations of abuse such as whip marks and cigarette burns or as blunt abdominal injury. Approximately one million children are reportedly abused and neglected each year, and this shocking fact is reflected by the number of injured children who require emergent and intensive care therapy annually (5). The majority of the children are less than 5 years old, and 5 to 20% of the victims die.

Falls are the third major category of injury to children. Tumbles down stairs and falls from upper story windows continue to occur with alarming frequency, especially in the urban setting. Infant walkers are used by nearly 80% of children and seem to have been responsible, in 1980 alone, for 24,000 injuries nationally, 8,600 which required hospital emergency room treatment (6). A majority of these injuries involved falling down stairs while in the walker. Falls frequently involve injuries to the cervical spine, skull, central nervous system (CNS), and face, with the obvious potential for respiratory compromise.

Another major category of injury to children includes thermal, chemical, and electrical burns. In this category, nearly 5000 children die annually, and at least 10 times this many suffer serious and frequently permanently disabling injuries. These injuries are often accompanied by airway burns, smoke inhalation, carbon monoxide poisoning, and profound fluid loss and present an emergent challenge with regard to their airway and anesthetic management.

The pediatric section of the Maryland Institute for Emergency Medical Services Systems is based at the Johns Hopkins Hospital and involves members of the Departments of Surgery, Pediatrics, Anesthesiology, and Critical Care Medicine. In 1988, 700 children were treated for trauma of multiple etiologies. Of these, 500 suffered motor vehicle accidents, 37 were knocked from their bikes, and 66 were abused. One hundred forty (20%) were admitted to the Pediatric Intensive Care Unit (PICU). Of those admitted to the PICU, 10% died, the overwhelming majority from head injury. Forty per cent of all PICU patients were intubated, and 30% required more than 5 days of intensive care. Anesthesiology services were involved in the management of approximately 40% of these children in the emergency room, intensive care unit, or operating room.

## THE ANESTHESIOLOGIST AND PEDIATRIC TRAUMA

In any well-organized trauma service, anesthesiologists familiar with the pediatric airway and pediatric cardiovascular physiology form a crucial part of the pediatric trauma team. The trauma team should consist of pediatric surgeons, pediatricians, pediatric intensivists, and, where possible, anesthesiologists with special experience in

the management of children. The anesthesiologist is frequently called upon for more than airway skills in the setting of pediatric trauma. His expertise is directed at minimizing both acute and long-term morbidity. Emergent stabilization, evaluation, and resuscitation must all occur concurrently. Frequently, the pediatric anesthesiologist must play a central role in coordinating the child's care during these crucial early minutes. Apart from the obvious airway skills that facilitate rapidly securing the airway and assuring ventilation and oxygenation, the special skills of the anesthesiologist with regard to vascular access and monitoring and support of the hemodynamic status of acutely injured children are paramount. Further issues of concern include the provision of safe and appropriate sedation and analgesia for children who are unable to maintain their airway, may be hemodynamically unstable, or may require maintenance of an artificial airway. Consultation on the use of these anesthetic agents and on muscle relaxant techniques to facilitate further investigative studies may be required. All of these may be necessary during the early acute period, and the anesthesiologists' pharmacologic and physiologic knowledge is crucial in avoiding iatrogenic disasters and ensuring optimal conditions for the ongoing resuscitation and diagnosis of critically ill children.

The anesthesiologist also plays an important role for children with trauma that is less life-threatening. For example, anesthesiologists may be required to provide analgesia and sedation for less cooperative children who require treatment for minor lacerations, fractures, or painful diagnostic procedures. Provision of appropriate sedation and general anesthesia may be necessary in a wide spectrum of settings that include urgent care for children with multiple anesthetic risks such as full stomachs, ocular injury, and internal injuries.

Advance planning is essential to provide anesthetic resources for injured children in an emergency facility. Performing painful procedures on children with fractures or who may require sutures with inadequate anesthetic techniques is clearly inhumane. Furthermore, the increasing public awareness and demand for safe, effective analgesia for acutely painful procedures in children (7), coupled with our understanding of the deleterious metabolic effects of painful and stressful procedures in children who do not receive adequate analgesia (8), will increasingly mandate expert anesthetic management for these children over the next few years. Therefore, anesthesiologists must be prepared to deal with the need for pain management in injured children, frequently in nontraditional settings.

## PHYSIOLOGY

### The Pediatric Airway

The common perception that children tolerate hypoxic and ischemic insults better than do adults is a dangerous myth. In fact, there is no reason to expect that this is so outside the perinatal period. Children have a slightly smaller functional residual capacity (FRC) (per unit body mass) than do adults and a higher oxygen consumption. Additionally, the percentage of vital capacity that is closing volume is increased in young children. This clearly will lead to a more rapid decrease in oxygen availability during apnea in children compared to adults. This critical situation is aggravated in the immediate posttraumatic state. An increase in oxygen consumption caused by stress and hypothermia and the potential for decreased FRC in trauma combine to form a serious threat. Rapid desaturation after apnea or airway obstruction with the rapid onset of hypoxemia expectedly occurs in young children. Additionally, there is absolutely no evidence to support the notion that, in this setting, the resultant hypoxemia is better tolerated in children. Indeed, the outcome of cardiopulmonary resuscitation in children is worse than in adults (9).

In addition to these differences in the respiratory system, the child's airway presents a host of unique challenges. Respira-tory difficulties that occur at the scene of injury, during resuscitation, in transit to the hospital, or in the emergency room may be extremely difficult to manage for practitioners who may be less competent and less experienced with managing these small airways. Frequently, the anesthesiologist is the only practitioner available who is experienced in pediatric airway management.

What are the key differences between the pediatric and the adult airways? As can be seen in Figure 11.1, the glottis is higher, at C4, as compared to approximately C6 and C7 in adults; the vocal cords tend to slant downward and anteriorly, making access to the trachea more difficult; finally, the tongue is relatively larger compared to the oral cavity and the nares are narrower. The anterior, cephalad placement of the larynx coupled with a relatively small jaw require a different intubation technique in infants and small children. Maintaining the head in a neutral rather than an extended position frequently facilitates intubation. In the child, the larger, longer, $\Omega$-shaped, floppy epiglottis frequently obscures the glottis unless specifically lifted from the airway by the laryngoscope blade. The epiglottis assumes the adult configuration after puberty but becomes less curved and relatively shorter after 2 years of age. Another crucial factor to remember when intubating the child's airway is that the narrowest part of the airway is not the glottic opening. It is, in fact, the firm, completely circumferential cricoid ring. Just because an endotracheal tube will go through the cords does not indicate that it will go past the cricoid ring. Damage by the use of too large a tube under these circumstances is not infrequent.

For these reasons, appropriate airway management equipment in children differs from that in adults. The emergent use of oral esophageal obturator airways in pediatrics is not recommended. These airways frequently obstruct the small, pliable larynx. Additionally, with poor placement of these airways or the use of oral airways that are too large, the child's large epiglottis can obstruct the glottis. Any pediatric emer-

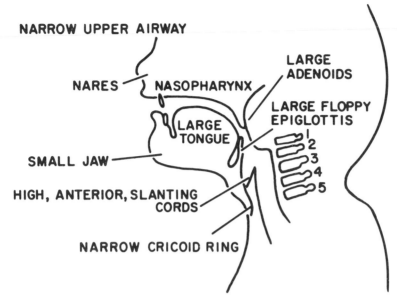

NARROW UPPER AIRWAY

NARES — NASOPHARYNX

LARGE ADENOIDS

LARGE FLOPPY EPIGLOTTIS

LARGE TONGUE

SMALL JAW

HIGH, ANTERIOR, SLANTING CORDS

NARROW CRICOID RING

**Figure 11.1   The pediatric airway.** This profile of the child's airway highlights the major differences between it and the adult's airway. The upper airway is narrowed by narrow nares and a narrow nasopharynx, which is partially occluded by large adenoids, and an oropharynx that is occluded by a large tongue. Further narrowing is due to the small jaw and a large, floppy Ω-shaped epiglottis. The cephalad, anterior displacement of the vocal cords, as well as the posterior-anterior slanting of the cords downward, makes visualization additionally difficult. The cricoid ring is the narrowest point in the pediatric airway, unlike the adult anatomy.

gency resuscitation area should contain a wide selection of sizes of oral and nasal airways, as well as pediatric face masks. Insertion of oral airways, unless cautiously done, may also obstruct the larynx by displacing the tongue. In addition, suctioning equipment both for the pharynx and for the endotracheal tubes of appropriate size should be available (Table 11.1). Frequently, the posttraumatic infant and small child has vomited, and debris may not only block the upper airway but also be subglottic. Adequate airway suctioning may be immediately necessary after tracheal intubation in critically injured children. A properly stocked pediatric airway resuscitation cart in the emergency triage area is essential. Only forward planning can prevent the disasters

**Table 11.1.   Sizes of Endotracheal Tubes and Suction Catheters Appropriate for Infants and Children**

| Age | Endotracheal Tube | | Suction Catheter |
| | I.D. | Length (oral) | |
| --- | --- | --- | --- |
| | *mm* | *mm* | *French* |
| Premature | 2.5–3.0 uncuffed | 9 | 6 |
| 0–6 mo | 3.0–3.5 uncuffed | 10–11 | 6 |
| 6–12 mo | 3.5–4.0 uncuffed | 12 | 8 |
| 1–2 yr | 4.0 uncuffed | 13 | 8 |
| 2–4 yr | 4.5 uncuffed | 14 | 8 |
| 4–6 yr | 5.0 uncuffed | 15 | 10 |
| 6–8 yr | 5.5 uncuffed | 16 | 10 |
| 8–10 yr | 6.0–6.5 cuff optional | 17 | 10–12 |
| 10–12 yr | 7.5–8.0 cuff optional | 18 | 12 |
| >1 yr | 7.5–8.0 cuffed | 19–22 | 12 |

associated with trying to resuscitate children with adult equipment. Some anesthesia departments provide a readily available pediatric resuscitation tackle box with necessary airway resuscitation equipment.

Selection of appropriate airways (oral or nasal) and endotracheal tubes is related to age (Table 11.1). Selection of the appropriate endotracheal tube can be guided initially by the well-known formula: (Age in years + 16)/4; however, we generally prefer to use the data in Table 11.1. Age is a more crucial factor. The airway continues to grow even when the child is small, and proper tube selection therefore depends on age. Because of concerns about subglottic trauma, only uncuffed endotracheal tubes are used in children under 8 years of age. For similar reasons, it is customary to ensure that the pressure at which air "leaks" around the endotracheal tube is less than 30 cm $H_2O$. The child is reintubated with the next half size smaller endotracheal tube if the leak occurs only at airway pressures greater than 30 cm $H_2O$ unless contraindicated by the child's clinical status. A leak pressure of less than 10 cm $H_2O$ indicates a need for a larger tube, as adequate ventilation cannot be assured with this size leak, especially if compliance is decreased. The tip of the endotracheal tube should be midway between the carina and larynx or at least 2 cm below the cords. Most pediatric endotracheal tubes have length marks at the tip to guide placement. Flexion and extension of the child's neck readily move the endotracheal tube further into or out of the trachea, respectively. One final warning about pediatric endotracheal tubes: their small diameter and the physical fact of Poiseuille's law make airway obstruction from increased resistance and plugging by mucus, blood, or food particles highly likely. This occurs much more readily than in adults, and appropriately sized suction catheters must be always available.

Classically, laryngoscopy in young children is performed with a straight blade, such as a Miller, Anderson-Magill, Wis-Hipple, Seward, or Robertshaw blade (Fig. 11.2). The anterior placement of the larynx coupled with a floppy epiglottis makes the best approach to extend the neck slightly, straightening out the airway axes, and elevate the epiglottis with the tip of the laryngoscopy blade, thus exposing the glottic opening. This maneuver is difficult with a curved blade placed in the vallecula in children less than 1 year of age. The straight blade approach with a Miller 0 or 1 blade is very effective in newborns and infants less than 2 months of age. In children over 1 year of age, a MacIntosh curved laryngoscopy blade (either a #2 or a #3 in older children) can be used with positioning similar to that for adults. In a traumatized child, special consideration must be given to the setting (e.g., neck injury) or specific complications of the injury (e.g., airway burns).

## Cardiovascular Physiology

Hemodynamically, children adapt remarkably well to stress. The child's cardiovascular system has intact homeostatic mechanisms to maintain central blood volume and perfusion at the expense of the periphery. These compensatory mechanisms, which operate in trauma, are fully mature at birth. One of the primary differences between adults and infants is that cardiac output in children is, in general, maintained by increases in heart rate rather than in stroke volume during stress (10). The infant's myocardium is less compliant, demonstrates a less well-organized myocardial structure, and is less extensively sympathetically innervated (11). The ability to augment stroke volume is therefore limited. On the other hand, increases in heart rate of up to 180 to 200 beats/minute occur quite readily in children. The fear of myocardial ischemia and preload limitation in children who have sinus tachycardia is minimal, and heart rates of up to 200 in children under 2 years are well tolerated. In children, tachycardia per se does not cause hypotension or poor perfusion. Anxiety over a marked sinus tachycardia is unnecessary. Any endeavor,

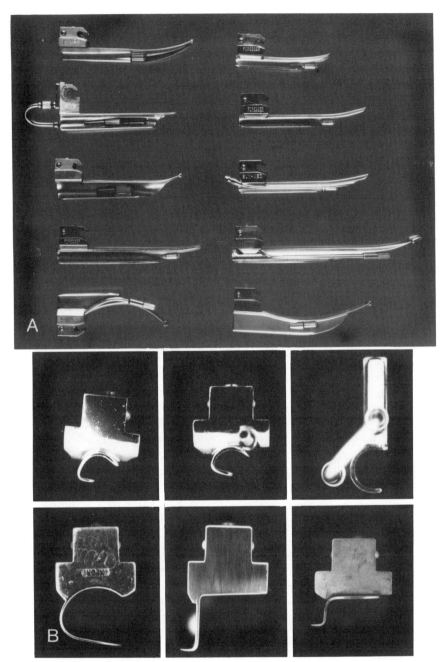

**Figure 11.2.   Pediatric laryngoscope blades. A,** *Left, top* to *bottom*: Seward, Anderson-Magill, Oxford, Wis-Hipple 1½, MacIntosh 1; *right, top* to *bottom*: Miller 0, Miller 1, Miller 1 with oxygen port, Miller 2, and MacIntosh 2. **B,** End-on views of the various blades showing airway access. *Top, left* to *right*: Miller 1, Miller 1 with oxygen port, Anderson-Magill; *bottom, left* to *right*: Oxford, MacIntosh, Seward.

other than treating the primary condition, to lower the heart rate, such as $\beta$-blockade, must be resisted vigorously or catastrophe

will result. Evidence of ST–T changes on electrocardiogram (ECG) in traumatized children most likely indicates a myocardial though these changes can also occur in the setting of severe head trauma (12).

Because children respond so thoroughly to intravascular volume contraction, the blood pressure is frequently maintained until there is a 30 or 40% decrease in intravascular volume. Intravascular blood volume is proportionally greater in children. In children younger than 2 years, the average blood volume is about 80 ml/kg; in those between 2 and 16 years of age, 70 ml/kg is more accurate. These volumes are in contrast to that of adults, which is nearer 60 ml/kg. Thus, a blood loss of 200 ml in a 10-kg child will reduce the blood volume by 25% (see Chapter 4). The blood pressure could be normal despite this severe hemorrhage and obvious anesthetic risk (13). Although the child may be cold and hypoperfused, with decreased capillary refill, decreased urine output, and acidosis, the blood pressure may still be within the normal range for age (Table 11.2). It is axiomatic that the blood pressure is the last thing to fall in children (13). For this reason, careful monitoring of the hemodynamic status by observation of peripheral perfusion, urine output, capillary refill, the central to peripheral temperature gradient, and the patient's level of consciousness is critical in assessing the hemodynamic status of the child (14). An adequate blood pressure does not exclude shock in children. In fact, dangerous volume contraction and shock can occur in the face of a normal blood pressure. This cannot be too strongly stressed. An adequate blood pressure does

**Table 11.2. Normal Pulse and Blood Pressure Ranges for Infants and Children**

| Age | Pulse | Blood Pressure | |
|-----|-------|----------|----------|
| | | Systolic | Diastolic |
| | *bpm* | *torr* | *torr* |
| Newborn | 100–200 | 60–90 | 40–60 |
| 1–6 mo | 80–160 | 70–150 | 45–60 |
| 6–12 mo | 70–140 | 75–110 | 55–75 |
| 1–3 yr | 70–120 | 75–115 | 55–75 |
| 3–5 yr | 70–110 | 85–120 | 50–75 |
| 5–10 yr | 70–100 | 85–125 | 50–75 |
| 10–15 yr | 70–90 | 85–125 | 50–75 |
| ≥15 yr | 60–80 | 90–130 | 55–85 |

not mean that sedation and the induction of anesthesia are safe. Evidence of decreased perfusion and tachycardia should indicate the need for volume expansion.

### Temperature Regulation

Because of the child's large ratio of surface area to volume, loss of core temperature occurs more readily than in the adult. In all injured patients there is a transient decrease in heat production due to deranged hypothalamic thermoregulation. In addition to this, infants have poor thermoregulatory capabilities, and hypothermia is a very common secondary insult in the injured child. In this situation the additional hypothalamic effects of general anesthesia can cause further deterioration. This secondary insult may prevent adequate cardiopulmonary resuscitation, prolong acidosis and obtundation, and make it difficult to obtain adequate hemodynamic function.

To ensure adequate maintenance of core body temperature, one must have an organized system to provide thermal protection for children at the scene of injury. Transportation in space blankets, tin foil, air bubble plastic, or even plastic bags provides an adequate means of preventing heat and fluid loss. All injured children should be well insulated during transport. On arrival in the emergency room, overhead warmers, a warm environment, and continuous attention to maintaining the child's core temperature are essential and require monitoring and forward planning. All intravenous fluids must be warmed, either through a pediatric blood warmer or, in the case of crystalloids, in a microwave oven. Preplanning is essential to ensure that critically injured children receive warm fluids—if they are not immediately available, they will not be given. The child who is critically injured and hypotensive will not be aided by being stripped, exposed to a cold room (made cold for the comfort of the physicians), and drowned in 16°C intravascular volume expansion. Core temperatures under these circumstances can readily fall der these circumstances can readily fall below 30°C, and resuscitative efforts then become incredibly difficult. Additionally, even moderate hypothermia drastically increases oxygen demand while at the same time impairing the release of oxygen from hemoglobin in the periphery (15, 16). In the child who is in shock with a critical limitation of oxygen delivery, this increase in oxygen demand can further stress a failing cardiovascular system and accentuate the vicious cycle of ischemia, hypoxemia, and acidosis. Despite the fact that temperature regulation in children is continually stressed strongly, it is frequently but inexcusably overlooked.

### The Glucose Question

Traumatized infants and children in shock may rapidly consume their gluconeogenic substrate (17). Although it is more usual for children with trauma to present with hyperglycemia and, indeed, glucose values of up to 800 mg/dl have been seen in critically ill children, hypoglycemia can occur. Frequently in small children and certainly in malnourished children, hypoglycemia may intervene. For this reason, all children who are critically injured should have a Dextrostix or a Chemstrip determination of blood glucose as soon as possible after admission. Hypoglycemia should be treated only when present. The use of large volumes of glucose-containing solutions to resuscitate children from hypovolemic shock may result in significant hyperglycemia, leading to an osmotic diuresis and presenting a serious potential for further neurologic injury (18). For these reasons, it is no longer recommended that during resuscitation the initial crystalloid resuscitation fluid contain 5% dextrose in children under 2 years of age. In children outside the neonatal age range, Ringer's lactate is the initial fluid of choice (19). In neonates a 10% dextrose solution is indicated. Of course, all patients comatose without an apparent cause should receive a bolus of glucose if hypoglycemia cannot be ruled out.

## PEDIATRIC CARDIOPULMONARY RESUSCITATION (CPR)

The anesthesiologist's role in the child with cardiac arrest is similar to that in the arrested adult; however, airway manipulations and drug dosages differ. The hierarchy of Airway, Breathing, and Circulation (ABCs) is just as mandatory in children as in adults (19). One of the child's physicians should attempt vascular access while the airway is intubated and ventilation is assured. The use of resuscitative drugs including atropine, lidocaine, bretylium, and epinephrine is based on the patient's assumed or measured weight (Table 11.3). In children the optimal dose of epinephrine and other vasopressors has not been conclusively defined. The recommended dose of 10 μ/kg every 10 minutes is probably on the low side, and a constant epinephrine infusion may be warranted (20). Defibrillation, although seldom necessary in the arrested child, is again dosed by weight (19). The use of bicarbonate is currently under severe attack, and its use in children bears the same caveats as those currently being discussed about its use in adults (20). One additional problem in children is the danger of inject-

**Table 11.3. Resuscitation Drugs and Techniques**

| Drug or Technique | Dose | Route |
|---|---|---|
| Epinephrine | 20 μg/kg (0.1 ml/kg of 1:10,000) | i.v. endotracheal intracardiac |
| Atropine | 20 μg/kg never < 150 μg | i.v endotracheal intramuscular |
| Bretylium | 5–10 mg/kg | i.v. over 10 min |
| Lidocaine | 1–2 mg/kg | i.v |
| Calcium chloride | 20 mg/kg (0.2 ml/kg, 10%) | i.v |
| Sodium bicarbonate | 1 mEq/kg (1 mEq/ml) | i.v |
| Defibrillation | 2–4 J/kg | infant: 4.5-cm paddles child: 8-cm paddles adult: 14-cm paddles |

ing hyperosmotic solutions in neonates; thus, sodium bicarbonate must be diluted to a concentration of 0.5 mEq/ml in infants. In children, cardiac arrest is usually due to respiratory failure or obstruction, and bicarbonate administration should await intubation and ventilation (21).

The performance of cardiac compression in infants and small children is different from the method in adults (18). The child's chest is dramatically different when compared with adults, both in geometric configuration and in compliance and pliability. Therefore, clinical experience in adults as well as research data in adult models of CPR are not necessarily applicable to infants and small children (21). What does seem clear from a wide variety of investigations is that conventional CPR with chest compression is more efficacious at increasing intrathoracic pressure and maintaining peripheral perfusion in younger animals (21). Thus, CPR is liable to be more efficacious in infants and small children than in adults. The technique for chest compression varies in small infants. The heart is located lower in the thorax in infants, and the site of compression is located by placing the finger one (adult) fingerbreadth below a line connecting the child's nipples. In young infants (0–6 months), two-fingered compression of the sternum 100 times/minute, retrograde by about 1 inch of the thoracic depth (which may directly compress the heart), is recommended (Fig. 11.3). In older infants (6–18 months), hands encircling the thorax with fingers posteriorly near the spine and the thumbs compressing the sternum is a comfortable and effective way of providing CPR (Fig. 11.4). In children over 18 months, conventional sternal compression with a two-handed technique is performed as in adults. The heel of the hand is placed two fingers above the xiphisternum. The sternum is depressed 1 to 1.5 inches at a rate of 80 compressions/minute (22).

Simultaneous chest compression and ventilation may not be efficacious in small children. Compression of the thorax can generate pressures of up to 80 torr, and the

addition of increased airway pressure does not seem to be advantageous. This is contrary to what has been suggested by adult models of CPR (19, 20). In infants and small children, a compression rate of 100/minute with ventilation approximately every fifth compression is indicated. In children over 8 years of age, chest compression is performed as in adults (19).

## EMERGENCY STABILIZATION

In the emergency room, success depends on an organized, systematic approach to the traumatized child. Thus, anesthesiologists should be involved in organizational decisions. When a child arrives, initial attention to the airway, breathing, and circulation is mandatory. The anesthesiologist will frequently be the best-trained individual for airway management and should be responsible for the identification and management of particular airway complications in the emergency room. The child arriving in the emergency room requires immediate airway assessment and endotracheal intubation if necessary. Particular notice of the anatomic differences and technical difficulties associated with instrumenting the child's airway is required. As in all trauma patients, children are assumed to have a full stomach and, until proven otherwise, a neck injury.

### Neck Stabilization

Children who suffer acceleration/deceleration injuries, as in motor vehicle accidents, are at extreme risk for cervical dislocations and upper cord lesions. Furthermore, children are more likely than adults to survive severe cervical spine injuries and present in the emergency room. Therefore, neck stabilization and immobilization (see Chapter 3) are routine for all injured children until x-ray films reveal no bony or soft tissue damage to the cervical spinal column. Rapid dislocation with subsequent relocation of the vertebra can occur in children because of marked ligamentous elasticity (23). The absence of bony injury, therefore, does not preclude significant CNS

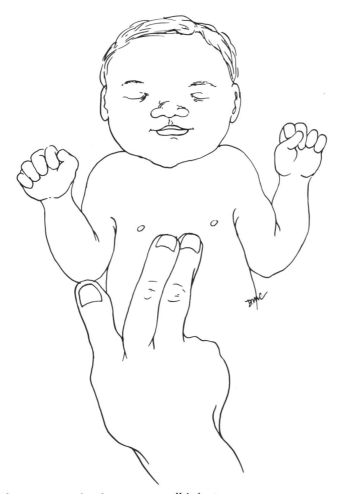

**Figure 11.3.  Chest compression in young, small infants.**

trauma. Soft tissue injury, such as ligamentous tears of the odontoid cruciate ligaments and paravertebral and spinous ligaments, can occur, causing instability even in the face of normal alignment of the vertebral bodies. In this case, careful examination for soft tissue swelling, increased intervertebral distances, and axial dislocation of the skull on the spinal column is required. Clearly, airway management and endotracheal intubation under these circumstances are very difficult and carry the risk of further CNS injury.

Securing the airway in the trauma setting requires skill and judgment. Debris such as blood and vomitus must be removed from the airway, and rapidly securing the airway to prevent aspiration is essential. In children

there is a high incidence of oral trauma, mandibular fractures, and facial trauma, which may complicate airway management and even necessitate primary cricothyroidotomy or tracheostomy. Several endotracheal intubating techniques are available, and the choice is between awake direct laryngoscopy, sedated direct laryngoscopy, sedated and paralyzed direct laryngoscopy, blind nasal intubation, and fiberoptic intubation. These will be dealt with separately.

In the presence of neck injury, direct laryngoscopy can safely be performed as long as there is a skillful assistant who knows how to provide cervical traction and stabilization during intubation. While another assistant holds the body, the assistant familiar with cervical stabilization holds the

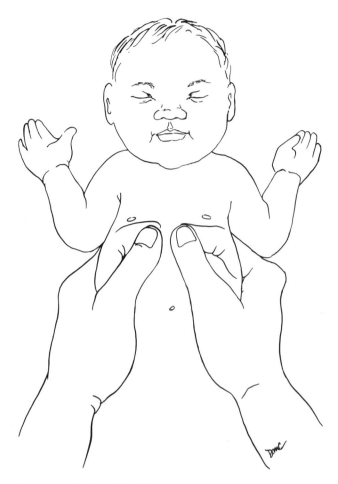

**Figure 11.4.    Chest compression in older infants.**

head and provides direct in-line axial traction while preventing rotation and extension of the neck during intubation. Intubation in the smallest infants in this position may be extremely difficult, as alignment of the airway axes with such positioning can be quite difficult. Extension cannot be permitted. In older children, the use of a curved blade can facilitate intubation. Because of the anterior cephalad placement of the larynx in children, blind intubation and intubation with traction and axial alignment of the neck are more difficult and require greater skill and experience. Although the risks of overextension during direct laryngoscopy are well described, its danger also must not be forgotten during blind nasal or awake intubations. During these procedures, the head is frequently flexed and extended to position the endotracheal tube through the cords. These maneuvers carry the same risk as they do during direct laryngoscopy. In children, blind nasal intubation is difficult and, in the setting of head injury, dangerous because of the potential for midfacial fractures and intracranial intubation. Fiberoptic intubation is also technically difficult in children; however, it is possible in children who are older than 3 or 4 years of age. Fiberoptic bronchoscopes will pass through a 4.0 endotracheal tube and thus allow intubation in smaller children. Fiberoptic intubation in children is a skill that requires much practice and familiarity; in the emergent situation, the immediate availability of equipment and personnel is difficult to assure without adequate advance planning. Finally, cricothyroidotomy, although difficult in children, is also a possible option. A large bore Teflon over-the-needle catheter can be introduced through the cricothyroid membrane to provide oxygenation for patients with severe upper airway injuries (24).

All injured persons have a full stomach. This is certainly true in children. Gastric decompression is mandatory before intubation in all but the most extreme emergencies. An orogastric tube is preferred as it is generally possible to use a larger bore orally, avoiding the use of a nasogastric tube in head trauma, with its risk of midfacial fractures. Performance of Sellick's maneuver during intubation, especially if obtundation and paralysis are induced, is mandatory. A skilled assistant who has been trained in this technique in children should always be present. In children the airway is more pliable, and overzealous cricoid pressure may totally occlude the airway, making intubation quite difficult or causing a fracture of the cricoid ring. In patients who are severely obtunded with no airway reflexes, intubation can be performed without sedation and paralysis and, if bulbar reflexes are lost, is urgently required to prevent aspiration.

In those children who are obtunded enough to require airway manipulation but are not cooperative enough to be intubated, sedation and paralysis may be necessary (see Chapter 6). Sedation in the emergent situation can be provided with fentanyl (2 to 4 µg/kg intravenously [i.v.]), a benzodiazepine (diazepam, 0.1 to 0.2 mg/kg i.v.; midazolam, 0.03 to 0.05 mg/kg i.v.), ketamine (1 to 2 mg/kg i.v.), or, in hemodynamically stable patients with suspected CNS injury, thiopental (3 to 5 mg/kg i.v.). Obviously, close monitoring during sedation in patients with potential hemodynamic instability is mandatory. The use of ketamine in patients with CNS injury is relatively contraindicated as it is associated with an increase in intracranial pressure (ICP) (25). In children with suspected elevated ICP, ventilation and oxygenation is of course mandatory. The stress of intubation

may be associated with an elevation in ICP (26). Sedation with thiopental and the use of lidocaine, which has been shown to blunt the rise in ICP with airway manipulation (27), is indicated under these circumstances in children. Cricoid pressure and a rapid sequence technique must always be used after preoxygenation, gastric suctioning, and, where possible, volume expansion.

## Muscle Relaxants

The use of muscle relaxants in critically ill children for endotracheal intubation has certain obvious difficulties. One must be assured of being able to manage the pediatric airway if paralysis is induced. With a few caveats, succinylcholine can be used to induce muscle relaxation for rapid airway intubation in the emergency setting. In young children there is a decreased sensitivity to succinylcholine, and a dose of 2 mg/kg is appropriate in children under 8 years of age. Although it is reported that fasciculations do not occur in young children, this is certainly not our common experience. Fasciculations occur in children as young as 1 year of age and can readily be seen. The presence of fasciculations is related to the major complications of the use of succinylcholine in children (28). The elevation of intraocular pressure, ICP, and intragastric pressure is related to the muscle depolarizing effect of succinylcholine. In addition, the possibility of dislocating compound fractures and accentuating trauma-induced myoglobinuria in children makes succinylcholine less than an optimal drug to use in the emergent, traumatized child (29). The use of a defasciculating dose of nondepolarizing muscle relaxant is beneficial; however, even small doses in critically injured children may cause critical airway compromise. Furthermore, the 3 to 5 minutes necessary to provide adequate defasciculation may not always be available. The concern that accompanies the use of succinylcholine in burn patients, trauma patients, and spinal cord lesion patients need not be considered in the acute situation but subsequently (> 24 hours after injury) is as important in children as in adults (see Chapters 6 and 9).

Use of nondepolarizing agents to provide relaxation for intubation is an alternative, albeit one associated with a degree of anxiety for most anesthesiologists. In children, pancuronium is the long-acting relaxant of choice. The tachycardia caused by this agent is not detrimental and may even lead to increased cardiac output in some children. The rapid onset (3 minutes, less in infants) of profound relaxation seen with pancuronium may make it acceptable for rapid sequence intubation. Hypotension, which may be seen with curare or atracurium, makes these agents dangerous in children who have suffered trauma. Needless to say, however, prolonged paralysis should only be used if airway intubation can be assured by the practitioner. In children, prolonged relaxation may facilitate further diagnostic workup and therapeutic maneuvers, such as thorough physical examination, peritoneal taps, bladder and arterial catheterization, computed tomographic scanning, magnetic resonance imaging, and the induction of hyperventilation in patients with head trauma.

## VASCULAR ACCESS

In the critically injured child, intravascular access is as crucial as in the adult. Vascular access, may be more difficult in children for simple reasons such as size and technical difficulty. In children the most frequent cause of hemodynamic catastrophe is hypovolemia. In this situation, all peripheral vessels and most central vessels are small and empty. Each practitioner must be familiar and facile with at least one means of accessing the child's circulation. Sites of access in children include peripheral vessels, long bones, the external and internal jugular veins, subclavian veins, femoral vessels, and the saphenous veins (both superficial saphenous and the saphenous vein at the ankle). The only necessity is that the access must be central to the site of bleeding; thus, in severe

abdominal trauma, a saphenous or femoral cutdown is not indicated if inferior vena caval integrity is suspect. A further difficulty occurs in the arrested child or the infant with severe shock. In this case, a cutdown on paired vessels can be difficult. The veins may all be contracted and difficult to identify, with the first vessel that is come across being an artery. For example, intended cutdown on a brachial vein is very difficult in the hypovolemic child. The brachial artery may be cannulated, leading to a vascular catastrophe, especially if catecholamines are given. Although fluid resuscitation through arteries can occur safely, it is best avoided because of the serious risk of retrograde perfusion of the cerebral circulation, and cannulation of an artery with subsequent vasoactive infusions can be catastrophic (30). For this reason, persons skilled at vascular access in small infants and children should be available in a pediatric trauma team. Although we generally use internal jugular or femoral venous access in critical situations, other institutions use other sites. For example, a recent report from Children's Hospital in Pittsburgh recommends the subclavian approach in children and reports a low incidence of complications (31). Table 11.4 is a guide to relative catheter size for large central vessels in children according to age.

Recently the intraosseous route for volume restitution and pharmacologic resuscitation has become popular (32). The intramedullary space of the tibia can readily be accessed through its anterior surface below the patella (see Chapter 4). A bone marrow needle with stylet and Luer lock can be twisted into the medulla of the bone, and fluids can be pumped into this space. As

**Table 11.4.   Appropriate Central Catheters for Age**

| Age | Diameter | Length |
|---|---|---|
| | | cm |
| newborn–6 mo | 3 F (20 gauge) | 5 |
| 16 mo–4 yr | 4 F (18 gauge) | 9 |
| 4–7 yr | 5 F (16 gauge) | 20 |
| >7 yr | as adults | |

there is direct venous communication through the marrow sinusoids, rapid volume expansion can be achieved. This technique is useful in the moribund, hypovolemic child who requires resuscitation within minutes.

One further means of vascular access in children in the emergent situation is the airway. Administration of atropine, epinephrine, and lidocaine via the endotracheal tube is effective during CPR in infants and small children without vascular access (33). Thus, in the arrested child, intubation rapidly followed by administration of oxygen and epinephrine via the endotracheal tube should be routine practice.

## MONITORING

The same principles that guide anesthetic monitoring in adults guide monitoring in children (see Chapter 6). Technical difficulties make the actual manipulation at times more difficult; however, they do not change the indications. Most of the technical difficulties of size have been overcome by advances in technology. Suitable ECG equipment, pulse oximeters, assorted precordial and esophageal stethoscopes, intravascular cannulas for arterial and central venous cannula monitoring, and Swan-Ganz catheters all exist in appropriate pediatric sizes. The monitoring of anesthesia for traumatized children should be identical to that in adults, with the addition of compulsive core temperature monitoring. Automated blood pressure devices are available for use in children; however, their reliability in hypovolemic shock is questionable.

If there is serious question about the patient's baseline hemodynamic status, invasive intraarterial pressure monitoring should be undertaken. The preferred site for this is a nondominant radial artery as in adults, followed in decreasing order of preference by the dorsal artery of the foot or the posterior tibial artery, the axillary artery, and finally the femoral artery. Percutaneous access to any of these sites is possible even in

small, premature infants. A 22 gauge cannula is appropriate for all infants full term or older. It should only occasionally be necessary to perform an arterial cutdown; however, where invasive arterial monitoring is indicated, this option is available. Central venous pressure (CVP) monitoring in children is of only limited value in the absence of preexisting heart disease. CVP very poorly reflects intravascular volume in children, and the main purpose of siting large central lines is to provide immediate central access for large volume infusion. A CVP of greater than 10 cm $H_2O$ in a previously well child probably indicates existing cardiac compromise, which in the setting of trauma could be myocardial contusion, profound acidosis or metabolic insult, or gross volume overload. In healthy children a CVP of below 5 cm $H_2O$ is maintained even with expanded intravascular volume. Attempts at elevating the cardiac output by pushing fluid until the CVP is 10 cm $H_2O$ will certainly be met with an increase in interstitial water, peripheral edema, and, in a setting of severe trauma or burns, pulmonary edema. A Foley catheter is a far better indication of volume status and perfusion than is a CVP line.

Intraoperatively, pulse oximetry, ECG, capnography, temperature, blood pressure, and urine output should be monitored routinely in injured children. Safety alarms such as circuit disconnect and $FIO_2$ alarms are, of course, also mandatory. Careful observation of the operation, perfusion, pulse, volume, and heart tones continues to be crucial to the detection of intraoperative deterioration. None of these monitoring techniques should be compromised in the setting of emergent trauma surgery, and all should clearly be assured for subsequent semi-elective trauma surgery in children.

If a child is suspected of having sustained significant head injury and presents with a Glasgow coma scale score of 7 or less, serious consideration should be given to whether ICP should be monitored intraoperatively. All anesthetics ablate the ability to monitor the neurologic status. If head injury with cerebral edema is suspected, ICP monitoring is advisable. If the child has a Glasgow coma scale score of less than 7 before the induction of anesthesia or at the last examination before muscle relaxation is given, we strongly advise intraoperative ICP monitoring. The placement of a Richmond bolt in the operating room after the patient is intubated, adequately ventilated, and hemodynamically stable need not delay urgent thoracoabdominal surgery; the bolt can be placed simultaneously with operation. A situation that requires surgery would be expected to cause hemodynamic instability, and alterations in pulse and blood pressure, respiratory rate, and eye signs are all lost during anesthesia. Thus, ICP measurement itself is the only way to detect sudden, potentially catastrophic changes in ICP. These changes in ICP may be due not only to cerebral edema, but also obviously to intracranial bleeding, such as subdural and subarachnoid hemorrhage.

Monitoring ICP intraoperatively in patients transferred in stable condition from the intensive care unit (ICU) for such operations as orthopedic procedures and burn grafting may also be necessary. If a child requires ICP monitoring in the ICU, this should necessarily be continued in the operating suite.

## OPERATIVE CARE

Clearly, management of the previously anesthetized, intubated, and paralyzed patient who requires surgery is essentially that of pediatric critical care with ongoing resuscitation. Attention must be given to providing relaxation and analgesia intraoperatively while constantly providing ongoing cardiorespiratory support in line with the general principles outlined elsewhere in this text. Ketamine remains a frequently used anesthetic in patients with hypovolemia and is particularly suited to children. In hemodynamically stable patients, the use of titrated doses of fentanyl and amnestic agents such as scopolamine, diazepam, or midazolam

provides suitable anesthesia in critically ill children.

Perhaps more difficult than the emergent anesthesia support for the surgery of acutely life-threatening injuries is that for urgent and semielective procedures. Children who have undergone multisystem trauma frequently require multiple visits to the operating room. Initially, stabilization, prevention of bleeding, and removal of ruptured viscus may occur. Open fractures may require reduction and closure. Skull fractures may require elevation. Subsequently, multiple orthopaedic procedures may be required during the subacute phase and, if the child is also a burn victim, burn grafting must begin early. The exact timing of these procedures requires careful consultation among the anesthesiologist, the surgical service, and the intensive care service to ensure that the child is in the optimal state before anesthesia. Almost all traumatized children require careful attention to the possibility of a full stomach and gastric aspiration; therefore, a rapid sequence induction should probably be considered, unless specifically contraindicated. The general caveats about the use of depolarizing muscle relaxants in burned and multiply traumatized patients, as mentioned elsewhere in this text, also apply to children (see Chapters 6 and 9).

Perhaps a more difficult group of patients are those children who are unable to cooperate with surgeons for minor operations and fracture reduction and who may require significant sedation and potentially general anesthesia to allow surgical attention. Children less than 7 years old infrequently cooperate for regional or field block anesthesia. Some form of sedation is almost always necessary. Multiple agents are used; however, the consideration of a full stomach in children who require laceration suture or fracture reduction remains ever present. The choices vary from intravenous ketamine with some preservation of airway protective reflexes to a rapid sequence intubation inhalational anesthetic with extubation delayed until the patient is fully awake and all airway protective reflexes have returned. The drugs that have recently proven most useful for providing sedation for minor procedures are midazolam and fentanyl. These agents generally allow quick recovery when given intravenously. They are also suitable to be given by other routes such as rectally or intramuscularly. Ketamine provides brief anesthesia; however, concern about aspiration of gastric contents must be ever present. The traditional DPT (Demerol, Phenergan, Thorazine) still is widely used to provide sedation for children. Chloral hydrate (either orally or rectally) may also provide adequate sedation to allow minor suturing.

For adequate sedation and potential general anesthesia in a completely safe situation, the anesthetizing location for these minor procedures should be as well equipped as a general operating room. Terrified, traumatized children (with full stomachs and anxious parents) who require minor procedures are as serious an anesthetic risk as children who require major procedures. In fact, because of the temptation to use sedation, hypotension, respiratory arrest, and loss of airway reflexes must constantly be guarded against.

Approaching children who are in pain, with either minor or major injuries, who will generally be unable to control themselves, and who may be accompanied by anxious and frightened parents who are unaware of the severity of the injury requires all of the skills a physician can offer. Calming the parents goes a long way to calm the child. Calming the child requires a candid, friendly, and honest approach from the anesthesiologist with continual reassurance and comfortable, assured communication. This is aided by complete preparation and preplanning to assure that the anesthesiologist has available all that may potentially be required before beginning to interact with the child. Delays and confusion with unnecessary waiting and anxiety for the child and family are unkind and do not make the anesthesiologist's job any easier.

## REGIONAL ANESTHESIA

In general, all forms of regional anesthetic techniques available for providing anesthesia in adults can also be used in children. Children, however, may require greater sedation, and at times general anesthesia may be required to allow blocks to be performed. A particularly useful approach in children is that of caudal epidural anesthesia. This can provide analgesia for procedures below the umbilicus, such as treatment of pelvic fractures and lower limb reductions. Epidural anesthesia has the additional advantage of providing some immobility and pain relief postoperatively. We almost always supplement our general anesthetic techniques with a regional anesthetic to provide postoperative pain relief. The use of regional anesthesia to supplement general anesthesia and provide postoperative pain relief in children has been extensively reviewed elsewhere (34).

Long-term pain relief for multiply traumatized children can be provided by repeated intravenous narcotics. It has recently become clear that prolonged analgesia may be provided by epidural or intrathecal narcotic agents. At present, we consider the administration of caudal epidural morphine to every multiply traumatized child admitted to a critical care unit in our hospital. Recent evidence indicates that, in children, prevention of the pain that may accompany trauma may decrease posttraumatic metabolic processes, encourage healing, and improve recovery outcomes (8). If this is so, continuous potent analgesia may be a therapy of great benefit in multiply traumatized children. The anesthesiologist may serve as the best source of guidance in pediatric critical care areas and other areas where injured children are treated.

## SUMMARY

The continuing epidemic of pediatric trauma requires anesthesiologists to be prepared to manage these children. Managing traumatized children can be extremely rewarding. Their resilience, once the crucial early hours of care have been expertly managed, is remarkable and frequently assures a good outcome even in cases of severe trauma. The key to successful emergent and anesthetic management is planning and preparation. Careful attention to physiologic, equipment, and fluid management and psychologic differences before the child arrives assures smooth, effective management of these technically and emotionally challenging patients.

## References

1. Guyer B, Gallagher SS. An approach to the epidemiology of childhood injuries. Pediatr Clin North Am 1985;32:5–15.
2. Yaster M, Haller JA. Multiple trauma in the pediatric patient. In Rogers MC (ed): Textbook of Pediatric Intensive Care. Baltimore, Williams & Wilkins, 1987, vol 2, ch 35, pp 1265–1322.
3. American Academy of Pediatrics, Committee on Research & Accident & Poison Prevention. Reducing the toll of injuries in childhood requires support for a focused research effort. Pediatrics 1983;72:736–737.
4. Solomon T. History and demography of child abuse. Pediatrics 1973;51:773–776.
5. Reece RM, Grodin MA. Recognition of nonaccidental injury. Pediatr Clin North Am 1985;32:41–60.
6. Garrettson LK, Gallagher SS. Falls in children and youth. Pediatr Clin North Am 1985;32:153–162.
7. Fischer A. Babies in pain. Redbook Oct 1987;124–185.
8. Anand KJS, Phil D, Hickey PR. Pain and its effects in the human neonate and fetus. N Engl J Med 1987;317:1321–1329.
9. Gillis J, Dickson D, Rieder M, Steward D, Edmonds J. Results of inpatient pediatric resuscitation. Crit Care Med 1986;14:469–471.
10. Friedman WF. The intrinsic physiologic properties of the developing heart. Prog Cardiovasc Dis 1972;15:87–111.
11. Casella ES, Rogers MC, Zahka KG. Developmental physiology of the cardiovascular system. In Rogers MC (ed): Textbook of Pediatric Intensive Care. Baltimore, Williams & Wilkins, 1987, vol 1, ch 11, pp 329–365.
12. Rogers MC, Wetzel RC, Deshpande JK. Unusual causes of pulmonary edema, myocardial ischemia, and cyanosis. In Rogers MC (ed): Textbook of Pediatric Intensive Care. Baltimore, Williams & Wilkins, 1987, vol 1, ch 12, pp 366–410.
13. Wetzel RC, Rogers MC. Dysrhythmias and their management. In Rogers MC (ed): Textbook of Pediatric Intensive Care. Baltimore, Williams & Wilkins, 1987, vol 1, ch 14, pp 459–482.
14. Wetzel RC, Rogers MC. Pediatric monitoring. In Shoemaker WC, Ayres S, Grenvik A, Holbrook PR, Thompson WL (eds): Textbook of Critical Care, ed 2. Philadelphia, WB Saunders, 1989, ch 22, pp 215–222.
15. Britt BA. Temperature regulation. In Gregory GA (ed): Pediatric Anesthesia. New York, Churchill Livingstone, 1983, vol 1, ch 7, pp 253–314.
16. Vale RJ. Normothermia: its place in operative and post-operative care. Anaesthesia 1973;28:241–245.
17. Kliegman RM, Fanaroff AA. Developmental metabolism and nutrition. In Gregory GA (ed): Pediatric Anesthesia. New York, Churchill Livingstone, 1983, vol 1, ch 6, pp 169–251.
18. Pulsinelli WA, Waldman S, Rawlinson D, Plum F. Moderate hyperglycemia augments ischemic brain damage: a neuropathologic study in the rat. Neurology 1982;32:1239–1246.
19. Part IV. Pediatric basic life support. JAMA 1986;255:2954–2960.
20. Schleien CL: Recent advances in pediatric CPR. Anesthesiology Rep 1988;1:6–20.
21. Schleien CL, Rogers MC. Cardiopulmonary resuscitation in infants and children. In Rogers MC (ed): Textbook of Pediatric Intensive Care. Baltimore, Williams & Wilkins, 1987, vol 1, ch 2, pp 7–56.
22. Part II. Adult basic life support. JAMA 1986;255:2915–2932.
23. Davis RJ, Dean JM, Goldberg AL, Carson BS, Rosenbaum AE, Rogers MC. Head and spinal cord injury. In Rogers MC (ed): Textbook of Pediatric Intensive Care. Baltimore, Williams & Wilkins, 1987, vol 1, ch 21, pp 649–699.
24. Backofen JE, Rogers MC. Emergency management of the airway. In Rogers MC (ed): Textbook of Pediatric Intensive Care. Baltimore, Williams & Wilkins, 1987, vol 1, ch 3, pp 57–79.
25. Shapiro HM, White SR, Harris AB. Ketamine anesthesia in patients with intracranial pathology. Br J Anaesth 1972;44:1200–1206.
26. Raju TNK, Vidyasagar D, Torres C, Grundy D, Bennett EJ. Intracranial pressure during intubation and anesthesia in infants. J Pediatr 1980;96:860–862.
27. Donegan MF, Bedford RF. Intravenously administered lidocaine prevents intracranial hypertension during endotracheal suctioning. Anesthesiology 1980;52:516–518.
28. Gregory GA. Pharmacology. In Gregory GA (ed): Pediatric Anesthesia. New York, Churchill Livingstone, 1983, vol 1, ch 8, pp 315–339.
29. Cook DR. Succinylcholine: an argument to abandon its elective use in pediatric anesthesia. Anesthesiology Rep 1988;1:84–88.
30. Prian GW, Wright GB, Rumach CM, O'Meara OP. Apparent cerebral embolization after temporal artery catheterization. J Pediatr 1978;93:115–118.

31. Venkataraman ST, Orr RA, Thompson AE. Percutaneous infraclavicular subclavian vein catheterization in critically ill infants and children. J Pediatr 1988;113:480–485.

32. Spivey WH, Lathers CM, Malone DR, Unger HD, Bhat S, McNamara RN, Schoffstall J, Tumer N. Comparison of intraosseous, central, and peripheral routes of sodium bicarbonate administration during CPR in pigs. Ann Emerg Med 1985; 14:1135–1140.

33. Ward JT Jr. Endotracheal drug therapy. Am J Emerg Med 1983;1:71–82.

34. Yaster M, Wetzel RC. Pediatric regional anesthesia. Anesthesiology Rep 1988;1:120–130.

# Regional Anesthesia for Trauma

*John I. Lauria*

> "The inseparability of anesthesia from the total care of the surgical patient is to us the compelling reason why surgeon and anesthetist, engaged as they are in a common task, cannot with profit pursue separate goals" (1). This quote from the foreword of Beecher and Todd's classic study applies with more meaning to the care of trauma patients perhaps than to other areas of surgical care.

Over the past four decades, the ever-increasing incidence of trauma has required that its treatment become more specialized and centralized in trauma centers. A common characteristic of many (but certainly not all) trauma patients is the presence of varying degrees of pain preoperatively. The presence of severe pain preoperatively is one factor that separates these patients from the routine elective surgery candidate. Circulatory instability secondary to hypovolemia and central nervous system depression secondary to head injury are also frequent complicating factors that require special attention. Regional anesthesia techniques may play an important role in addressing some of the problems complicating the initial and long-term care of trauma patients. Regional anesthetic techniques have been the focus of renewed attention nation-

ally and internationally over the past few years. Regional anesthesia for trauma surgery has a history dating back much farther than most present-day physicians realize. Beecher's classic paper addressed the issue in 1946 (2). Besides pointing out the utility of various regional techniques to relieve pain and provide anesthesia for surgery, Beecher described the enigmatic nature of pain in casualties. Some victims experience little or no pain from their injuries, whereas others seem to be overwhelmed by their pain. Beecher also pointed out the role that anxiety played in escalating the reaction to injury, which can be mistaken for pain. Ancient Chinese warriors were reported to suffer little or no pain when shot through with arrows in various sites of their anatomy. This fact has been cited as a possible basis for the early establishment of acupuncture points. The expression of reaction to pain is a very complex phenomenon having a great deal to do with biologic factors such as the site and mechanism of injury as well as social and personal factors. Although we may not understand completely the underlying basis of the personal reaction to pain, we acknowledge the protective as well as the deleterious nature of pain and recognize the benefits of relieving it. Perhaps Beecher's greater contribution to the care of trauma patients was his observation of the dangers of narcotics indiscriminately administered to battle casualties. He recognized, without elaborate laboratory equipment, the toll of severe respiratory depression paid by wounded troops. Recent advances in technique, equipment design, and pharmacology have led to wider application of regional techniques during the perioperative period and in trauma victims.

Often the attention of the anesthesia surgical team is focused entirely upon the cardiopulmonary resuscitation of trauma victims to the complete exclusion of regional techniques of analgesia or anesthesia that may be of some benefit in the patient's overall management.

## EARLY PAIN RELIEF AND ASSESSMENT

Early management of pain in trauma victims beginning at the scene of the accident has been suggested. Bridenbaugh's statement that "the role of regional anesthesia in the early and late treatment of trauma patients is under-appreciated and under-utilized" (3) should stimulate the present generation of anesthesiologists to seek better understanding of the problem. The early relief of pain at the scene of the accident has some appeal. The reality of providing sufficiently trained manpower looms as a great obstacle. As long as the vast majority of scene-of-the-accident care is provided by volunteers with little or no extensive training, the provision of analgesia must await the next level of care. In emergency room settings, however, the use of regional techniques to relieve pain should be given more attention. Properly used local anesthetics can provide more satisfactory analgesia/anesthesia with less impairment of the state of consciousness and respiration than is provided by narcotics administered parenterally (4).

The demonstration of specific opioid receptors in the dorsal horn of the grey matter of the spinal cord (5) and the isolation of endogenous opioid-like peptides (6) have revolutionized our ability to utilize regional techniques to provide analgesia. Both the subarachnoid and the epidural routes are now used routinely to administer narcotics in combination with local anesthetics. The dose of narcotic required to provide excellent analgesia via these routes is far below that required by parenteral administration.

Careful attention to total dose and the avoidance of intravascular injection should eliminate the possibility of local anesthetic toxicity. Bearing in mind the probable lower maximal safe dose of local anesthetics in those who are volume-depleted should allow the skilled practitioner to apply the techniques with less risk than presented by parenteral narcotics. Standards of practice for the use of regional anesthesia in the operating room should apply to the emergency room as well. The patient must have a secure intravenous line in place, there must be a full complement of resuscitation equipment, and drugs must be immediately at hand. All personnel allowed to use local anesthetics must know the maximal safe dose of each drug used and the minimal effective concentration of that drug for each block. One must be able to calculate instantly the total dose when injecting a given volume of a given concentration. Recalling that 1 ml of a 1% solution contains 10 mg is very useful in converting volume and concentration to total dose. Without such knowledge of the drugs and the techniques, one is doomed to either provide inadequate blocks or overdose patients, producing systemic toxic reactions.

## LOCAL ANESTHETIC TOXICITY

### Manifestation

Classically, local anesthetic toxicity is manifested by central nervous system irritability. Early signs and symptoms may be irritability, restlessness, shivering, and slurred speech. Full-blown jacksonian-type epileptic seizures may follow. The systemic toxicity of some local anesthetics, notably lidocaine and procaine, may progress to central nervous system depression with somnolence and unconsciousness without a preceding seizure. Cardiovascular depression may also be seen as a result of the direct depressant effect on the myocardium or as a result of massive central nervous system depression in a postictal state marked by unconsciousness and apnea. Cardiovascular depression may also be noted as a result of the sympatholytic effects when local anesthetics are inadvertently injected into the subarachnoid space or epidural space when performing blocks in those portions of the anatomy in which this is possible.

### Prevention

Whenever a significant dose of local anesthetic is injected, the possibility of systemic toxic reactions must be kept in mind. Whether it occurs depends on the plasma level achieved, which in turn is related to the site of injection, the rate of absorption, and the volume of distribution. Injection into highly vascular areas may result in inadvertent intravenous injection. Application of topical anesthetics to the tracheal bronchial mucosa may result in rapid absorption approaching the rate of intravenously administered drug. What constitutes a significant dose of local anesthetic? The author believes that one-half of the recommended safe dose constitutes a significant dose. The primary step in prevention is to use the smallest volume of the lowest concentration of the drug that will do the job. Repeated aspiration during injection should always be practiced to avoid intravascular or intrathecal injection. The use of the immobile needle (that is, a needle held in place in an immobile fashion while the injection is made by another person through an extension tube connected to the needle) also helps prevent intravascular injection by maintaining accurate placement of the needle.

### Treatment

Once a toxic reaction is recognized, it should be of little consequence if promptly and properly treated. Anyone who is given a significant dose should have a reliable intravenous line in place and be appropriately monitored. Appropriate monitoring at a minimum should consist of a pulse oximeter, blood pressure cuff, and electrocardiogram (see Chapter 6). The patient should be in a setting, preferably on an operating room table, that allows respiratory support, tracheal intubation, and ventilation to be achieved easily

Central nervous system irritability or outright seizures should be terminated with a short-acting barbiturate such as thiopental, 1 to 2 mg/kg, or valium, 5 to 10 mg depending on severity. Should the intravenous line be lost during a seizure, the patient should be paralyzed with intramuscular succinylcholine, 1.5 mg/kg. The trachea should then be intubated and ventilation controlled while the patient is further assessed. Reestablishing an intravenous route while the patient is relaxed will allow further therapy with fluids and vasopressors, should they be needed.

The use of a benzodiazepam derivative before performance of the block procedure, either orally or parenterally, will increase the seizure threshold. These drugs, however, should not be used as substitutes for good technique and will not prevent the potential cardiovascular toxicity.

After recovery from a toxic reaction manifested by seizure activity, the patient should be closely monitored for some hours in an appropriate recovery room setting. In the trauma patient, it is especially wise to reassess at this time the patient's volume status.

## HYPERSENSITIVITY REACTION

True hypersensitivity reaction to local anesthetic drugs is rare. The ester derivatives, such as procaine and tetracaine, are most commonly involved because there may be cross-hypersensitivity to other commonly used drugs, such as sulfonamides, which are ester derivatives. True hypersensitivity to the amide-based drugs is extremely rare. It is not uncommon to encounter a patient who claims to be allergic to Novocain, having been given a local anesthetic in a dentist's office. Frequently, Novocain is used as a generic term for all anesthetics by dentists speaking with their patients. It is seldom used by dentists any more. Many of these patients will describe a syndrome that is consistent with the pharmacologic response to epinephrine, which was commonly used in rather high concentrations in some dental preparations of local anesthetics. If a patient is truly hypersensitive to one of the ester derivatives, as determined by skin testing, one should consider the use of an amide drug as probably safe but would be well-advised to skin test for the amide preparation before administering it.

## ADVANTAGES OF REGIONAL TECHNIQUES OF ANALGESIA OVER NARCOTICS

The use of appropriately applied regional anesthetic techniques gives the opportunity to provide excellent analgesia without paying the price of the respiratory depression and alteration of consciousness that may be associated with the use of parenteral narcotics. The degree of pain relief with regional anesthesia is greater, often being associated with a completely pain-free situation. The evaluation of the trauma patient may be facilitated by having the patient totally conscious and free of respiratory depression. At times, the cardiovascular response to pain or the anxiety accompanying injury may complicate evaluation of the patient's volume status. The advantages of regional anesthesia over narcotics are probably best exemplified by the use of intercostal blocks for the relief of pain from multiple rib fractures. The patient who has respiratory dysfunction because of splinting secondary to pain often has significant improvement in respiratory function after relief of the pain using local anesthesia. Although intubation may still be required in the patient with multiple rib fractures to ensure adequate ventilation, it would then be mandated by the injuries and not by the drugs used to treat the pain. Thoracic epidural anesthesia has been used to treat chest trauma with similar beneficial effects on ventilation (4).

## REGIONAL ANESTHETIC TECHNIQUES AND NERVE BLOCKS USEFUL IN THE TRAUMA PATIENT

Rather than provide detailed descriptions and accurate diagrams of the anatomy involved in each technique, the author advises the reader to obtain one or more of the excellent texts on the subject. Winnie's *Plexus Anesthesia* (7) has become a favorite in many training programs and one frequently referred to by staff when refreshing their techniques. The quality of the anatomic diagrams is excellent. Moore's *Regional Block* (8), although dated, remains a classic reference source in most departments.

In contemplating the use of regional anesthetic techniques for surgery, one must appreciate the time necessary for various blocks to become fully effective. It is not uncommon for a particular block to take 15 to 30 minutes, depending upon the drug used, to become fully effective. An anesthesiologist performing the block must be capable of reassuring both the patient and the surgeon while waiting for the block to take effect and must have a predetermined plan to rescue the incomplete or totally ineffective block. Sedation with small doses of short-acting narcotics may be all that is required. At other times, additional injections at the initial or other sites of skin infiltration may be required. Impatience on the part of the surgeon or the anesthesiologist will be appreciated by the patient and will only add to the patient's anxiety and possible ineffectiveness of the technique.

In providing regional anesthesia, particularly for prolonged procedures on the extremities, one must realize that, although the block may achieve complete anesthesia of the part of the anatomy required, the patient may become very uncomfortable on the operating room table, and the patient's restlessness may interfere with the operation. It is very important to ensure that the patient is comfortably situated on the table. A small amount of flexion of the table in the lumbar area and at the knees will avoid the back pain that patients frequently develop while lying flat on their backs on a firm table. A calm atmosphere in the operating room, smoothing music, and a comfortable temperature all contribute to successful regional anesthesia.

**Upper Extremity**

In caring for upper extremity injuries, one must become expert in both a supraclavicular technique and the more commonly applied axillary approach to the brachial plexus. The axillary approach seems to have become the standard for hand surgery. The major drawback of this approach is the occasional failure to achieve anesthesia of the musculocutaneous nerve, which gives rise to the lateral cutaneous nerve of the forearm which innervates the dorsum of the wrist. This problem is avoided by paying particular attention to applying pressure distal to the injection site so that the bolus of local anesthetic solution is forced proximal in the fascial sheath surrounding the neurovascular bundle. Incomplete blocks of the forearm can easily be rescued by blocking the appropriate nerves peripherally, resulting in a complete anesthesia of the forearm. If one uses this block, therefore, it is necessary to become familiar with the anatomy of the nerves peripherally. The

popularity of the axillary approach is explained by absence of the possibility of producing a pneumothorax.

To provide complete regional anesthesia for the upper extremity, one must make use of one of the supraclavicular approaches. The most popular supraclavicular approach practiced during the 1950s was associated with a significant incidence of pneumothorax, which became more and more unacceptable as the litigious climate in which we practice became more focused on such events. The interscalene approach, in which the local anesthetic is deposited at the roots of the brachial plexus at the C6 level, provides brachial plexus anesthesia with much less potential for pneumothorax (9). The landmark for this block, the groove between the anterior and the medial scalene muscles, can be identified well with practice. In making injections in the cervical area close to the spine, there is always the potential for an inadvertent intrathecal injection. The possibility of injection into the intervertebral artery also exists. The use of proper technique, direction of the needle caudad, and aspiration before injection avoid these problems. A well-executed interscalene block produces good operating conditions about the shoulder, the upper arm, and the elbow. Occasionally, caudad spread of the anesthetic is incomplete, and distal portions of the upper extremity are not completely anesthetized. This problem can be avoided by proper positioning of the patient in a head-up position before injection to allow more caudad spread of the solution. As with the axillary block, appropriate block of the nerves distally, commonly the ulnar, can rescue this situation.

Simple aspiration of hematomas and injection around fracture sites of the hand, wrist, and elbow can be used to provide analgesia in the emergency room.

An intravenous or Bier block of the upper extremity is a very easily accomplished block (10). An anesthetic solution is injected into the venous system of either the upper or the lower extremity after most of the blood of the extremity has been removed by elevation and wrapping with an Esmarch bandage. Two tourniquets are applied to the extremity, and the anesthetic solution is administered through a previously placed intravenous catheter with the proximal tourniquet inflated. Anesthesia of the entire limb is provided up to the proximal tourniquet. After the establishment of anesthesia, the distal tourniquet is inflated. When the patient complains of discomfort from the upper proximal tourniquet, it may be deflated. The patient then remains with the lower, distal tourniquet inflated in an anesthetized portion of the arm. The anesthesia from this technique is terminated upon release of the tourniquet. This is a serious disadvantage of the technique. Another disadvantage of this technique is the very ease with which the anesthesia is produced, which may encourage untrained individuals to apply it. Although the technique is simple, proper knowledge of all of the equipment and drugs involved is required. Fifty milliliters of 0.5% lidocaine or 0.25% bupivacaine are utilized most frequently to anesthetize the arm. One hundred milliliters of the same drugs are used for the leg.

The use of buffered 0.5% chloroprocaine should be considered for intravenous regional anesthesia. A seldom-noted report (11) indicates that it is more effective and safer than Xylocaine and has the added advantage of providing anesthesia that persists beyond the time of tourniquet release. Chloroprocaine has previously been considered unsuitable because of the incidence of thrombophlebitis associated with its intravenous injection. Thrombophlebitis was not observed with the buffered 0.5% preparation. There is a small incidence of toxic reaction after an intravenous block because of tourniquet failure or inadvertent release. Despite the ease with which this block is accomplished, individuals should be credentialed to perform it with the same standards of care that apply to the performance of other regional techniques.

## Lower Extremity

The use of spinal or epidural anesthesia for fractures of the hip has stood the test of time. There is ample evidence to indicate that the incidence of postoperative complications is less than with general anesthesia (12, 13). The obvious advantage of spinal anesthesia is the ease with which it can be produced and the consistency of results. The epidural route requires more finesse and has a higher incidence of failure. Both techniques of anesthesia are associated with sympathetic block, which may result in severe hypotension, particularly in the hypovolemic patient. Volume loading before performance of spinal or epidural anesthesia, however, can avoid much of the problem. In the case of the trauma patient, one should probably reconsider the use of isobaric or hypobaric techniques of spinal anesthesia in which the patient can be placed in a slightly head-down position to enhance venous return and diminish the circulatory effects of the sympathetic block (14).

Lumbar plexus block, by either of the two accepted routes, should also be considered for producing analgesia or anesthesia for surgical procedures on the upper leg, although it must be combined with obturator block to anesthetize the thigh completely.

The femoral nerve block, which is easily accomplished as the femoral nerve passes under the inguinal ligament lateral to the femoral artery, provides excellent analgesia in patients who have severe pain after open reduction and internal fixation of the femur. It should be equally effective in the early management of the pain of femur fractures.

Combined femoral and sciatic nerve block can provide excellent anesthesia for the leg below the knee and is frequently the choice in patients in whom spinal anesthesia may not be appropriate.

The well-described ankle block can consistently provide excellent analgesia and good operating conditions for the ankle and foot.

All of these blocks can be performed with reasonable volumes of local anesthetics and require modest experience for consistent results.

## Thorax and Abdomen

Multiple intercostal blocks can provide excellent surgical anesthesia of the upper abdominal wall and can be used to provide analgesia for rib fractures (15). In the performance of intercostal blocks, strict attention to the details of the technique should avoid the major complications of intravascular injection and pneumothorax.

The use of thoracic epidural block has also been reported for the care of multiple rib fractures but has not obtained widespread use (4). Many anesthesiologists remain reluctant to perform epidural anesthesia in the thoracic area for benign conditions.

The most significant recent advance in regional anesthesia technique that can be applied to the trauma patient is interpleural regional anesthesia. This route of local anesthetic administration was discovered accidentally during investigation of the use of continuous intercostal nerve blocks for postoperative pain relief (16). The technique is easier to learn and apply than is thoracic epidural anesthesia. It has obvious advantages over multiple intercostal nerve blocks because it involves a single needle stick. There are also other advantages over the epidural and intercostal routes. There is less sympathetic block and, therefore, less potential for circulatory side effects than with the epidural approach. There is less concern for high local anesthetic plasma levels than with the intercostal approach. The side effects seen with epidural opioids—respiratory depression, nausea, drowsiness, itching, and urinary retention—have not been observed after interpleural local anesthetic administration.

As with many other regional anesthetic techniques, the interpleural approach has met with a high degree of success among those who are enthusiastic about it and who were early innovators in the field. Very strict attention to the details of the recommended technique in regard to needle placement and positioning of the patient is associated with a very high degree of success, which should make this technique well accepted and applied widely for traumatic chest injuries, postoperative pain relief, and chronic pain syndromes. It has also been successfully used for surgical procedures such as breast surgery, nephrostomy, nephrolithotomy, and other procedures on the lateral aspects of the chest (17, 18).

An interpleural catheter may be introduced either percutaneously or intraoperatively in open chest procedures. The percutaneous placement is accomplished with the patient lying in the horizontal lateral decubitius position, with the affected side up. A Tuohy needle is introduced at an angle of 40° to 60° through the skin of the 4th to 8th intercostal space, 8 to 10 cm from the posterior midline. The needle is introduced in a manner that will direct it to the upper surface of the lower rib of the interspace to avoid the neurovascular bundle in the intercostal groove of the lower surface of the upper rib of a given interspace. As the needle is walked off the top of the rib, the caudal membrane is encountered and offers resistance. The technique then used is somewhat like the loss of resistance in the placement of an epidural catheter, although in reverse. The stylet is removed from the Tuohy needle, and a glass syringe with a moistened barrel containing 3 or 4 ml of air is attached to the hub of the needle. The syringe and needle are then advanced as a unit through the membrane toward the parietal pleura. When the parietal pleura is perforated, a clicking sensation may be noted. Because the interpleural pressure is negative, the freely mobile barrel of the syringe will then advance. Obviously, the syringe needle unit is held by the barrel of the syringe and the needle shaft, with no pressure on the plunger. After appreciating the presence of the negative interpleural pressure, one can assume that the space has been identified. The syringe is removed, and an epidural catheter is advanced 5 to 7 cm into the interpleural space. The Tuohy needle is then removed over the catheter. A catheter is never withdrawn from a Tuohy needle because of the possibility of shearing it off and losing the distal portion. Aspiration is carried out to ensure that the catheter has not entered a blood vessel and/or the lung parenchyma. The catheter is then taped in place as with epidural catheters, with appropriate strain relief loops and a small cushion-like dressing at the puncture site to avoid kinking. A local anesthetic solution is then injected through a micro-filter—20 to 30 ml of 0.5% bupivacaine has been used very successfully.

Placement of the catheter in an open chest after thoracotomy is quite simple. The surgeon can insert the catheter through a Tuohy needle over the rib immediately below the incision. The epidural catheter can then be placed in the thoracic cavity in the paravertebral gutter as close to the midline as possible. It is important to maintain the catheter in a position posteriorly and medially as high as possible in the chest cavity. Placement of a loose absorbable suture around the catheter to hold it in place facilitates maintenance of the proper position. The incidence of infection encountered with this technique has been extremely low.

Patients who are given this form of regional anesthesia after cholecystectomy experience complete pain relief for 6 to 26 hours (19). Topping up the dose on the average of every 8 to 9 hours has been reported to provide an almost pain-free 48 hours immediately postoperative.

In patients with chest injuries involving multiple rib fractures, this technique has been used very successfully (20) and is undergoing further study at a number of centers. If the patient has a chest tube in place, the chest tube should be clamped for 10 to 20 minutes after the drug is injected initially and with each top-up dose. It is important that the patient be maintained in a supine position with the affected side up while the drug is injected and for 10 to 20 minutes afterward to ensure spread to the posterior superior aspects of the thoracic cavity. Utilizing this technique, patients with multiple rib fractures who might otherwise splint and hypoventilate may be treated without a ventilator.

The major complication associated with this technique is obviously pneumothorax. However, appropriate use of the glass syringe to detect negative interpleural pressure and use of the rather blunt Tuohy needle will avoid this. Chest x-ray films should be obtained after applying this technique, however. Frequently, a small collection of air will be noted over the apex of the lung. This small collection is the air that enters while changing over from the air-filled glass syringe to the syringe used to inject the local anesthetic. It is of no consequence but may be upsetting to x-ray personnel who are not aware of the preceding event. The incidence of pneumothorax reported in several thousand patients in studies around the world has been less than 5%.

Although the amount of sympathetic blockade with this technique is less than with an epidural anesthetic, the vital signs should be monitored for a couple of hours after the initial placement and each top-up dose.

The contraindications to placement of an interpleural catheter are several. Obviously, catheters should not be introduced through infected skin or into someone who has pneumonia. An inflamed pleura may result in very rapid absorption of the anesthetic solution and a toxic reaction. Other pulmonary conditions associated with a thickened pleura are relative contraindications. The risk to a patient with bullous emphysema of entering the pulmonary parenchyma should be considered.

Over the past few years, various narcotics have been introduced with local anesthetics, epidurally and intrathecally, to provide prolonged analgesia. The addition of morphine or fentanyl to spinal and epidural anesthetics extends the pain-free period for 10 to 12 hours postinjection, long after the sympatholytic effects of the local anesthetics have disappeared. Much smaller doses of the narcotics are effective when given by these routes than would be necessary to achieve the same level of analgesia when injected parenterally (21).

General anesthesia for abdominal surgery is frequently combined with the placement of an epidural catheter to provide postoperative analgesia. This practice has proven safe and effective in managing pain in extensive elective surgical procedures and should be equally advantageous for patients requiring extensive surgery for trauma. The catheters can be placed pre- or postoperatively. As experience is gained in these techniques, the obvious advantage of pain-free recovery without narcotic-induced central nervous system depression speaks for itself.

## CONTINUOUS SPINAL ANESTHESIA

Continuous spinal anesthesia has been practiced for many years. Enthusiasm for the technique has not been high because of the high incidence of headache associated with the placement of the then-available catheters. At present, a 32 gauge catheter is available, which can be safely placed through a 25 or 26 gauge needle (22). Use of the smaller catheters is associated with an acceptable incidence of headache. Apparently, the catheters are structurally capable of withstanding the stresses applied to them without breaking off in the subarachnoid space. This technique should provide a reasonable alternative for those who are insecure about the placement of epidural catheters because of inconsistent results.

## SECONDARY BENEFITS OF REGIONAL ANESTHETIC TECHNIQUES IN TRAUMA PATIENTS

The sympathetic blocks associated with the use of regional techniques, particularly for hand surgery, substantially contribute to preservation of the blood supply by preventing or reversing the vasospasm due to injury and surgery. The reflex sympathetic

dystrophies observed in the extremities after injury respond well to appropriate sympathetic blocks. It may well be that the use of regional anesthesia is effective in preventing the development of these dystrophies (23).

The psychologic benefit of recovering from major trauma or surgery in a relatively pain-free, awake state provided by regional techniques may contribute substantially to a patient's early recovery.

There is evidence that the metabolic responses to pain and stress may be detrimental to recovery (24). The selective use of various drugs administered via regional anesthetic techniques may be effective in reducing or eliminating the deleterious metabolic responses to injury.

## ADJUNCTS TO SUCCESSFUL REGIONAL ANESTHETIC TECHNIQUE

Doppler flow probes may prove particularly useful in providing regional anesthesia for trauma patients. Blocks that require identification of vascular landmarks may be facilitated by identifying the artery with a Doppler probe. Swelling, pain, and tenderness may preclude positive identification of a landmark by palpation. The probe is especially useful in identifying the brachial artery for the axillary approach to the brachial plexus and can also be very useful in identifying the neurovascular bundle along the lower rib margin, either in approaching it or in trying to avoid it.

Nerve stimulators have also found a place in assisting proper needle placement close to the appropriate nervous structure. This can be particularly useful in a short, thick-necked individual in whom an interscalene block of the brachial plexus is attempted.

## SUMMARY

In summary, well-developed and accepted techniques of regional anesthesia are capable of providing excellent operating conditions for many of the surgical procedures required in trauma victims. The use of these regional techniques to provide analgesia during the perioperative period has significant advantages over the use of systemically administered narcotics in that central nervous system depression may be avoided. Also, the quality of the anesthesia/analgesia produced is far superior in a given area than that which can be achieved with the use of narcotics. The use of catheters to introduce local anesthetics allows prolonged maintenance of analgesia. The regional introduction of narcotics with local anesthetics has proven effective and safe for prolonging the anesthetic action. There are other secondary benefits to the provision of anesthesia by regional techniques.

## References

1. Beecher HK, Todd DP. A Study of the Deaths Associated with Anesthesia and Surgery. Springfield, IL, Charles C Thomas, 1954.
2. Beecher HK. Pain in men wounded in battle. Ann Surg 1946;123:96–105.
3. Bridenbaugh PO. Regional Anesthesia for the Trauma Patient. ASA Refresher Course Lectures, 1987, p 232.
4. Worthley LI. Thoracic epidural in the management of chest trauma: a study of 161 cases. Intensive Care Med 1985;11(6):312–315.
5. Pert CB, Snyder SH. Opiate receptor: demonstration in nervous tissue. Science 1973;179:1001–1004.
6. Hughes J, Smith TW, Kosterlitz HW, Fothergill LA, Morgan BA, Morris HR. Identification of two related pentapeptides from the brain with potent opiate agonist activity. Nature 1975;258:577–579.
7. Winnie AP. Plexus Anesthesia, Volume 1, Perivascular Technique of Brachial Plexus Block. Philadelphia, WB Saunders, 1984.
8. Moore DC. *Regional Block*, ed 4. Springfield, IL, Charles C Thomas, 1979.
9. Ward MG. The interscalene approach to the brachial plexus. Anesthesia 1974;29:147–157.
10. Farrell RG. Safe and effective i.v. regional anesthesia for use in the emergency department. Ann Emerg Med A April 14, 1985;4:288–292.
11. Yudenfreund SM, Bansal P, Watson WA. Evaluation of pH buffered chloroprocaine for intravenous anesthesia. In Anesthesiology 1986;65:A209.
12. Modig J, Borg T, Karlstrom G, Maripuu E, Sahlstedt. Thromboembolism after total hip replacement: role of epidural and general anesthesia. Anesth Analg 1983;62:174–180.
13. McKenzie PJ, Wishart HY, Dewar KMS, Gray I, Smith G. Comparison of the effects of spinal anaesthesia and general anaesthesia on postoperative oxygenation and perioperative mortality. Br J Anaesth 1980;52:49–54.
14. Donaghy GE. Modern anesthesia for war surgery. Milit Surg June 1960;86:577–581.
15. Murphy DF. Continuous intercostal nerve blockade: an anatomical study to elucidate its mode of action. Br J Anaesth 1984;56:627–630.
16. Reiestad F. Interpleural Regional Analgesia—A New Method for Pain Relief in Various Acute and Chronic Pain Conditions. Ulleval University Hospital, Oslo, Norway, thesis summary, 1989.
17. Schlesinger TM, Laurito CE, Baughman UL, Carranza CO. Interpleural bupivacaine for mammography during needle localization and breast biopsy. Anesth Analg 1989;68:394–395.
18. Narendra ST, Robalino J, Shevda K. Intrapleural block: a new technique for regional anesthesia during percutaneous nephrostomy and nephrolithotomy. Regional Anesth 1989;14:S48.
19. Murphy DF. Continuous intercostal nerve blockade for pain relief following cholecystectomy. Br J Anesth 1983;55:521–525.
20. Rocco S, Reiestad F, Gudman J, McKay W. Intrapleural administration of local anesthetics for pain relief in patients with multiple rib fractures. Regional Anesth 1987;12:10–14.
21. Cousins MJ, Mather LE. Intrathecal and epidural administration of opioids. Anesthesiology 1984;61:276–310.
22. Hurley RJ. Continuous Spinal Anesthesia. International Anesthesiology Clinics, Vol 27. Boston, Little, Brown, 1989.
23. Rosenblatt R, Pepitone, Rockwell F. Continuous axillary analgesia for traumatic hand injury. Anesthesiology 1979;51:565–566.
24. Fellows IW, Woolfson AMJ. Effects of therapeutic interventions on the metabolic responses to injury. Br Med Bull 1985;41(3):287–294.

# Hypothermia and Hyperthermia in Trauma Patients

*Murray A. Kalish*

Hypothermia and hyperthermia are two complications of special significance in the care of the trauma patient. In this chapter, we explore their importance in relation to pathophysiology, prevention, treatment, effects on organs, and complications. We also outline the epidemiology, inheritance, incidence, diagnosis, and anesthetic management of malignant hyperthermia and compare the neuroleptic malignant syndrome with malignant hyperthermia.

## HYPOTHERMIA

Medical literature from antiquity described cases of total body hypothermia. The Hippocrates school in the 4th and 5th centuries BC, for example, recommended systemic hypothermia to treat tetanus and convulsions (1). Subsequently, additional therapeutic uses for hypothermia came into use. However, there are profound adverse effects of hypothermia. Although limited in therapeutic use in modern medical practice, hypothermia, defined as core temperature below 36°C, is an everyday unplanned occurrence in most operating rooms (2)

(Table 13.1). Accidental hypothermia is particularly prevalent in the trauma patient population.

### Pathophysiology

Humans, being homeothermic, maintain temperature regulation within narrow limits (36.0° to 37.5°C) (3). The preoptic anterior region of the hypothalamus controls the thermoregulatory center, which in turn controls heat loss and production (1–3). Heat loss is partially controlled by thermoreceptors in the skin and subcutaneous tissue, leading to vasodilation or vasoconstriction. On the other hand, heat production is increased by an increased level of catecholamines and thyroid hormones, which produce "nonshivering" thermogenesis. Catecholamines cause mobilization of free fatty acids from adipose tissue and, through cyclic adenosine monophosphate (cAMP), initiate heat production in brown adipose tissue (4). However, the most important cause of increased heat production is skeletal muscle shivering. When the thermoregulatory system is depressed or

Table 13.1.  **Factors Precipitating Inadvertent Hypothermia**[a]

Ambient operating room service
Exposed sedated patient
Intravenous infusions
General anesthesia
  Central nervous system depression
  Decreased metabolic rate
  Vasodilation
  Abolishment of shivering
  Controlled ventilation
Surgical intervention
  Cold surgical preparation solutions
  Nasogastric tube, Foley catheter
  Open body cavities
  Fluid and blood loss

[a] From Fallacaro MD, Fallacaro NA, Radel TJ. Inadvertent hypothermia: etiology, effects, and prevention. AORN J 1986;44(1):54–57, 60–61.

overwhelmed, humans become poikilothermic, i.e., dependent on their external environment to maintain body temperature.

Heat loss occurs in one of four ways: radiation, convection, evaporation, and conduction (2, 5) (Fig. 13.1). Radiation, which refers to the transfer of energy between objects through electromagnetic waves, accounts for 40 to 50% of the body's total heat loss in the operating room. Radiant heat loss is proportional to the temperature difference between the patient and the environment (6). Convection, which refers to the direct transfer of energy by collisions between body surface molecules and moving air molecules, accounts for 25 to 35% of the total heat loss in the undressed patient lying in a properly air-conditioned operating room. Ambient temperature, air velocity, and surface area are the main determinants of heat loss via convection (6).

Evaporative heat loss refers to the vaporization of water or volatile skin preparation solutions, which demands heat. Evaporative heat loss is also caused by insensible perspiration plus evaporation from the respiratory tract. This is approximately 25 kcal/hr, which can be reduced to 10 to 15 kcal/hr by using moist, warm inspired gases (6).

Finally, conduction, which refers to the transfer of heat by direct contact between objects, plays a minor role (<10%) in intraoperative cooling as a result of low specific heat and conductivity of drapes and mattresses (6).

Thermogenesis has two components: shivering and nonshivering. Shivering is a centrally mediated neural response that consists of involuntary rhythmic contractions of skeletal muscle; it is not a function of the sympathetic nervous system. Shivering increases heat production by the con-

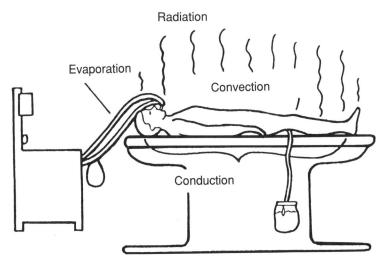

**Figure 13.1  Four mechanisms of intraoperative heat loss.** (From Fallacaro MD, Fallacaro NA, Radel TJ. Inadvertent hypothermia: etiology, effects, and prevention. AORN J 1986;44(1):54–57, 60–61.)

tracting muscles; however, it also increases convective and radiative heat loss by increasing muscle movement and blood flow. Nonshivering thermogenesis is caused by an increase in the combustion of fatty acids and glucose. The most active metabolic areas in humans are the liver and skeletal muscle. In the neonate, the highly vascular and visibly innervated brown fat plays the major role in thermogenesis. Epinephrine and thyroxine are important in the efficiency of norepinephrine-induced thermogenesis (5, 6).

Many environmental factors affect the body temperature of the surgical patient. The temperature in a modern operating room ranges from 19 to 24°C (7). This ambient temperature plays an important role, as do the humidity of the operating room, the number of room air exchanges per hour, and the presence of laminar airflow devices. These factors keep the staff comfortable and decrease growth of bacteria. The duration of exposure to the operating room temperature will vary according to the length of the surgical procedure (3). A study conducted by Morris showed the following: (a) there was a significant correlation between operating room temperature and the patient's temperature; (b) the greatest fall in temperature occurred during the initial hour of anesthesia, and neither the patient's age nor the site of operation influenced the temperature decline; (c) 70% of the patients maintained normal temperature when the operating room temperature was between 21° and 24°C; and (d) the critical ambient operating room temperature was 21°C (8).

Body weight and surface area contribute to temperature variability. Children have poor thermal insulation (i.e., thin skin and subcutaneous fat layer), small body size, large ratio of surface area to body weight, and increased curvature of the body (effects heat loss by radiation), all increasing heat loss (9). Obese patients take longer to cool (10). The opening of peritoneal and pleural body cavities, along with cold irrigants, contributes to hypothermia.

General anesthetics contribute to hypothermia in a number of ways. First, anesthe-

sia depresses the thermoregulating centers. Second, anesthetic agents are potent vasodilators and therefore contribute to heat loss by radiation and conduction. Third, the heat regulatory center of the brain becomes depressed and inefficient. Finally, shivering is abolished by muscle relaxants, and alterations of sweating occur (10) (Table 13.2). Anesthetic-induced hypothermia begins before the patient arrives at the operating room if preoperative medications are given (7). Metabolic demand decreases 6.5% for each 1°C drop in temperature from 37° to 28°C (11).

Hypothermia may be divided into three degrees: mild, 36° to 32°C (96° to 90°F); moderate, 32° to 30°C (90° to 85°F); and severe, 30° to 27°C (85° to 80°F). Normal body temperature ranges from 35.8° to 37.4°C (96.5° to 99.3°F) (7).

The volume and type of fluid replacement are important in temperature control. One unit of cold blood decreases the body

**Table 13.2. Heat Loss Data[a]**

Mechanisms of heat loss during anesthesia
  Loss of muscle tone: anesthetic agent, muscle relaxant
  Peripheral vasodilation
  Depressed temperature-regulating center (halothane)
  Shivering abolished
  Sweating altered
Factors affecting changes in body temperature
  Temperature in operating room
  Humidity
  Duration of anesthesia
  Patient's weight
  Surface area exposed
  Site of operation
  Blood and fluid replacement
  Patient's age
  Anesthetic agent
  Muscle relaxants
Manifestations of low body temperature in recovery room
  Slow respiratory rate
  Cyanosis of extremities
  Diminished blood pressure
  Bradycardia
  Lethargy
  Delay in metabolism of muscle relaxants

[a] From Klingensmith W. Inadvertent hypothermia during surgery. Tex Med 1971;67(5):52–55.

temperature by 0.5° to 1.0°C. Unwarmed intravenous fluids, blood, irrigating fluids, and antiseptic solutions all contribute to lower body temperature.

Preexisting medical conditions such as hypothyroidism, hypoadrenalism, circulatory failure, central nervous system disorders, and protein malnutrition also cause hypothermia (2).

The application of a plaster jacket caused significant hypothermia in one patient (11). The heat of the exothermic chemical reaction occurs only briefly and amounts to only a small number of calories, but the heat necessary for drying the plaster must be provided over a period of 24 to 28 hours. If this is not available from the environment, the heat must come from the patient. Basal heat production for a 51-kg man would be 50 kcal/hr, and 17 kcal/hr is required to dry the plaster (12).

Heat regulation in the normal, unanesthetized patient, as described above, occurs via three mechanisms: (*a*) dilation and constriction of the cutaneous blood vessels, which control heat loss; (*b*) shivering, which generates heat in the muscles; and (*c*) sweating, which also controls heat loss. There is a 1.0% increase in temperature for every 13% increase in metabolism (7). The large tissue masses, including muscle, liver, and glands, generate the greatest proportion of body heat (7).

Vasodilation of superficial blood vessels over body surface area in the skin exposes large volumes of extracellular fluid to cooler surface temperature. The respiratory tract also has significant evaporative heat loss (7).

Older patients have decreased amounts of subcutaneous fat, reduced muscle mass (i.e., atrophy), and damaged heat regulatory mechanisms in the brain secondary to age (13). In 1973, Exton-Smith found that 20% of the people older than 65 living at home in winter in Portsmouth, England, demonstrated a poikilothermic response (14). Watts, in 1971, confirmed a limited decrease in sensitivity to cold in the aged (15). Fox et al., describing a study by the Royal College of Surgeons, reported that 9000 patients

(mostly elderly) were admitted to hospitals for hypothermia in 1966 (16).

Infants and children have small body mass, less developed muscular activity, increased ratio of surface area to weight, and immature heat-regulating mechanisms. Small infants can mobilize brown fat, a nonshivering thermogenesis, to increase heat production, but this thermogenesis can be overwhelmed by heat loss to the environment. These factors place the very old and the very young at increased risk of developing hypothermia.

**Prevention**

Hypothermia occurs more frequently than expected. Routine temperature monitoring will reveal frequent hypothermia. Klingensmith studied 3127 consecutive patients admitted to a recovery room over a 6-month period by obtaining rectal temperature records (10). Occasionally, axillary temperature was substituted. Of 43 patients (1%) with temperatures above 100°F (37.8°C), most underwent surgical procedures for septic processes (10). Of another 347 patients (11%) entering the recovery room with temperatures below 97°F (36.1°C), 33 had body temperatures below 95°F (35°C) (10).

There are a number of methods with which to monitor temperature. The rectal thermometer is convenient but does not always indicate the true core body temperature. The presence of stool, position of the thermometer, and pathologic conditions can alter the reading. The axillae are easily accessible sites that give an index of the core temperature, but they are exposed to the environment (2).

Nasopharyngeal and esophageal measurements give representative core temperature (2). Some physicians say the best monitor for core temperature is an esophageal temperature probe inserted 37 to 38 cm past the patient's teeth to locate the tip near the heart (11). Cork et al. (17) and Fallacaro et al. (2) showed that bladder temperatures obtained with Foley catheter sensors compare favorably with other methods. Benzinger showed that the tympanic membrane temperature is the most reliable measurement of core temperature (18). However, Wallace et al. reported perforations of the tympanic membrane (19). The use of cutaneous liquid crystal thermography (adhesive temperature strips) is another way to monitor temperature (20), but skin temperature may not rapidly reflect changes in core temperature.

The prevention of intraoperative heat loss is multifactorial. The operating room temperature should be maintained at 21°C. Even at this temperature, an exposed patient's convective heat loss can be 80 kcal/hr. By reducing both the velocity and the volume of interacting air, surgical draping decreases this loss to about 20 kcal/hr (6).

Radiant heat loss is a direct function of the temperature difference between the patient and the ambient temperature (6). Therefore, the use of a reflecting blanket, which reflects 80% of radiated heat, in a 21°C operating room can reduce heat loss from 100 to 40 kcal/hr. Bourke et al. recommend using a reflective blanket when more than 60% body surface can be covered and when the procedure will take longer

than 2 hours (6). Reflective blankets are lightweight, clean, and disposable; they cannot burn patients and are not subject to mechanical or electrical failure. In addition, these blankets do not interfere with radiologic procedures, do not trap moisture that could condense and cause skin maceration, and do not increase risk associated with undetected electrocautery dispersion plate faults (6).

Tollofsrud et al. studied hypothermia prevention by using a warming blanket/ heating mattress (21). They studied 80 patients undergoing abdominal aortic or extraabdominal vascular surgery. They compared the fall in temperature during surgery when no active warming was used (Fig. 13.2) to the temperature course when the inspired anesthetic gases were heated and humidified (Fig. 13.3) (21). Inspired anesthetic gases were heated and humidified using a Bennett cascade humidifier with the airway temperature, monitored close to the endotracheal tube, kept between 37° and 48°C. A warming blanket (Gorman Rupp-type, 45 × 60 cm) was placed under the patient and covered with two layers of cotton sheets (21). Figure 13.4 shows that the combination of heated and humidified inspired gas and a warming blanket was

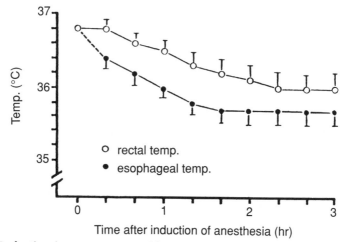

Figure 13.2.   **Reduction in temperature with no active warming.** Mean temperatures (±SE) of patients undergoing extraabdominal vascular surgery on lower extremities. (From Tollofsrud SG, Gundersen Y, Anderson R. Perioperative hypothermia. Acta Anaesthesiol Scand 1984;28(5): 511–515.)

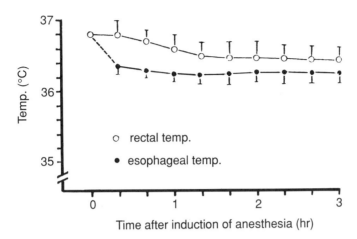

Figure 13.3.    **Reduction in temperature with use of heated and humidified inspired gases.** Mean temperatures (±SE) for patients undergoing extraabdominal surgery. (From Tollofsrud SG, Gundersen Y, Anderson R. Perioperative hypothermia. Acta Anaesthesiol Scand 1984;28(5): 511–515.)

significantly better than no active warming or the use of a warming blanket alone (21). This combination gave results that were significantly different from those with heated and humidified gases alone.

Kristensen et al. in Denmark used a specially constructed double-lumen esophageal thermal tube (GK-tube) (22). In this closed system, 41.7°C water was circulated through the tube with a speed of 3 liters/min and a maximal pressure of 23.3 kPa (177 mm Hg). The 20 patients warmed with the GK-tube had a median end-temperature of 36.8°C (36.1° to 37.0°C), whereas the group of 20 without any warming device had a median end-temperature of 34.9°C (34.6° to 35.8°C), a statistically significant difference. Two risks are associated with this procedure. First, the water may cause thermal injuries in the esophagus if the temperature exceeds 42°C for an extended length of time. Second, there is a possible risk of the tube leaking, thus filling the stomach with water (22).

Prevention of hypothermia can also be achieved with humidification of anesthetic gases. This can be done by several types of humidifiers such as the Bennett cascade, the Fisher-Paykel (F-P) MR 418, and the SERVO 150 heat and moisture exchanger. A study of 30 patients undergoing major intraabdominal surgery found heated humidification by the F-P MR 418 and SERVO 150 to have only marginal effects on body temperature compared with the control group (23). However, the authors noted that heated humidification reduced postoperative shivering (23). Another study showed that patients can be warmed actively by heated humidification (20). When the body temperature was well preserved in the control group because of the use of metallized plastic sheeting, warmed intravenous fluids, and a heat and moisture exchanger, heated airway humidification was only marginally effective (23).

Burch showed that hyperventilation increases the cooling effect of inspiratory gases at room temperature (24), and Morrison et al. showed that an increased warming effect occurred with heated and humidified gases (25). The consensus seems to be that heated humidification provides no additional advantage to prevent excessive heat loss when surfaces are insulated, intravenous fluids are warmed, hyperventilation is avoided, and a heat and moisture exchanger is used.

As previously mentioned, the following are effective for preventing hypothermia: (*a*) Cover the patient as much as possible and use thermal blankets during transfer (3). (*b*)

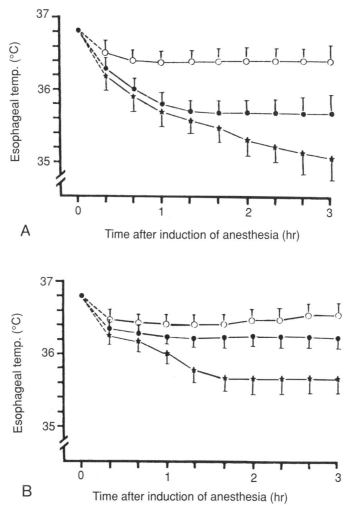

**Figure 13.4.   Temperature reductions in patients undergoing surgery on the abdominal aorta (A) or extraabdominal vascular surgery on the lower limbs (B).** The values at time 0 are rectal temperatures; the means and standard errors were calculated from esophageal temperatures. *Open circles,* combination of warming blanket and heated and humidified gases; *solid circles,* heated and humidified inspired gases; *stars,* no active warming. The plots of data for patients having no active warming and those having only a warming blanket were virtually identical; in both **A** and **B** they are represented by the *lowest curve.* (From Tollofsrud SG, Gundersen Y, Anderson R. Perioperative hypothermia. Acta Anaesthesiol Scand 1984;28(5):511—515.)

Warm intravenous fluids, including blood. (*c*) Protect and warm exposed viscera with warmed saline packs or irrigating fluids. (*d*) Run warm fluids through the nasogastric tube (26).

Additional methods of preventing hypothermia include variations in anesthetic circuits. Closed and to-and-fro circuits (Water's cannisters) and low flows are effective in reducing heat loss (6). Radiant heaters effectively maintain body temperature, especially in children, who have a greater ratio of body surface to volume. These have adjustable height and temperature settings, but they must be warmed before use, the same as warming blankets (6, 9).

In practical terms, there are three main ways of preventing hypothermia. (*a*) Increase the ambient operating room temperature, as is commonly done with neonates and small infants only. (*b*) Use anesthetic agents with minimal vasodilatory effects. (*c*) Use expeditious surgical techniques to avoid lengthy procedures (27).

## Effects on Organs/Complications

There are numerous intraoperative consequences of moderate to severe hypothermia (temperature < 33°C) in paralyzed, ventilated patients. The cardiovascular system is the most critical. The cardiac output initially increases as temperature decreases below 37°C, but below 32°C it starts to decline (23, 28). At 30°C, the cardiac output has decreased by 30 to 40% and sinus bradycardia is seen (27). This occurs in spite of a shift of blood to the central compartment. At 31°C, cardiac conduction abnormalities start to appear, atrial arrhythmias first followed by ventricular arrhythmias at 30°C (2, 11, 28). These atrial arrhythmias, including atrial fibrillation, may be secondary to atrial distension (2). At 28°C the onset of ventricular fibrillation occurs. However, ventricular fibrillation may occur at a higher temperature in the presence of a diseased or ischemic myocardium or with such stimuli as the insertion of a central venous pressure line, Swan-Ganz catheter, or endotracheal tube (1, 28). J-waves, pathognomonic of hypothermia, begin to appear at 30°C.

A secondary effect of cardiovascular problems is decreased blood flow to the extremities. This leads to stress, postoperative venous thrombosis, and the possibility of pulmonary embolism (2, 29). With hypothermia, cardiopulmonary resuscitation becomes very difficult because the severely depressed myocardium is relatively unresponsive to inotropic stimulation by catecholamines and intolerant of both acute volume loss and overload (30).

The respiratory system shows no clinically significant changes in respiratory mechanics in the temperature range of 30° to 36°C in the ventilated patient. The respiratory drive does not cease until a temperature of 24°C is reached. However, the respiratory rate increases with the initiation of hypothermia and then gradually declines (12, 28). Nunn concluded that there is no bronchodilation in humans and therefore no increased dead space (31). This was in contrast to the opposite findings of Severinghaus and Stupfel in dogs (32).

Benumof and Wahrenbrock determined that hypoxic pulmonary vasoconstriction is impaired in dogs with even mild hypothermia. They found that the hypoxic response at 31°C was less than half that at 40°C (33).

With decreasing temperature, the inhalational agents become more soluble but, despite decreasing partial pressures, they are more potent because patients are more sensitive to their effects. Induction is slowed by the slower rate of increase of anesthetic partial pressure in the alveoli. On the other hand, hypothermia reduces minimal alveolar concentration. This reduction per degree change in body temperature varies from agent to agent. The net effect is that minimal alveolar concentration is achieved at roughly the same rate at all temperatures (28, 34).

In a similar manner, carbon dioxide and oxygen increase in solubility with hypothermia, lowering $PCO_2$ and $PO_2$ and raising pH. Blood gas tensions and pH value are measured in the laboratory at a temperature of 37° and traditionally corrected with nomograms to determine $PCO_2$ and pH at the patient's temperature (28, 35).

Rahn et al. hypothesized from both laboratory work and observations of hibernating animals that the rising pH and dropping $PCO_2$, which occur as body temperature is lowered, maintain a constant ionic charge on proteins (36). Ream et al. argued that the best method of managing the acid-base status of hypothermic patients is to use uncorrected values measured at 37°C (37). The temperature changes in pH and $PCO_2$ are reversible and occur identically in vivo and in vitro, so interpretation can be performed at only one temperature. Because most anesthesiologists know the appropriate values of pH and $PCO_2$ at 37°C, they can treat the patient's ventilatory status using pH and $PCO_2$ values read directly from the blood gas analyzer.

Hypothermia will affect the hemoglobin-oxygen dissociation curve by shifting it to the left. Therefore, at any given partial pressure of $O_2$, hemoglobin will have greater affinity for oxygen and will not release oxygen as readily at the tissue level (2). Therefore, tissue hypoxia with anaerobic metabolism and lactic acidosis will occur. The hemoglobin saturation remains constant with decreasing temperature. As blood cools, the oxygen solubility increases, dropping its partial pressure. The correction factor for $PO_2$ depends on the level of hemoglobin saturation. When the saturation is below 90%, $PO_2$ decreases by 7.2%/1°C decrease; when $PO_2$ is above 500 mm Hg and hemoglobin saturation is 100%, the $PO_2$ decreases by 1.3%/1°C decrease. In the practical range of saturation (90 to 100%), nomograms or equations must be used (4).

The central nervous system effects of hypothermia include a 7% reduction in cerebral blood flow per degree Celsius decrease in temperature (28). This results from three factors: decreased cardiac output, increased viscosity, and increased cerebrovascular resistance. In addition, the cerebral metabolic rate decreases.

Low-grade hypothermia (34°C) may exert a cerebral protective effect. However, below 34°C, the potential cerebrovascular complications outweigh any protective benefit (28). At 32°C, cerebration is impaired, reflexes are sluggish, thinking is impaired, and there is loss of coordination (13, 38). At 30°C, loss of consciousness and pupillary dilation supervene (28).

The metabolic and endocrine systems are changed by hypothermia. (a) The basal metabolic rate declines 5 to 7%/1°C. There is a slower metabolism of drugs via the liver and excreted by the kidney (38). (b) At 32°C, hyperglycemia can occur, partly due to decreased insulin release and impaired utilization of glucose. (c) Plasma catecholamines are elevated secondary to an initial sympathetic response. In deeply anesthe-tized animals, this response is minimal (28, 39).

A second complication of hypothermia is a restriction of insulin secretion by inhibition of the pancreatic secreting process (40). Baum and Porte reported that inhibition of insulin secretion could be reversed under conditions of deep hypothermia, suggesting that hypothermia is not the sole factor responsible (41). Diminished pancreatic blood flow could also decrease insulin secretion. The cardiac output is redistributed during deep hypothermia, with little decrease in cerebral and coronary flow but with a morbid decrease in splanchnic, including pancreatic, flow. Lower levels of insulin have been recorded during periods of hypothermia and low perfusion rate (40).

The musculoskeletal system is affected by prolonged hypothermia, which augments neuromuscular blockade by two mechanisms. During a rapid drop in temperature, the neuromuscular junction may exhibit an initial resistance to nondepolarizing relaxants because of an increase in the amount of acetylcholine released. However, after 20 minutes, the readily available stores of acetylcholine become depleted, thus augmenting neuromuscular blockade. Miller and Rodericks found that the serum clearance rate of curare and pancuronium decreases with decreasing temperature (42). Finally, the breakdown of atracurium is temperature-dependent; therefore, a reduction in temperature from 37° to 26°C increases its half-life twofold (43).

Finally, there are changes in the renal-hematopoietic/gastrointestinal systems. The glomerular filtration rate progressively declines with cooling to reach 50% of normal at 30°C. The urine flow is not reduced until 20°C because of the early depression of tubular reabsorption. Hypothermia impairs renal tubular secretion, and eventually sodium, water, and potassium are lost in the urine. Blood viscosity increases, which becomes clinically important if the temperature falls below 30°C. There is platelet sequestration if the temperature falls below 32°C, with a decrease in platelet count (7, 28). This normalizes with rewarming. Below 34°C, intestinal mobility frequently decreases, with the occurrence of an ileus (7, 28). There have been several reports concerning decreased host resistance with hypothermia, a sequela of immunologic depression (38).

A number of additional potential complications are associated with hypothermia. First, there is the problem of cold agglutinins (both specific and nonspecific), which are serum antibodies activated at reduced temperatures to produce red blood cell agglutination and hemolysis. Cold agglutinin antibodies have three characteristics: a specific thermal amplitude, which is the temperature below which antibody activation occurs; an exponential increase in antibody activity on cooling below the thermal amplitude; and rapid reversibility of antibody activation and red blood cell agglutination on rewarming (44).

The cold autoimmune decreases may be primary, acquired, or the result of naturally occurring cold autoantibodies. Two diseases, cold hemagglutinin disease and cryoglobulinemia, may be precipitated by the range of temperature associated with mild to moderate hypothermia. These may be problems in controlled hypothermia, as for cardiopulmonary bypass surgery (45). A case report by Guena and Addei presented a 67-year-old woman who underwent elective abdominal surgery. The patient had a history of chronic anemia due to cold agglutinin disease. The operative time was 2 hours 25 minutes, after which studies revealed a hemolytic crisis (46). To produce hemolysis, there must be an overlap of the cold agglutinin and complement activities. Usually this occurs at 22°C in patients with thermal amplitudes of 32°C (44). Cold agglutination aggregates of red blood cells are reversed immediately on rewarming. However, perioperative myocardial infarction, hemolytic anemia with cardiac failure, persistent postoperative hemolysis with hemoglobinemia, and immune complex nephritis with renal failure have been reported (45).

## Postoperative Complications of Hypothermia

Further complications are shivering, peripheral vasoconstriction, and delayed drug clearance (28). Shivering can produce a 400 to 500% increase in metabolic rate within skeletal muscles (28). Roe et al. studied 24 patients and related body temperature to early postoperative $O_2$ consumption (47). In 20 of 24 patients whose temperatures decreased at least 0.2°C (average fall, 1.1°C), the average increase in postoperative $O_2$ consumption was 80% over basal levels (13, 47).

Goldberg and Roe studied 100 patients to determine the factors related to temperature changes. They found that decreased temperature varied directly with age and duration of surgery (48). Temperature decreases were less significant if the peritoneal cavity was not opened, and changes were unrelated to the type of inhalational anesthetic used but were twice as large if muscle relaxants were used. Finally, the temperature decrease was not related to ambient temperatures. This last result is very questionable, as shown in later studies (48).

Debilitated, elderly patients have limited cardiovascular and respiratory reserves in the face of increased postoperative $O_2$ consumption. This may lead to hypoxemia and cardiac failure.

The study by Rodriguez et al. confirmed that postoperative patients who shiver as a result of hypothermia have increased $O_2$ consumption and $CO_2$ production (49). Shivering also led to increased heart rate, rate pressure product, and mean arterial pressure, suggesting increasing myocardial $O_2$ consumption and therefore increased myocardial work (10). Burton and Bazett pointed out that shivering leads to increased heat loss and therefore is a poor method of maintaining body temperature (50). Horvath et al. estimated that shivering was approximately 11% efficient in protecting against a reduction in body temperature (51). Rodriguez et al. showed an increase in the $O_2$ cost of rewarming, verifying that shivering is an important adaptive response

(49). They also demonstrated that suppression of shivering is associated with a lower $O_2$ consumption (49); however, the use of muscle relaxants may extend the rewarming process.

Slotman et al. showed that elderly patients become hypothermic more frequently than younger patients (1). These age-related effects are due to hypothermic thermoregulatory failure, limited cardiopulmonary reserves, and protein-calorie malnutrition (1). These investigators evaluated 100 consecutive, general surgical patients admitted postoperatively to a surgical intensive care unit. Hypothermia (temperature less than 97°F) was present in 77% of the patients intraoperatively, in 53% at the end of surgery, and in 21% at 4 hours after surgery. Mortality was increased with patient age greater than 55 years; emergency surgery; operative blood pressure less than 100 mm Hg; operative fluid requirements greater than 1500 ml/hour; temperature less than 97°F at 2, 4, and 8 hours postoperatively; and presence of postoperative complications. Slotman and colleagues thought that hypothermic patients with mortality risk factors should be rewarmed aggressively after surgery (1).

Rodriguez et al. advocated postoperative respiratory treatment with muscle relaxants and/or high doses of morphine to avoid the ill effects of hypothermia (52). The work of Henneberg et al. showed that postoperative external heating with a thermal ceiling reduced oxygen consumption and shivering significantly in moderate hypothermia (4). This reduced plasma catecholamine levels and, at the same time, increased the comfort of the patient.

Increased $O_2$ consumption and carbon dioxide production raise ventilatory requirements when gas exchange may be impaired by residual drugs, partial upper airway obstruction, pain, or intrinsic lung disease.

Another complication of intraoperative hypothermia, which becomes a problem postoperatively, is peripheral vasoconstriction. This may be a cause of unexplained hypertension postoperatively. In addition, this vasoconstriction may mask hypovolemia as the patient gradually warms and vasodilates with a sudden drop in blood pressure.

Intraoperative hypothermia causes delayed drug clearance in patients who already suffer from insufficient clearance mechanisms. The maximal rate of renal excretion of a drug can decline by 10%/0.6°C decrease in body temperature (28). Hepatic detoxifying processes are delayed significantly with even a 3° to 4°C drop. This affects narcotics and barbiturates (28). The effects of hypothermia on the actions of nondepolarizing relaxants have been discussed previously.

Lunn's data implied that the incidence of deep venous thrombosis and pulmonary embolism increases in hypothermic patients (53). On the other hand, hypothermia activates the thrombotic and thrombolysis system, leading to disseminated intravascular coagulopathy (54).

### Therapeutic Hypothermia

Relative profound hypothermia is used frequently in cardiovascular surgery, specifically pediatric open heart surgery (55–61). Hypothermia has also been used for major hepatic tumor resection in children (27).

Reasbeck et al. reported that a 7-year-old with a ventricular septal defect who presented with untreatable right ventricular failure after open heart surgery responded to moderate whole-body hypothermia (54). Hypothermia had a depressant effect on heart rate, allowing improved ventricular filling, which had a positive effect on cardiac function.

Hypothermia is used on many occasions in neurologic surgical procedures. Depending on the degree of hypothermia, it will decrease cerebral metabolism, cerebral blood flow, and cerebrospinal fluid pressure. Matsuki and Oyama successfully used hypothermia in a pregnant woman with an intracranial arteriovenous malformation (34). Strange and Halldin reported the use of hypothermia during resection of a posterior fossa tumor (35).

Walton and Rawstron described the effect of local hypothermia on blood loss during transurethral resection of the prostate (29). This small reduction in blood loss was not statistically significant and agrees with data collected by Cockett et al. (62). On the other hand, Serrao et al. reported that blood loss was reduced almost sixfold (29, 63), and Robson and Sales reported a 53% reduction in blood loss (64).

Donders et al. reported the use of hypothermia in carotid endarterectomy (65). The patient's temperature fell to 29.5°C, and occlusion of the common carotid artery was tolerated for 5 minutes without significant deterioration of the electroencephalogram. Provided that arterial blood pressure and partial pressure of $CO_2$ can be maintained within normal limits, cerebral hypoxia is better tolerated under hypothermic conditions than at 37°C (65), especially by those in whom the collateral circulation of the cerebrum is reduced by obstruction of the contralateral internal carotid artery.

## MALIGNANT HYPERTHERMIA

In 1962, Denborough et al. first described malignant hyperthermia (66). Their account concerned a 21-year-old student with a compound fracture of the right leg who was reluctant to be anesthetized because 10 of 24 relatives who had received general anesthesia had died (66).

### Epidemiology, Inheritance, and Incidence

Malignant hyperthermia crisis occurs predominantly in humans and pigs. Cases have rarely occurred in cattle, greyhounds, racehorses, and giraffes (67). In humans, the greatest incidence is in patients between the ages of 3 and 30 years, but the condition has been documented in newborns and in the elderly up to age 78 (67). The possession of the trait for malignant hyperthermia is equal in males and females; however, malignant hyperthermia crises are more common in

males than in females (67), probably because men have larger, stronger muscles and take part in more high-risk sports. Thus, they present with more injuries that require surgery and anesthesia. Men are also involved in more vehicle trauma, again requiring more frequent surgery and anesthesia.

A history of a normal episode of anesthesia does not rule out the possibility of a future malignant hyperthermia reaction. One patient had 12 previous normal anesthetic inductions with triggering agents but had a fatal reaction during the thirteenth (67). Fifty per cent of patients in whom malignant hyperthermia develops have had prior anesthetics without difficulty.

Malignant hyperthermia is found in all racial groups. It is common in whites and Orientals but rarely seen in blacks. The highest reported incidence in children is 1 in 15,000, and the incidence in adults ranges from 1 in 40,000 to 1 in 100,000 (67–70). Why malignant hyperthermia is more common in children is unknown.

The inheritance pattern has been described as predominantly autosomal dominant with one or more weaker background modifying genes (69). McPherson and Taylor studied 93 families and found 50% autosomal dominant, 3% with associated known myopathy, and 20% with either recessive or multifactorial inheritance (69, 71).

According to Denborough, all susceptible individuals have an underlying muscle disease (72). The following disorders have been associated with malignant hyperthermia: arthrogryposis, central core disease, cramp fasciculation syndrome, Duchenne's dystrophy, King-Denborough syndrome (lordosis, pectus deformity, cryptorchidism, hypotonia, webbed neck), myotonia congenita, neuroleptic malignant syndrome, and osteogenesis imperfecta (69, 73, 74).

Other muscular dystrophies, pheochromocytoma, and sudden infant death syndrome have been linked to malignant hyperthermia (69, 74). Children with short stature, facial and spinal abnormalities, scoliosis, hernia, squint, ptosis, and undescended testes are at risk for malignant hyperthermia (68, 73).

Ording from Denmark showed fulminant malignant hyperthermia in approximately 1 in 260,000 general anesthesia episodes and 1 in 60,000 when succinylcholine was used (75). If nonspecific signs of malignant hyperthermia such as masseter muscle rigidity are included, the incidence increases to 1 in 12,000 anesthetic episodes. If unexplained tachycardia and fever are added, the incidence increases to 1 in 5,000.

·Denborough et al. found that 5 of 15 parents of children who had died from sudden infant death syndrome had increased muscle contractility with the halothane and caffeine tests (76); therefore, there may be a relationship of malignant hyperthermia with sudden death syndrome in infants (76). Stanton et al. incriminated overheating as a factor in some unexplained infant deaths (77). A study performed in Newcastle and Gateshead showed that 7 of 34 infants who had died from sudden infant death syndrome were unusually hot when found dead, and 4 others were noticed to be hot shortly before death. Pathologically, 8 of 33 victims of sudden infant death syndrome showed histologic changes in the small intestine similar to heat stroke, which has been associated with malignant hyperthermia (77).

Reynolds et al. showed that malignant hyperthermia was not related to physical exercise by studying seven survivors of malignant hyperthermia (78). They were put through a standardized, multistage treadmill exercise protocol. No patient developed signs of malignant hyperthermia.

## Pathophysiology

Malignant hyperthermia is a widespread membrane deficit involving both different membranes within the same cell type and membranes of different cell types (67). The most common cell type is skeletal muscle, with lesser degrees found in heart muscle, smooth muscle, motor nerves, brain cells, platelets, lymphocytes, erythrocytes, and cells of the islets of Langerhans (67).

Thiagarajah presented two explanations for the mechanism of malignant hyperthermia: first, reuptake of calcium from the myoplasm by the sarcoplasmic reticulum is decreased and, second, there is a deficit in the excitation and contraction coupling mechanism in the release of calcium ions into myoplasm, which involves contraction of muscles (79).

As reported by Stanec and Stefano, the precipitating cause of malignant hyperthermia is a sudden rise in the concentration of calcium in myoplasm (80). The mechanism can be abnormal accumulation of calcium by sarcoplasmic reticulum, defective accumulations by mitochondria, or passive calcium diffusion or exaggerated metabolism with fragile sarcolemma. Plasma cAMP concentrations obtained before exercise in malignant hyperthermia groups were consistently higher, although not significantly (Fig. 13.5). In patients susceptible to malignant hyperthermia, the cAMP concentration remained higher after exercise and returned slower to control values. In addition, the rapidity of development of generalized fatigue with a feeling of exhaustion in malignant-hyperthermia-susceptible individuals was statistically significant (80).

Britt thinks that the abnormality is latent until activated by environmental triggers (81), i.e., drugs or stresses. The drugs include inhalational anesthetics, skeletal muscle relaxants, amide local anesthetics, caffeine, and sympathomimetic compounds. The stresses that precipitate malignant hyperthermia are strenuous and prolonged exercise, excessively hot weather, shivering, emotional lability, massive muscle trauma, and concomitant infection. These factors cause a release of calcium from storage membranes (sarcoplasmic reticulum, mitochondria, and/or sarcolemma) to the cytoplasm (81).

Gronert concluded that alteration in calcium control results in skeletal muscle dysfunction when the individual is exposed to certain stimuli (82). Calcium ions affect

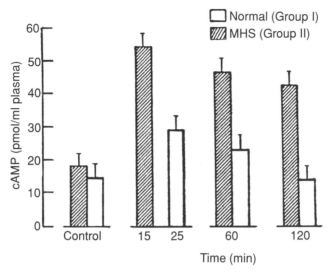

**Figure 13.5.** Cyclic AMP concentrations at rest (control), at the peak (15 and 25 min), and at 60 to 120 min after the peak of the treadmill exercise test in malignant-hyperthermia-susceptible (*MHS*) and normal individuals. (From Stanec A, Stefano G. Cyclic AMP in normal and malignant hyperpyrexia susceptible individuals following exercise. Br J Anaesth 1984;56(11):1243–1246.)

the permeability and control of both excitable and unexcitable tissues. A generalized alteration in membrane properties or permeability can affect skeletal muscle membranes; enzyme systems; mitochondria and sarcoplasmic reticulum; heart; central nervous system; liver; blood cells, including platelets; endocrine-pancreas; thyroid; and bone (82).

Recently, using calcium ion electrodes, Lopez and colleagues documented an increase in cellular calcium levels in malignant-hyperthermia-susceptible swine during a malignant hyperthermia crisis; that increase was reversed with dantrolene (83). The question of the site and mechanism(s) of calcium release remains. There are conflicting data concerning the accentuation of the calcium-induced calcium release process (69).

Phospholipase $A_2$ activity is elevated in human muscle preparation. Phospholipid breakdown leads to release of free fatty acids, which may release calcium from the sarcoplasmic reticulum. Finally, malignant hyperthermia may result from abnormalities at several sites that all contribute to calcium release from storage organelles (84).

Heffron thought that the regulation of

intracellular free calcium in skeletal muscle is defective in those with the malignant hyperthermia syndrome (Table 13.3) (85–92). Of the three cellular organelles known to regulate calcium (sarcoplasmic reticulum, mitochondria, and sarcolemma), the sarcolemma seems to be the leading candidate (85).

Cheah suggested an abnormality in excitation-contraction coupling and an abnormal increase in membrane permeability to calcium, resulting in an increased level of calcium ion, the principal defect (84). Enhanced endogenous phospholipase $A_2$ activity and calmodulin could be involved with the syndrome (84).

Nelson et al. thought that a defective protein combines with the anesthetic (triggering agent) to keep channels open in the membrane of the sarcoplasmic reticulum (93).

Calmodulin, a calcium-regulating protein responsible for enhanced phospholipase $A_2$ activity, results in excess release of calcium. The increased level of sarcoplasmic calcium is then responsible for muscle hyperrigidity and an enhanced rate of glycolysis in mitochondria (84).

Allen et al. thought that the primary

**Table 13.3.    Some Properties of Ca²⁺-transporting Membrane Systems of Skeletal Muscle Susceptible to Malignant Hyperthermia[a]**

| Property | Reference |
|---|---|
| Sarcoplasmic reticulum | |
| Decreased initial rate of Ca²⁺ uptake and capacity | Gronert et al. (86) |
| | Cheah and Cheah (87) |
| Spontaneous Ca²⁺ efflux not altered; dantrolene had no effect on Ca²⁺ efflux | Gronert et al. (86) |
| | White et al. (88) |
| Mitochondria | |
| Increased levels of endogenous fatty acids and Ca²⁺ content; decreased Ca²⁺ loading capacity at 40°C | Cheah and Cheah (89) |
| Sarcolemma | |
| Decreased membrane potential (5 to 10 mV) in the presence of 2% halothane | Gallant et al. (90) |
| Decreased K⁺-contracture threshold | Gallant et al. (91) |
| Increased adenylate cyclase activity | Willner et al. (92) |

[a] From Heffron JJ. Mitochondrial and plasma membrane changes in skeletal muscle in the malignant hyperthermia syndrome. Biochem Soc Trans 1984;12(3):360–362.

lesions were manifested by a functional biochemical defect of skeletal muscle (94). Kim and Sreter established that calcium transport in malignant hyperthermia skeletal muscle sarcoplasmic reticulum is abnormal (95). Lopez et al. noted that baseline-free intracellular calcium ions were four times more abundant in malignant hyperthermia muscle compared with normal muscle (83). They also reported that, with the onset of malignant hyperthermia, calcium measurements revealed a 20× elevation, which returned rapidly to a resting level with the intravenous administration of dantrolene.

Britt observed that the cause of the acute catabolic crisis seems to be a sudden rise in the concentration of myoplasmic calcium (96) (Figs. 13.6 and 13.7). This hypothesis is supported by the observation that drugs like lidocaine, caffeine, and cardiac glycosides, which raise myoplasmic calcium, will worsen the prognosis of malignant hyperthermia reactions. On the other hand, drugs such as dantrolene sodium, procaine, and verapamil, which lower myoplasmic cal-

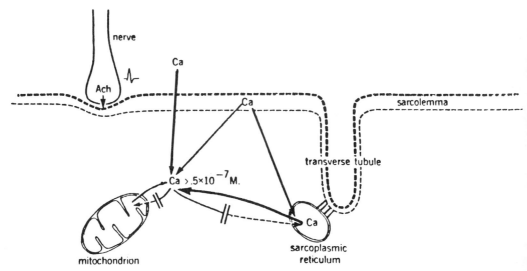

**Figure 13.6.    Possible source of excess myoplasmic calcium during malignant hyperthermia.** (From Britt BA. Etiology and pathophysiology of malignant hyperthermia. Fed Proc 1979;38(1):44–48.)

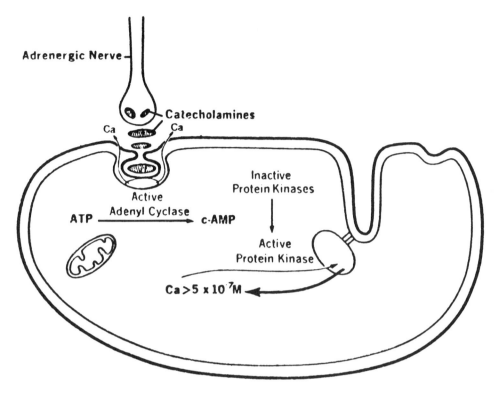

**Figure 13.7. Possible sources of excess myoplasmic calcium during malignant hyperthermia reaction—catecholamine innervation.** (From Britt BA. Etiology and pathophysiology of malignant hyperthermia. Fed Proc 1979;38(1):44–48.)

cium, will improve survival with malignant hyperthermia. Britt suggested the following possibilities for the rapid rise in myoplasmic calcium: (*a*) defective accumulation of calcium in the sarcoplasmic reticulum, (*b*) defective accumulation of calcium in the mitochondria, (*c*) excessively fragile sarcolemma with passive diffusion of calcium into the myoplasm from the extracellular site, (*d*) exaggeration of catecholamine innervation with multiple indirect effects on myoplasmic calcium, and (*e*) decreased sensitivity of myofibrillar adenosine triphosphatase (ATPase) to calcium (Figs. 13.8 and 13.9) (96).

The elevated myoplasmic calcium exerts a number of heat-producing effects because of (*a*) increased catabolism of muscle glycogen and liver lactate, (*b*) accelerated hydrolysis of ATP by myosin ATPase, and (*c*) uncoupling of oxidative phosphorylation of calcium. In addition, there is a decrease in heat loss due to peripheral vasoconstriction (96).

### Diagnosis

Diagnosing malignant hyperthermia before anesthesia is the best way to avoid a malignant hyperthermia reaction during anesthesia (67, 96). History and physical examination play a major role in diagnosis. Some patients report or present with ptosis and strabismus in childhood; kyphoscoliosis or lumbar lordosis; clubfoot; various kinds of hernias (inguinal, hiatal, umbilical); joint hypermobility with occasionally repeated joint dislocations; winged scapulae; undescended testes; calcium stones in ureter or gallbladder; or poor enamel and/or misshapen and misplaced teeth. Skeletal muscle hypertrophy is seen along with, less often, atrophic muscles. Malignant hyperthermia patients may have associated Duchenne's muscle dystrophy, limb girdle muscular

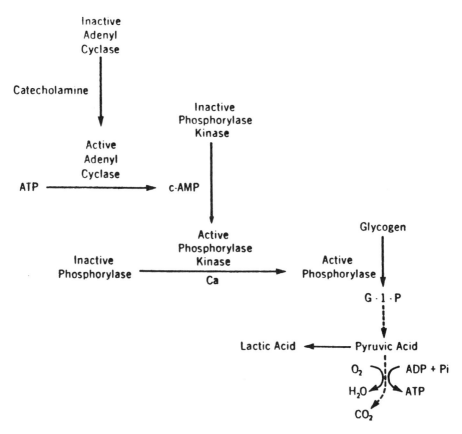

**Figure 13.8.   Effect of excess myoplasmic calcium and excess catecholamines on glycogen catabolism.** (From Britt BA. Etiology and pathophysiology of malignant hyperthermia. Fed Proc 1979;38(1):44–48.)

dystrophy, or central core disease (67, 96). Intermittent muscular cramps may be a nonspecific sign of malignant hyperthermia.

Aldrete found an elevated creatine phosphokinase (CPK) level in 70% of malignant-hyperthermia-susceptible patients (97). Tan et al. measured a normal CPK concentration in 60% of the patients with otherwise proven susceptibility to malignant hyperthermia (98). Paasuke and Brownell noted that serum CPK levels, as determined routinely, presented too many false-positive and false-negative results (99). The elevated CPK level does not identify malignant-hyperthermia-susceptible individuals, but it may indicate the presence of muscle disease. Britt noted that about 60% of malignant hyperthermia patients have normal CPK levels part of the time (67). In 10% of normal patients, CPK levels are elevated! In malig-

nant hyperthermia patients, rest produces a greater reduction in CPK levels than in normal patients and exercise produces a greater elevation. CPK levels are higher in blacks and Orientals than in whites. CPK levels are elevated in patients with hypothyroidism, paranoid schizophrenia, recent neurologic injury, myocardial infarction, major skeletal muscle trauma, other myopathies, chronic alcoholism (67), pulmonary emboli, and polymyositis. Elevated CPK levels are associated with strenuous exercise and muscular injections (97). The study by Amaranath et al. suggested a connection between the concentration of CPK, CPK isoenzymes, and the syndrome of malignant hyperthermia (100).

Currently, the diagnosis can be made only by means of a muscle biopsy, generally from the quadriceps muscle. A number of

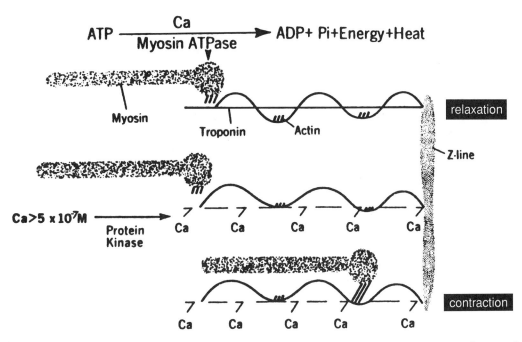

**Figure 13.9.   Effect of excess myoplasmic calcium in myofibrils.** (From Britt BA. Etiology and pathophysiology of malignant hyperthermia. Fed Proc 1979;38(1):44–48.)

tests are performed by different laboratories: caffeine skinned fiber test, caffeine and halothane contracture test, radioactive calcium uptake in muscle, platelet function, ATP depletion, and microscopy (structural, histochemical, and ultrastructural stains).

Lewis and Cattran recommended using the musculus vastus lateralis with spinal anesthesia induced by tetracaine or femoral and lateral femoral cutaneous nerve blocks effected by 2-chloroprocaine (101). Britt recommended general anesthesia because more muscle can be removed for more testing (102). Also, regional anesthesia causes a considerable amount of supplementary sedation, which depresses respiration, thereby increasing $PaCO_2$ and decreasing $O_2$ in tissues and thus causing changes in the muscle.

The caffeine and halothane contracture tests were first done by Kalow et al. (103) and Ellis et al. (104), respectively. Kalow and coworkers observed that skeletal muscles from susceptible patients undergo hypercontracture or an accentuated contracture response to caffeine and that halothane potentiates this effect (103). Caffeine causes

release of calcium from microplasmic reticulum. The caffeine-halothane contracture test is the most accurate and reliable test for malignant hyperthermia. The parameter upon which the test depends is resting tension or contracture (69, 73, 103, 105). In normal muscle, halothane does not increase resting tension but, in severely affected malignant hyperthermia muscle, it alone induces a contracture of several minutes' duration.

In 1978, Wood described the simplified method for preparing single, chemically skinned skeletal muscle fibers (106). This procedure, named the caffeine skinned fiber tension test, has several advantages over the caffeine-halothane contracture test: the volume of muscle required is smaller and the fibers prepared can be stored for several months in a freezer and still be viable to recheck experimental data. Britt et al. showed that the test should be used only to complement the caffeine-halothane contracture test (107). Other advantages of this test are that more is learned about the site and nature of the malignant hyperthermia defect and that muscle can be mailed to other laboratories for confirmation.

The next series of tests advocated for malignant hyperthermia patients concern platelets, e.g., the platelet halothane bioassay test, platelet caffeine-aggregation test, and platelet ATP depletion. Platelets are known to contain contractile elements like muscle (108). Abnormalities of platelet metabolism and aggregations were reported by Solomons et al. (109) and Zsigmond et al. (110) in association with malignant hyperthermia. The in vitro study by Ranklev et al. showed that heat was produced by exposing small specimens of muscle to halothane and exposing platelets to halothane and caffeine (108). The malignant hyperthermia patients showed the greatest increase in heat production, but the difference was too small to be significant. However, halothane has a tendency to make platelets aggregate, which in itself can produce heat (108).

The platelet is appropriate for the study of a muscle-based genetic defect because of its calcium-ATP-actinomycin contractile triggering system, interval calcium storage, and presence of glycolytic and oxidative pathways for the production of ATP. The platelet ATP depletion or platelet bioassay measures the content of high-energy phosphate after exposure of isolated platelets to halothane. This was advocated as a diagnostic test by Solomons et al. (111), but others have failed to confirm it. Solomons and coworkers found a significant reduction in adenine incorporated into nucleotides by the influence of halothane; i.e., a significant reduction is obtained in the ratio incorporated: (ATP + ADP)/AMP (111, 112). Furthermore, Solomons and Masson stated that exposure to halothane produces a significant reduction of platelet pool ATP and a significant increase in the hypoxanthine pool (112), but Verburg et al. showed this to be nonconclusive (113).

Finally, the last major type of test is the calcium uptake test. This measures the uptake of calcium into frozen thin slices of skeletal muscle and of calcium ATPase (69).

Additional tests, such as the tourniquet twitch test, have marginal value (81). Other reports have mentioned cAMP levels with exercise (80) and myoadenylate deaminase deficiency. Myoadenylate deaminase deficiency is the most common known enzyme deficiency of skeletal muscle, with an incidence of 1 to 2% in most muscle biopsies. Patients with this deficiency and the carrier state may be at increased risk of malignant hyperthermia when subjected to anesthesia (114). Klip et al. have advocated the Quin-2 method for lymphocytes (115). The parent compound of Quin-2, a quinoline derivative, enters the lymphocyte and is converted to the negatively charged Quin-2. This Quin-2 binds to calcium to form a fluorescent product. The addition of halothane in normal patients produces no significant increase in myoplasmic calcium, whereas it does in the malignant-hyperthermia-susceptible patient (67, 115).

Most patients have minor skeletal muscle and other connective tissue abnormalities (69). The initial typical and consistent early sign is tachycardia (67). However, with the use of end-tidal $CO_2$ analyzers, the earliest observable sign is a rising expired $CO_2$ tension, up to three to four times normal (67, 116). Other early signs are unstable blood pressure (generally an upward trend), increasing cardiac output (hypermetabolic state), and ventricular arrhythmia (67). Unexplained tachycardia, occasional ventricular extrasystole, bigeminy, and ventricular tachycardia may be signs of malignant hyperthermia (78, 82). Studies of serial electrocardiograms on 93 consecutive patients with proven susceptibility to malignant hyperthermia by caffeine contracture and ATP depletion test without prior history of pyrexia crisis were abnormal in 26 cases (82, 117): conduction defect in 14, repolarization abnormalities or Q waves in 9, and increased voltage suggestive of left ventricular hypertrophy with the absence of MBP in 3. Those investigators concluded that an abnormal electrocardiogram in a young patient may reflect malignant hyperthermia susceptibility. The conduction defects were seen as right bundle branch block and left anterior fascicular block (118). The cardiac manifestations were due to defective cellular membrane function. Cardiac catheterization showed abnormal left ventricular wall motion and mitral valve prolapse. There were clinical, electrocardiographic, biochemical, hemodynamic, and myocardial image changes (118).

Rigidity is the most unique of all signs, but it is not always present or may not develop until late after a gradual onset (67). Most typically, rigidity begins immediately and rapidly after the infusion of succinylcholine, with masseter jaw spasm (67). Masseter spasm may be the only abnormality observed, especially in children, in a mild or rapidly aborted malignant hyperthermia reaction (67). On the other hand, adults may show a mild reaction characterized by only moderate bradycardia and fever with no rigidity (67).

Profuse sweating and a bright red blushing of the skin may be followed by a peculiar mottled cyanosis due to an intense peripheral vasoconstriction and widening of the arterial-venous oxygen tension gradient. If the patient is breathing spontaneously, tachypnea is seen and the soda lime becomes hot and discolored and must be replaced. Fever, as a finding, develops late as the result of various biochemical derangements in the muscles. The time of onset of fever and its rate of rise are variable; fever onset may occur a few minutes after induction to several hours after the patient leaves the recovery room.

The onset of malignant hyperthermia is quite variable. The study by Kolb et al. showed that 25% of cases of malignant hyperthermia developed during the first 15 minutes, more than 50% at 1 to 2 hours after induction, and 20% after several hours (73, 119). Twenty-five per cent of malignant hyperthermia episodes were present after recovery from anesthesia, with 25% recurrence after the initial episode (74). Souliere et al. noted a marked delay of postoperative malignant hyperthermia reaction of 11 hours after a routine tonsillectomy and adenoidectomy (120).

A number of laboratory changes are associated with malignant hyperthermia. The serum calcium and potassium levels rise early, followed by serum phosphorus and magnesium and blood glucose levels. There is a rise in metabolism with metabolic acidosis, respiratory acidosis, and increased oxygen consumption (67, 82). Later, one sees myoglobinemia followed by myoglobinuria with a rising blood urea nitrogen. Serum CPK and other muscle enzymes rise late. If CPK is greater than 15,000, there is an 88% likelihood of malignant hyperthermia susceptibility (69).

The late complications are renal failure, acute pulmonary edema, consumption coagulopathy, encephalopathy with cerebral edema, skeletal muscle edema, and generalized muscle pain (67).

## Anesthetic Management

### PREMEDICATION

Some consultants have recommended the heavy use of premedications to avoid excessive emotional and physical stress. Rosenberg and Fletcher think that narcotics, benzodiazepines, ataractics, barbiturates, and antihistamines are safe for malignant-hyperthermia-susceptible patients (69). Phenothiazines should be avoided because of the similarities between malignant hyperthermia and neuroleptic malignant syndrome (69). Britt stated that parasympatholytic agents may induce or aggravate malignant hyperthermia (67), and Rosenberg and Fletcher have used intravenous atropine to reverse nondepolarizing relaxants (69).

### ANESTHESIA

Rosenberg and Fletcher recommended four procedures concerning the anesthesia machine: (*a*) use of a disposable anesthesia circuit, (*b*) removal or drainage and disconnection of vaporizers, (*c*) change of carbon dioxide absorbants, and (*d*) stabilization of flow $O_2$ at 3 to 5 liters/min for 12 to 24 hours (69).

End tidal $CO_2$ should be monitored in all malignant-hyperthermia-susceptible patients because the earliest sign of a malignant hyperthermia reaction is an increase in $CO_2$ production (69).

Regional, local, or major conduction anesthesia is recommended but may be associated with increased temperatures in susceptible patients (69, 82). The esters, such as chloroprocaine, procaine, piperocaine, and tetracaine, are recommended over the amides, such as lidocaine or mepivacaine (121). Rosenberg and Fletcher stated that amide local anesthetics are safe to use (69). If general anesthesia is the method of choice, then the following is recommended: a thiopental induction followed by a nitrous oxide-oxygen/pancuronium/narcotic anesthetic (68, 69). Midazolam, diazepam, droperidol, and althesin have not been implicated in malignant hyperthermia. The other nondepolarizing muscle relaxants such as vecuronium and D-tubocurare, as well as atracurium, seem safe (69).

Nitrous oxide has been implicated in two cases—a dental case reported by Waite et al. (122) and one case reported by Ruhland and Hinkle (123). The volatile inhalational agents, including isoflurane, should be avoided. Jenson et al. reported a fatal case of malignant hyperthermia subsequent to the administration of isoflurane to a 28-year-old for suturing of the left Achilles tendon (124). The depolarizing muscle relaxant succinylcholine, potassium supplements, calcium supplements, and ketamine should be avoided in malignant-hyperthermia-susceptible patients (69, 82).

## Treatment of Acute Malignant Hyperthermia

Early detection of malignant hyperthermia is important for successful treatment. There are both specific and symptomatic treatments. The specific treatment is rapidly eliminating the triggering agents and changing anesthesia machines, anesthesia circuits, and fluid administration sets if intravenous drugs are being used. The next step is administration of 100% oxygen and intravenous administration of dantrolene, which lowers the myoplasmic calcium. Some recommend the administration of steroids, which are useful in stress situations but have not been proven effective. Procainamide is useful for treating arrhythmia. With procainamide, procaine is released, which increases calcium transfer from the sarcolemma of muscle cells into the sarcoplasmic reticulum, a membrane-stabilizing effect (67, 69, 82).

Symptomatic treatment includes cooling the patient—on the surface, intravenously, gastrically, rectally, intraperitoneally (if the abdomen is open), by peritoneal dialysis, and even by cardiopulmonary bypass if necessary. The cooling process should stop when the temperature falls below 38°C. Lloyd and Scott stated that cooling with ice causes peripheral vasoconstriction; therefore, it is better to use a fine spray of warm water and to blow hot air over the patient (125). The hot air maintains vasodilation by perceived warmth on the skin, whereas the very low thermal capacity of air causes negligible heat input. The patient being treated by Lloyd and Scott was placed on a net stretcher suspended over a trough, thus maximizing the surface area for evaporation. One should treat metabolic acidosis with sodium bicarbonate and suspected respiratory acidosis by increased hyperventilation. Hyperkalemia should be treated with insulin and 50% glucose, whereas arrhythmia can be treated with propranolol, edrophonium, verapamil, or procainamide. The use of lidocaine is questioned because of its ability to accelerate release of calcium from the terminal sacs of the sarcoplasmic reticulum. The patient should be observed for 48 hours, and dantrolene should be continued for 24 hours. Several drugs are contraindicated in the treatment of malignant hyperthermia: the cardiac glycosides, quinidine analogs, parasympatholytics, sympathomimetics, and calcium salts (67, 69, 82).

A number of complications must be prevented or treated appropriately. First, the vigorous cooling should cease at 38°C to prevent inadvertent hypothermia leading to arrhythmias. Second, acute renal failure due to rhabdomyolysis with massive myoglobin release can be prevented by maintaining vigorous diuresis with mannitol and furosemide. Third, disseminated intravenous coagulation can occur and should be treated appropriately. Fourth, pulmonary edema and cerebral edema with neurologic sequelae can occur and should be treated appropriately. Finally, recrudescence is occasionally seen after appropriate treatment of the acute episode. Therefore, the patient must be monitored appropriately, and dantrolene should be continued for at least 24 hours after the incident. Significant muscle weakness may follow a malignant hyperthermia episode in combination with dantrolene (67, 69, 82).

The agent of choice for the treatment of malignant hyperthermia is dantrolene. It acts directly on the contractile mechanism of skeletal muscle by interfering with the release of calcium from the sarcoplasmic reticulum. The most serious reaction with oral administration has been hepatotoxicity, with prolonged high doses leading to hepatic necrosis. In all cases studied, liver function returned to normal after withdrawal of the drug. Petuseusky et al. noted chronic pleural effusion in three patients, one of whom also developed acute pericarditis (126). A fourth patient developed both pleural and pericardial effusions. Resolution occurred after discontinuance of dantrolene. Long-term, high-dose dantrolene therapy causes a fine cuneiform rash over the face and back (127, 128).

More common side effects, which largely subside after a few days, include dizziness; diplopia; dysarthria; a sensation of swelling of the eyeballs and tongue; a feeling that limb muscles are rubbery, spaghetti-like, and weak; uncertainty of location of feet when ascending or descending stairs; nausea; epigastric discomfort; and diarrhea (127, 128).

Dantrolene is marketed in a freeze-dried form and must be reconstituted with sterile water. The treatment for malignant hyperthermia is a rapid intravenous push, starting with 1 mg/kg and continuing until symptoms have begun to subside, the temperature begins to fall, muscle stiffness starts to subside, and/or the heart rate begins to decline or to a maximal single dose of 10 mg/kg. If symptoms recur, this dose can be repeated every 15 minutes. Even in the absence of reaction recurrence, the loading dose(s) should be followed by a maintenance infusion of 1.0 to 2.0 mg/kg during each 3- to 4-hour period until all evidence of an active malignant hyperthermia crisis has disappeared.

Oral dantrolene has been used extensively in preanesthetic prophylaxis of malignant-hyperthermia-susceptible patients. The recommended dosage is 4.0 mg/kg for 24 to 48 hours before the surgical procedure (67, 90, 128). One patient was treated with 3.0 mg/kg for 48 hours and developed a malignant hyperthermia reaction during anesthesia with droperidol, fentanyl, thiopental, pancuronium, and cocaine (128). Some clinicians recommend not to use oral dantrolene prophylactically (68, 69).

## Comparison with Neuroleptic Malignant Syndrome (NMS)

NMS is characterized by muscular rigidity, hyperthermia, altered consciousness, and autonomic dysfunction. It was first described in the French psychiatric literature in the 1960s (129). The incidence is unknown but was stated by Delpy and Deniker, who named the syndrome, to be 0.5 to 1.0% (130, 131).

The clinical characteristics are described as generalized "lead pipe" or "plastic" rigidity plus akinesia with an elevated temperature. Consciousness fluctuates from an alert but dazed mutism to stupor and coma. Sialorrhea, dyskinesia, and dysphagia are noted. The autonomic nervous system is affected and produces severe tachycardia, a labile blood pressure, disordered cardiac conduction, profuse diaphoresis, dyspnea, and urinary incontinence. All of this leads to secondary respiratory distress (129, 132, 133).

Laboratory results are nondiagnostic and

include leukocytosis (15,000 to 30,000), elevated CPK (as high as 15,000 IU), and generalized encephalographic abnormalities. NMS has developed within hours or from days to months after initial exposure. Prior exposure may occur without the syndrome, or the syndrome can occur with reexposure causing no recurrence of the syndrome. The physiologic state of the patient at the time of drug exposure may be important (129, 132, 133).

Most cases occurred after the administration of haloperidol, thiothixone, or piperazine phenothiazines (129, 131). Thioridazine, neuroleptics with lithium, and the combination of monoamine oxidative inhibitors and tricyclic antidepressants have also been implicated (129, 132, 133).

All ages and both sexes are involved, but young adult males predominate by a 2:1 margin. Eighty per cent of the patients are younger than 40 years old (range, 3 to 61 years). Patients with organic brain syndrome are at high risk (129, 132, 133).

The NMS is a self-limited entity that generally lasts 5 to 10 days after cessation of oral neuroleptic but lasts two to three times longer after long-acting depot injection. In a case report, Allan and White noted that decreased signs of NMS coincided with a fall in urinary concentrations of fluphenazine breakdown products (129, 131–134).

Fatalities have occurred 3 to 30 days after the onset of NMS and are secondary to respiratory or renal failure, cardiovascular collapse, or arrhythmia. The mortality rate is 20% (129, 131). There are two theories concerning pathophysiology (69). First, the NMS is related to dopamine-receptor blockade by the pharmacologic agent. Second, the NMS is related to skeletal muscle abnormalities similar to those of malignant hyperthermia. In a number of cases the response to halothane of muscle biopsied from NMS patients is similar to that of malignant-hyperthermia-susceptible patients (70, 129, 135). Also, the uptake of calcium by the sarcoplasmic reticulum can be inhibited by phenothiazines in very high concentrations (129).

The treatment consists of early recognition, immediate discontinuation of psychotropic medication, and prompt institution of intensive, supportive medical and nursing care. Dantrolene is effective in NMS treatment, but not all patients respond, and the use of dopamine agonists (e.g., bromocriptine) is not always effective (70, 129). The differential diagnosis has included all of the following: infectious disease processes of the central nervous system (e.g., acute viral encephalitis), tetanus, postinfectious encephalopathies, akinetic mutism, "locked-in" syndrome, central hyperthermia, collagen-vascular disorders (e.g., polymyositis), basal ganglion disorders (e.g., Parkinson's disease), disorders of muscular hypertoxicity, catatonia, and heat stroke. Tollefson stated that perhaps the NMS is a variant of the drug-induced malignant hyperthermia syndrome (131).

Included in the differential diagnosis are the muscle-related disorders (e.g., myotonia dystrophy) that will give an elevated CPK, but not a fever, during anesthesia. Extensive rhabdomyolysis treatable with dantrolene may be secondary to nonanesthetic triggers (such as severe infection, alcohol, and exercise) and phenothiazine drugs (136). Finally, thyrotoxicosis or malignant hyperthyroidism may also present very similar to malignant hyperthermia and be associated with stress and sudden death. Thyrotoxicosis produces decreased CPK levels, whereas malignant hyperthermia produces increased levels in 70% of the patients.

The trauma patient is usually a young, healthy man, often with orthopedic and other severe system injuries, who gives a negative family history of anesthetic difficulty or previous anesthetic experiences. The patient undergoes emergency surgery without family members available. The patient is considered to have a full stomach and undergoes rapid sequence induction and intubation with succinylcholine, the most commonly used muscle relaxant. The patient may already be tachycardiac and hypovolemic from the initial trauma, blood loss, and pain. Fever is not an early finding because the patient may be hypotensive and hypothermic. The first finding consistent with malignant hyperthermia may be a rising $PaCO_2$, but this may rise just with the initial injury, particularly with lung pathology. Therefore, one must have a high index of suspicion.

## Medicolegal Considerations

The mortality rate should be close to zero according to Rosenberg and Fletcher (69). Certain themes lend themselves to litigation.
1. Failure to obtain a thorough personal and family history suggestive of malignant hyperthermia as well as a history of unexplained perioperative problems
2. Failure to monitor temperature continuously
3. Failure to have adequate supplies of dantrolene and a treatment plan
4. Failure to investigate unexplained increases in body temperature, muscle tone, and jaw muscle rigidity, particularly when associated with tachycardia, arrhythmia, and rising end tidal $CO_2$

## Support Services

Support services are available for patients and families with malignant hyperthermia and for physicians who want to learn more about the syndrome. The Malignant Hyperthermia Association of Canada can be contacted at Room 314, Elizabeth Wayne, Toronto General Hospital, 101 College St, Toronto, Ontario, Canada M5G 1L7. The address of the Malignant Hyperthermia Association of the United States (MHAUS) is Box 3231, Darien, CT 06820. The Medic Alert Foundation, International, has worked with the MHAUS to establish a hotline for physicians (209-634-4917, request index zero).

## SUMMARY

The trauma patient may be faced with a number of complications related to hypothermia and hyperthermia. Prevention is the key to avoiding hypothermia. It may be accomplished via many strategies, but an important precaution is to warm the trauma patient immediately.

With malignant hyperthermia, the key to a safe outcome of anesthesia is a high index of suspicion. Once the diagnosis is made, the appropriate treatment must be instituted quickly to reduce the morbidity and mortality.

## References

1. Slotman GJ, Jed EH, Burchard KW. Adverse effects of hypothermia in postoperative patients. Am J Surg 1985;149(4):495–501.
2. Fallacaro MD, Fallacaro NA, Radel TJ. Inadvertent hypothermia: etiology, effects, and prevention. AORN J 1986;44(1):54–57, 60–61.
3. Dienes RS Jr. Inadvertent hypothermia in the operating room. Plast Reconstr Surg 1981; 67(2):253–254.
4. Henneberg S, Eklund A, Joachimsson PO, Stjernstrom H, Wikluno L. Effects of a thermal ceiling on postoperative hypothermia. Acta Anaesthesiol Scand 1985;29(6):602–606.
5. Spampinato N, Stassano P, Gagliardi C, Tufano R, Iorio D. Massive air embolism during cardiopulmonary bypass: successful treatment with immediate hypothermia and circulatory support. Ann Thorac Surg 1981;32(6):602–603.
6. Bourke DL, Wurm H, Rosenberg M, Russell J. Intraoperative heat conservation using a reflective blanket. Anesthesiology 1984;60(2):151–154.
7. Welch TC. Hypothermia: a nursing concern for surgical patients. Today's OR Nurse 1986; 8(4):20–22.
8. Morris RH. Operating room temperature and the anesthetized, paralyzed patient. Arch Surg 1971; 102:95–97.
9. Gauntlett I, Barnes J, Brown TC, Bell RJ. Temperature maintenance in infants undergoing anaesthesia and surgery. Anaesth Intensive Care 1985;13(3):300–304.
10. Klingensmith W. Inadvertent hypothermia during surgery. Tex Med 1971;67(5):52–55.
11. Kruse DH. Postoperative hypothermia. Focus Crit Care 1983;10(2):48–50.
12. Vale R. Post-operative accidental hypothermia. Anaesthesia 1969;24(3):449–452.
13. Heymann AD. The effect of incidental hypothermia on elderly surgical patient. J Gerontol 1977;32(1):46–48.
14. Exton-Smith AN. Accidental hypothermia. Br Med J 1973;4:727–729.
15. Watts AJ. Hypothermia in the aged. A study of the rise of cold sensitivity. Environ Res 1971; 5:119–126.

16. Fox RH, MacGibon R, Opvigs L, Woodward PM. Problem of the old and the cold. Br Med J 1973;1:21–24.

17. Cork RC, Vaughan RW, Humphrey LS. Precision and accuracy of intraoperative temperature monitoring. Anesth Analg 1983;62:211–214.

18. Benzinger M. Tympanic thermometry in surgery and anesthesia. JAMA 1969;209:1207–1211.

19. Wallace CT, Marks WE Jr, Adkins WY, Mahaffey JE. Perforation of the tympanic membrane: a complication of tympanic thermometry during anesthesia. Anesthesiology 1974;41:290–291.

20. Stone DR, Downs JB, Paul WL, Perkins HM. Adult body temperature and heated humidification of anesthetic gases during general anesthesia. Anesth Analg 1981;60:736–741.

21. Tollofsrud SG, Gundersen Y, Andersen R. Perioperative hypothermia. Acta Anaesthesiol Scand 1984;28(5):511–515.

22. Kristensen G, Guldager H, Gravesen H. Prevention of perioperative hypothermia in abdominal surgery. Acta Anaesthesiol Scand 1986;30(4):314–316.

23. Linko K, Honravaara P, Nieminen MT. Heated humidification in major abdominal surgery. Eur J Anaesthesiol 1984;1:285–291.

24. Burch GE. Rate of water and heat loss from the respiratory tract of normal subjects in a subtropical climate. Arch Intern Med 1945;76:315–327.

25. Morrison JB, Conn ML, Hayward JS. Thermal increment provided by inhalation rewarming from hypothermia. J Appl Physiol 1979;46:1061–1065.

26. Bar Z. "Central heating" for intraoperative hypothermia. Crit Care Med 1984;12(12):1082 (letter).

27. Ein SH, Shandling B, Williams WG, Trusler G. Major hepatic tumor resection using profound hypothermia and circulation arrest. J Pediatr Surg 1981;16(3):339–342.

28. Morley-Forster PK. Unintentional hypothermia in the operating room. Can Anaesth Soc J 1986;33(4):515–528.

29. Walton JK, Rawstron RE. The effect of local hypothermia on blood loss during transurethral resection of the prostate. Br J Urol 1981;53(3):258–260.

30. Belopavlovic M, Buchthal A. Cardiac arrest during moderate hypothermia for cerebrovascular surgery. Anaesthesia 1980;35(4):368–371.

31. Nunn JF. The distribution of inspired gas during thoracic surgery. Ann R Coll Surg Engl 1961;28:223–237.

32. Severinghaus JW, Stupfel M. Respiratory dead space increase following atropine in man and atropine, vagal or ganglionic blockage and hypothermia in dogs. J Appl Physiol 1955;8:81–87.

33. Benumof JL, Wahrenbrock EA. Dependency of hypoxic pulmonary vasoconstriction on temperature. J Appl Physiol 1977;42:56–58.

34. Matsuki A, Oyama T. Operation under hypothermia in a pregnant woman with an intracranial arteriovenous malformation. Can Anaesth Soc 1972;19(2):184–191.

35. Strange K, Halldin M. Hypothermia in pregnancy. Anesthesiology 1983;58(5):460–461.

36. Rahn H, Reeves RB, Howell BJ. Hydrogen ion regulation temperature and evolution. Am Re Respir Dis 1975;112:165–172.

37. Ream AK, Reitz BA, Silverberg G. Temperature correction of $PCO_2$ and pH in estimating acid-base status. Anesthesiology 1982;56:41–44.

38. Marta MR. Intraoperative hypothermia. a review of measure to protect patients. AORN J 1985;42(2):240–242.

39. August RV. Hypnotic induction of hypothermia an additional approach to postoperative control of cancer recurrence. Am J Clin Hypn 1975;18(1):52–55.

40. Benzing G 3rd, Francis PD, Kaplan S, Helmsworth JA, Sperling MA. Glucose and insulin changes in infants and children undergoing hypothermic open heart surgery. Am J Cardio 1983;52(1):133–136.

41. Baum P, Porte D Jr. Alpha-adrenergic inhibition of immunoreactive insulin release during deep hypothermia. Am J Physiol 1971;221:303–311.

42. Miller RD, Rodericks LL. Pancuronium-induced neuromuscular blockage and its antagonism by neostigmine at 29, 37 and 41°C. Anesthesiology 1977;46:333–335.

43. Flynn PJ, Hughes R, Walton B. Use of atracurium in cardiac surgery involving cardiopulmonary bypass with induced hypothermia. Br J Anaesth 1984;56:967–972.

44. Moore RA, Geller EA, Mathews ES, Botros SB, Jose AB, Clark DL. The effect of hypothermia cardiopulmonary bypass on patients with low-titer, nonspecific cold agglutinins. Ann Thorac Surg 1984;37(3):233–238.

45. Diaz JH, Cooper ES, Ochsner JL. Cold hemagglutination pathophysiology: evaluation and management of patients undergoing cardiac surgery with induced hypothermia. Arch Intern Med 1984;144(8):1639–1641.

46. Guena L, Addei KA. Intraoperative hypothermia in a patient with cold agglutinin disease. J Natl Med Assoc 1982;74(7):691–692.

47. Roe CF, Goldberg MJ, Blair CS, Kinney JM. The influence of body temperature on early postoperative oxygen consumption. Surgery 1966;60:85–92.

48. Goldberg MJ, Roe CF. Temperature changes during anesthesia and operations. Arch Surg 1966;93:365–369.

49. Rodriguez JL, Weissman C, Damask MC, Askanazi J, Hyman AI, Kinney JM. Physiologic requirements during rewarming: suppression of

the shivering response. Crit Care Med 1983; 11(7):490–497.

50. Burton AC, Bazett HC. A study of the average temperature of the tissues, of the exchanges of heat and vasomotor responses in man by means of a bath calorimeter. Am J Physiol 1936; 117:36–54.

51. Horvath GB, Spurr GB, Hutt BK, Hamilton LH. Metabolic cost of shivering. J Appl Physiol 1956;8:595–602.

52. Rodriguez JL, Weisman C, Damask MC, Askanazi J, Hyman AI, Kinney JM. Morphine and postoperative rewarming in critically ill patients. Circulation 1983;68:1238–1246.

53. Lunn NF. Observations on heat gain and loss in surgery. Guy's Hosp Rep 1969;18:117–127.

54. Reasbeck PG, Edwards JC, Monro JL. The treatment of intractable myocardial failure after open-heart surgery by whole body hypothermia. J Cardiovasc Surg 1980;21(1):91–94.

55. Cohen ME, Olszowka JS, Subramanian S. Electroencephalographic and neurological correlates of deep hypothermia and circulatory arrest in infants. Ann Thorac Surg 1977;23(3):238–244.

56. Brunberg JA, Reilly EL, Doty DB. Central nervous system consequences in infants of cardiac surgery using deep hypothermia and circulatory arrest. Circulation 1974;50(2)(suppl II):60–68.

57. Chandler KW, Rozas CJ, Kory RC, Goldman AL. Bilateral diaphragmatic paralysis complicating local cardiac hypothermia during open heart surgery. Am J Med 1984;77(2):243–249.

58. Engedal H, Skagseth E, Saetersdal TS, Myklebust R. Cardiac hypothermia evaluated by ultrastructural studies in man. J Thorac Cardiovasc Surg 1978;75(4):548–554.

59. Brunberg JA, Doty DB, Reilly EL. Choreoathetosis in infants following cardiac surgery with deep hypothermia and circulatory arrest. J Pediatr 1974;84(2):232–235.

60. Benjamin JJ, Cascade PN, Rubenfire M, Wajszczuk W, Kerin NZ. Left lower lobe atelectasis and consolidation following cardiac surgery: the effect of topical cooling on the phrenic nerve. Radiology 1982;142(1):11–14.

61. Silverman AK, Michels EH, Rasmussen JE. Subcutaneous fat necrosis in an infant, occurring after hypothermic cardiac surgery: case report and analysis of etiologic factors. J Am Acad Dermatol 1986;15(2 pt 2):331–336.

62. Cockett ATK, Schultz J, Franks O. Use of refrigerated solutions during transurethral surgery. J Urol 1961;85:632–635.

63. Serrao A, Mallik MK, Jones PA, Hendry WF, Wickham JEA. Hypothermic prostate resection. Br J Urol 1976;48:685–687.

64. Robson CJ, Sales JL. The effect of local hypothermia on blood loss during transurethral resection of the prostate. J Urol 1966;95: 393–395.

65. Donders HP, Jager JN, Solleveld H. Controlled hypothermia in carotid endarterectomy. J Cardiovasc Surg 1986;27(2):175–179.

66. Denborough MA, Foster JEA, Lovell RRH, Mapleston PA, Villiers JO. Anesthetic deaths in a family. Br J Anaesth 1962;34:395–396.

67. Britt BA. Malignant hyperthermia. Can Anaesth Soc J 1985;32(6):666–678.

68. Rosenberg H. Malignant hyperthermia. Hosp Pract 1985;20(3):139, 144–145, 148.

69. Rosenberg H, Fletcher JE. Malignant hyperthermia. In Barash PG (ed): Refresher Courses in Anesthesiology. 5. Philadelphia, JB Lippincott, 1986, vol 14, ch 5, pp 207–216.

70. Dodd MJ, Phattiyakul P, Silpasuvan S. Suspected malignant hyperthermia in a strabismus patient: a case report. Arch Ophthalmol 1981;99(7): 1247–1250.

71. McPherson EW, Taylor CA. The genetics of malignant hyperthermia: evidence for heterogeneity. Am J Med Genet 1982;11:273–285.

72. Denborough MA. The pathopharmacology of malignant hyperpyrexia. Pharmacol Ther 1980; 9(3):357–365.

73. Runciman WB. Malignant hyperthermia recognition, prevention and management. Dent Anaesth Sedat 1984;13(2):54–59.

74. Steenson AJ, Torkelson RD. King's syndrome with malignant hyperthermia. Am J Dis Child 1987;141:271–273.

75. Ording H. Incidence of malignant hyperthermia in Denmark. Anesth Analg 1985;64:700–704.

76. Denborough MA, Galloway GJ, Hopkinson KC. Malignant hyperpyrexia and sudden infant death. Lancet 1982;2(8307):1068–1069.

77. Stanton AN, Scott DJ, Downham MAPS. Is overheating a factor in some unexpected infant deaths? Lancet 1980;1:1054–1057.

78. Reynolds AC, Reynolds EV, Henschel EO. Physical exercise in malignant hyperthermia screening. Lancet 1981;2(8241):303 (letter).

79. Thiagarajah S. Management of an unsuspected case of malignant hyperpyrexia. Middle East J Anesthesiol 1986;8(4):269–275.

80. Stanec A, Stefano G. Cyclic AMP in normal and malignant hyperpyrexia susceptible individuals following exercise. Br J Anaesth 1984;56(11): 1243–1246.

81. Britt BA. Malignant hyperthermia. Can Anaesth Soc J 1985;32:S40–S41.

82. Gronert GA. Malignant hyperthermia. Anesthesiology 1980;53(5):395–423.

83. Lopez JR, Alamo L, Caputo C, Wikinski J, Ledezma D. Intracellular ionized calcium concentration in muscles from humans with malignant hyperthermia. Muscle Nerve 1985; 8:355–358.

84. Cheah KS. Skeletal muscle mitochondria and phospholipase $A_2$ in malignant hyperthermia. Biochem Soc Trans 1984;12(3):358–360.

85. Heffron JJ. Mitochondrial and plasma membrane changes in skeletal muscle in the malignant hyperthermia syndrome. Biochem Soc Trans 1984;12(3):360–362.

86. Gronert GA, Heffron JJA, Taylor SR. Skeletal muscle sarcoplasmic reticulum in porcine malignant hyperthermia. Eur J Pharmacol 1979;58:179–187.

87. Cheah KS, Cheah AM. Skeletal muscle mitochondrial phospholipase $A_2$ and the interaction of mitochondrial and sarcoplasmic reticulum in porcine malignant hyperthermia. Biochem Biophys Acta 1981;638:40–49.

88. White MD, Collins JG, Denborough MA. The effect of dantrolene on skeletal-muscle sarcoplasmic reticulum formation in malignant hyperthermia in pigs. Biochem J 1983;212:399–405.

89. Cheah KS, Cheah AM. Mitochondrial $CA^{++}$ transport and $Ca^{++}$ activated phospholipase in porcine malignant hyperthermia. Biochem Biophys Acta 1981;634:70–74.

90. Gallant EM, Godt RE, Gronert GA. Role of plasma membrane defect of skeletal muscle in malignant hyperthermia. Muscle Nerve 1979;2:491–494.

91. Gallant EM, Gronert GA, Taylor SR. Cellular membrane potentials and contractile threshold in mammalian skeletal muscle susceptible to malignant hyperthermia. Neurosci Lett 1982;28:181–186.

92. Willner JH, Cerri CG, Wood DS. High skeletal muscle adenylate cyclase in malignant hyperthermia. J Clin Invest 1981;68:1119–1124.

93. Nelson TE, Flewellen EH, Belt MW, Kennamer DL, Winsett OE. Comparison of $Ca^{++}$ uptake and spontaneous $Ca^{++}$ release from sarcoplasmic reticulum vesicles isolated from muscle of malignant hyperthermia diagnostic patients. J Pharmacol Exp Ther 1987;240(3):785–788.

94. Allen PD, Ryan JF, Jones DE, Mabuchi K, Virga A, Roberts J, Sreter F. Sarcoplasmic reticulum calcium uptake in cryostat sections of skeletal muscle from malignant hyperthermia patients and controls. Muscle Nerve 1986;9(5):474–475 (letter).

95. Kim OH, Sreter FA. Kinetic studies of $Ca^{++}$ release from sarcoplasmic reticulum of normal and malignant hyperthermia susceptible pig muscle. Biochem Biophys Acta 1984;775:320–327.

96. Britt BA. Etiology and pathophysiology of malignant hyperthermia. Fed Proc 1979;38(1):44–48.

97. Aldrete JA. Advances in the diagnosis and treatment of malignant hyperthermia. Acta Anaesthesiol Scand 1981;25(6):477–483.

98. Tan S, Aldrete JA, Solomons CC. Correlation of serum creatine phosphokinase and pyrophosphate during surgery in patients with malignant hyperthermia susceptibility. In Aldrete JA, Britt BA (eds): Second International Symposium on Malignant Hyperthermia. New York, Grune & Stratton, 1978, p 389.

99. Paasuke RT, Brownell AK. Serum creatine kinase level as a screening test for susceptibility to malignant hyperthermia. JAMA 1986;255(6):769–771.

100. Amaranath L, Lavin TJ, Trusso RA, Boutros AR. Evaluation of creatinine phosphokinase screening as a predictor of malignant hyperthermia: a prospective study. Br J Anaesth 1983;55(6):531–533.

101. Lewis GW, Cattran C. Malignant hyperthermia: choice of anaesthesia for muscle biopsy. Can Anaesth Soc J 1986;33:419–420 (letter).

102. Britt BA (ed). Malignant hyperthermia. International Anesthesiology Clinics. Boston, Little, Brown & Co, 1979;17(3).

103. Kalow W, Britt BA, Terreau ME, Haist C. Metabolic error of muscle metabolism after recovery from MH. Lancet 1970;2:895–898.

104. Ellis FR, Keaney ND, Kyei-Mensah K, Tyrrell JH. Halothane-induced muscle contracture as a cause of hyperpyrexia. Br J Anaesth 1971;43:721–722.

105. Ellis FR. European malignant hyperpyrexia group. Br J Anaesth 1984;56(11):1181–1182 (editorial).

106. Wood DS. Human skeletal muscle: analysis of $Ca^{+2}$ regulation in skinned fibers using caffeine. Exp Neurol 1978;58:218–230.

107. Britt BA, Frodis W, Scott E, Clements MJ, Endrenyi L. Comparison of the caffeine skinned fibre tension (CSFT) test with the caffeine halothane contracture (CHC) test in the diagnosis of malignant hyperthermia. Can Anaesth Soc J 1982;29(6):550–562.

108. Ranklev E, Monti M, Fletcher R. Microcalorimetric studies in malignant hyperpyrexia susceptible individuals. Br J Anaesth 1985;57(10):991–993.

109. Solomons CC, Tan S, Aldrete JA. Platelet metabolism and malignant hyperthermia. In Aldrete JA, Britt BA (eds): Second International Symposium on Malignant Hyperthermia. New York, Grune & Stratton, 1978, pp 221–225.

110. Zsigmond EK, Penner J, Kothary SP. Normal erythrocyte fragility and abnormal platelet aggregation in MH families: a pilot study. In Aldrete JA, Britt BA (eds): Second International Symposium on Malignant Hyperthermia. New York, Grune & Stratton, 1978, pp 213–219.

111. Solomons CC, McDermott N, Mahowald M. Screening for malignant hyperthermia with a platelet bioassay. N Engl J Med 1980;303(11):642 (letter).

112. Solomons CC, Masson NC. Platelet model for halothane-induced effects on nucleotide metabolism applied to malignant hyperthermia. Acta Anaesthesiol Scand 1984;28(2):185–190.

113. Verburg MP, VanBennekom CA, Oerlemans FT, De Bruyn CH. Malignant hyperthermia adenine

incorporation and adenine metabolism in human platelets, influenced by halothane. Adv Exp Med Biol 1984;165:443–446.

114. Fishbein WN, Muldoon SM, Deuster PA, Armbrustmacher VW. Myoadenylate deaminase deficiency and malignant hyperthermia susceptibility: is there a relationship? Biochem Med 1985;34(3):344–354.

115. Klip A, Britt BA, Elliott ME, Pegg W, Frodis W, Scott E. Anaesthetic-induced increase in ionized calcium in blood mononuclear cells from malignant hyperthermia patients. Lancet 1987;1(8531):463–466.

116. Armen R, Kanel G, Reynolds T. Phencyclidine-induced malignant hyperthermia causing submassive liver necrosis. Am J Med 1984;77(1):167–172.

117. Denborough MA. Heat stroke and malignant hyperpyrexia. Med J Aust 1982;1(5):204–205 (letter).

118. Huckell VF, Stahniloff HM, Britt BA, Waxman MB, Morch JE. Cardiac manifestations of malignant hyperthermia susceptibility. Circulation 1978;58(5):916–925.

119. Kolb ME, Horne ML, Martz R. Dantrolene in human malignant hyperthermia. Anesthesiology 1982;56(4):254–262.

120. Souliere CR Jr, Weintraub SJ, Kirchner JC. Markedly delayed postoperative malignant hyperthermia. Arch Otolaryngol Head Neck Surg 1986;112(5):564–566.

121. Paasuke RT, Brownell AK. Amide local anesthetics and malignant hyperthermia. Can Anaesth Soc J 1986;33(2):126–129 (editorial).

122. Waite PD, Ballard JB, Yonfa A. Malignant hyperthermia in a patient receiving nitrous oxide. J Oral Maxillofac Surg 1985;43(11):907–909.

123. Ruhland G, Hinkle A. Malignant hyperthermia after oral and intravenous pretreatment with dantrolene in a patient susceptible to MH. Anesthesiology 1984;60:159–160.

124. Jenson AG, Bach V, Werner MU, Nielsen HK, Jensen MH. A fatal case of malignant hyperthermia following isoflurane anaesthesia. Acta Anaesthesiol Scand 1986;30(4):293–294.

125. Lloyd EL, Scott DHT. Cooling technique for malignant hyperthermia. Lancet 1985;2:97 (letter).

126. Petuseusky ML, Faling LJ, Rocklin RE, Snider GL. Pleuropericardial reaction to treatment with dantrolene. JAMA 1979;242:2772–2774.

127. Abramowicz M. Dantrolene for malignant hyperthermia during anesthesia. Med Lett Drugs Ther 1980;22(15):61–62.

128. Britt BA. Dantrolene. Can Anaesth Soc J 1984;31(1):61–75.

129. Caroff SN. The neuroleptic malignant syndrome. J Clin Psychiatry 1980;41(3):79–83.

130. Delpy J, Deniker P. Drug-induced extrapyramidal syndromes. In Vinken PJ, Bruyn GW (eds): Handbook of Clinical Neurology. Amsterdam, North-Holland Publishing, 1968, vol 6, pp 248–266.

131. Tollefson G. Case of neuroleptic malignant syndrome: in vitro muscle comparison with malignant hyperthermia. J Clin Pharmacol 1982;2(4):266–270.

132. Guzie BH, Baxter CR Jr. Current concepts: neuroleptic malignant syndrome. N Engl J Med 1985;313(3):163–166.

133. Gibb WR, Lee AJ. The neuroleptic malignant syndrome: a review. Q J Med 1985;56(220):421–429.

134. Allan R, White HD. Side effects of parenteral long acting phenothiazine. Br Med J 1972;1:221–222.

135. Caroff S, Rosenberg H, Gerber JC. Neuroleptic malignant syndrome and malignant hyperthermia. Lancet 1983;1:244 (letter).

136. Denborough MA, Collins SP, Hopkinson KC. Rhabdomyolysis and malignant hyperpyrexia. Br Med J 1984;288(6434):1878.

# Hyperbaric Medicine: A Trauma Perspective

*Christopher M. Grande and Roy A. M. Myers*

## INTRODUCTION: TRAUMA, HYPERBARIC MEDICINE, AND THE ANESTHESIOLOGIST

Hyperbaric medicine (HM) has an integral role in generally all phases of comprehensive trauma care: resuscitation, definitive therapy, and subsequent recovery. After one becomes familiar with the concepts and theory behind the clinical practice of HM (the gas laws and patterns of gaseous uptake and distribution throughout the body, for example), inclusion of the Trauma Anesthesia/Critical Care Specialist (TA/CCS) as part of the HM team will seem natural. After all, the TA/CCS deals with these principles, which are basic to the practice of anesthesiology, on a daily basis. To be truly capable as a "Life Support Physician" for the trauma patient, the TA/CCS must be knowledgeable and facile in HM (see Chapter 1).

Because the body of literature dealing with HM is substantial, it is necessary that this chapter focus on specific aspects. The reader will be introduced to the types of hyperbaric chambers that exist today, to the terminology inherent to HM, to the four gas laws that govern the usefulness of HM and their physiologic effects, to the medical conditions that deserve special considerations before the application of HM, and to the use of HM for nine selected traumatic diseases. Because this chapter is directed at the TA/CCS, special considerations regarding continuance of critical care within the chamber as well as anesthetic management at depth will be addressed.

Simply stated, HM involves the clinical application of pressure upon the body and the use of oxygen specifically as a drug (1, 2). HM is used as the primary mode of treatment for some disorders and as an important therapeutic adjunct for others. Table 14.1 shows all indications presently accepted by the Undersea and Hyperbaric Medical Society (UHMS) for the use of HM (3). This list is easily related to familiar trauma scenarios: the victim of chemical trauma, the burn patient with smoke inhalation and assumed carbon monoxide poisoning, the victim of physical trauma, the scuba diver with either decompression sickness or arterial gas embolism.

Practitioners from a wide range of medical subspecialties are represented in HM. Surgeons, anesthesiologists, internists, emergency physicians, and military physicians, as well as nonclinical personnel (physiologists), are involved in its daily practice. At present there is no universally recognized governing board for the practice of HM, but one is desperately needed. Standards and guidelines for clinical practice must be defined and enforced to ensure efficacy, safety, and quality. As with anesthesia, if HM is used improperly, serious consequences may be incurred at the cost of the patient.

Until now, the UHMS in Bethesda, Maryland, has assumed the role of a steering committee for HM (4). Third-party payers (i.e., insurance carriers, Medicaid) generally follow the recommendations of the UHMS and use the society's list of "accepted

**Table 14.1.   Conditions That Can Be Treated with Hyperbaric Therapy**

Accepted conditions
  * Air or gas embolism (acute)
  * Amputation stumps (nonhealing)
    Arterial insufficiency (acute peripheral)
  * Carbon monoxide poisoning, acute smoke inhalation, and assumed carbon monoxide/cyanide poisoning
  * Crush injury, compartment syndrome, and other acute traumatic ischemias
  * Cyanide poisoning (acute)
  * Decompression sickness
    Enhancement of healing in selected problem wounds (e.g., diabetic wounds)
  * Exceptional blood loss (anemia)
  * Gas gangrene (clostridial)
    Necrotizing soft tissue infections (e.g., subcutaneous tissue, muscle, fascia)
  * Osteomyelitis (refractory)
    Radiation necrosis: osteoradionecrosis and soft tissue radiation necrosis, caries in radiated bones
  * Skin grafts of flaps (compromised)
Special consideration
  * Burns (thermal)
Investigative indications
  * Anaerobic and mixed aerobic, anaerobic brain abscesses
    Carbon tetrachloride poisoning (acute) and poisoning by other liver toxins
    Cerebrovascular accident (acute thrombotic or embolic)
  * Head injury (cerebral edema)
  * Fracture healing and bone grafting
    Hydrogen sulfide poisoning
    Lepromatous leprosy
    Meningitis
    Multiple sclerosis
    Pyoderma gangrenosum
    Pseudomembranous colitis (antimicrobial agent-induced colitis)
    Radiation enteritis and proctitis
    Radiation myelitis
    Retinal (central) artery insufficiency, acute
    Selected refractory mycoses: mucormycosis, canibolus coronato, invasive aspergillosis
  * Sepsis (chronic), intraabdominal abscesses
    Sickle cell anemia crises
    Spider bite (brown recluse, *Loxosceles reclusa*)
  * Spinal cord injury

* Conditions that may be related to trauma.

conditions" for reimbursement payments regarding HM (3). The Safety Committee of the UHMS and the College of Undersea and Hyperbaric Medicine presently serve as a peer pressure group to raise the level of adherence to safety guidelines and ethical practice. However, the UHMS does not have absolute authority; thus, many of the therapeutic uses of HM in the general medical community still have no sound scientific basis.

For a full appreciation of the application of HM, one must be aware of the continuum of pressure that may affect the human, more so than any other mammal. Humans are the only animal that can alter the pressure of their surroundings to such a large extent. A person may be exposed to the hypobaric environment of mountains such as Mount Everest or to even greater extremes of high altitude, as in high-performance aircraft or space vehicles. Alternatively, hyperbaric environments are trespassed regularly, for instance, in deep-sea diving operations or in the hyperbaric chamber. The limits of these extremes will continue to extend as technology inevitably progresses. Conceivably, the concepts that pertain to the physiologic effects of pressure on humans will become less "exotic" until a point is reached at which topics to be discussed in this chapter will be included as part of a regular medical school curriculum.

The study and application of diving and aviation medicine (hyperbaric and hypobaric medicine) are not new (5, 6). There are records of the use of HM from as far back as 1662. However, scientific investigations in this area really did not begin until the 1930s (7). In fact, there have been periods in history (for example, during the middle 1800s) when HM was in "vogue" (8, 9). The 1980s have shown a resurgence of interest in the use of hyperbaric environments as part of the therapy for medical diseases (10). This resurgence is now tempered with conservatism. Key physician-scientists interested in the continued development of HM, along with the UHMS, are particularly careful to ensure that its clinical use is based upon sound reasoning. Generally, this would mean that at least a beneficial relationship between HM and a given condition must be appreciated and that a research protocol is written. This is partly

the reason for the various classifications of the present indications for HM (i.e., accepted, investigative) (1). Great care is being exercised to avoid the labeling of HM as "quackery" or charlatanism (11–14). The authors fully endorse this approach. The use of HM is slowly achieving prominence and general acceptability. The United States Navy and Air Force, long-time investigators and practitioners of HM, are engaged in large-scale projects to set up huge multiplace chambers at several installations (15). The facility at Wright-Patterson Air Force Base (Fig. 14.1A) is one of these.

## HYPERBARIC CHAMBERS

There are two basic types of hyperbaric chambers: the multiplace and the monoplace (16–18). The multiplace chamber, as the name suggests, is designed to hold several people at the same time. This may include up to 22 patients, as well as the medical personnel accompanying the patients during their dive, referred to as inside "tenders" (Navy terminology) or "observers" (Air Force terminology) (Fig. 14.1B). Multiplace chambers are used at major research/treatment centers such as the Department of Hyperbaric Medicine at the Maryland Institute for Emergency Medical Services Systems (MIEMSS) in Baltimore, Maryland (Fig. 14.1E); the F. G. Hall Hyperbaric Center at Duke University Medical Center, North Carolina (Fig. 14.1D); the U.S. Air Force School of Aerospace Medicine at Brooks Air Force Base in San Antonio, Texas; the U.S. Navy Experimental Diving Unit at Panama City, Florida; and the National Hyperbaric Center in Aberdeen, Scotland. These vessels are constructed with airlocks so that additional personnel and materials may be pressurized to the same depth as the main chamber to permit entry and exit during an emergency. Smaller locks may be built as part of the chamber system to facilitate exchange of items (e.g., blood gas samples, medications) between inside and outside. Some of these chambers were used as operating rooms functioning at pressure. In

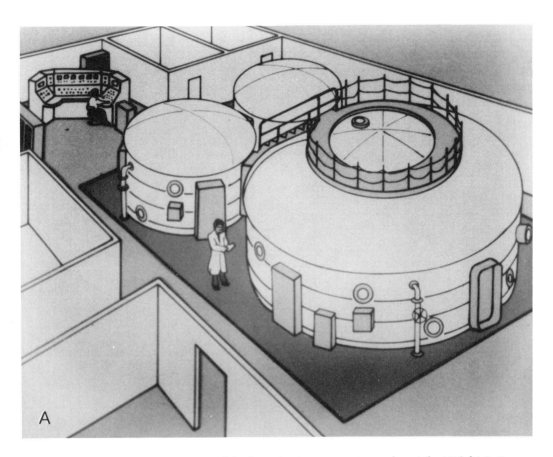

**Figure 14.1.** **A, Artist's conception of the hyperbaric treatment complex at the Wright-Patterson Air Force Base.** Note the one large and two small "igloo"-shaped multiplace chambers, which are interconnected, and the control console. **B, Hyperbaric treatment in progress.** Note the use of built-in breathing devices and the two inside tenders/observers. **C, Hyperbaricist and support personnel at the control console** monitor progress of the dive. (Courtesy of the Department of the Air Force.) **D, Artist's rendition of the F. G. Hall Hyperbaric and Hypobaric Facility of Duke University Medical Center.** Note the three treatment chambers (one with an operating table), "pass through" locks, and control console. (Courtesy of Enrico M. Camporesi, M.D., Department of Anesthesiology, Upstate Medical Center, State University of New York.) **E, Multiplace hyperbaric chamber at the Shock Trauma Center of the Maryland Institute for Emergency Medical Services Systems.** (Courtesy of the Maryland Institute for Emergency Medical Services Systems.)

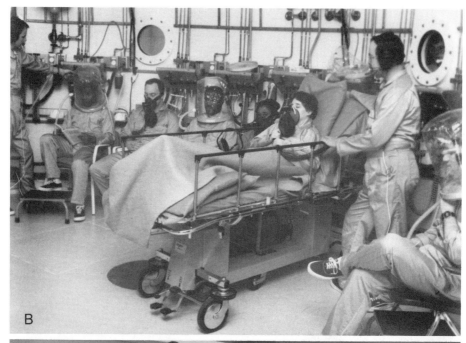

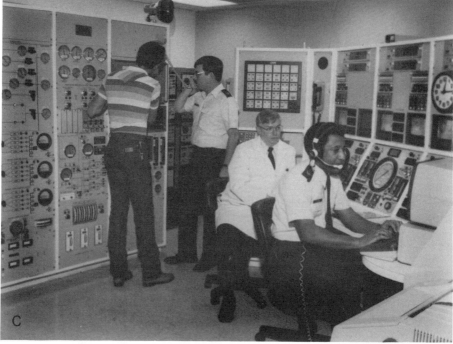

**Figure 14.1.    B** and **C.**

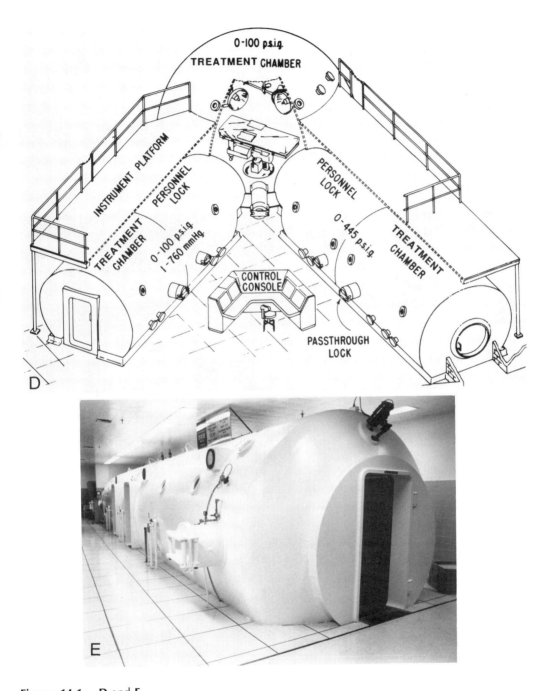

**Figure 14.1.** D and E.

the early 1960s large HM facilities were built to undertake open heart surgery; with the advent of simpler alternatives such as cardiac bypass equipment, this practice has become obsolete.

Smaller multiplace chambers also exist. The chamber must accommodate at least two persons to be classified a multiplace chamber. One of the smallest multiplace chambers is configured in the shape of an L (Fig. 14.2A). In such chambers, one patient (or the "tender") is in the sitting position with the head and torso in the chamber's vertical portion while the lower half of the body remains horizontal. The second patient is placed in the supine position with his or her head between the seated person's legs. This is a cramped situation and is less than ideal. However, this configuration does allow an inside "tender" or an "observer" to accompany the patient on a dive.

Monoplace chambers are designed to

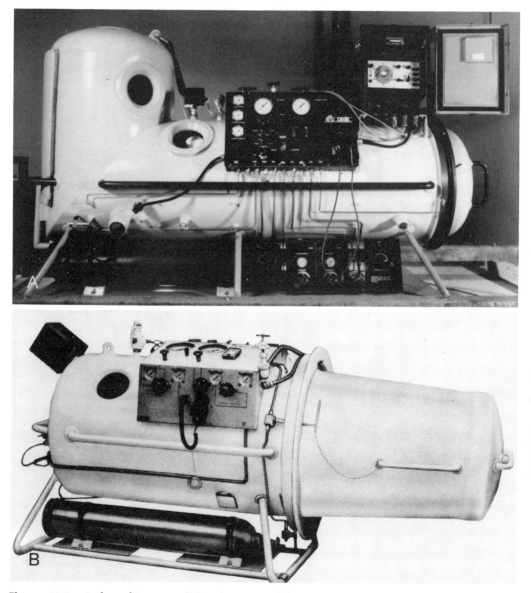

**Figure 14.2.   L-shaped two-man (A) and one-man (B) emergency transfer chambers** designed for treatment/transfer in remote locations. (Courtesy of Environmental Tectonics Corporation.)

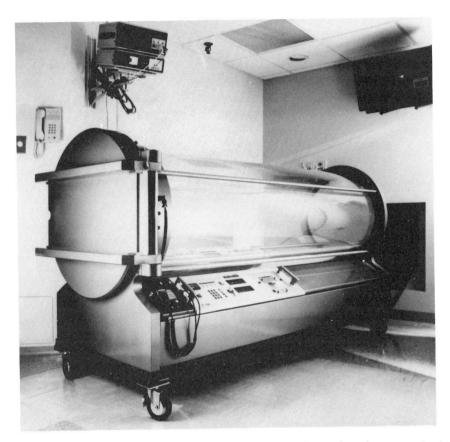

**Figure 14.3. Acrylic monoplace chamber.** Note the control panel and communication set. (Courtesy of Environmental Tectonics Corporation.)

accommodate only one person (Figs. 14.2**B** and 14.3). The cost of such apparatus presently approximates $100,000, which is fairly inexpensive compared with most medical equipment. Monoplace chambers do not require much space for operation. Because of the diminished cost in operating and logistics, monoplace chambers have become increasingly popular. It is not unusual to find a monoplace chamber in a community hospital. In these settings, the monoplace chambers are purchased and operated as a group effort, sometimes by practitioners from various specialties (e.g., family practice, emergency medicine, internal medicine, and surgery). Typically, these chambers are used to treat chronic diseases for which there may be a recognized indication for hyperbaric oxygen (HBO) therapy (e.g., chronic diabetic foot ulcers). These chambers are also used occasionally

for the treatment of decompression sickness, arterial gas embolism, and carbon monoxide poisoning. Certain ramifications of the treatment of an emergency in a monoplace chamber must be understood (18). For example, the physician is prevented from "laying on hands" and, if an emergency situation develops at depth, must stand by while decompression is accomplished.

## TERMINOLOGY USED IN HYPERBARIC OPERATIONS

Before any discussion of the concepts involved in hyperbaric operations (as well as hypobaric operations), certain terms must be defined. Pressure is defined as the force (weight) extended over a given area. It is described commonly in the English system as pounds per square inch (psi). In discussions of HM, customary units of pressure are

**Table 14.2.   Units of Measurement for Pressure[a]**

| Barometric English System | Hydrostatic | | | Atmospheric | |
|---|---|---|---|---|---|
| mm Hg | fsw | ATA | ATg | psia | psig |
| 760 | 0 | 1 | 0 | 14.7 | 0 |
| 1452 | 33 | 2 | 1 | 29.4 | 14.7 |
| 2280 | 66 | 3 | 2 | 44.1 | 29.4 |
| 3040 | 99 | 4 | 3 | 59.8 | 44.1 |
| 3800 | 132 | 5 | 4 | 73.5 | 59.8 |
| 4560 | 165 | 6 | 5 | 88.2 | 73.5 |

[a] Abbreviations: mm Hg = millimeters of mercury; fsw = feet of sea water; ATA = atmosphere absolute; ATg = atmospheres (gauge); psia = pounds per square inch absolute; psig = pounds per square inch (gauge).
From Camporesi EM, Moon RE, Grande CM. Hyperbaric medicine: an integral part of trauma care. Crit Care Clin 1990;6:203–219.

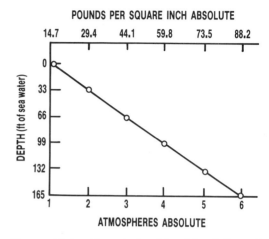

**Figure 14.4.   The relationship of depth (feet of sea water) and pressure** (in both pounds per square inch and atmospheres absolute).

atmospheres (atm), millimeters of mercury (mm Hg), and feet of sea water (fsw), as shown in Table 14.2 (19, 20).

One atmosphere of pressure is the weight of all gas particles of the earth's atmosphere when measured at sea level. This pressure is equivalent to 14.7 psi. When one travels below sea level or into any body of sea water, a depth of 33 feet (34 feet for fresh water) must be reached before an additional 14.7 psi will be measured. Thus, at sea level, 1 atm (14.7 psi) is equivalent to 0 fsw. At 33 fsw, 2 atm of pressure (29.4 psi) will be experienced. For each additional 33 fsw one descends, an additional atmosphere of pressure will be gained (Table 14.2 and Fig. 14.4).

Both atmospheres and pounds per square inch are measured on gauges. When used for diving operations, gauges are often calibrated to read 0 at the surface (sea level), ignoring the fact that 1 atm or 14.7 psi exists already. These measurements are designated "gauge pressures" (i.e., the pressure read from a gauge calibrated to zero at the surface). When surface pressures are included in measurements, they are called "absolute pressures." Gauge pressure is denoted by the placement of the letter "g" after the unit of pressure (i.e., ATg or psig) and by saying the word "gauge" after the unit in the spoken language (i.e., "atmospheres gauge" or "psi gauge"). Similarly,

absolute pressures are denoted with an "A" following the written word (i.e., ATA or psia) or by saying the word "absolute" after the unit (i.e., "atmospheres absolute" or "psi absolute"). To convert from gauge to absolute pressure, one simply adds one atmosphere and vice versa. Such differences in denotation for measurement of fsw also exist, but operationally the use of "fsw" is assumed to represent the gauge pressure.

## GAS LAWS

### Charles' Law

Charles' law, which describes the pressure-temperature relationship, is expressed mathematically as

$$P1/P2 = T1/T2$$

This law states that, at any given pressure, the volume of a constant mass of gas will be proportional to its absolute temperature (20–24). With regard to hyperbaric chambers, volume is held constant and pressure is varied; thus, changes in temperature occur. Charles' law accounts for the increase in ambient temperature (adiabatic heating) within the chamber that is appreciated during compression and for the cooling experienced during surfacing. As gases are added to the chamber (a constant-volume container) during diving, pressure increases and so does temperature.

## Boyle's Law

Boyle's law describes the pressure-volume relationship:

$$P1/P2 = V2/V1$$

This relationship shows that, at a constant temperature, the given volume of gas is inversely proportional to its pressure (20–24). In both "wet" (in water) and "dry" (chamber operations) diving, the greatest changes in volume occur just below the surface. As indicated in Table 14.3, within the first ATA of additional pressure, the relative volume of a theoretic gas bubble will decrease by 50%. Beyond the second ATA, incremental decreases in volume gradually will be smaller. This fact accounts for the difficulty in adjustment with respect to the middle ear and sinuses during early portions of a dive (21). If a patient can tolerate the initial part of the descent, it is likely that there will be no such problems during the remainder of the dive.

## Dalton's Law

Dalton's law of partial pressures states that, in a mixture of gases, the pressure exerted by each gas is the same that would be exerted if that gas alone occupied the

**Table 14.3. Bubble Volume and Diameter Changes Related to Increases in Pressure[a]**

| Depth | Pressure | Relative Volume | | Relative Diameter |
|---|---|---|---|---|
| feet | ATA | % | | % |
| 0 | 1 | 100 | ○ | 100 |
| 33 | 2 | 50 | ○ | 79.3 |
| 66 | 3 | 33.3 | ○ | 69.3 |
| 99 | 4 | 25 | ○ | 63 |
| 132 | 5 | 20 | ○ | 58.5 |
| 165 | 6 | 16.6 | ○ | 55 |
| 297 | 10 | 10 | ○ | 46.2 |

[a] Modified from Bassett BE, Bennett PB. Introduction to the physical and physiological bases of hyperbaric therapy. In Davis JC, Hunt TK (eds): Hyperbaric Oxygen Therapy. Bethesda, Maryland, Undersea and Hyperbaric Medical Society, 1977, pp 11–24.

same volume and that the total pressure is the sum of the partial pressures of the component gases (20–24). Stated mathematically, Dalton's law is

$$PTotal = P_{O_2} + P_{N_2} + P_{other\ gases}$$

The ambient atmosphere, or air, consists of 78.08% nitrogen, 20.95% oxygen, 0.93% argon, 0.03% carbon dioxide, and traces of other gases. For practical purposes, this may be simplified to 79% nitrogen and 21% oxygen ($FO_2 = 0.21$). The relative percentage of each of these gases does not change with varying degrees of pressure, regardless of a hypobaric or hyperbaric environment. However, the relative pressure of each gas will change according to the changes in the ambient absolute atmospheric pressure, but the fraction of the overall pressure exerted by any given contributing gas will remain constant, according to Dalton's law. Thus, as total atmospheric pressure increases, the absolute partial pressures of both oxygen and nitrogen increase, but the relative partial pressures remain in a 21:79 ratio (Table 14.4). Conversely, diminutions in all pressures occur with preservation of the partial pressure ratios as higher altitudes are achieved in a hypobaric setting (see Chapter 15).

At a depth of 124 fsw in an air environment, at a total pressure of 4.76 ATA, the $PO_2$ is 760 mm Hg or 1 ATA, which corresponds to breathing "100%" oxygen at sea level.

## Henry's Law

Henry's law states that the mass of a gas that will dissolve in a given volume of solvent at a given temperature is proportional to the pressure of the gas with which it is in equilibrium (20–24). Therefore, during hyperbaric operations using air, increasing amounts of both nitrogen and oxygen are dissolved in the body. This concept is important for understanding the therapeutic mechanisms of HM and the development of decompression sickness.

**Table 14.4. Partial Pressures of Gases in Compressed Air at Various Chamber Depths**

| Depth | Total Pressure | Oxygen Partial Pressure | | Nitrogen Partial Pressure | |
|---|---|---|---|---|---|
| | | mm Hg | ATA | mm Hg | ATA |
| *fsw* | *ATA* | | | | |
| 0 | 1 | 160 | 0.21 | 600 | 0.79 |
| 33 | 2 | 320 | 0.42 | 1200 | 1.58 |
| 66 | 3 | 480 | 0.63 | 1801 | 2.37 |
| 99 | 4 | 640 | 0.84 | 2402 | 3.16 |
| 124 | 4.76 | 760 | 1.00 | 2858 | 3.76 |
| 132 | 5 | 800 | 1.05 | 3002 | 3.95 |
| 165 | 6 | 960 | 1.26 | 3602 | 4.74 |

## EFFECTS OF PRESSURE ON THE BODY

### Mechanical Effects

When discussing the effects of pressure, a simplistic approach is to regard the body as being composed of structures that are either liquid-filled (e.g., tissues and bones) or air-filled (e.g., lungs, bowels, sinuses, and middle ear) (20–24). Liquids are considered to be unaffected by additional pressure (i.e., they are incompressible) and are thus unaffected by the hyperbaric environment. Conversely, the air spaces are influenced by pressure changes: as pressure in the hyperbaric chamber increases, the pressure within the air spaces also increases.

Usually the pressure within all of the aforementioned anatomic cavities equilibrates with the ambient chamber pressure. Problems arise when equilibration is prevented, usually because of a defect in the communication systems between the air spaces and the exterior. Regarding the middle ear, as pressure grows within the external auditory canal during diving, the tympanic membrane is forced inward (24, 25). Normally, the air space in the middle ear is permitted to equilibrate via the eustachian tube. If the eustachian tube is blocked, perhaps because of congestion, the pressure in the external canal eventually will cause the tympanic membrane to *im*plode. Alternatively, the eustachian tube may be patent during descent but may become blocked during surfacing. Thus, the air within the middle ear will become trapped

and continue to expand during ascent until the tympanic membrane system ruptures outwardly, or *ex*plodes. This same type of relationship may be described for the other cavities within the body such as the perinasal sinuses, the lungs, and even carious teeth or those with poorly placed fillings.

### Special Considerations

Problems due to faulty equilibration of air spaces are most serious in the lungs during ascent. The incidence of these problems will be reduced by using treatments that favor oxygen as a breathing medium as opposed to air. Three conditions deserve special attention.

#### ASTHMA (BRONCHOSPASM) (25–27)

Persons with reactive airway disease may suffer a bronchospastic reaction after having had an uneventful descent. Stress, cold, and dry air may induce bronchoconstriction, and these factors may be plentiful within the hyperbaric chamber; thus, "air trapping" may occur within the small airways. According to Henry's law and Dalton's law, as depth increases, the partial pressure of nitrogen will increase during diving with air mixtures. The nitrogen will diffuse into air spaces according to existing gradients and thus enlarge them upon ascent. As ascent proceeds, these air spaces will continue to enlarge. Air trapped in the distal airways may eventually cause a type II pneumothorax and possibly an arterial gas embolism. Thus, there are stringent recommendations to exclude persons with even a remote history of asthma from "wet" diving and, to a lesser extent, from hyperbaric treatments. These considerations also apply to the patient with a history of chronic obstructive lung disease (COPD, emphysema) with a bronchospastic component.

#### PREVIOUS THORACIC SURGERY (25–27)

When any surgery is performed, the possibility of residual air or surgical emphysema of some degree, as well as scarring and adhesions, exists. As stated above, according to Dalton's and Henry's laws, during hyperbaric treatments, diffusion occurs into these air spaces. If the original air spaces were placed "strategically," the possibility of pneumothorax or other complications exists. Patients who have had thoracic surgery are also excluded from most types of diving but may receive special consideration when HBO treatment is warranted.

## PNEUMOTHORAX (25–27)

The presence of a pneumothorax at depth from any cause will serve as a "sink" for the collection of more nitrogen molecules during diving. During ascent, the air space will enlarge, eventually causing a tension pneumothorax and/or arterial gas embolism. (A simple 15% pneumothorax at 3 ATA will enlarge to almost 50% at the surface.) Thus, the hyperbaricist must be vigilant for such conditions and must evaluate the chest thoroughly by physical examination and review of x-ray films before diving. If a pneumothorax is present, it must be treated definitively with intercostal tube thoracostomy before descent. Likewise, the hyperbaric physician must always maintain a high degree of clinical suspicion for the acute development of pneumothorax at depth and be prepared to treat such an eventuality within the chamber. If a chest tube cannot be placed, then at least a large-bore intravenous catheter should be inserted into the second or third intercostal space along the midclavicular line.

## EFFECTS OF ELEVATED PARTIAL PRESSURES OF GASES

### Physical Effects of Hyperbaric Oxygen

#### CARDIOVASCULAR

HBO simultaneously induces peripheral vasoconstriction and bradycardia, with no significant changes in blood pressure (19, 28). Although the bradycardia may cause a 10 to 20% reduction in cardiac output, it is well compensated by the increase in afterload. The vasoconstrictive effect is greater in the vasculature of certain organs, such as the kidney and brain. Because of these effects in the kidney, antidiuretic hormone release is suppressed and diuresis may occur (29). This may become an important factor after HBO therapy, when the patient has been returned to the intensive care unit (ICU) and the vasoconstrictive effect diminishes as oxygen tensions fall. Hemodynamically unstable patients may then exhibit hypotension, which usually responds to fluid replacement with an isotonic crystalloid solution.

The aforementioned vasoconstrictor effect is often desirable in a number of conditions for which HBO is indicated. Its effect on the cerebral vasculature results in reduction of intracranial pressure, which may be of value in patients with head injury (30). In cases of burns and other peripheral trauma, the vasoconstrictive effect reduces tissue edema without sacrificing oxygenation (see below) (31).

#### CARBON DIOXIDE RETENTION

When HBO is used to the point at which the hemoglobin in venous blood is fully saturated, venous pH and $PCO_2$ may be elevated because fewer binding sites for carbon dioxide are available on the hemoglobin and the Bohr effect is less active. In most cases, this phenomenon is inconsequential. However, patients with previously compromised respiratory exchange (i.e., carbon dioxide retention) deserve close attention.

#### OXYGEN TOXICITY

The concept of oxygen toxicity is familiar to anesthesiologists and intensivists (Fig. 14.5). In a normal ICU environment at sea level, this complication may develop after prolonged exposure to high fractional concentrations of oxygen, usually greater than 50%. This toxicity is most commonly associated with the pulmonary system (Lorrain-Smith effect), beginning as tracheitis and progressing eventually to a full-blown adult respiratory distress syndrome-like picture (23, 32, 33). The time frame for such developments varies with the actual $FO_2$, but it may begin as early as 6 to 12 hours after therapy using 100% oxygen is initi-

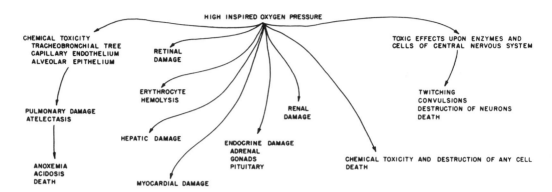

**Figure 14.5.    The various effects of oxygen toxicity.** (From Clark JM. The toxicity of oxygen. Am Rev Respir Dis 1974;110:40–50.)

ated. Typically, the highest $FO_2$ that a clinician could hope to administer at sea level is 1.0. However, once the hyperbaric realm is entered, oxygen can be delivered in excess of 1 ATA. As the $PO_2$ is raised by increasing pressure, the onset time for pulmonary signs and symptoms decreases (Fig. 14.6) (34).

The "rate-limiting factor" in the hyperbaric environment is not the pulmonary oxygen toxicity but its untoward effect on the central nervous system, which does not

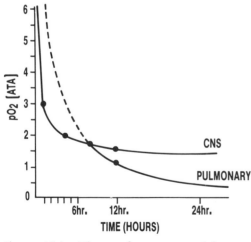

**Figure 14.6.    Time and oxygen partial pressure relationships as they affect the pulmonary system and CNS.** (Modified from Morris L (ed): Physics of the hyperbaric environment. In Hyperbaric Chamber Operations. Air Force Pamphlet 161–27. Washington, DC, Department of the Air Force, Headquarters, US Air Force, 1983, pp 10–17.)

occur in a normobaric environment (Fig. 14.6) (23, 35). This central nervous system (CNS) oxygen toxicity (Paul-Bert effect) will usually occur during exposures to oxygen approximating 2 ATA (33 fsw). The signs and symptoms of CNS oxygen toxicity include circumoral numbness and tingling and motor twitching and will eventually proceed to loss of consciousness, generalized seizures, and respiratory arrest. At the MIEMSS hyperbaric facility, the most common signs and symptoms of CNS oxygen toxicity during a total of almost 15,000 dives were nausea and vomiting (0.37%) and seizures (0.21%) (1). The use of "air breaks," or intermittent periods of air breathing, reduces the incidence of CNS oxygen toxicity. These air breaks, usually 5 minutes long, interspersed during HBO treatment (during which oxygen is breathed usually for periods of 20 minutes), reduce the total cumulative time of exposure to oxygen. There is a relationship between exercising and an increased incidence of oxygen toxicity seizures (possibly based on local tissue pH changes) (23). Thus, all patients should be advised not to engage in any unnecessary movement (35). Elevated $PCO_2$ has been implicated as a causative or contributory factor in these seizures, so adequate ventilation must be maintained (23).

The treatment of oxygen toxicity seizures is generally supportive and rests mainly upon lowering the ambient oxygen $PO_2$. Ambient, $PO_2$ is reduced by "venting" the chamber (i.e., allowing air to replace the

100% oxygen environment) or removing the oxygen mask/hood, but *not* by reducing the chamber pressure (35, 36). Such a reduction in chamber pressure could be detrimental with regard to intrapulmonary pressure, as the glottis may be closed (i.e., Valsalva maneuver). A reduction in chamber pressure under these conditions might result in barotrauma to the lung by expanding the air held within the sealed pulmonary system, along with all of the possible sequelae of such a complication (e.g., arterial gas embolism). The seizure itself is managed like any other seizure: by preventing aspiration, maintaining an airway, keeping the tongue from being bitten (e.g., inserting an oral airway), and protecting the patient from self-injury caused by flailing limbs (35, 36).

The seizures are short-lived and clear quickly once the partial pressure of oxygen is diminished. It is not known whether a history of a seizure disorder predisposes the patient to oxygen toxicity seizures. If the patient is taking anticonvulsants, efficacious levels should be maintained. The use of short-acting barbiturates or benzodiazepines for the control of seizures in the hyperbaric chamber is not well described in the literature but is thought to be effective.

This raises an interesting point with regard to the patient experiencing oxygen seizures in a monoplace chamber. As stated above, monoplace chambers are pressurized using 100% oxygen, and there is no method by which to "vent" such chambers to reduce

the partial pressure of oxygen (although recent developments may soon permit pressurization with air). Further, decompression is not a viable alternative because of the possibility of a closed glottis (see above). Thus, there is no alternative except to wait for the seizures to end spontaneously before beginning emergency decompression (36).

## Physiologic Effects of Hyperbaric Nitrogen: Nitrogen Narcosis

Nitrogen, the other major gas in air, is considered inert in the normobaric environment. At sea level this is indeed the fact; however, as the partial pressure of nitrogen rises during hyperbaric operations, nitrogen narcosis ("rapture of the deep") is encountered (23, 35, 37). The mechanism of nitrogen narcosis seems to be related to the same processes (Meyer-Overton theory) by which anesthesia is induced by inhalational anesthetics (e.g., isoflurane, halothane). In fact, all of the so-called "rare" elemental gases of the periodic table (e.g., argon, krypton, xenon, helium) possess the ability to produce the anesthetic state once an idiosyncratic partial pressure of the respective gas is reached (Table 14.5) (23, 37). The anesthetic abilities of a gas are dependent upon its molecular weight and lipid solubility characteristics. Generally the narcotic potency correlates to the degree of lipid solubility (23, 37). Argon, which is present at a level of almost 1% in air, may begin to

**Table 14.5. Correlation of Narcotic Potency of the Inert Gases with Lipid Solubility and Other Physical Characteristics**

| Gas | Molecular Weight | Solubility in Lipid | Temperature | Oil:Water Solubility Ratio | Relative Narcotic Potency |
|---|---|---|---|---|---|
| | | | °C | | |
| | | | | | (least narcotic) |
| He | 4 | 0.015 | 37 | 1.7 | 4.26 |
| Ne | 20 | 0.019 | 37.6 | 2.07 | 3.58 |
| $H_2$ | 2 | 0.036 | 37 | 2.1 | 1.83 |
| $N_2$ | 28 | 0.067 | 37 | 5.2 | 1 |
| Ar | 40 | 0.14 | 37 | 5.3 | 0.43 |
| Kr | 83.7 | 0.43 | 37 | 9.6 | 0.14 |
| Xe | 131.3 | 1.7 | 37 | 20.0 | 0.039 |
| | | | | | (most narcotic) |

**Table 14.6.   Effects of Compressed Air (Nitrogen Narcosis)**

| ATA | Effect |
|---|---|
| 2–4 | Mild impairment of performance on unpracticed tasks |
| | Mild euphoria |
| 4 | Reasoning and immediate memory affected more than motor coordination and choice reactions |
| | Delayed response to visual and auditory stimuli |
| 4–6 | Laughter and loquacity may be overcome by self control |
| | Idea fixation and overconfidence |
| | Calculation errors |
| 6 | Sleepiness, hallucinations, impaired judgement |
| 6–8[a] | Convival group atmosphere |
| | May be terror reactions in some |
| | Talkativeness |
| | Dizziness reported occasionally |
| | Uncontrolled laughter approaching hysteria in some |
| 8–10 | Severe impairment of intellectual performance; manual dexterity less affected |
| 10 | Stupefaction |
| | Severe impairment of practical activity and judgment |
| | Mental abnormalities and memory defects |
| | Deterioration in handwriting, euphoria, hyperexcitability |
| | Almost total loss of intellectual and perceptive faculties |
| | Hallucinogenic experiences (similar to the effects of hallucinogenic drugs rather than alcohol) |
| | Unconsciousness |
| | Death |

[a] Maximal depth for clinical diving (U.S. Air Force and most civilian centers).

exert its narcotic effect once sufficient depths are reached during air diving.

The signs and symptoms of nitrogen narcosis (Table 14.6) are commonly first noticed at depths approaching 100 fsw (although some individuals are prone to nitrogen effects at lesser depths), which corresponds to an inspired $PN_2$ of approximately 2400 mm Hg. Studies show that the majority of persons cannot concentrate or perform goal-directed tasks at 200 fsw (35). The onset of narcosis will occur after reaching a depth idiosyncratic to the particular person and is not usually progressive. Habituation, training, and experience allow chamber personnel to accommodate to the effects of nitrogen toxicity and quickly recognize its symptoms (35). Almost all persons are incapacitated at depths of 300 fsw. In chamber operations, the greatest detriment is that inside medical attendants affected by nitrogen narcosis are unable to be responsible for the safety of their patients. Thus, a maximal depth of 165 fsw is enforced for most clinical diving. An overview of the effects of exposure to hyperbaric air (i.e., nitrogen) is presented in Tables 14.6 and 14.7.

Methods to prevent nitrogen narcosis include altering the gaseous mixture within the chamber in an effort to reduce or eliminate the amount of nitrogen present. Alternatives include using solely oxygen

**Table 14.7.   Signs and Symptoms of Nitrogen Narcosis**

Common
  Delayed response to sight, sound, and smell
  Euphoria
  Fatigue
  Idea fixation
  Impairment of learning
  Inability to reason normally
  Laughter
  Loss of fine movement
  Loss of judgment
  Overconfidence
  Recent memory impairment
Serious
  Hallucinations
  Loss of consciousness
  Numbness and paresthesia
  Dizziness and vertigo
  Muscular weakness

(which is impractical for any significant depths or lengths of time because of the probability of oxygen toxicity); using nitrogen and oxygen mixtures in which the fraction of nitrogen is reduced (0.68, 0.60, 0.50 Nitrox); and using oxygen in combination with another gas such as helium (Heliox), which has a less pronounced narcotic effect (23, 37). The use of "oxygen-enriched mixtures" such as Nitrox raises the possibility of oxygen toxicity.

## Scientific Rationale of Hyperbaric Therapy

### PRESSURE

The effects of pressure can be divided into two categories: (*a*) direct, immediate and (*b*) indirect, delayed (3). Treatment of arterial gas embolism provides an example of direct, immediate effects. When ambient pressure is increased in a hyperbaric chamber, gas bubbles (and, for that matter, all air spaces) in the patient will be affected. According to Table 14.3, the volume and size of the bubble will decrease. Immediate reduction of bubble size relieves most of the problems associated with systemic gas embolism (e.g., intracardiac ventricular outflow obstruction, small vessel obstruction).

The indirect, delayed effects on air bubble size are due to the increased partial pressure of nitrogen as predicted by Henry's law. The higher partial pressure of the nitrogen within the bubble causes a higher rate of "off-gassing" of nitrogen from the bubble into solution. This pressure gradient for nitrogen can be enhanced by breathing 100% oxygen, when no additional nitrogen is supplied to the system. Eventually, a size

is reached at which a "critical diameter" is achieved. Then the dynamics of surface tension dictate that the smaller bubble will collapse or coalesce to form a larger, more stable bubble (38). These larger bubbles are then reduced by a combination of direct and indirect effects until virtually all bubbles are eliminated as the gas is dissolved into solution (i.e., the blood).

### OXYGEN

Under normobaric conditions, oxygen is both bound to hemoglobin (the majority) and dissolved (a smaller percentage). The amount of dissolved oxygen is usually 3.0 ml/100 ml of whole blood (0.31 vol%) in the presence of a $PaO_2$ of 100 mm Hg (39). As shown in Table 14.8, when ambient pressure is increased, the alveolar oxygen pressure, the amount of dissolved oxygen and thus the total $PaO_2$ (total $O_2 = HbO_2$ plus dissolved $O_2$) will increase linearly (Fig. 14.7). The alveolar oxygen pressure at any depth may be calculated by the following equation:

$$PAO_2 = FIO_2 (P_b - PAH_2O) - PACO_2$$

What is the therapeutic basis for such elevated levels of oxygen tension? Apparently, in a large number of varied conditions, either the oxygen carrying mechanism is defective (e.g., carbon monoxide poisoning) or the delivery scheme is compromised at some point (e.g., microvascular disease). HBO bypasses the specific oxygen carrying mechanisms by overloading the amount of dissolved oxygen to a point at which the presence of hemoglobin is superfluous. In fact, studies have demonstrated that animals may be sustained at extreme levels of

**Table 14.8.   Alveolar Oxygen Pressure and Oxygen Content of Blood Up to Depths of 3 ATA**

| Depth | Pressure | $PAO_2$ Breathing Air | $PAO_2$ Breathing 100% Oxygen | Breathing Air | Breathing 100% $O_2$ |
|---|---|---|---|---|---|
| *feet* | *ATA* | *mm Hg* | *mm Hg* | *vol%* | *vol%* |
| 0 | 1 | 102 | 673 | 0.31 | 2.09 |
| 30 | 1.91 | 247 | 1365 | 0.77 | 4.23 |
| 33 | 2 | 262 | 1433 | 0.81 | 4.44 |
| 45 | 2.36 | 319 | 1707 | 0.99 | 5.29 |
| 60 | 2.82 | 377 | 2056 | 1.17 | 6.37 |
| 66 | 3 | 422 | 2193 | 1.31 | 6.80 |

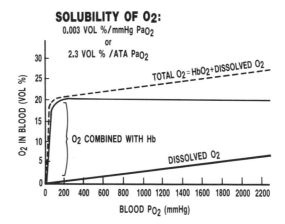

**Figure 14.7.   Solubility of oxygen (O₂) as a function of atmospheric pressure.** $Hb$ = hemoglobin, $ATA$ = atmosphere absolute. (Modified from Lanphier EH, Brown IW. Fundamentals of Hyperbaric Medicine. Publication No. 1298. Washington, DC, National Academy of Sciences, National Research Council, 1966.)

anemia through the use of HBO (See "Exceptional Blood Loss/Anemia") (40). HBO will overcome poor microvascular supply by increasing the amount of oxygen to such an extent that relatively avascular areas will be supplied with oxygen by gaseous diffusion. The ability of HBO to oxygenate relatively ischemic areas becomes important in conditions associated with chronic diseases such as diabetes and diabetic foot ulcers, osteomyelitis, or osteonecrosis (1, 2, 4, 15).

Normal tissue activity such as fibroblast proliferation and collagen production requires that a threshold local oxygen tension be present (20 to 40 mm Hg) (41, 42). Increased fibroblastic activity and collagen production provide a matrix for capillary budding and neovascularization. Raising local oxygen tension above these threshold levels (i.e., 40 to 50 mm Hg) will stimulate a greater degree of neovascularization, which may favor long-term rehabilitation of the area.

Also, in the case of certain anaerobic or microaerophilic infections, the mere presence of oxygen is bactericidal. Susceptible organisms lack the essential enzymes (e.g., superoxide dismutase) to permit their existence in highly oxygenated environments (43). Conversely, the ability of neutrophils to kill bacteria depends upon their intracel-

lular metabolism of oxygen molecules to various free radicals (e.g., superoxide, hydrogen peroxide) (44). Oxygen itself present in high tensions will inactivate bacterial toxins (e.g., clostridial alphatoxin). Also, oxygen is required for the transport of antimicrobials (such as the aminoglycosides) into bacteria (1).

## Treatment Tables

The majority of early work on diving and hyperbaric medicine was performed within the military establishments of various countries, most notably England, Canada, and the United States. Through original animal and human testing, as well as empirically, various standardized diving profiles that describe the depth and duration and the gas mixtures for a given hyperbaric treatment were developed (45). These diving profiles are known as decompression tables, recompression tables, or treatment tables (Fig. 14.8). Early on, most centers in the United States, both military and civilian, used the U.S. Navy (USN) Treatment Tables, which actually were developed to treat complications of diving (i.e., decompression sickness and gas embolism). For conditions other than those related to diving (e.g., carbon monoxide poisoning), clinical and research experience has dictated that treatment need

TIME IN MINUTES

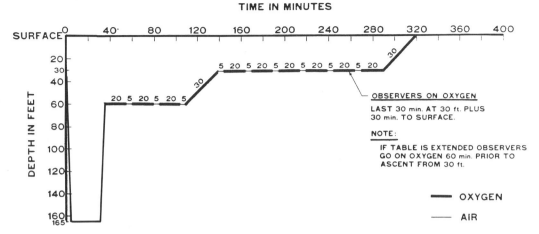

**Figure 14.8.   U.S. Navy Treatment Table 6A.**

not follow these Navy protocols. Different sets of protocols emphasize HBO therapy and not air recompression. Various diving profiles will be described in more detail in conjunction with the conditions for which they are indicated.

## HYPERBARIC THERAPY FOR SPECIFIC CONDITIONS RELATED TO TRAUMA

### Carbon Monoxide Poisoning

The clear, colorless, odorless gas carbon monoxide (CO) is often the product of incomplete combustion of hydrocarbons, whatever the source: automobile fumes, fires, or explosions (46). When inhaled, this compound binds directly to hemoglobin to form carboxyhemoglobin. CO competes directly with oxygen for these hemoglobin binding sites but has an affinity more than 200 times greater. CO can also combine with the cytochrome oxidase system at a cellular level and thus may interfere with mitochondrial respiration (47).

In the treatment of CO poisoning, HBO therapy can serve at least three functions. First, oxygen can be delivered to the cell independently of hemoglobin. Second, the oxygen levels are raised to such a degree that the competition of oxygen with CO for binding sites on both hemoglobin and the cytochrome oxidase chain becomes feasible. In this way, carbon monoxide elimination

half-time is greatly reduced compared with surface oxygen therapy (Table 14.9). Third, HBO reduces the degree of cerebral edema caused by CO poisoning because of its effect on the cerebral vasculature (see below) (30, 48).

The diminution in CO elimination half-time requires further discussion. For patients who have undergone a short, intense exposure to CO but who have been transported for an extensive period while breathing 100% oxygen, HBO may not have much to offer. Shown in Table 14.9 are the corresponding CO elimination half-times associated with breathing various partial pressures of oxygen. If, for example, a patient is treated with a nonrebreathing apparatus and arrives at the trauma center 2 hours after injury, the value of HBO is questionable. Alternatively, if the transport time is 20 or 30 minutes, HBO may be beneficial.

The decision to use or withhold HBO

**Table 14.9.   Carbon Monoxide Elimination Half-Time in Relation to Various Oxygen Treatments**[a]

| Depth | Treatment | CO Elimination (min) |
|---|---|---|
| Surface | Air (0.21 ATA) | 320 |
| Surface | Nonrebreather (0.95 ATA) | 80 |
| 33 fsw | Oxygen (2 ATA) | 56 |
| 66 fsw | Oxygen (3 ATA) | 23 |

[a] Abbreviations: fsw = feet of sea water (gauge); ATA = atmospheres absolute.

therapy should be tempered by consideration of at least three additional factors (49, 50): The first of these is the serum CO levels. Generally, various levels of CO may correspond to the signs and symptoms listed in Table 14.10. The second factor is the arterial pH as determined by blood gas analysis (51). If the patient is shown to be acidotic (pH < 7.30), HBO therapy should be instituted. The third factor is the finding of psychometric testing, which becomes important when considering the various "exposure profiles" that a smoke inhalation victim may experience (e.g., long versus short).

One of the tissues most affected by residual CO levels is the brain. If abnormalities are not readily apparent by casual observation, examination of the patient, or serum CO levels, they may be elucidated by detailed psychometric testing, usually requiring less than 25 minutes to be completed (50). Even exposure victims who have normal CO levels may receive HBO if psychometric testing is abnormal. HBO therapy will be repeated if necessary. Two other factors that should also receive consideration are age (greater than 60) and medical history (e.g., the presence of cardiovascular disease, especially coronary artery pathology).

## TREATMENT

One of the most popular treatment tables for CO poisoning recommends immediately compressing the patient to 66 fsw (3 ATA) and remaining at this depth for two 23-minute periods of HBO separated by a 5-minute air break. After the second oxygen breathing period, an ascent to 33 fsw is made with a 5-minute air break. The patient remains at 33 fsw for two treatment periods of 25 minutes each, separated by a 5-minute air break. At this point the patient is clinically assessed. If additional treatment is deemed necessary, the patient remains at 33 fsw for oxygen therapy, with air breaks interposed; otherwise, an ascent is made to the surface (30). The protocol at the MIEMSS hyperbaric department consists of diving to 60 fsw for 46 minutes with a second dive at 6 hours to 33 fsw for 90 minutes. Treatments are then repeated twice daily as necessary. Psychometric testing within the chamber, performed by the inside observer, may be useful in this decision-making process.

### Arterial Gas Embolism (AGE)

AGE is a possible complication in the trauma patient. It may develop not only in the compromised diver but also in a hypovolemic patient who may have a greatly reduced central venous pressure and is undergoing rapid and hectic intravenous line placement and receiving positive-pressure ventilation in the face of a concurrent unvented pneumothorax or in a patient who has received a penetrating chest injury. In fact, systemic AGE, thought to be rare, may occur in up to approximately 14% of all major thoracic injuries, the incidence being three times greater in association with penetrating injuries versus blunt trauma

**Table 14.10. Clinical Manifestations of Carbon Monoxide Poisoning Associated with Varying Levels of Blood Carboxyhemoglobin (COHb)**

| Blood COHb Concentration | Signs and Symptoms |
|---|---|
| % | |
| 0–10 | None (angina may be noted in patients with coronary artery disease) |
| 10–20 | Slight headache<br>Exercise-induced angina<br>Dyspnea on vigorous exertion |
| 20–30 | Throbbing headache<br>Dyspnea on moderate exertion |
| 30–40 | Severe headache<br>Nausea/vomiting<br>Weakness<br>Visual disturbance<br>Impaired judgment |
| 40–50 | Syncope<br>Tachycardia<br>Tachypnea/dyspnea at rest |
| 50–60 | Coma<br>Convulsions<br>Cheyne-Stokes respiration |
| 60–70 | Compromised cardiorespiratory function |
| 70–80 | Death |

(52). It may occur either on the venous side of the circulation (affecting right heart stroke volume, obstructing pulmonary outflow, or causing pulmonary hypertension) or on the left side of the heart (resulting in coronary artery embolization, cerebrovascular embolization, or peripheral AGE). Most often the injury occurs as a result of invasive lines, open heart surgery, dialysis, or lung trauma with either open pulmonary vasculature or bronchopulmonary venous fistulas. For example, an open pneumothorax may lead to air entrainment through an open pulmonary vein, or positive-pressure ventilation may lead to AGE in a closed chest, tracheobronchial injury. Additionally, AGE may occur due to an open skull fracture with exposed diploic veins. Hypovolemia and positive-pressure ventilation are predisposing factors.

As with other conditions described in this section, a high degree of clinical suspicion is necessary. Suggestive scenarios are (a) the sudden, unexplained deterioration of a trauma patient with severe chest trauma, (b) the trauma patient who has no obvious head trauma but who has localized findings on neurologic examination such as paraplegia or hemiplegia, and (c) sudden hemodynamic collapse after endotracheal intubation and the initiation of positive-pressure ventilation. Associated signs include hemoptysis, air visualized in the retinal veins during funduscopic examination, or froth obtained during aspiration of arterial blood for blood gas analysis (52).

Treatment of suspected AGE involves emergency thoracotomy without delay and/or immediate compression in a hyperbaric chamber and subsequent hyperoxygenation. Overall mortality (immediate and delayed) is extremely high (52).

## TREATMENT

Hyperbaric therapy is the *only* definitive treatment for AGE (1, 53). However, when considering treatment for AGE, one must be aware of not only the secondary problem, the AGE itself, but of the causative, initial (primary) problem, which may or may not

still be active. For example, if the primary problem was a pneumothorax, this must be attended to immediately by the placement of a thoracostomy tube or at least a large-bore intravenous catheter. Because of the urgency of the treatment of AGE, this should be done, if possible, during compression, depending upon the size of the chamber and the capability of the inside observer or physician.

On the other hand, if the primary problem was entrainment of air through an intravascular port in a central vein with a subatmospheric pressure, then a tertiary problem may need to be addressed (for example, a collection of air in the right ventricle, which can obstruct pulmonary artery outflow). Such an air collection may have to be evacuated by a percutaneous needle puncture, the passage of a central line, or a formal thoracostomy.

Regarding the HBO treatment itself (which may vary from center to center), USN Treatment Table 6A, which includes both hyperbaric air and oxygen, is most commonly followed (Fig. 14.8). It involves rapid compression using air to 165 fsw (6 ATA) for 30 minutes. After 30 minutes the patient is reevaluated and a further decision is made (53).

If the patient has made no improvement after 30 minutes at 165 fsw, the treatment at this depth can be extended for a total of 2 hours maximum at 165 fsw. This is considered an "exceptional exposure" dive (referring to the amount of nitrogen saturation) and, hence, a "modified" USN Treatment Table 6A is followed (53). If, at 165 fsw, the patient has progressed or is no worse, an ascent is made to 60 fsw and the rest of USN Table 6A is followed, with the entire table totaling 320 minutes (oxygen and air breaks interspersed). The efficacy of the treatment can be enhanced by using a 50:50 Nitrox mixtype during the portion of the dive between 66 and 165 fsw (30). However, if the patient has worsened at 60 fsw, a saturation dive may be undertaken or the patient can be brought out and dived on a repetitive basis, maximizing $O_2$ exposures with the repetitive diving (54).

At least one author advocates placing the patient in a modified Trendelenburg position (head down 10° degrees in the left lateral decubitus position, known as the Durant position) during the dive, as this will increase the venous return to the cranial vasculature and possibly dilate the vessels (55). This may improve passage of trapped bubbles. Further, the use of Heliox mixtures has been advocated to provide a maximal gradient for nitrogen "off-gassing" and bubble reduction (30). However, this may work to a disadvantage, as helium may diffuse into the previously helium-free bubbles.

The use of steroids in the treatment of AGE is controversial (30, 56). Dexamethasone (10 mg every 6 hours) may be given for the first 48 to 72 hours in an effort to reduce cerebral edema and stabilize cell membranes. At this point steroids should be tapered.

If symptoms remain after the initial treatment, daily treatments of HBO can be maintained. If repetitive dives are necessary, one might consider the use of prophylactic anticonvulsants for those patients receiving exogenous steroids, although this point is not well defined (30).

### Decompression Sickness (DCS)

DCS, along with AGE, is one of the "dysbaric conditions" that occur due to pressure effects. Generally, DCS can be seen in persons involved with "wet" or "dry" diving. This includes, of course, the scuba diver as well as observers working in the HM environment. In most cases, a differential diagnosis of DCS versus AGE is entertained and may be difficult to define. As described above, AGE is usually of sudden onset and confined to neural dysfunction. On the other hand, DCS usually develops more slowly and can be limited to complaints concerning the musculoskeletal system but also can involve neural dysfunction.

Most cases of DCS will manifest within 2 to 4 hours after a dive, although the

presentation of signs and symptoms may be delayed for 24 hours. Beyond 24 hours, the likelihood of DCS is diminished (57, 58). The signs and symptoms of DCS are listed in Table 14.11.

Another important distinction between AGE and DCS is the pattern of distribution of paralysis. In DCS the distribution is usually transverse (e.g., from the waist down). In AGE, it is usually vertical (e.g., divided at the longitudinal midline).

If the hyperbaricist can determine that a scuba diver has made a "nonstandard" dive or that an accidental explosive decompression to the surface occurred, then the differential diagnosis will be clearer. Depth and length of dive are important, as there must be a sufficient length of exposure to an adequate depth (usually depths greater than 33 fsw) to allow accumulation of nitrogen. AGE can occur in as little as 4 feet of water, almost instantaneously. DCS would also be likely in a sea-level-acclimatized aviator or passenger who has experienced decompression (in a nonpressured cabin) to an altitude greater than 18,000 feet, based on Haldane's 2-to-1 rule (see below). Flying less than 12 to 24 hours after diving can also cause DCS (57). DCS has even been reported in persons driving home through mountainous areas of relatively low altitude (e.g., 5000 feet) after diving (57, 59).

In 1906, the concept of "critical supersaturation" was described by the British

**Table 14.11.   Signs and Symptoms of Decompression Sickness**

Type I
  90% of cases involve pain
  Pain usually located in an extremity, usually a joint (i.e., knee, elbow)
Type II
  25% of cases involve neurologic derangements:
    Extremity paresthesia/paresis
    Vertigo
    Visual disturbances/blindness
  2% of cases involve respiratory system (chokes):
    Wheezing
    Substernal pain
    Nonproductive cough
    Burning pain on inspiration
  May also involve the skin or cardiac system

physiologist J. S. Haldane. This theorem proposed a relationship between ambient pressure changes, bubble formation, and the development of DCS. Although no longer used in its original simplistic form, the basic concept that DCS would not develop if the critical supersaturation ratios of pressure reductions were limited to less than 2:1 is still roughly correct (45). Thus, according to the theory, one can essentially experience an abrupt ascent from 2 to 1 ATA without the development of DCS. One can also ascend quickly from sea level (1 ATA) to 18,000 feet (0.5 ATA) with minimal risk.

The diagnosis of DCS is divided into two major categories: type I and type II. Type I DCS, also known as the "bends" and caisson disease (because of early observations of the bent-over posture of caisson workers, whose extremity joints had been affected) or "pain-only" DCS, is limited to complaints of pain (60). Fifteen to twenty per cent of type I DCS symptoms will present as pain in an area other than the extremities (57). Eighty to eighty-five per cent of this pain affects areas of the extremities, particularly the joints (57). Because of mechanical shearing forces, limb joints creating negative hydrostatic pressures, and/or the turbulent blood flow in the vascular plexuses surrounding these joints, these are primary areas for the collection of bubbles. Exercise in these areas also increases the incidence of bubble development. It is still not clear at which point relative to diving exercise becomes important in the development of bubbles. Exercise at depth or after surfacing seems to be a fairly certain promoter of bubble development. Theoretically, if exercise occurs before diving, then bubbles that are formed should be compressed back into solution during a dive (60, 61).

In addition to pain, type II DCS exhibits manifestations in one or more of the following systems: neurologic, circulatory, respiratory, or skin (62). Type II DCS involving the respiratory system (also known as "chokes" because victims appear to be asphyxiating) is due to an overload of the pulmonary capillary vasculature with air

bubbles. Normally, small amounts of air passing through the lungs can be equilibrated with the atmosphere. However, the massive accumulation of bubbles that occurs during type II DCS with a respiratory component leads to large degrees of shunting and eventual circulatory collapse. This collapse is due not only to interference with the cardiopulmonary system (e.g., by reductions of venous return to the left heart) but also possibly to other direct effects of the bubbles on the vasomotor regulatory center and vessel endothelial damage (63).

Neurologic manifestations of type II DCS can involve either the central or peripheral systems or both. Regarding central involvement, an interesting association is made between aviators with DCS, who usually develop brain abnormalities, and divers, who usually show symptoms of spinal cord lesions (58). Possible central manifestations include convulsions, unconsciousness, nausea and vomiting, visual disturbances, dizziness, vertigo, headache, aphasia, restlessness, confusion, and personality changes. Peripheral nervous system problems may involve the cranial nerves, the spinal nerves, or the autonomic system. Signs and symptoms include numbness, paresthesia, paresis, paralysis, and muscular weakness or twitching (57).

Skin manifestations are usually minor and may include itching or peripheral edema (due to bubble blockage of the lymphatics) (57).

## TREATMENT

Transport of a patient with suspected DCS (and AGE) is discussed below and in Chapter 15. In this section it will be assumed that the patient is already present at a hyperbaric treatment facility capable of a 6-ATA dive.

Regardless of whether the differential diagnosis between AGE and DCS is unclear or not or, for that matter, whether the DCS diagnosis alone is unclear, hyperbaric therapy should commence as quickly as possible. Before diving, patients should receive 100% oxygen on the surface and an intravenous port should be established with hydration under way (54).

Patients with type I DCS usually are treated according to USN Table 5, which involves immediate compression to 60 fsw on 100% oxygen (30, 56, 62). If pain persists at this depth, then the plan changes to USN Table 6 (discussed below). If not, two 20-minute oxygen-breathing periods with air breaks occur at this depth and then ascent to 30 fsw, on oxygen, takes place over 30 minutes. Oxygen breathing is continuous at this new depth and then is followed by a 30-minute ascent to the surface on oxygen.

Cases of type II DCS will usually be treated according to USN Table 6. This table also involves compression to 60 fsw on oxygen, where three oxygen breathing periods occur with intermittent air breaks. A 30-minute ascent to 30 fsw on oxygen will then occur. At 30 fsw, six oxygen breathing periods, with corresponding air breaks, occur. A 30-minute ascent to surface on oxygen follows. In extremely serious cases, USN Table 6 can be lengthened by adding another oxygen-breathing period at 60 fsw, another hour of oxygen breathing at 30 fsw, or both. If the patient fails to improve or fully recover after Table 6 is followed, one might resort to saturation diving or another alternative (54). The most common reasons for failure of hyperbaric therapy in the treatment of dysbaric conditions are related to the errors listed in Table 14.12.

In addition to the hyperbaric treatment, it is also important to hydrate the patient (54). Normally, this begins with a crystalloid solution. A urinary output of 1 ml/kg/hr is usually a sign of adequate hydration. If shock is present, as in some patients with

**Table 14.12. Most Frequent Errors Related to Emergency Hyperbaric Therapy**

Patient delays in reporting symptoms
Serious symptoms not recognized
Delay in treatment
Inadequate treatment
Patient not kept near chamber after initial treatment
Hesitancy to treat doubtful cases
Patients within chamber allowed to assume positions that interfere with blood circulation

type II DCS, a colloid solution and blood products should be infused as necessary. Presently, there is some ongoing controversy regarding the use of dextran, which has the ultimate goal of stabilizing the surface of red blood cells and preventing rouleaux formation (62). It is not clear whether dextran 40 or 70 (molecular weight) serves these purposes better.

Another controversy is related to the use of steroids (62). One concern here is the possibility of steroid-induced exacerbation of oxygen toxicity. As yet, there have been no reports of oxygen toxicity in divers undergoing the treatment of USN Tables 5 or 6. Thus, dexamethasone (20 to 40 mg intravenously followed by 40 mg intramuscularly every 6 hours) may be instituted for 72 hours. Heparin may also be useful in cases of DCS in an effort to prevent thromboembolism, but it should not be used in cases of vestibular bends or air embolism (62). Diuretics such as glycerol, mannitol, and lasix may be useful in reducing cerebral and peripheral edema, but, according to the literature, no definite recommendations can be offered (30, 56). The same situation applies to the use of aspirin and other antinflammatory agents. Aspirin would have the additional benefit of preventing platelet aggregation.

## TRANSPORT OF PATIENTS NEEDING HYPERBARIC THERAPY

It is not unusual for persons suffering from type I or type II DCS or AGE to be in need of transportation from a remote location, where their injury occurred, to a hyperbaric facility. Examples of these patients include the sport diver, using SCUBA, on a resort island (a scenario becoming more common with the increasing number of sport divers) and the diver who has unwisely made an airplane flight too soon after his or her last dive. Usually there is a degree of urgency associated with this type of transport, especially in cases of AGE. This urgency will translate to the use of flying vehicles, either a helicopter or a fixed-wing aircraft, for medical evacuation. Currently, there exist small one- or two-person hyperbaric chambers that are either built into a helicopter or carried by cables below (Fig. 14.2). These chambers usually can be "docked" with a larger, stationary chamber at a treatment facility where the patient who has undergone "transfer-under-pressure" (TUP) is moved into the larger chamber.

Unless a highly specialized TUP vehicle can be obtained, an important interplay of altitude and pressure effects must be controlled. Fortunately, the differences in bubble volume are not as pronounced with altitudes above sea level as they are below sea level (Fig. 15.6). However, it is still important to maintain the lowest possible altitude, with those below 1000 feet being best (55). The real concerns in these cases are the pressure effects of the hypobaric high-altitude environment and not those of hypoxia, as additional oxygen can be supplied. If geographic obstacles to low-level flight are not a concern, then transportation problems are reduced to vehicular range and refueling. If the trip must be made over a mountain range or other aeronautical obstruction, special arrangements may be needed. This might include obtaining a fixed-wing aircraft capable of maintaining a cabin pressure of 1 ATA, even at high altitudes (e.g., a Lear jet). Alternatively, a small multiplace or monoplace chamber could be brought to the patient's location for the initial treatments.

If satisfactory transport can be arranged, the patient should be placed in the supine position. In cases of DCS or AGE with a cerebral edema component, the patient should be oriented in the vehicle with the head toward the rear of the plane to avoid increases in intracranial pressure due to the acceleration forces during take-off (which are less easily controlled than the deceleration forces that occur during landing [see Chapter 15]). The patient should be wearing a tight-fitting face mask (100% $O_2$). One of the goals here is denitrogenation, in addition to oxygenation.

Advice regarding movement and treatment of these isolated patients can be sought through the Divers Alert Network, whose National Center is headquartered at Duke University Medical Center (telephone 919-684-8111), or one of the six regional centers, such as MIEMSS (northeastern United States, 301-328-7814), all of which provide telephone consultations. Alternatively, military personnel or civilians in distress usually can seek medical advice from the U.S. Air Force Hyperbaric Center at the School of Aerospace Medicine at Brooks Air Force Base in San Antonio, Texas. Another option would be to contact the U.S. Navy Experimental Diving Unit in Panama City, Florida (telephone 904-234-4351) or the Naval Medical Research Institute in Bethesda, Maryland (telephone 202-295-1859).

### Crush Injury/Compartment Syndrome

In both crush injury and the compartment syndrome, the vascular integrity and supply to the affected areas are compromised. Although HBO will have little value if the blood supply to the area is completely interrupted, in most cases HBO can exert a beneficial effect and improve outcome (1). Presurgically, the most important factor relating to the prognostic ability of HBO in these conditions is the interval between injury and the institution of hyperbaric treatment. In the case of compartment syndrome, if HBO is begun early enough, fasciotomy for compartmental decompression may be avoided (64). HBO can also be used as a temporizing maneuver if surgical decompression is, for some reason, impossible at the time (30). In crush injury, postoperative tissue viability will be improved by the early use of HBO. Benefits are due not only to the effects of improved oxygenation but also to the intense vasoconstrictor effect of oxygen. Tissue edema will then be less severe, and perfusion will be better. Ideally, treatment must begin within 5 to 6 hours after the injury (30).

Postoperatively, in all of these cases, neovascularization is encouraged. Ischemic areas will thus have a better prognosis, and the degree of muscle necrosis will be reduced. This is particularly important in cases of reimplantation of digits or extremities.

## TREATMENT

A variety of protocols exist for this condition. It is the authors' opinion that long oxygen exposures during the first 48 to 72 hours are crucial. At the MIEMSS hyperbaric facility, HBO is given over 2 to 3 hours every 4 hours for the first 48 hours and then twice daily in 90- to 120-minute increments.

### Exceptional Blood Loss (Anemia) (Investigative—Special Situation)

Thoughts regarding the usefulness of HBO treatment in trauma patients with exceptional blood loss trace back to a paper published by Boerema et al. in 1960 (40). It was shown that, in an oxygen environment of 3 ATA, the oxygen content of the serum (6.7 vol%) would be sufficient to obviate the need for oxygen transport by red blood cells. Also, the arteriovenous oxygen extraction difference is very close to this same 6.7 vol%. Theoretically, a solution with a colloid oncotic pressure similar to that of whole blood could support life in the presence of HBO. This concept has interesting implications in cases of religious objections (e.g., Jehovah's Witnesses) or medical objections (e.g., hemolytic crisis without available compatible blood) to blood transfusion for anemia or in those cases in which blood for massive transfusion is unavailable (e.g., severe trauma, disasters). Several case reports have been published regarding HBO treatment for similar situations (65–67).

## TREATMENT

Obviously, patients requiring this course of therapy for anemia must be in extremis. In the case reports cited above, patients treated with HBO had hemoglobin levels of 1 to 3 g/dl (65–67). Therefore, a full complement of critical care diagnostic and therapeutic equipment should already be in place (i.e., electrocardiogram [ECG], arterial line, central venous pressure monitoring).

Close observation of the patient with surveillance for signs (e.g., ST segment depression or T wave changes on ECG) and symptoms (e.g., substernal chest pain) of ischemia is required. A delicate balance is maintained in these patients between the ischemia, due to anemia, and the possibility of oxygen toxicity due to excessive exposure to HBO. One author recommends that HBO be used in the acute situation at 2.5 ATA every hour (or treatments at 2 ATA for 1 to 2 hours) (31). Surface intervals may be for 2 to 6 hours. The treatment schedule is then individualized for the patient, depending upon the response to treatment and the course on the surface (e.g., ECG changes).

### Burns

Suggestions regarding the usefulness of HBO for burn patients were derived from observations that the burn wounds of patients undergoing hyperbaric treatment for CO poisoning seemed to heal better. Although there is some degree of variance in results and some controversy, a number of studies of HBO for burn patients show accelerated and improved wound healing; a reduction in fluid requirement; a reduced incidence of paralytic ileus, cerebral edema, and burn encephalopathy; and a reduction in overall mortality (31, 68, 69). A summary of the proposed uses of HBO in burn patients is shown in Table 14.13.

## TREATMENT

The treatment regimen for HBO therapy in burn patients is HBO therapy at 2.0 to 2.4 ATA for 90 to 120 minutes on a three-times-daily basis for the first 24 hours and then on a twice-daily basis until healing/coverage is achieved (31). If HBO is used, an important consideration is the avoidance of mafenide (Sulfamylon) (31). In cases where this agent is used, it must be removed before HBO treatments. This topical antimicrobial agent for burn wounds induces peripheral vasodilation because of its carbonic anhydrase inhibitory action. When coupled with the central vasoconstrictor effects of HBO, worse results are produced. Silver sulfadia-

**Table 14.13.   Proposed Functions of Hyperbaric Oxygen Treatments in Patients with Thermal Injury**

| Phase I (Immediate Considerations) | Phase II (Delayed Considerations) |
|---|---|
| Treat carbon monoxide poisoning | Improve adult respiratory distress syndrome secondary to smoke inhalation. |
| Reduce severity of tissue edema, thus improving microcirculation and reducing stasis. | Accelerate revascularization of burn wound. |
| Improve oxygenation of salvageable cells at burn wound. | Improve graft viability. |
| | Reduce contractures and hypertrophic scarring. |
| | Prevent/reduce cerebral edema. |
| | Prevent/improve paralytic ileus. |

zine (Silvadine) may be applied to the burn wound instead.

## Cerebral Edema (Investigative)

In most patients with head trauma, cerebral edema will occur. Because of the "closed box" characteristics of the cranial vault, cerebral edema will result in increases in intracranial pressure (ICP) (see Chapter 7). These increases may result in the herniation of brain contents through the foramen magnum or regional ischemia of the brain due to localized decreases in cerebral perfusion pressure. HBO is thought to exert beneficial effects by improving oxygenation (which indirectly limits the subsequent development of cerebral edema) and by directly reducing ICP (probably due to the direct vasoconstrictor properties of oxygen). Various investigators have shown that the electroencephalogram (EEG) is significantly improved if HBO is instituted soon after the injury (within 12 hours) (30). These desirable EEG changes are less dramatic the longer HBO is delayed. Conversely, HBO may be detrimental to head-injured patients who have cerebral vasomotor paralysis. This is probably because of a loss of protective effect of vasoconstriction with regard to oxygen toxicity. Likewise, HBO is thought not to be helpful in head-injured patients in whom the ICP is unresponsive to hyperventilation (30, 48, 70, 71).

### TREATMENT

Recommended treatment protocols vary, but HBO should be started within 12 hours of injury. Dives to 1.5 to 2.0 ATA intermittently for up to 5 days may follow on a 4-, 6-, 8-, or 12-hour basis. It is very helpful in head trauma cases to institute monitoring of ICP, which can be used as a guide to the effectiveness of HBO treatments.

## Spinal Cord Injury (Investigative)

The theoretic usefulness of HBO in acute spinal cord trauma rests upon the concept that a large proportion of these injuries are not complete anatomic transections (72). It is postulated that the cord edema and regional ischemia that accompany this type of injury, within the confines of the narrow spinal canal, account for much of the morbidity. If HBO can be started within a fairly well-defined period (approximately 4 hours), it may be possible to diminish the degree of edema and ischemia. This injury-improving effect has been demonstrated in a number of animal studies (72, 73). The difficulty with the clinical application of this concept involves the time constraints and logistics imposed by the transportation of the trauma patient and the subsequent diagnostic and therapeutic procedures that must be performed (e.g., resuscitation, roentgenography, CT scanning, application of skeletal traction, reduction of the fracture and/or dislocation, myelography, and possibly surgery).

### TREATMENT

If the trauma patient can be prepared to receive HBO within a reasonable amount of time, then the following schedule is used. All dives are to 2.0 ATA for 2 hours. The regimen begins with one dive every 2 hours for four cycles, followed by four more dives, one every 6 hours. If the patient demonstrates improved function at the end of these eight dives, then HBO treatment is continued on a twice-a-day basis for 5 days. If the patient shows no functional recovery, then the HBO is discontinued (72).

### Nonhealing Wounds/Amputated Stumps

It is not uncommon in trauma patients for a number of compromising factors (e.g., infection, ischemia, poor nutrition) to result in delayed or poor healing of wounds. This is particularly true in previously impaired patients, for example, diabetics or other patients with chronic vascular stasis. As described above, the physiologic basis for HBO in these patients rests upon its ability to raise the local tissue oxygen tension in ischemic areas and thus induce collagen synthesis and neovascularization.

#### TREATMENT

The effectiveness, or lack thereof, of all HBO treatments for these conditions should be documented with serial measurements of transcutaneous oxygen tensions, the "magic number" being in the range of 40 to 50 mm Hg (41). An initial transcutaneous $PO_2$ level, before HBO therapy, of less than 20 mm Hg may indicate a poor prognosis, even with the addition of hyperbaric therapy (30). If, after 10 to 14 days of daily or twice-daily treatments to 2.4 ATA for 90 minutes, there is no appreciable improvement either in the transcutaneous $PO_2$ levels or in the proliferation of granulation tissue, then treatments should be discontinued. Hyperbaric treatments should be complemented with close observation of the wounds, which should be aggressively debrided to remove all necrotic tissue.

Wound treatment tables vary from center to center. One popular table involves a treatment depth of 45 fsw for 120 minutes. Ten-minute air breaks can be given every 30 minutes, with a total of three oxygen-breathing periods and a 10-minute ascent. If the patient demonstrates signs and symptoms of oxygen toxicity, the same bottom time (i.e., total time at maximal depth) can be utilized, with oxygen-breathing periods reduced to 20 minutes and 5-minute air breaks.

### CRITICAL CARE IN THE HYPERBARIC CHAMBER (16, 27, 74, 75)

The physician involved in the care of critically ill patients in the hyperbaric environment must possess a solid foundation in critical care doctrine and trauma management. The same level of understanding of the principles and practices of hyperbaric medicine is essential. This background will afford the hyperbaricist the ability to function with the same degree of effectiveness within the hyperbaric chamber as have intensivists in critical care areas on the surface. The same level of care that occurs in conventional ICUs, including most forms of physiologic monitoring, is presently possible within the hyperbaric chamber (76). All forms of vasoactive infusions can and should be maintained and adjusted according to the appropriate, monitored parameters, and mechanical ventilation can be continued. However, because of differences between the hyperbaric and normobaric environments, modifications in certain critical care equipment or procedures require special attention (Table 14.14).

The "typical" ICU patient in a major trauma center has at least one intravenous port and possibly has one or more intravascular pressure-monitoring systems (e.g., arterial line, pulmonary artery catheter) in place, as well as the associated high-pressure "flushing" systems. These intravascular pressures, as well as the ECG, must be monitored continuously in the chamber. Frequently such patients will be mechanically ventilated by an endotracheal or a tracheostomy tube. If the patient has sustained chest trauma and has a pneumothorax or pneumohemothorax, at least one thoracostomy tube will be attached to underwater suction.

Regarding intravenous, central venous, and intraarterial ports, one must be absolutely certain that no air is introduced into these systems, as the consequences may be

**Table 14.14. Critical Care Equipment or Procedures Requiring Special Attention or Modification before Use in Multiplace Hyperbaric Chamber**

| | |
|---|---|
| Intravenous (i.v.) infusion equipment | |
| Glass i.v. bottles | Avoid, or vent must extend all the way to the bottom of jar. |
| i.v. infusion pump | Frequent alarming; must disarm "anti-infiltration" switch. Readjust at depth. |
| Tubing | Ensure absolutely no air entrainment. Avoid puncturing rubber injection sites (use 3-way stopcocks) (especially monoplace). Safeguard against disconnection (especially monoplace). |
| Intravascular pressure monitoring systems (e.g., intraarterial pressure) | |
| Pressure bladder | Must adjust volume of air in bladder during ascent/descent. |
| Tubing | Avoid air entrainment (because it may be injected into patient or interfere with signal transmission). |
| Monitoring equipment | Avoid using portable monitors at depths greater than 3 ATA (cathode ray tubes may implode). Consider purging interiors continuously with nitrogen to avoid ignition. |
| | Cardiac output computers must be specially adjusted. Function of pulse oximeters/capnographs may be unreliable. For blood gas analysis, must either use specially adjusted equipment within chamber or expect spurious results from samples dispatched through airlock and analyzed at surface (due to "off-gassing"). |
| Central line placement | Avoid subclavian puncture. Use femoral or internal jugular veins. |
| Pulmonary artery catheters | Ensure that balloon at catheter tip is deflated and balloon port is left open. |
| | Obtaining wedge pressures during the dive is not recommended. |
| Airway equipment | |
| Endotracheal/tracheal tubes | Must adjust volume of air in cuff during ascent/descent using aneroid manometer or replace air with saline or water |
| Mechanical ventilator systems | |
| Ventilator | Must monitor "set" tidal volume vs. "delivered" tidal volume and make appropriate adjustments during ascent/descent using respirometer (must also adjust). Positive end-expiratory pressure may be used. Recommended ventilators (volume-cycled preferred): |
| | Penlon Oxford |
| | Siemens 900 B, C, D |
| | Sechrist (for monoplace only) |
| | Bird Mark 14 |
| | Ensure that humidification devices remain in upright position. |
| Wright respirometer | Must recalibrate at various depths due to varying gas densities with depth or formulate conversion on chart. |
| Chest tube drainage systems | Must have thoracostomy apparatus ready within vicinity of chamber for emergency procedures. |
| Pleurevac | Maintain suction, monitor air-fluid levels during ascent/descent. |
| | May substitute one-way valve (e.g., Heimlich valve). Must repeat balancing/calibration of transducers after any depth change. If possible, connect transducers to monitors outside the chamber via hull penetrators. |
| Injections | |
| Intramuscular/subcutaneous | Avoid because of delayed/erratic absorption (due to vasoconstriction secondary to HBO). |
| Defibrillation | Must maintain $FIO_2 < 0.23$. Have fire suppression equipment ready. Recommend external trigger. Place nonconducting pad beneath patient. Operator should stand on nonconducting surface. |
| Nasogastric tubes | Leave unclamped or on intermittent suction. |
| Oxygen breathing device (built-in breathing device) | Use of all oxygen within chamber must be controlled carefully (use only tight-fitting aviator masks or hoods or endotracheal/tracheostomy tubes). |
| | Only aqueous solutions should be used because of fire hazards. |

*Table continues next page*

**Table 14.14.    Continued**

| | |
|---|---|
| Suction devices | Several systems are available that utilize interior/exterior pressure differential. Use in-line trap and vacuum regulator. |
| Indwelling urinary catheter | Ensure that balloon is inflated with water/saline. |
| Sphygmomanometer | Do not use mercury-filled type. (If broken, it will contaminate the chamber). |
| Clothing/fabric | Wearing street clothes or shoes is prohibited. (Oil on street shoes may contaminate chamber.) Recommend "Durette Gold" fabric or cotton as an alternative. |

disastrous (e.g., systemic embolism). If there is an indwelling pulmonary artery catheter, one must be certain that the balloon at the tip is deflated and that the balloon port is left open. Expansion of the balloon to the point of breaking during decompression could lead to pulmonary artery rupture and air embolism. Also, because there is a good likelihood that air will be introduced unknowingly during the placement of such lines, no new central lines should be placed during a dive, unless absolutely necessary. All lines should be inspected before a dive is begun. Similarly, if one decides that a new line may be necessary for therapeutic or diagnostic purposes, it should be placed before the dive, not during it. If an emergency occurs at depth and intravenous access is inadequate, most resuscitation drugs can be given via the intratracheal tube. When the insertion of a new central line during a dive is absolutely mandatory, the subclavian route should be avoided at all costs because of the association with a high incidence of pneumothorax. Viable alternatives for vascular access include the femoral venous or possibly the internal jugular route.

In all cases of recently placed central venous lines, a chest roentgenogram should be obtained before diving and evaluated for the presence of pneumothorax. If there are signs that the lung has been punctured, a chest tube must be inserted and then placed on continuous suction.

In patients with a thoracostomy tube, several points must be remembered:
1. It should be ensured that the entire intrapleural suction drainage system is patent and that the thoracostomy tube itself, connectors, and other apparatus are securely fastened to avoid dislodgement.
2. Constant suction can be maintained by any one of several systems that function well at depth and are described elsewhere.
3. Alternatively, in cases where suction is unavailable, the exterior end of the thoracostomy tube may be fitted with a one-way valve (e.g., Heimlich valve, McSwain dart).
4. If a water suction system is used, the level of the water in the drainage canisters must be kept below the level of the chest so that backflow is prevented. Thus, the possibility of intrapleural contamination and hydrothorax is minimized.

Special considerations must be given to intravascular systems: (a) Compression bags (which prevent backflow in arterial lines or raise the infusion pressure of intravenous fluids such as blood) must have bladder volumes adjusted according to the depth. If air is not added during diving, the bladder will be compressed and deflated and then backflow may occur in an arterial line. Alternatively, if air is not bled during decompression, the air bladder of the bag may rupture. (b) The connections on the intravenous lines must be secured, especially in a monoplace chamber. An accidental disconnection could be disastrous, as blood will flow freely from the compressed patient to the relatively hypobaric chamber exterior. Likewise, using stopcocks for injection rather than rubber injection ports, which will leak after being punctured, will prove more convenient.

If patients are being mechanically ventilated via an endotracheal/tracheostomy tube, the cuff must be filled with water or saline instead of air; thus, readjustments due to volume variation secondary to pressure effects are unnecessary. The inability to remove all of the fluid from the cuffs before extubation may become a problem, but this should be rare.

Mechanical ventilation should be continued, usually at the same settings that are in use in the ICU. Listed in Table 14.14 are some of the special considerations regarding mechanical ventilators used in hyperbaric chambers. Several models have been found to function well at depth and are recommended. The ideal mechanical ventilator for use in hyperbaric operations should be nonelectrically powered, volume-cycled, and unaffected by pressure.

It is usually a wise idea to confirm that the delivered ventilatory variables (e.g., tidal volume) are closely related to the predetermined parameters that have been set on the ventilator. This can be done by using the self-contained monitors that are part of some ventilators or a Wright respirometer. Because of varying gas densities at depth, these respirometers themselves must be recalibrated, or conversion charts must be used to interpret the readings at a given depth.

Electrical monitoring equipment (e.g., cathode ray tubes) should be kept outside the chamber, connected to the sensors by a "hull penetrator," and positioned so that the displays may be observed through a viewport. This is not a closely followed rule at some centers. If such equipment is brought into the chamber, potential fire hazards can be reduced in several ways. First, solid-state equipment should be chosen. Second, all equipment should be inspected thoroughly by the biomedical engineering shop. Third, a secure ground should be provided. Last, a continuous "nitrogen purge" should be used and be directed either within the monitor cabinet itself or into the general area. This will reduce the regional $FO_2$ and reduce the likelihood of ignition.

Several types of monitors do not function well or function imprecisely at depth. These include transcutaneous pulse oximeters, capnographs, and cardiac output computers, from which spurious results may be obtained. It is possible to adjust some of this equipment for hyperbaric operation.

Several companies manufacture blood gas analyzers specifically for use within the chamber. If such a machine is not obtained, the sample must be sent out through the airlock for analysis at the surface. Again, spurious results may be obtained because of "off-gassing" as the sample is decompressed.

Other miscellaneous points regarding care of the critically ill patient during chamber operations include the following: (a) In the unconscious patient or one who is unable to control gastric insufflation, a nasogastric or orogastric tube should be inserted to decompress the stomach. The tube should be left unclamped to gravity drainage or attached to suction. Several companies manufacture suction devices for use within the chamber. These make use of the pressure differential between the chamber interior and the external environment. Thus, any regular suctioning of the trachea or pharynx should proceed as normal, and chest tube suction may also be continued. (b) When oxygen is breathed in the multiplace chamber, the exhaust of this oxygen must be controlled tightly. The ambient $FIO_2$ must not rise above 0.23. This means that a tight-fitting aviator's mask or hood should be worn, with the exhaust directly exiting the chamber (generally referred to as a built-in breathing device). (c) Oil-based topical ointments and antiseptics must be avoided, as they pose fire hazards. (d) The balloon tips on indwelling Foley catheters must also be filled with water or saline. (e) Because of the possibility of ignition of fabric during a chamber fire, most clothing, sheets, pillowcases, etc., are now made of flame-retardant material such as Durette Gold. If this is not available, cotton may be used. (f) Patients who are receiving one of the agents listed in Table 14.15 (e.g. continuous infusion of ethanol for the prevention of alcoholic withdrawal syndrome) may manifest some of the changes caused by hyperbaric effects on pharmacologic actions.

**Table 14.15. Interactions: Pharmacology and the Hyperbaric Environment**

| Drug | Hyperbaric Effect |
|------|-------------------|
| Ethanol | Increased incidence of type I decompression sickness (presumably secondary to dehydration) |
| Steroids | May exacerbate oxygen toxicity Consider prophylactic anticonvulsants (especially for seizure-prone patients) |
| Narcotics | May exacerbate oxygen toxicity (presumably secondary to hypercarbia due to respiratory depression) |

## CONTRAINDICATIONS TO HYPERBARIC THERAPY

As listed in Table 14.16, a number of conditions require special considerations before allowing the patient to receive hyperbaric therapy. Of all of these conditions, only one is literally an absolute contraindication in a monoplace chamber: a pneumothorax. For reasons already reviewed, the hyperbaricist must determine if the pneumothorax is present before a dive and, if the dive is necessary, ensure that the pneumothorax is treated properly. The other conditions listed in Table 14.16 should be thought of more as indicators for special scrutiny than as contraindications per se.

With regard to the conditions that are respiratory or pulmonary in nature, asthma and chronic obstructive pulmonary disease (COPD) were discussed earlier in this chapter, and concerns here are related to "air trapping" in the distal small airways. One might consider the prophylactic use of bronchodilators in these patients, ensuring that therapeutic serum levels exist for those already receiving maintenance bronchodilator therapy (e.g., theophylline). Those patients with COPD who exhibit carbon dioxide retention and are dependent upon hypoxic ventilatory drive may develop complications during diving because of the ability of HBO therapy to affect pH, $PO_2$, and $PCO_2$ (in these cases, raising serum $O_2$ levels and removing hypoxic drive) (74). The hyperbaricist must be aware of these problems and consult with other physicians involved in the overall care of the patient to

**Table 14.16. Medical Conditions Requiring Special Consideration before HBO Therapy**

Respiratory
   Chronic obstructive lung disease (emphysema)
   Asthma
   Upper respiratory infection
   History of thoracic surgery
   History of spontaneous pneumothorax
   Pneumothorax
   Chest x-ray film with asymptomatic pulmonary lesions
Otolaryngologic
   Chronic sinusitis
   History of ear surgery
Ophthalmologic
   History of optic neuritis
Neurologic
   Seizure disorder
Hematologic
   Congenital spherocytosis
Systemic
   Viral infections
   Hyperthermia (uncontrolled high fever)
   Untreated/metastatic malignancy (controversial)
Miscellaneous
   Pregnancy

delineate the cost/benefit scheme for each given patient. If HBO therapy is strongly indicated, in some cases prophylactic intubation and mechanical ventilation may be necessary (74).

Patients with previous thoracic surgery and unidentified chest lesions on x-ray must be evaluated individually (74). Slow decompression (possibly while breathing oxygen) is recommended.

Careful consideration is always necessary for those patients with a history of spontaneous pneumothorax (especially those receiving positive-pressure ventilation). Review of the chest roentgenogram is essential, and in certain instances one might consider the prophylactic placement of chest tubes.

Upper respiratory infections and chronic sinusitis fall in the same category. There is a possibility that patients with such conditions may be unable to "clear" their ears or the paranasal sinuses. Decongestants may be tried; if they are unsuccessful, myringotomy with or without the placement of polyethylene (PE) tubes may be performed (26, 74).

Prior consultation with an otolaryngologist should be sought if implants have been inserted and there is a risk of dislodgement from pressure changes (74). A workable solution may be obtained by the prophylactic placement of PE tubes through the tympanic membrane. The risk/benefit must be determined.

Also mentioned earlier is the fact that persons with a history of seizure disorder may be more prone to the development of oxygen toxicity seizures. If such patients are receiving maintenance anticonvulsant therapy, therapeutic serum levels should be confirmed and regular dosing should be maintained throughout the diving schedule. The acute management of oxygen toxicity seizures has already been discussed.

Increased body temperature may also increase the incidence of oxygen seizures (36). The continuance of HBO therapy in febrile patients must be for reasons such as the treatment of a soft tissue infection that is responsible for the fever; otherwise, diving should be discontinued until defervescence (36). All appropriate methods of lowering body temperature should be utilized as necessary (e.g., antipyretics, cooling blankets). Prophylactic anticonvulsant therapy should be considered.

Premature closure of a patent ductus arteriosis secondary to the high oxygen tensions of the pulmonary vein and the development of retrolental fibroplasia in the fetus are of theoretic concern with respect to the pregnant female undergoing HBO. Research, the majority of which has been done in the Soviet Union, has documented no adverse effects (74, 77).

Another concern has been that HBO may enhance tumor growth in patients with untreated malignancy or metastases (74). This has not been proven in clinical or animal studies.

## ANESTHETIC MANAGEMENT DURING HYPERBARIC OPERATIONS

With the advent of complete cardiopulmonary bypass, the need for surgery and general anesthesia in conjunction with hyperbaric operations has become almost nonexistent. There is very little published in the English language literature relating to anesthesia and hyperbaric medicine. The majority of the available information is concerned more with the provision of medical and surgical care to deep sea divers involved with offshore oil exploration than with conventional hospitalized patients (78–81). This information raises several important points, especially for the European TA/CCS who may be in command of an emergency medical team assigned to cover a diving operation, for example, in the North Sea.

In large-scale offshore diving operations, professional divers frequently utilize "saturation diving" (82, 83). Because of the great depths at which much of the work is conducted (e.g., in excess of 1000 fsw) and the time involved for both decompression and safe compression to these depths, complex saturation diving systems have been devised (Fig. 14.9). There are sound economic and physiologic reasons for the saturation diving technique. These systems usually consist of a large multiplace hyperbaric chamber located at the surface (on either an oil rig or a ship) and an attached diving bell capable of being compressed to an identical pressure as the hyperbaric chamber and then of being detached and lowered to the operational depth with the divers inside (a "hyperbaric elevator") (Fig. 14.9C). Using the saturation diving system, divers can remain at the operational pressure for extended periods (usually up to 2 weeks). They travel in the diving bell to the depth at which work is being performed and live in the hyperbaric chamber. Compression and decompression must then occur only once. Compression to common operational depths may require several hours (e.g., 2 hours to 15 ATA, 4 hours to 24 ATA) because of the possibility of high-pressure nervous syndrome (disorientation, tremor, loss of fine movement control), which may develop if compression is too rapid (84).

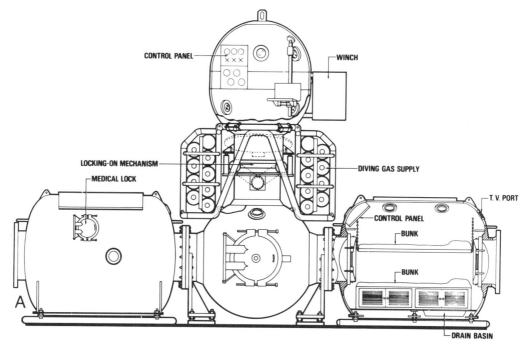

**Figure 14.9.    A, Saturation diving system.** Note living area, medical chamber, and transfer chamber (attached at top). **B,   Artist's conception of the U.S. Navy Mark II deep-diving system,** part of a larger system, and located beneath the deck of a salvage ship. (Courtesy of U.S. Navy. Also from Vorosmarti J. Saturation diving. In Strauss RH (ed): Diving Medicine. Orlando, FL, Grune & Stratton, 1976, pp 287–301.) **C,   Operating sequence of a deep (saturation) diving system.** *DDC* = deck decompression chamber, *PTC* = personnel transfer capsule. Divers living in the DDC enter the PTC and are transported to and from their work depth. (From *U.S. Navy Diving Manual.* Washington, DC, Department of the Navy.)

Decompression from these depths may require as much as a week.

Problems with the delivery of health care arise when a diver is injured while at these tremendous depths, either in the water or in the hyperbaric chamber. Frequently, sophisticated medical care, which in these instances would include a physician, is several hours away by helicopter flight. Initial care must be provided by personnel (e.g., other divers, diving medical technicians) already at these depths. Communication between the divers in the chamber and the outside tender is possible, as is communication between the oil rig and designated hospitals on shore. Verbal medical guidance can thus be provided. Depending upon the seriousness of the injury, a medical team may be dispatched to the rig by helicopter or fast boat. Simultaneously, decompression will begin. When the medical team arrives at the rig, it must be decided whether to "lock-in" the medical team through a secondary attached chamber (Fig. 14.9). This may require several hours. The cost/benefit of committing the medical team to such an emergency operation must be considered. Will the medical team have an appreciable influence upon the outcome by the time they reach the depth? Will space limitations prevent the use of medical equipment? How will the outcome be affected by the extraordinarily long decompression time, which will delay evacuation? Should limited medical assets be irrevocably committed to this particular operation?

Alternatively, the injured diver and possibly an inside tender may be moved into a small transport chamber (Fig. 14.2) and undergo TUP via helicopter to shore. Similar considerations regarding compressing the medical team will apply in this situation.

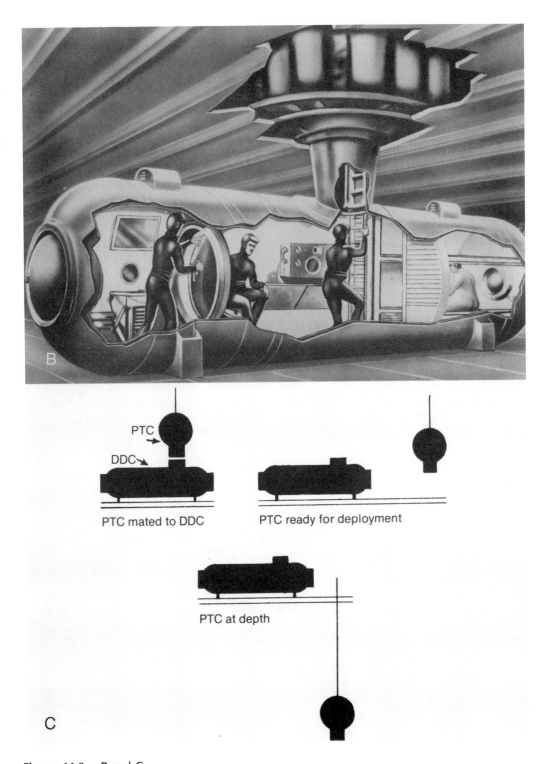

**Figure 14.9. B** and **C.**

Normally, intravenous sedation with an anxiolytic (e.g., midazolam) is sufficient to maintain the patient in a comfortable state.

However, if it does become necessary to provide HBO therapy emergently and there is a simultaneous need for operative general anesthesia (e.g., for major trauma with concurrent AGE), it can be provided. Generally, there are no known appreciable effects upon the action of anesthetic agents by increasing pressure until an extremely high pressure is reached. Normal interindividual variability of effects of these drugs may make it appear otherwise. The effects of high pressure on anesthetic agents are not well studied. Several in vitro animal studies have shown varied effects of pressure upon different drugs (85–88). Indeed, varying pressure with respect to a single drug may reveal opposite results. One human study using alphaxalone/alphadolone (Althesin) at 31 ATA showed a 30% increase in anesthetic requirement (79).

In almost all instances, an intravenous (balanced) anesthetic technique is preferred to an inhalational technique (Table 14.17). This preference is explained by the following facts (39, 78–81, 89–91).

1. Additional bulky equipment must be brought into the already cramped confines of the chamber.
2. The potential fire hazards within the chamber may be increased by the addition of equipment necessary for the inhalation of general anesthesia.
3. There is a potential for contamination of the chamber atmosphere by the additional oxygen and/or anesthetic agent. Because most halogenated anesthetics do not undergo a significant degree of metabolism under normal conditions, this is not a major concern. However, consideration must be given to the flammability characteristics of these agents.
4. The use of any intravenous or inhalational anesthesia or analgesia that could suppress mentation or the perception of pain may interfere with the patient's appreciation and reporting of the signs or symptoms of decompression sickness or AGE during decompression. Monitoring the EEG potentials if general anesthesia is chosen may aid in the diagnosis of these conditions and surveillance for oxygen toxicity seizures, which might not otherwise be detected in the presence of unconsciousness and muscle relaxation. Attempts to elicit Chvostek's sign may be of limited usefulness in these patients.
5. Another problem concerns modification of the anesthesia machine. As ambient pressure increases, gas densities become an issue in terms of the accuracy of flowmeters. This problem can be overcome by applying differently calibrated scales that correspond to specific depths and fit over the flowmeters.

If it is decided to use an inhalational technique, nitrous oxide should be avoided for several reasons: First is its potential to aggravate conditions such as AGE or pneumothorax because of bubble formation and inward diffusion of the gas upon decompression. (Theoretically, this could be

**Table 14.17.  Anesthetic Equipment and Procedures Requiring Special Attention or Modification for Use in Hyperbaric Chamber Operations[a]**

| | |
|---|---|
| Anesthetic gas supply | |
| Individual gas cylinder | Should function satisfactorily |
| Central supply outlet | Reducing valve will function satisfactorily providing gas supply pressure is greater than 60 psi. |
| Anesthetic gas delivery | |
| Flowmeters | Should be recalibrated for each specific depth because of varying gas density |
| Vaporizers | Theoretically, no adjustment is necessary; practically, there is variability depending upon actual model. |
| | Filter plugs should be left open during change in ambient pressure to avoid the danger of explosion. |
| Regional anesthesia | Must avoid air entrapment/injection while performing technique. |
| Inhalational anesthesia | Avoid nitrous oxide (potential to enlarge air emboli or pneumothorax) |

[a] Refer to Table 14.14 for other items that may also apply.

avoided by a prolonged washout of nitrous oxide at the maximal depth before decompression.) Second, the outflow of nitrous oxide into the alveoli during eduction could result in a profound "diffusion hypoxia/anoxia."

Alternatively, one may choose to utilize a regional anesthetic technique: spinal, epidural, or major nerve block. Entrainment and injection of air into these areas must be avoided because of the potential complication of bubble enlargement during decompression. Also, the local anesthetic fluid (the containers of which must be opened before descent to avoid explosion) may contain a higher partial pressure of gas. This gas may then form bubbles in the tissue space during decompression.

Another problem, usually limited to saturation divers living in unusually humid environments, concerns the concomitant alteration in bacterial skin flora, with a great increase in Gram-negative organisms, especially *Proteus* and *Pseudomonas* (78). In the same vein, contaminants in the chamber atmosphere may be forced into the opened local anesthetic ampules with ambient pressure increases.

Despite the fact that the availability of cardiopulmonary bypass has drastically reduced the number of hyperbaric operations performed, some surgeons still believe that there are definite advantages gained by having high tissue oxygen levels during surgery. For example, when abdominal aortic aneurysms are repaired in a hyperbaric environment, subsequent "reperfusion" injury is rare. Carotid endarterectomies with significant bilateral stenosis (generally done within 30 minutes) performed at depth do not require the placement of shunts (WH Bensky, J Jacobson, C Pierce, personal communication; Hyperbaric Medical Staff, the Mount Sinai Medical Center, New York, NY, December 29, 1988).

Anesthesia under hyperbaric conditions is also very popular for performing pulmonary lavage in cases of pulmonary alveolar proteinosis. On the surface it is very difficult to perform repeated lavages of one lung while ventilating via the other diseased lung. Clinicians at Duke University Medical Center routinely provide anesthesia at depth (2–4 ATA) using intravenous ketamine infusions (92).

## SUMMARY

A perspective in which hyperbaric medicine is seen as a reliable, efficacious mode of therapy for several traumatically induced conditions has been proposed. The basic physics of gas behavior, the physiologic basis of hyperbaric medicine, the clinical application of pressures and oxygen, and the special medical care problems encountered in the hyperbaric environment were presented. When learning about hyperbaric medicine, one should seek a more global perspective and simultaneously acquire knowledge of hypobaric medicine (aviation medicine, transport medicine), presented in this book in Chapter 15. Highly motivated anesthetic care providers who are dedicated to trauma care are encouraged to enhance their contribution to and active participation in the field of hyperbaric medicine.

### References

1. Myers RAM, Marzella L. Hyperbaric medicine: what is it; how is it used? Md Med J 1988; 37:559–564.
2. Norkool M. Current concepts of hyperbaric oxygenation and its application in critical care. Heart Lung 1979;8:728–735.
3. Committee on Hyperbaric Oxygenation. Hyperbaric Oxygen Therapy: A Committee Report. Bethesda, MD, Undersea and Hyperbaric Medical Society, 1986, pp 30–103.
4. Myers RAM, Baker TL, Cowley RA. Hyperbaric medicine, state-of-the-art, 1979. Am Surg 1982; 48:487–494.
5. Jacobson JH, Morsch JHC, Rendell-Baker L. The historical perspective of hyperbaric therapy. Ann NY Acad Sci 1965;117:651–670.
6. Behnke AR. A brief history of hyperbaric medicine. In Davis JC, Hunt TK (eds): Hyperbaric Oxygen Therapy. Bethesda, MD, Undersea Medical Society, 1977, pp 3–10.
7. Behnke AR Jr. High atmospheric pressure, physiological effects of increased and decreased pressure; applications of these findings to clinical medicine. Ann Intern Med 1940;13:2217–2228.

8. Williams ET. The compound air bath and its uses in the treatment of disease. Br Med J 1985;1:769, 824, 936.

9. Corning JL. The use of compressed air in conjunction with medicinal solutions in the treatment of nervous and mental affections, being a new system of cerebrospinal therapeutics. Med Record 1981;40:225–232.

10. Bryant M. Breathing new life into old wounds, hyperbaric oxygen chambers grow in popularity. Washington Post, April 19, 1988.

11. Cunningham CJ. Oxygen therapy by means of compressed air. Anesth Analg, April 27, 1927: 64–66.

12. American Medical Association Bureau of Investigation. The Cunningham "tank treatment": the alleged value of compressed air in the treatment of diabetes mellitus. JAMA 1928;90:1494–1496.

13. Gabb G, Robin ED. Hyperbaric oxygen: a therapy in search of diseases. Chest 1987;92:1075–1082.

14. Robin ED, James PB, Krigbaum EM, Keim LW, Runciman WB, Gorman DF, Webb RK, Russel WJ, Gilligan JE, Parsons JE, Davis JC, Koch GH. Differing opinions on hyperbaric oxygen therapy. Chest 1988;94:667–674.

15. Workman WT, Calcote RD. Hyperbaric oxygen therapy and combat casualty care: a viable potential. Milit Med 1989;54:111–115.

16. Sheffield PJ, Davis JC, Bell GC, Gallagher TJ. Hyperbaric chamber clinical support: multiplace. In Davis JC, Hunt TK (eds): Hyperbaric Oxygen Therapy. Bethesda, MD, Undersea Medical Society, 1977, pp 25–39.

17. Hart GB, Kindwall EP. Hyperbaric chamber clinical support: monoplace. In Davis JC, Hunt TK (eds): Hyperbaric Oxygen Therapy. Bethesda, MD, Undersea Medical Society, 1977, pp 41–46.

18. Miller JW (ed). Hyperbaric chambers. In NOAA Diving Manual, ed 2. Washington, DC, US Government Printing Office, 1979, pp 16-1-16-22.

19. Bassett BE, Bennett PB. Introduction to the physical and physiological bases of hyperbaric therapy. In Davis JC, Hunt TK (eds): Hyperbaric Oxygen Therapy. Bethesda, MD, Undersea Medical Society, 1977, pp 11–23.

20. Somers LH. Diving physics. In Bone AA, Davis JC (eds): Diving Medicine. Philadelphia, WB Saunders, 1990, pp 9–18.

21. Miller JW (ed). The physics of diving. In NOAA Diving Manual, ed 2. Washington, DC, US Government Printing Office, 1979, pp 1-1-1-15.

22. Naval Sea Systems Command. Underwater physics. In US Navy Diving Manual, Volume 1, Air Diving, Revision 1 (NAVSEA 0994-LP-001-9010). Washington, DC, Navy Department, 1985, pp 2-1-2-24.

23. Shilling CW, Faiman MD. Physics and physical effects of diving. In Shilling CW, Cartston CB,

Mathias RA (eds): The Physician's Guide to Diving Medicine. New York, Plenum, 1984, pp 35–69.

24. Miller JW (ed). Air diving and decompression. In NOAA Diving Manual, ed 2. Washington, DC, US Government Printing Office, 1979, pp 10-1-10-18.

25. Miller JW (ed). Diving physiology. In NOAA Diving Manual, ed 2. Washington, DC, US Government Printing Office, 1979, pp 2-1-2-24.

26. Morris L (ed). Mechanical effects of pressure changes. In Hyperbaric Chamber Operations. Air Force Pamphlet 161-27. Washington, DC, Department of the Air Force, Headquarters US Air Force, 1983, pp 18–21.

27. Davis JC, Dunn JM, Heimbach RD. Hyperbaric medicine: patient selection, treatment procedures and side-effects. In Davis JC, Hunt TK (eds): Problem Wounds: The Role of Oxygen. New York, Elsevier, 1988, pp 225–235.

28. Lundgren CEG, Pasche AJ. Immersion effects: physiology of diving. In Shilling CW, Carlston CA, Mathias RA (eds): The Physician's Guide to Diving Medicine. New York, Plenum, 1988, pp 99–107.

29. Evans DE. Cardiovascular effects: physiology of diving. In Shilling CW, Carlston CR, Mathias RA (eds): The Physician's Guide to Diving Medicine. New York, Plenum, 1986, pp 85–97.

30. Kindwall EP, Goldmann RW. Currently accepted hyperbarically treated disorders. In Kindwall EP, Goldmann RW (eds): Hyperbaric Medicine Procedures. Milwaukee, St Luke's Hospital, 1984, pp 75–164.

31. Kindwall EP, Goldmann RW. Special considerations. In Kindwall EP, Goldmann RW (eds): Hyperbaric Medicine Procedures. Milwaukee, St Luke's Hospital, 1984, pp 166–180.

32. Clark JM. Oxygen toxicity. In Bennett PB, Elliot DH (eds): The Physiology and Medicine of Diving, ed 3. San Pedro, CA, Best Publishing Co, 1982, pp 200–238.

33. Lorrain-Smith J. The pathological effects due to increase of oxygen tension in the air breathed. J Physiol 1899;34:19–35.

34. Clark JM, Lambertsen CJ. Rate of development of pulmonary $O_2$ toxicity in normal men at 2ATA ambient. Fed Proc 1966;25:566.

35. Morris L (ed). Effects of elevated partial pressures. In Hyperbaric Chamber Operations. Air Force Pamphlet 161-27. Washington, DC, Department of the Air Force, Headquarters US Air Force, 1983, pp 23–27.

36. Kindwall EP, Goldmann RW. Procedures, equipment and drugs. In Kindwall EP, Goldmann RW (eds): Hyperbaric Medicine Procedures. Milwaukee, St Luke's Hospital, 1984, pp 23–75.

37. Bennett PB. Inert gas narcosis. In Bennett PB, Elliot DH (eds): The Physiology and Medicine of Diving, ed 3. San Pedro, CA, Best Publishing Co, 1982, pp 239–261.

38. Morris L (ed). Physiologic basis of hyperbaric

therapy. In Hyperbaric Chamber Operations. Air Force Pamphlet 161-27. Washington, DC, Department of the Air Force, Headquarters US Air Force, 1983, pp 28–36.

39. Churchill-Davidson HC. Hyperbaric physiology and medicine. In Churchill Davidson HC (ed): A Practice of Anaesthesia, ed 5. Chicago, Year Book, 1984, pp 145–165.

40. Boerema I, Merjne WM, Brummelkamp S, et al. Life without blood: a study of the influence of high atmosphere pressure and hypothermia on dilution of blood. J Cardiovasc Surg 1960;1: 133–146.

41. Sheffield PJ. Tissue oxygen measurements. In Davis JC, Hunt TK (eds): Problem Wounds: The Role of Oxygen. New York, Elsevier, 1988, pp 17–51.

42. Niinikoski J, Hunt TK. Oxygen tension in human wounds. J Surg Res 1972;12:77–82.

43. McCord JM, Keele BB, Fridovich I. An enzyme-based theory of obligate anaerobiosis: the physiological function of superoxide dismutase. Proc Natl Acad Sci USA 1971;68:1024–1027.

44. Mader JT, Brown GL, Guckian JC, et al. A mechanism for the amelioration of hyperbaric oxygen of experimental staphylococcal osteomyelitis in rabbits. J Infect Dis 1980;142:915–922.

45. Hempleman HV. History of evaluation of decompression procedures. In Bennet PB, Elliot DH (eds): The Physiology and Medicine of Diving, ed 3. San Pedro, CA, Best Publishing Co, 1982, pp 319–351.

46. Kindwall EP. Carbon monoxide and cyanide poisoning. In Hyperbaric Oxygen Therapy. Bethesda, MD, Undersea Medical Society, 1977, pp 177–190.

47. Goldbaum LR, Ramirez RG, Absalim KB. What is the mechanism of carbonic monoxide toxicity? Aviat Space Environ Med 1978;46:1289–1291.

48. Suckoff M, Hollin SA, Jacobson JH. The protective effect of hyperbaric oxygenation in experimentally produced cerebral edema and compression. Surgery 1967;62:42–46.

49. Marzella L, Myers RAM. Carbon monoxide poisoning. Am Fam Physician 1986;34:186–194.

50. Myers RAM. Planning an effective strategy for carbon monoxide poisoning. Emerg Med Rep 1987;8:195–200.

51. Myers RAM, Britten JS. Are arterial blood gases of value in treatment decisions for carbon monoxide? Crit Care Med 1989;17:139–142.

52. Trunkey DD. Air embolism. In Trunkey DD, Lewis FR (eds): Current Therapy of Trauma-2. Philadelphia, BC Decker, 1986, pp 247–248.

53. Morris, L (ed). The diagnosis and treatment of air embolism. In Hyperbaric Chamber Operations. Air Force Pamphlet 161-27. Washington, DC, Department of the Air Force, Headquarters US Air Force, 1983, pp 72–75.

54. Davis JC. Treatment of decompression sickness

55. Mebane GY, Dick AP. DAN Underwater Diving Accident Manual. Durham, NC, National Divers Alert Network, Duke University, 1985, pp 11–13.

56. Bove AA. The basis for drug therapy in decompression sickness. Underwater Biomed Res 1982; 9:91–111.

57. Morris L (ed). Decompression sickness. In Hyperbaric Chamber Operations. Air Force Pamphlet 161-27. Washington, DC, Department of the Air Force, Headquarters US Air Force, 1983, pp 58–71.

58. Elliott DH, Kindwall EP. Manifestations of the decompression disorders. In Bennett PB, Elliot DH (eds): The Physiology and Medicine of Diving, ed 3. San Pedro, CA, Best Publishing Co, 1982, pp 461–472.

59. Edel PO, Carrall JJ, Homaker RW, Beckman EL. Interval at sea level pressure required to prevent decompression sickness in humans who fly in commercial aircrafts after diving. Aerospace Med 1969;40:1105–1110.

60. Smith AH. Caisson disease. Med Record 1984; 45:130–133.

61. Vann RD. Decompression theory and application. In Bennett PB, Elliot DH (eds): The Physiology and Medicine of Diving ed 3. San Pedro, CA, Best Publishing Co, 1962, pp 352–382.

62. Kindwall EP. Decompression sickness. In Davis JC, Hunt TK (eds): Hyperbaric Oxygen Therapy. Bethesda, MD, Undersea Medical Society, 1977, pp 125–140.

63. Hallenbeck JM, Andersen JC. Pathogenesis of the decompression disorder. In Bennett PB, Elliot DH (eds): The Physiology and Medicine of Diving, ed 3. San Pedro, CA, Best Publishing Co, 1982, pp 435–460.

64. Strauss MC. Role of hyperbaric oxygen therapy in acute ischemias and crush injuries—an orthopedic perspective. HBO Rev 1981;2:87–106.

65. Myking O, Schreiner A. Hyperbaric oxygen in hemolytic crisis. JAMA 1974;227:1161–1162.

66. Amonic RS, Cockett ATK, Lorhan PH, Thompson JC. Hyperbaric oxygen therapy in chronic hemorrhagic shock. JAMA 1969;208:2051–2054.

67. Hart GB. Exceptional blood loss and anemia: treatment with hyperbaric oxygen. JAMA 1974; 228:1028–1029.

68. Ketchum SA III, Zubrin JR, Thomas AN, Hall AD. Effect of hyperbaric oxygen on small first second and third degree burns. Surg Forum 1967; 18:65–67.

69. Hart GB, O'Reilly RR, Broussard ND, Cave RH, Goodman DB, Yanda RL. Treatment of burns with hyperbaric oxygen. Surg Gynecol Obstet 1974; 139:693–696.

70. Kanschepolsky J. Early and delayed oxygenation

in experimental brain edema. Bull Los Angeles Neurol Soc 1972;37:84–89.

71. Moody RA, Mead CO, Ruamsuke S, Mullen S. Therapeutic value of oxygen at normal and hyperbaric pressure in experimental head injury. J Neurosurg 1970;32:51–54.

72. Kindwall EP, Goldmann RW. Experimental. In Kindwall EP, Goldmann RW (eds): Hyperbaric Medicine Procedures. Milwaukee, St Luke's Hospital, 1984, pp 181–203.

73. Yeo JD, Stabback S, McKenzie B. A study of the effects of hyperbaric oxygen on the experimental spinal cord injury. Med J Aust 1977;2:145–147.

74. Kindwall EP, Goldmann RW. Introduction. In Kindwall EP, Goldmann RW (eds): Hyperbaric Medicine Procedures. Milwaukee, St Luke's Hospital, 1984, pp 3–22.

75. Holcomb JR, Matos-Navarro AY, Goldmann RW. Critical care in the hyperbaric chamber. In Davis JC, Hunt TK (eds): Problem Wounds: The Role of Oxygen. New York, Elsevier, 1988, pp 187–209.

76. Dauphinee K, Gross CE, Myers RAM. The spectrum of monitoring in the multiplace hyperbaric chamber. Hyperbaric Oxygen Rev 1985; 6:169–181.

77. Van Hoesen KB, Camporesi EM, Moon RE, Hage ML, Piantadosi CA. Should hyperbaric oxygen be used to treat the pregnant patient for acute carbon monoxide poisoning? JAMA 1989;261: 1039–1044.

78. Cox J, Robinson DJ. Anaesthesia at depth. Br J Hosp Med 1980;23:144, 147, 150, 151.

79. Dundas CR. Alphaxalone/alphadolone in diving-chamber anaethesia. Lancet 1979;1:378.

80. Editorial. High pressure medicine. Br Med J 1975;4:541–542.

81. Nicodemus HF. Anesthesia for emergency surgery under high pressure. In Shilling CW, Carlston CB, Mathias RA (eds): The Physician's Guide to Diving Medicine. New York, Plenum, 1984, pp 460–487.

82. Miller JW (ed). Saturation diving. In NOAA Diving Manual, ed 2. Washington, DC, US Government Printing Office, 1979, pp 12-1–12-19.

83. Beven J. Commercial diving practice and equipment. In Bennett PB, Elliot DH (eds): The Physiology and Medicine of Diving, ed 3. San Pedro, CA, Best Publishing Co, 1982, pp 46–54.

84. Bennett PB. The high pressure nervous syndrome in man. In Bennett PB, Elliot DH (eds): The Physiology and Medicine of Diving, ed 3. San Pedro, CA, Best Publishing Co, 1982, pp 262–296.

85. Johnson FH, Flagler EA. Hydrostatic pressure reversal of narcosis in tadpoles. Science 1950; 112:91–92.

86. Lever MJ, Miller KW, Paton WDM, Smith EB. Pressure reversal of anaesthesia. Nature 1971; 231:368–371.

87. Roth SK, Smith RA, Paton WDM. Pressure antagonism of anaesthetic-induced conduction failure. Br J Anaesthesia 1976;48:621–628.

88. Johnson FH, Brown DES, Marsland DA. Pressure reversal of the action of certain narcotics. J Cell Comp Physiol 1942;20:269–276.

89. Severinghaus JH. Anesthesia and related drug effects. In Fundamentals of Hyperbaric Medicine. Washington, DC, National Academy of Sciences Publication 1298, 1966, pp 115–127.

90. McDowell DG. Anaesthesia in a pressure chamber. Anaesthesia 1964;19:321–336.

91. Correa JG, Camporesi EM. Anesthesia in the hyperbaric environment. In Jain TM (ed): Hyperbaric Oxygen Therapy, ed 2. New York, Springer-Verlag (in press).

92. Camporesi EM, Moon RE, Grande CM. Hyperbaric medicine: an integral part of trauma care. Crit Care Clin 1990;6:203–219.

# Critical Care Transport: Mobile Management of the Trauma Patient Inside and Outside the Trauma Center

*Christopher M. Grande, Deborah Williams,*
*and Mark McCauley*

## Introduction: The Role of the Anesthesiologist in the New Subspecialty of Critical Care Transport

Movement of the trauma patient (TP) from one location to another is essential for maximal medical management. In its most basic form, critical care transport (CCT) involves evacuating the TP from the scene of injury to a skilled-care trauma center (TC). As medical care has become more sophisticated, so has CCT. Because of the ability to provide a high level of ongoing care during mobile operations, interhospital CCT permits seriously ill patients to be transferred routinely. The same patient may undergo several trips each day between hospitals as the need arises for special diagnostic and therapeutic procedures (e.g., hyperbaric oxygen therapy, magnetic resonance imaging) not normally available at many centers.

Medical transport programs with highly equipped and professionally staffed vehicles (e.g., boats, hovercraft, helicopters, small jets, and land-based assets) have been developed at specialized centers around the country (1–3). An entire industry (i.e., vehicles, pilots, paramedics, flight nurses, flight physicians) concerned with extrahospital transport now exists (4, 5). Some groups of patients who are in critical condition and who benefit daily from the special attributes of modern CCT programs include women with high-risk pregnancies, neonates, unstable cardiac patients in need of open heart surgery or some other procedure, and trauma patients (e.g., burn victims). The level of sophistication of CCT is such that a cardiac patient with an intraaortic balloon pump may be transported safely, with no interruption in therapy (6).

Physiologic changes occur with each type of CCT. The range of possible interventions varies depending upon logistics (e.g., space, electrical power, equipment available). Ideally, for each condition the physician involved in CCT should gauge the level of care being provided during transport to be of the same sophistication and quality as would occur in a fixed intensive care unit.

What is the role of the anesthesiologist in the new subspecialty of CCT? As described later in this chapter, much of what happens to the patient during transport is of a pathophysiologic nature, and interventions may be required. Within most TCs, a physician accompanies a critically ill patient during intrahospital transports. Thus, the physician may (a) monitor the physiologic data presented by the array of surveillance equipment available (e.g., electrocardiogram, blood pressure, intravascular pressures), (b) ensure that the critical care equipment is maintained properly (e.g., endotracheal tubes, efficacy of ventilation), and (c) render sophisticated intervention when suboptimal conditions are present. These functions are being assumed increasingly by anesthesiologists who have been trained as critical care physicians (7, 8). For example, the anesthesiologist with special additional training in hyperbaric medicine (see Chapter 14) may be called upon to provide coverage for the transport of an injured diver in the field. The anesthesiologist who performs this type of CCT must have special knowledge and training in aviation medicine and the physiologic effects of flight. Ideally, such a physician should possess the skills and knowledge of the fully trained trauma anesthesiologist/critical care specialist (see Table 15.1 and Chapter 1). This type of anesthesiologist has much to offer the injured patient who is in pain and must undergo transport. To quote one prominent traumatologist, "the organized utilization of aeromedical evacuation by both helicopter and fixed-wing vehicles further extends the 'Golden Period' in which better resuscitation and definitive care can be made more readily available to the critically ill and injured" (2) (see also Chapter 4). On the other hand, another author says, "the majority of missions flown are presently manned by medical personnel who are inadequately trained to care for patients in the aviation environment" (9).

**Table 15.1.    Prehospital Aeromedical Treatment[a]**

Oral intubation
Nasal intubation
Cricothyroidotomy
Open venous catheter placement
Central venous catheter placement
Arterial catheter placement
Transvenous cardiac pacemaker placement
Transthoracic cardiac pacemaker placement
Thoracostomy tube placement
Open thoractomy
    Open cardiac compression
    Aortic cross-clamp placement

[a] From Baxt WG. Prehospital treatment and transport of the trauma patient. In Baxt WG (ed): Trauma: The First Hour. East Norwalk, CT, Appleton-Century-Crofts, 1985, pp. 293–303.

The concept of the physician in the field is certainly not new. This is one of the oldest facets of medical practice, beginning with the "house-call." With the increased modernization of medicine as a whole and trauma care in particular, there has been a general tendency to limit medical care by physicians to the hospital or office. Surely, there is some justification for this modus operandi, such as the improved facilities and support personnel at these locations. The same type of thinking has led to the "scoop and run" and "load and go" philosophies in trauma and emergency care, which basically uses "primary responder" units. These systems operate on the premise that it is most important to limit the amount of time between injury and arrival at a definitive care facility. However, the only parameter that is under the control of these units is the time between their arrival on the scene and their arrival at the TC.

Theoretically, this creates at least two problems: (*a*) A variable amount of time may have elapsed between the accident and the arrival of the primary responder units on the scene. (*b*) Examination of some of the most highly organized medical evacuation systems shows that, in the best of circumstances, the time between the arrival of the primary responder unit on the scene and its arrival at the definitive care center is significant. (In Viet Nam transport took up to 35 minutes once the patient was loaded

on the helicopter, in the West German system 90% of the population is within 15 minutes of a TC, and in the Swedish system 93% of the urban population is also within 15 minutes of a TC [10–15].)

These two problems become significant when one considers their implications in relation to the "golden hour." The golden hour concept is that, if a TP with a survivable injury who is in clinical shock does not receive the definitive care necessary to reverse the process within 1 hour after entering the shock state, long-term survivability has dropped below 10%, no matter how good the care is after that 60 minutes have elapsed. Transport time, even in the best of situations, may unavoidably consume more than 50% of the golden hour. One author reports that, for every 30 minutes of delay in the treatment of a severely injured patient, the mortality rate increases by 300%. Civilian transport ranges from 3 minutes to 2.5 hours, with an average of 40 minutes (16).

Many articles have examined the contributions of including a physician in the primary responder team, as well as having the physician remain at the scene long enough to "stabilize" the TP, with the goal of reducing morbidity and mortality. Careful review of the majority of these articles will show deficiencies in almost all of them, whether their results were "pro" or "con" in regard to the physician in the field (12–15, 17–27). Indeed, it would be very difficult to perform a definitive, randomized, prospective study to examine this subject.

The argument can be summarized in several points. First, the physician should not be strictly excluded from a field team, as has been done in some systems (28–30). However, it would be wasteful to include a physician with every primary responder unit, as his or her expertise would not be utilized in the majority of cases. Thus, a scheme must be developed that permits rapid delivery of the CCT physician to the scene as needed. For example, in a metropolitan area this might be done by keeping a helicopter on standby at a central facility from which the physician can be deployed as needed. Because of the speed and maneuverability of the helicopter, a short trip to a location close to the scene, if not to the scene itself, could be managed. Once again, the *physician must be properly trained and qualified* (i.e., not junior residents or interns, but experienced senior residents or attending physicians) (31). There are definite situations where rapid transport is warranted (32–33), but even in some of these cases temporary maneuvers performed by trained physicians, such as an emergency thoracotomy for the application of an aortic clamp or open cardiac massage, may be important (33).

Second, there is an intraspecialty power struggle among surgeons, emergency medicine physicians, and other groups (34). Most of the studies finding that the physician should not be deployed to the field were performed by surgeons. Surgeons may take this view because, for the most part, they have been trained in the security of a sophisticated operating room with all of the support available (35, 36). Also, there is a misconception, again reinforced mostly by surgeons, that a surgeon is necessary for the majority of trauma cases, which is certainly not true (see Chapter 1). In a 1980 survey, 46% of surgical program directors reported that more than 10% of all cases were trauma. However, in the same year, 95% of surgical residents reported that less than 5% of their experience was in the treatment of trauma. Further, 47% stated that they had managed less than 20 trauma cases during their residencies, while 18% had handled fewer than 10 cases (37).

Issues that cannot be ignored when the decision is made to deploy a physician to the field include fiscal considerations, the development of an appropriate scheme for the optimal deployment of the physician to the field, and the logistics involved in selecting, training, and maintaining the appropriate physicians for such a task (22). Whether a physician ultimately will be deployed to the field depends upon the commitment and ability of a given community to support this venture.

Situations in which it will be imperative for physicians to travel to the field include mass casualty and disaster (man-made and natural) situations and cases in which trauma victims are entrapped and the field teams are unable to extricate them (38, 39). In the latter instances, an anesthesiologist may be expected to provide anesthesia until extrication can be achieved and/or a surgeon will be required to perform an amputation/disarticulation of an entrapped limb.

## PHYSIOLOGIC EFFECTS OF MOVEMENT

### Extrahospital Transport

#### GENERAL CONSIDERATIONS

As the human body (with intact sensory and effector neural systems) is subjected to movement (translational, vertical, or a combination), physiologic changes occur (Fig. 15.1). Normally, the movement is detected by integrated sensorineural complexes such as the vestibular, vasomotor, and proprioception systems. Once the particular movement and its physiologic effect are appreciated, the servo-control feedback mechanisms will be activated to maintain homeostasis. An example is seen in the physiologic response to movement from the supine to the standing position. Usually, as an individual stands after having been lying down for a period, transient changes in heart rate and blood pressure occur. The body, which has acclimated to the supine position, will then receive sensory information, and adjustments will be made via the servo-controlled feedback circuits until a new equilibrium is reached in the standing position.

If the degree of movement or change in orientation is too exaggerated (e.g., a sharp turn in a high performance jet, which produces extreme gravitational [G] forces), the body may not be able to compensate or adjust (40). Homeostasis will not be maintained and pathophysiologic signs and symptoms will be manifested. The same

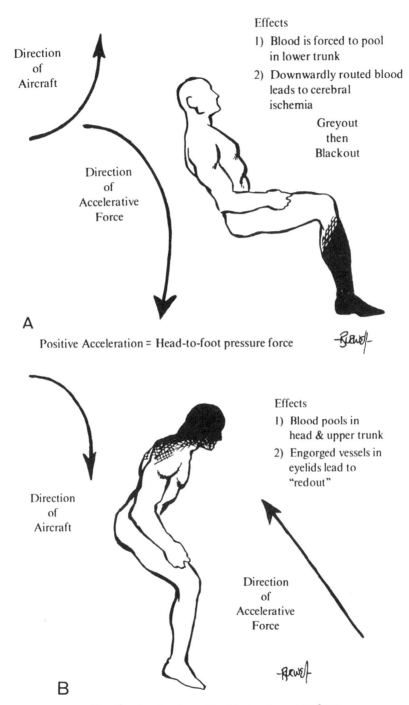

Direction
of
Aircraft

Effects
1) Blood is forced to pool
   in lower trunk
2) Downwardly routed blood
   leads to cerebral
   ischemia

Greyout
then
Blackout

Direction
of
Accelerative
Force

**A**

Positive Acceleration = Head-to-foot pressure force

Direction
of
Aircraft

Effects
1) Blood pools in
   head & upper trunk
2) Engorged vessels in
   eyelids lead to
   "redout"

Direction
of
Accelerative
Force

**B**

Negative Acceleration = Foot-to-head pressure force

**Figure 15.1. Effects of three-dimensional acceleration on the human body. (From Skedl DM. Acceleration.** In Skredl DM (ed): Airborne Patient Care Management: A Multidisciplinary Approach. St Louis, MO, Medical Research Associates Publications, 1983, pp. 74–88.)

types of considerations apply to the seriously ill TP. A TP who is in class I or II shock (i.e., up to 15% of blood volume lost with hypotension barely discernible when measured by sphygmomanometer) and who is moved abruptly from the supine to the upright position before resuscitation will demonstrate profound postural hypotension. In cases of sufficient hypovolemia, cardiac arrest may ensue.

The CCT physician must develop a conceptual understanding of physical and physiologic factors involved in movement and learn to anticipate and avoid detrimental situations. In the following sections, physical characteristics most prominent for each type of transport environment will be discussed (e.g., acceleration and deceleration forces in fixed-wing aircraft during take off and landing, the generation of centrifugal forces secondary to a high-speed turn in a land ambulance). Many of these characteristics apply to all transport situations to varying degrees. Therefore, the reader is advised to regard the entire range of physical effects and secondary physiologic changes as a continuous spectrum and to

apply these concepts to various CCT situations as they arise.

## AVIATION OPERATIONS

### Helicopter versus Fixed-Wing Aircraft

Currently, two forms of aircraft (i.e., rotary-wing/helicopter and fixed-wing/airplane or jet) are used for aerial CCT (evacuation, med-evac, transfer) of patients from one location to another. In military situations, this may involve moving a TP from one field location to another (e.g., combat area to a MASH facility) or from a field location to a large, fixed facility in a relatively nonthreatened (rear) area (Fig. 15.2). In a civilian situation, TPs are usually evacuated from the site of the incident to a level I, II, or III TC. To which location the TP will be brought depends upon evaluation of the injury, triage protocols for a given community, capabilities of the aircraft, meteorologic conditions, and the capabilities of

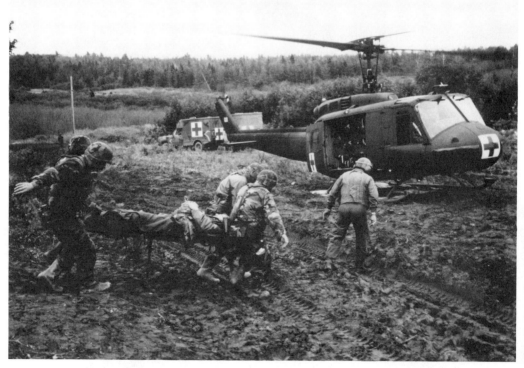

**Figure 15.2.    Medical team prepares for helicopter evacuation of an injured soldier aboard a UH-IV ("Huey").** (Courtesy of Col. William N. Bernhard, M.D. Director of Anesthesia, MIEMSS).

a particular TC to accept various aircraft. For example, the CCT program at Stanford University Medical Center in Palo Alto, California, one of the most sophisticated in the world, is designed to accept patients from the immediate geographic area who are transported by helicopter to the heliport adjacent to the hospital (7). This center can also accept patients who have undergone long-range transport from all parts of the globe at the U.S. Air Force facility at Moffett Field. Patients are then transported from Moffett Field to the medical center by land ambulance (approximately a 10-minute trip).

Another example of sophisticated aerial CCT limited to rotorcraft operations is found in the new R Adams Cowley Shock Trauma Center of the Maryland Institute for Emergency Medical Services Systems in Baltimore, which opened in February 1989. This ultramodern facility is capable of accepting four helicopters simultaneously at its roof-top heliport (Fig. 15.3**A**). TPs are then transported on a gurney by elevator to the resuscitation areas and the operating rooms just below (Fig. 15.3**B**).

There are several differences in the capabilities of rotary-wing and fixed-wing aircraft as well as in their physical environments (5, 41). Helicopters have the ability to take off and land vertically. Thus, they are more flexible for extracting patients from remote areas as well as delivering them to medical centers in urban areas (e.g., roof-top heliports). They can be thought of as "obstacle jumpers." Their most prominent limitations compared with fixed-wing aircraft are (a) relatively short ranges of flight (normally 100 to 150 miles, 300 to 500 miles round trip maximum) secondary to fuel supply (Fig. 15.4) and consumption rate (maximal operating time, 2 to 3 hours); (b) fairly small passenger treatment compartments and limited payloads, except for large military helicopters such as the UH-1V (Huey, Iroquois), UH-60A (Blackhawk), or CH-47 (Chinook), which are not commonly used in the civilian sphere; (c) noticeable vibration and noise, which make simple tasks such as auscultation of breath sounds difficult; (d) limitations in flight capabilities (i.e., altitude and meteorologic conditions), which may prevent their use across high mountain ranges or in poor visibility due to lack of instrument flight capabilities; and (e) inability to pressurize the cabin for special conditions (e.g., med-evac of an injured diver with air embolism or decompression sickness). Currently, few models of rotary-wing aircraft have pressurizing capability.

On the other hand, fixed-wing aircraft carry their own set of limitations: (a) They generally require an airfield for takeoff and landing; however, some planes can land or take off from a minimally prepared airstrip or from airstrips shorter than normally desired (short takeoff/landing aircraft). These aircraft are usually reserved for dire emergencies. It would not be desirable to expose a TP to the pronounced physical forces produced by a bumpy takeoff or the exaggerated slope of ascent during a short-field "climb-out." (b) Because of inherent requirements for adequate landing and takeoff sites, refueling considerations, and other logistic problems, the use of fixed-wing aircraft demands more intense coordination and planning. The use of fixed-wing aircraft for evacuation across international borders may require additional planning to avoid problems with immigration and customs services of various countries (42).

### High-Altitude Pressure-Volume Changes and Hypoxic Hypoxia

In both rotary-wing and fixed-wing aircraft, prime medical considerations must be the maximal altitude achieved by the aircraft (i.e., the cruising altitude) and the ability to "pressurize" the passenger compartment. Similar (but opposite) to the way the partial pressure of oxygen increases with depth during hyperbaric operations, the absolute amount of oxygen available diminishes as higher altitudes are traversed (43, 44). This is why CCT and aviation medicine can be considered related to hypobaric medicine and a part of the continuum that includes hyperbaric medicine as well. Con-

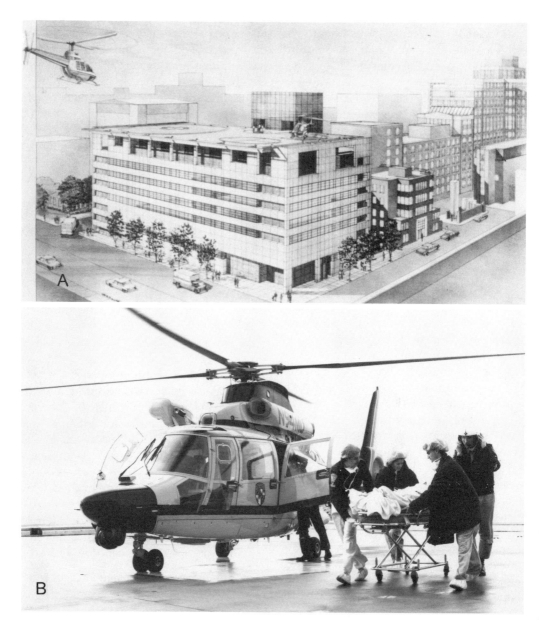

**Figure 15.3.   A, Artist's conception of a med-evac helicopter arriving at the new R Adams Cowley Shock Trauma Center of the MIEMSS. B,** Trauma patient and CCT team on the rooftop helipad at the MIEMSS Shock Trauma Center. A Maryland State Police Aerospatiale Dauphin med-evac helicopter is seen. (Courtesy of MIEMSS.)

sistent with this concept is the fact that, as altitude increases, both total ambient pressure and partial pressure of oxygen fall. This gives rise to two considerations: (a) the effects of changes in the size of airspaces in the body (e.g., pleural cavity, systemic arterial gas embolism) and (b) the effects of hypoxia.

Figure 15.5 shows the relationship of total pressure and altitude. At 18,000 feet

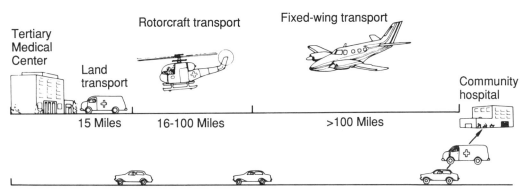

**Figure 15.4.    The spectrum of CCT using land ambulances, helicopters, and fixed-wing aircraft.** (From Baxt WG. Prehospital treatment and transport of the trauma patient. In Baxt WG (ed): Trauma: The First Hour. East Norwalk, CT, Appleton-Century-Crofts, 1985, pp. 293–303.)

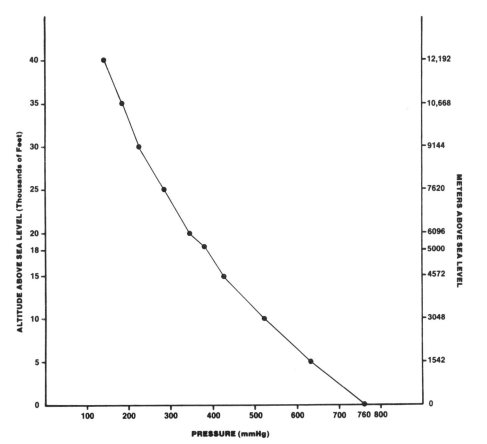

**Figure 15.5.    Atmospheric pressure versus altitude above sea level (in both thousands of feet and meters).** (From Grande CM. Critical care transport: a trauma perspective. Crit Care Clin 1990;6:165–183.)

above sea level (ASL), the atmospheric pressure is 380 mm Hg, which is half that at sea level (760 mm Hg). In terms of pressure-related phenomena, in the normal human being, according to the "two-to-one rule" (see Chapter 14), at this altitude one would expect spontaneous bubble formation to begin. Of course, in the TP undergoing CCT because of a dysbarism (i.e., arterial gas embolism [AGE] or decompression sickness), changes in bubbles that are already formed occur with each foot that the altitude is increased. At 18,000 feet, a given bubble theoretically would have increased its volume by a factor of 2 (Fig. 15.6). For the TP with a cerebral AGE and an evolving secondary area of cerebral ischemia, such increases in bubble size could be disastrous.

Figure 15.7 shows the relationship of the partial pressure of atmospheric, alveolar, and arterial oxygen to altitude. The "magic number" here is 8,000 feet ASL. Above this altitude, the partial pressure of atmospheric oxygen has fallen to such a degree that the intraarterial oxygen tension, the true focus of concern, is 55 mm Hg, which is clinically defined as hypoxia (44). Persons who become acclimated to these extremely low levels of oxygen through mechanisms such as polycythemia may extend travel as high as 12,000 ASL without supplementary oxygen. Experienced mountaineers are able to venture to the range of 18,000 feet ASL, sometimes with the sporadic use of supplemental oxygen. However, the stresses of such feats are well documented and obviously cannot be sustained by an unconditioned individual, let alone a TP.

Although the average healthy person may extend travel to 8000 feet ASL without the need for supplemental oxygen, steps must be taken to support the patient undergoing an aerial CCT. One method is to "pressurize" the passenger compartment. In aircraft with this capability, a compressor is used to force air into the passenger compartment. This concept is very similar to the operation of a hyperbaric chamber. Thus, a pressurized aircraft may be thought of as a mobile hyperbaric chamber at altitude. Since a more sturdy aircraft design is required and a more powerful pressurization system is needed as altitude increases, not all aircraft that are capable of pressurizing are capable of doing it to the same degree. An acceptable level of pressurization is found in those aircraft pressurizing to a simulated altitude of 8000 feet ASL (43–47). An aircraft with this capability would be able to maintain a cabin pressure equivalent to the atmospheric pressure found at 8000 feet ASL ("equivalent alti-

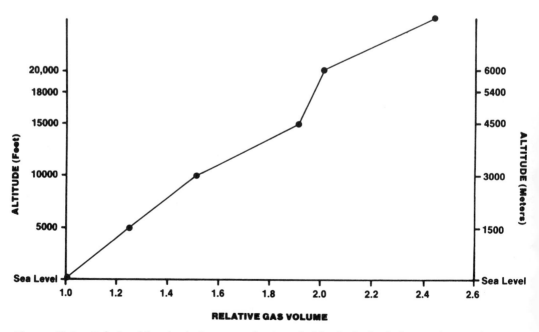

**Figure 15.6.   Relationship of relative gas volume and altitude (in both feet and meters).** (From Grande CM. Critical care transport: a trauma perspective. Crit Care Clin 1990;6:165–183.)

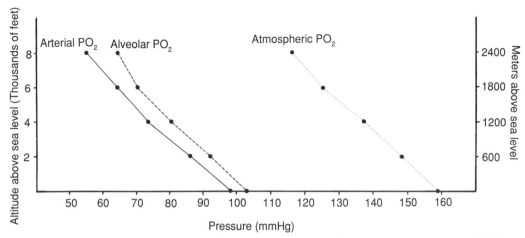

**Figure 15.7.** Relationship of arterial, alveolar, and atmospheric oxygen partial pressure (PO$_2$) to each other and to altitude above sea level (in both thousands of feet and meters). (From Grande CM. Critical care transport: a trauma perspective. Crit Care Clin 1990;6:165–183.)

tude") while flying at its prescribed cruising altitude. This would afford a minimally acceptable level of atmospheric oxygen in the cabin and thus a minimally acceptable arterial oxygen tension. A few exceptional aircraft are capable of pressurizing to "sea level" or "1 atm."

When discussing the capabilities of an aircraft to pressurize to a given level, the factor of greatest importance is the structural ability of the vehicle to withstand the differential in pressure between the inside cabin pressure and the outside atmospheric pressure. If the engineering limitations of the aircraft are exceeded by this pressure differential, cabin explosion ("blow-out") becomes very probable (43). Thus, the risks and benefits of pressurizing to a certain

altitude versus applying supplemental oxygenation become an issue. The CCT physician can use a hand-held altimeter to ascertain the "equivalent altitude" at a given moment and adjust the oxygen therapy as needed (44).

Transport of a critical TP in an aircraft not capable of pressurizing or capable of pressurizing only to 8000 feet ASL requires the use of supplemental oxygen. Table 15.2 shows the amount of supplemental oxygen needed to maintain the PaO$_2$ at 100 mm Hg. Based on the FIO$_2$ needed to saturate the patient, in some cases elective intubation and/or positive-pressure ventilation may be necessary to prevent significant desaturation as altitudes higher than 6000 feet are reached.

**Table 15.2. Oxygen Supplementation Required to Maintain a PaO$_2$ of 100 mm Hg up to Altitudes of 3000 Meters (10,000 Feet)**[a]

|  | 0 m/0 ft | 400 m/ 2,000 ft | 1,200 m/ 4,000 ft | 1,800 m/ 6,000 ft | 2,400 m/ 8,000 ft | 3,000 m/ 10,000 ft |
|---|---|---|---|---|---|---|
| | 21 | 23 | 25 | 27 | 29 | 32 |
| | 30 | 33 | 35 | 38 | 42 | 45 |
| | 40 | 44 | 47 | 51 | 55 | 60 |
| | 50 | 54 | 59 | 64 | 69 | 75 |
| FiO$_2$ | 60 | 65 | 70 | 76 | 83 | 90 |
| | 70 | 76 | 82 | 90 | 97 | 100 |
| | 80 | 87 | 94 | 100 | | |
| | 90 | 98 | 100 | positive pressure required | | |
| | 100 | 100 | | | | |

[a] From McNeil EL. Airborne Care of the Ill and Injured. New York, Springer-Verlag, 1983, p 121.

For this reason and for the rationale outlined above for pressure-volume changes, an attempt is always made to fly at the lowest possible altitude. This is usually more easily accomplished when using a helicopter. Although fixed-wing aircraft can fly at low altitudes, fuel consumption rates increase dramatically. This consideration will be important for long-range evacuation, during which refueling is a problem. Meteorologic considerations may force the plane or jet to fly "above the weather." Terrain features (e.g., high mountains) may require that a certain altitude be maintained to afford a safe crossing.

**Translational Forces Associated with Flight**

When an aircraft maneuvers, whether in two or three dimensions, certain forces are generated. Most notably, these forces occur during takeoff, landing, and turns (48). For example, if a limited amount of airstrip is available for takeoff or landing, the pilot must accelerate or decelerate to a greater degree to execute these maneuvers. Conversely, if adequate runway exists, the pilot may be able to maximize use of the length and accelerate or decelerate more gradually. Preflight communication with the pilot when marginal patients are being transported may prevent sharp turns or flight at altitudes at which turbulence exists (44).

All of these considerations of the translational forces of flight may affect the outcome of patients with certain conditions, and prior knowledge and understanding may help to avoid them or to modify conditions so as to minimize them. For example, a TP with a head injury and a raised intracranial pressure (ICP) should be placed with feet toward the tail of the aircraft during takeoff. Thus, additional increases in ICP due to venous blood pooling in the head will be avoided. Ideally, the patient's orientation should be changed during the flight so that the head is rearward, for similar reasons, upon landing (44, 49).

A rotary-wing aircraft that is capable of vertical takeoff and landing will minimize horizontal acceleration and deceleration forces. However, helicopters have their own set of idiosyncratic maneuvers that can generate combinations of these forces (for example, mixed horizontal and vertical deceleration during the "flare" before "touchdown").

**Physical Considerations of the Aircraft Cabin**

The air within an aircraft at altitude is extremely dry (50, 51). This affects long-range, fixed-wing aircraft more than helicopters. Such considerations become important when transporting patients whose conditions may deteriorate because of lack of moisture (e.g., patients with pneumonia whose mucous membranes become desiccated and secretions inspissated). As altitude increases, both the relative and the absolute humidity of the ambient atmosphere are reduced. Because of the reduced humidity of the environment, heat loss is also accelerated (50–52). This problem is aggravated because virtually all aircraft cabins are cold at altitude. Careful consideration must then be given to monitoring the temperature and maintaining it at a normal level.

Other considerations that can be categorized in the cognitive or psychologic category include the increased level of visual, auditory, and olfactory stimuli in the aircraft environment (Table 15.3). Patients who are conscious and have never flown before may be apprehensive or frightened (53). These emotions can adversely affect outcome because of adrenergic stimulation. It is well documented that emotional stress can be a significant contributor to the evolution of a myocardial infarction. Certain patients may become combative, belligerent, or irrational and thereby endanger themselves and crew members. It is wise to sedate these patients moderately, as is consistent with hemodynamic considerations.

High levels of noise and vibration in the aircraft environment can contribute insidiously to the psychologic and physical degradation of both the patient and the crew (e.g., diminished motor coordination, fatigue, irritability, diminished concentration)

**Table 15.3.   Characteristics of Aerial Critical Care Transport[a]**

Subject to sudden three-dimensional forces
Subject to gravitational and centrifugal forces
Gas space expansion/contraction coincident with alterations in altitude
Subject to rapid and extreme temperature changes
Increased and varied visual, audio, and olfactory stimuli
Increased vibration
Limited cabin space with secondary difficulties in patient care (cabin room and floor space)
Limitations in amount of electrical power (especially during engine shutdown) and in the type of electrical equipment that can be used (e.g., interface with avionics equipment)
Diminished levels of ambient partial pressure of oxygen in the cabin (dependent upon cabin pressurization)
Limitations in payload and thus in weight and bulk of passengers and supplies
Access doors may be small, have steps, or be high above the ground, making it difficult to move patients in and out of the aircraft

[a] From Grande CM. Critical care transport: a trauma perspective. Crit Care Clin 1990;6:165–183.

(54). Noise in the aviation environment is caused by sources outside (e.g., engines, propellers, rotors, exhaust streams) and inside (e.g., air conditioning, pressurization systems, or any medical equipment in operation) the plane. Helicopters produce the worst vibration and the most excessive noise of all aircraft.

Turbulence can make simple medical maneuvers difficult and contributes to the deterioration of patients with certain conditions (50). Except in aircraft specifically designed for aeromedical transport (e.g., U.S. Air Force C9-A Nightingale), the lighting within the cabin may be inadequate (46). This factor will make caring for a patient difficult in terms of methods of observation (e.g., reading monitors and recognizing skin pallor or cyanosis) and the medical attendant's ability (e.g., drowsiness). Other problems, particularly in long-range transports, are changing time zones and climates and their effect on the function of medical personnel.

**LAND-BASED OPERATIONS**

Ground vehicles in a CCT system are generally used in one of three ways: (a) in the vicinity of a TC (50-mile radius) in a conventional, short-term, rapid-response fashion to evacuate the ill and injured from a scene; (b) to provide tertiary care, such as interhospital transfers from referring centers, usually for distances up to 250 miles (but as far as 500 miles is reasonable); and (c) in support of aerial CCT to transport the patient either to or from a remote heliport or airport (1–5).

A system such as that described in the first example is referred to as a "primary responder." The primary responder units may perform measures such as extrication and begin resuscitation and transport for a large variety of patients. The equipment, expertise, and time necessary to complete resuscitation and stabilization of the patient may not be available within this type of scheme. In the more sophisticated systems these units are either deployed in the field, "orbiting" within a specified geographic zone, or garaged in a variety of locations from which they may respond to a call, usually with a response time goal of several minutes.

"Secondary responder" systems may be more cumbersome to activate, especially if the particular system handles various types of specialty patient populations (e.g., burns, pediatrics), as different teams of specialists must be assembled with their respective equipment. In larger metropolitan areas such teams are usually preformed and are devoted to one patient population (e.g., a burn team, a neonatal team). Often these teams are based at various centers throughout a given city and are coordinated through a central dispatching/communication facility.

The personnel staffing each of these types of land-based transport vehicles vary greatly throughout the United States and from country to country throughout the world. The number and expertise of these persons range from two minimally qualified persons (e.g., driver and medical attendant) to a full-scale team (e.g., driver, emergency medical technician or paramedic, CCT nurse, and CCT physician). The extent to which physicians are utilized in this area of CCT was explained previously.

Regardless of whether a ground ambulance will be used as a primary or a secondary responder, it must meet certain minimal standards. These standards include enough physical space to permit access to the patient and room to perform resuscitation and other maintenance procedures. Good lighting, climate control, and soundproofing are desirable (55–57). Thus, older ambulances, which were classically derived from converted hearses or station wagons, are no longer acceptable (5). Today, a wide range of vehicles designed specifically for CCT ("purpose-built") is available in the form of vans or trucks (55–57). Some emergency medical systems have even designed and outfitted motor homes and buses as mobile operating rooms and intensive care units (Fig. 15.8). These vehicles are usually reserved for special situations such as mass casualties or disasters. Other systems use specialty vehicles (for example,

motorcycles) to negotiate the traffic in major metropolitan areas (58).

Many of the same considerations encountered in the aircraft environment (such as noise and other forms of increased sensory stimulation) also apply to land-based vehicles. A different set of factors also arises, such as sirens and car horns. Many evasive and defensive driving maneuvers, such as the high-speed "S" turn, will generate gravitational and centrifugal forces. In fact, a significant number of motor vehicle accidents involve ambulances on emergency runs (5). As is the case with an aircraft pilot, prior communication and coordination with the ambulance driver may avoid some of these problems. In certain circumstances, for example, during transport of a cardiac patient, it may be more beneficial to forgo the use of the siren and maintain a smoother driving pattern to minimize the patient's anxiety level, at the cost of taking a longer time to reach the hospital.

As is the case with aerial CCT, the same

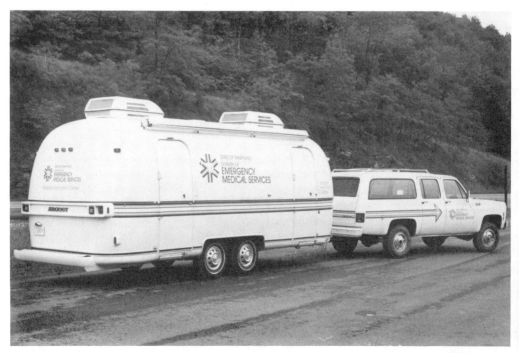

**Figure 15.8.    Converted trailer home that serves as a mobile operating room/intensive care unit for mass casualty/disaster situations.** (Courtesy of MIEMSS.)

level of critical care therapy must be maintained during a land ambulance mission. This includes the full gamut of monitoring and therapeutic techniques although, again, these capabilities would be more commonly used among long-range secondary responder units rather than the "load and go" primary responders. An important premise that applies to all CCT is to resuscitate and stabilize whenever possible before beginning the transfer.

### Physiologic Effects of Land-based Critical Care Transport

Many of the physiologic changes seen in TPs transported in a land ambulance correlate with those in patients transported in aircraft. However, there may be some differences. For example, because land ambulances are underpowered in relation to their gross weight, acceleration is usually more gradual than deceleration (59). Thus, the effect on venous pooling would be more significant during braking. The movement of abdominal viscera against the diaphragm might cause further respiratory embarrassment in patients with thoracic trauma or dyspnea. Thus, a head-aft position is recommended (60, 61).

Vibration transmitted through the chassis from the motor and vertical acceleration/deceleration induced by traveling along a bumpy road in land ambulances can also correlate with physiologic changes in transported patients (62–64). Improved suspension and automobiles designed specifically for function as ambulances have been suggested in a number of articles (55–57). These concerns also led to the development of the concept of the "floating" stretcher (65). One article examined these devices and showed a significant improvement in the quality of the ride. It was also suggested that a floating stretcher package should be used to upgrade a non-purpose-built ambulance at a lesser cost than that of replacing the entire ambulance (65).

It is also important to note that many patients being admitted from the field or after ambulance transport will be hypothermic (66).

### Intrahospital Transport

#### GENERAL CONSIDERATIONS

Transport within the TC is as important as transport outside the TC and, to a large extent, has been neglected in the discussion of transport medicine. Within the TC, patients are transported routinely from one area of the hospital to another (e.g., computed tomography (CT) to angiography suite). Consider the number of times the location of a TP may be changed: from gurney to bed, bed to gurney, gurney to x-ray table, x-ray table to gurney, gurney to operating room (OR) table, and so on. These changes are also plausible on a larger scale: from ambulance to resuscitation area (trauma room), from resuscitation area to the CT suite, from the CT suite to the elevator, from the elevator to the OR, from the OR to the intensive care unit (ICU), and so on (Table 15.4). The position of a TP also may change on a small scale: from supine to upright-seated, from seated to Trendelenburg, etc. These seemingly small differences actually have significant effects on hemodynamics and ultimately on the outcome of treatment (67–69). Thus, transportation can be extremely hazardous because of both the complexity of injuries involved and the difficulty of providing appropriate support en route. The success of intrahospital transport depends basically on two factors: the preparedness and experience of the transporting team and the availability of the necessary equipment.

**Table 15.4.  Destinations for the Intrahospital Critical Care Transport Team**

OR
Hyperbaric chamber
Another unit within facility
CT scanner
X-ray, tomography suite
Nuclear medicine
Whirlpool therapy
Radiation therapy
Helipad/ambulance loading dock

One author who examined this issue stated

the incidence of serious effects due to intrahospital movement in critically ill patients was much higher than that previously seen during ambulance transport of similar patients. This may be partly due to a willingness to move patients within the hospital who would be considered too moribund to subject to an ambulance journey. It is probably due also to less thorough preparation and less adequate maintenance of treatment during movement. In the ambulance study every possible care was taken to stabilize the patient and then maintain treatment throughout the journey. When simply wheeling a patient along a corridor it is tempting to imagine that there is less opportunity for misfortune and that a few minutes gap in treatment will do no harm (65).

Movement of patients may upset the compensatory mechanisms that have previously kept them stable. For example, blood loss can be accelerated by moving the TP. Additionally, it is thought that secondary effects (centrifugal forces) occur because of rapid acceleration or deceleration when a patient is rolled down a hallway or around a corner. Such movements may also lead to acute gravitational disturbances of an insufficient amount of fluid within an essentially empty vascular tree; circulatory collapse may ensue because of reduced venous return.

The solutions to these problems are in part: (a) recognition of the potential consequences of altering that position in which the TP has become relatively stable; (b) prevention of these effects through gently controlled handling and the use of assisting devices (rollers, mobilizers); (c) an attempt to provide the same level of care in a mobile environment as had been rendered in the previous stable one (i.e., using portable ventilators); (d) surveillance for and anticipation of these effects (i.e., using proper monitoring); and (e) rapid correction of compromising factors and active treatment of problems when they occur.

Three basic questions should be asked *before* moving a TP: (a) Is it *necessary* to the TP? Or can other arrangements be made to allow the TP to remain where he or she is (e.g., using a portable x-ray machine versus moving to the x-ray suite)? Minimizing the need for patient transport is a feature of ultraspecialized level I TCs (or accident hospitals) (see Chapter 1), which are built "around the TP." (b) Is the TP *stable*? If not, can stability be increased before the move? Or is the reason for transport crucial to improving the patient's status (e.g., from emergency room to OR)? (c) Have the *preparations* for the move been maximized? (Is all equipment functioning? Does the bed roll easily? Has the elevator been summoned and is it standing by? Has the "receiving end" been notified of an imminent transfer and are they ready for the TP)?

## THE CRITICAL CARE TRANSPORT TEAM

The CCT team members individually and collectively play key roles. Once the decision has been reached to transport a patient requiring ongoing critical care, action should begin promptly but safely. The team as a whole should be skilled in hemodynamic monitoring, ventilatory support, pharmacologic intervention, and cardiopulmonary resuscitation; in addition, each care giver must also be skilled in functioning as a team member to provide optimal patient support. At the Maryland Institute for Emergency Medical Services Systems (MIEMSS) Shock Trauma Center, the CCT team may consist of a physician, a nurse, a respiratory therapist, and one or more attendants, depending on individual patient needs.

Facilitation of safe transport and management of the patient requires a physician who is knowledgeable about the patient's injuries, current condition, and potential problems. Intervention by means of physical presence or verbal orders may be necessary. The physician's responsibilities include directing the team's resuscitative efforts in the event of cardiac/respiratory arrest, reestablishing the airway in the event of accidental extubation or other loss of airway, and ordering, in advance, any drugs necessary for resuscitation or maintenance during transport.

Guidelines should be established by individual units as to the need for a physician during transport. Multisystem failure victims are at the highest risk and may require the most consideration. If the patient's status has been considered fairly stable, the transport may be handled by the nurse and ancillary personnel without the physician.

### The Nurse

It is the nurse's responsibility to organize the entire transport process—inform all team members needed for transport, check essential equipment, advise the destination site personnel of needs, and, primarily, prepare the patient for the journey. To accomplish these objectives, the transport nurse must have exceptional communication skills as well as expertise in patient care. Through advance planning, the nurse can help ensure the patient's safety throughout the transport.

### The Respiratory Therapist

Airway management is of utmost importance during patient transport; ventilation, manual or mechanical, must be uninterrupted, carefully monitored, and designated the primary responsibility for a certain member(s) of the team. This responsibility can be shared by the anesthesiologist, the nurse anesthetist (CRNA), and/or the respiratory therapist, depending upon the particular situation, the institution, and the availability of personnel. In addition to being experienced in adult critical care medicine, anesthesia personnel and the respiratory therapists must be aware of the capabilities and limitations of all available equipment to be used on transport and at the destination site.

### The Attendants

The attendants will provide the majority of the labor necessary during the transport, not "hands-on" patient care. They are responsible for obtaining and handling equipment to be used during transport, such as cardiac and blood pressure monitors, oxygen cylinders, and the resuscitation cart/ pack. (The crash cart represents the patient's "lifeline" and must be moved along with the patient throughout the transport.)

The authors have recently been implementing the use of a "soft pack" (carry-bag) resuscitation bag as opposed to the standard bulky resuscitation cart. It contains the necessary drugs, intravenous fluids, and equipment and an airway tray, but it is small and lightweight.

### EQUIPMENT

Modern technology has much to offer in terms of small, self-contained, portable equipment that is ideal for transport. However, one must not rely solely upon electronic monitoring devices; basic essentials, such as stethoscopes and blood pressure cuffs, must accompany any transport. In addition, the care giver's senses—sight, hearing, and touch—should be relied upon heavily; for optimal patient benefits, these findings must be communicated on a continuing basis to the entire team.

Battery-powered oscilloscopes display electrocardiograms (ECGs) and have the ability to monitor information from intraarterial lines, pulmonary artery catheters, intracranial monitors, and capnographs on up to three other channels contained within the same unit. At least two articles have alluded to the inaccuracy of blood pressure measurements made by all but invasive methods of measurement (e.g., Korotkoff sounds, Doppler) in the CCT environment (70, 71). Thus, in marginal patients direct measurement of hemodynamic parameters may be warranted. An ECG/defibrillator combination may be especially useful. Pulse oximeters can also be used during transport; these devices now possess characteristics that enable them to be useful in these activities. Intravenous pumps can be included in this category as well and may be desirable in the care of TPs whose survival is dependent upon careful, continuous administration of vasoactive substances. All intravenous systems should be examined before transport to ensure that fluid bags are full and lines are functioning. Emergency drugs (bicarbonate, antiarrhythmics, vasopressor bolus) should accompany the patient during transport. It may be prudent to leave medical antishock trousers (MAST) in place during transport if they have already been applied, in case the need to inflate them arises.

## VENTILATOR SYSTEMS

With regard to respiratory support, several ventilator systems with characteristics valued in transport equipment are available and others are under development.

### Siemens Ventilator System

The most seriously injured patients require complex ventilation patterns that may not be achievable with manual "bagging." The authors have had experience with the use of the Siemens Servo Ventilator 900C and the Siemens Power Pack 160. Figure 15.9 illustrates this system accompanied by "E" cylinders of oxygen with gauging to provide the 50-psi source gas. This system provides continuous ventilation without interruption of previous ventilatory patterns. At the MIEMSS Shock Trauma Center, a wheeled cart holds the ventilator, battery pack, and cylinders and makes the system a portable unit for mobilization throughout the center (Fig. 15.9).

The Power Pack 160 supplies the electronic power to the 900C ventilator through a 12-volt DC that converts to 110 AC of 50 to 60 Hz. To maintain the 160 Power Pack's battery, one must plug the unit into an electrical outlet between transports. This battery has both an optical (a red light) and an acoustic alarm signal to indicate that only a limited amount of time (approximately 2 hours) remains to the battery charge.

If the use of this "ideal" equipment is not possible or deemed necessary, the patient may be manually "bagged" or ventilated while being transported to the destination site.

### Puritan Manual Resuscitator

The authors have had the most experience on transports with the use of the Puritan Manual Resuscitator PMR-2 Bag.

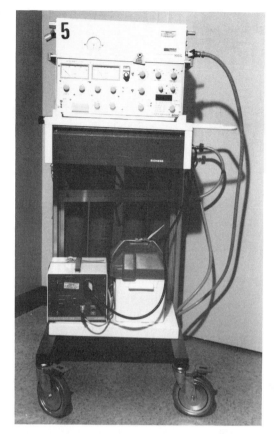

**Figure 15.9.** Portable system for intrahospital CCT, which includes the ventilator (Siemens Servo Ventilator 900C), battery pack (Siemens Power Pack 160), and gas cylinders.

This device can deliver supplemental oxygen, and an accumulator can be attached to the bag-fill valve to provide higher concentrations of oxygen. The accumulator serves as a reservoir of oxygen while the bag is squeezed, providing as much as 95% oxygen concentration for adult ventilation, as well as adequate flow (Fig. 15.10A).

If the accumulator attachment is not available, the oxygen source may be attached directly to the tubing connection in the center of the bag-fill valve. However, the oxygen concentration will then be reduced to approximately 45%, with a flow of 15 liters of source gas per min (Fig. 15.10B).

This system also offers an accessory that can deliver adequate positive end-expira-

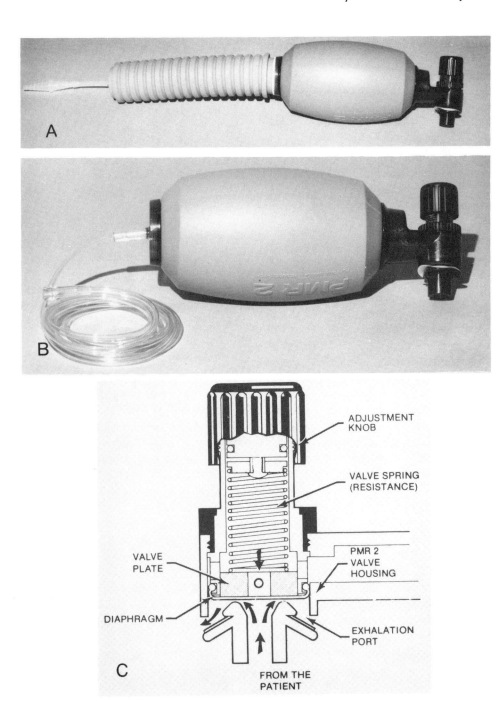

**Figure 15.10.   A, Puritan Manual Resuscitator Bag (PMR-2). Accumulator at the end serves as an oxygen reservoir, providing oxygen concentrations as high as 95%. B**, PMR-2 without the accumulator, which delivers oxygen concentrations of approximately 45%. Note the accessory that replaces the nonrebreathing valve on the PMR-2 to provide PEEP. **C**, PEEP valve of the PMR-2.

tory pressure (PEEP). The PEEP accessory replaces the nonbreathing valve for the PMR-2 resuscitator and may, by simple adjustment, deliver 4 to 14 cm $H_2O$ of PEEP. (Reference marks are approximate indicators of PEEP levels. For exact values, use of a manometer or airway pressure gauge is recommended by the Operating and Maintenance Instruction Manual of the PEEP accessory.) Figure 15.10C illustrates this accessory's operating principle. During exhalation, the diaphragm closes against the valve plate and exhaled air passes through the exhalation port. Acting on the valve plate, a spring creates a resistance to air flow out through the exhalation port in proportion to the setting of the adjustment knob.

### Other Systems

Several resuscitator bags are available today (e.g., Laerdal, Ambu, Penlon, Hope). Each should be evaluated on percentage of oxygen delivery capability, self-inflation time, and volume. (Again, the PMR-2 has the advantage of its accessory PEEP valve.) Whichever system is selected, it is of paramount importance that the team member responsible for patient ventilation during transport have full knowledge of the capabilities and incapabilities of the available resuscitator bag. It is possible to "hand-bag" a patient continuously during transport with the resuscitator bag; however, such a procedure requires adequate oxygen supply and a certain amount of stamina on the part of the "bagger" (for example, when a patient requires hyperventilation and increased PEEP levels).

Alternatively, a "Mapelson D" system connected to an oxygen tank may be used and can maintain PEEP. When hand-operated self-inflating bags are utilized, there is a tendency to hyperventilate the patient. Hyperventilation results in hypocarbia and unwanted respiratory alkalosis. This problem can be prevented by attaching a spirometer to monitor the minute volume. Conversely, after extended periods, the hands of the person squeezing the bag will tire and hypoventilation will occur. In a "worst case scenario," the person responsible for hand-bagging the TP may become engrossed with another aspect of care and neglect to ventilate the TP. However, such manual backup equipment is still necessary whenever a mechanical ventilator is used.

Attention must be given to maintenance of the airway at all times and to protection of the cervical spine if it is in jeopardy. The endotracheal or tracheostomy tube must be secured and connecting tubing checked so that there is no accidental dislodging or disconnection. In case of accidental dislodgement, emergency airway equipment is also essential for the transport. For example, the team should also transport an "intubation tray" that includes such essentials as oral airways, a functioning laryngoscope, and a varied but simple selection of endotracheal tubes and blades. Extra oxygen tanks may also be useful. Chest tubes must be protected so they are not accidentally pulled out; changes in their position may cause a fenestration to become extrathoracic and thus useless. Suction drainage should be continued or reinstituted as soon as possible.

### INTEGRATED INTRAHOSPITAL CRITICAL CARE TRANSPORT SYSTEMS

A number of integrated intrahospital transport systems incorporate all of the above elements (i.e., monitoring and therapeutic equipment such as ventilator, infusion pumps, rechargeable battery packs, and intravenous poles). Some transport beds or "trolleys" are motorized (because of the high gross weights of the systems), have "crash bars" for protection in the event of collisions with other objects or walls, and may be compatible with extrahospital transport systems such as land ambulances (72–74). Some of the designs even act to minimize vibration.

Perhaps the most important factor in intrahospital CCT is that a physician familiar with transport protocol and problems, as well as proper resuscitation procedures, must accompany the TP. In many TCs this role is already filled by the anesthesiologist because muscle relaxants, sedation, Entonox (Nitronox), or other planned therapy may be necessary. There can be no laxity in vigilance, as during the CT scan itself, and extra care must be instituted because conditions are suboptimal outside the OR or ICU (e.g., poor lighting and ventilation, cramped space). If the transport phase will be prolonged, efforts should be made to prevent heat loss (e.g., using aluminum/reflective sheets to cover the body) and the TP's temperature should be checked regularly. Last, the patient records should go with the patient during transport; they should be updated at the end of the trip as well with a description of the continued care. Ideally, hand-held two-way radios should be available so that the transport team may contact the support element at the "base" (ICU, OR) instantaneously if the need arises (e.g., in a hallway or elevator).

Equipment designed to facilitate quick transportation is essential; however, without *caring, cooperative,* and *communicative* personnel, transport is unlikely to go well. Realistically, members of the team are not simply standing by for the "big move"; they have other responsibilities to be carried out. Therefore, the transportation of a critically injured patient must be planned and followed through in a timely fashion with consideration of all involved.

## PUBLIC HEALTH AND ADMINISTRATIVE CONSIDERATIONS OF CRITICAL CARE TRANSPORT

Several administrative issues arise with a CCT: (*a*) cost, (*b*) in-flight death, (*c*) long-range retrieval and repatriation, (*d*) communicable disease, (*e*) limited availability of electrical power, (*f*) medical equipment, and (*g*) documentation (42, 74). Not all of these factors may be active in every case, but eventually the aeromedical physician will deal with each of them (4, 42, 74).

### Cost

A conservative estimate of the cost of an international CCT is $15,000. For example, for the medical evacuation of an injured sports scuba diver from a resort island in the Caribbean back to the United States, this fee would cover only the cost of transport itself

and not any of the medical treatment en route or at the final destination. Several groups and insurance companies working in conjunction (e.g., Divers Alert Network, see Chapter 14) offer "package deals" to members/policy holders, which make emergency funds available to meet these expenses. If a person does not have the required insurance, adequate monies, or collateral when queried by the various transport companies, the transport may be refused.

### In-flight Death

In-flight deaths of patients undergoing CCT may cause administrative and medical-legal problems. First, it may be difficult to assign a specific geographic location for the death. If the location can be determined, the aircraft may have to land within that jurisdiction to confer with local authorities and obtain certification for the death. If a death occurs over international waters, the jurisdiction may coincide with the country that issued registration to the particular aircraft. Second, as in any emergency medical situation, the likelihood of a lawsuit is automatically raised because of the conglomeration of circumstances (e.g., poor development of the physician-patient relationship) (see Chapter 18).

### Long-Range Retrieval and Repatriation

When the CCT team is requested to retrieve a patient being maintained in a foreign country, special considerations apply. The specific condition of the patient, the special equipment or medical specialist that may be needed ("care-to-patient" missions), administrative procedures for clearing customs, and the need for a translator must be anticipated. If the CCT team is carrying any controlled substances (e.g., narcotics), special arrangements must be made ahead of time. Local authorities may have to be warned so that the team is not detained or arrested and so that the drugs are not seized (74).

## Communicable Diseases

Before agreeing to perform a CCT, the medical director (flight surgeon, aeromedical physician, CCT physician) must ascertain the presence of any communicable diseases. Because of the heating and pressurization systems currently used, most aircraft condition and recirculate cabin air. Thus, unless special filter systems are used or other individually worn devices are supplied, crew members may become infected. Immunizations for the CCT team may be necessary before commencing the trip (74).

## Electrical Power

Another consideration is the availability of electrical power, the type of electrically powered equipment brought along on a CCT, and the electromagnetic interference caused by this equipment with regard to the communication and navigational equipment of the aircraft. An aircraft may be able to supply only a certain amount of electrical power when the engines are running at full. This level of power may drop when the aircraft is taxiing or is parked. If the engines are totally shut down, the amount of power is even further reduced. In fact, if a generator is not onboard, the continued use of electronic medical equipment (e.g., ventilators) may quickly drain the batteries of the aircraft. It may be possible for an external generator to be brought to the plane at its parking space to provide power for medical equipment; planning and coordination with airport authorities are required to make these arrangements. It is also wise to carry battery packs for each piece of equipment in case of an emergency.

Another consideration is the compatibility of the plug on the medical equipment and the configuration of the electrical outlet of the aircraft (50). Differences between the two would be especially likely if the equipment and the aircraft were manufactured and used primarily in different countries. This is also an important point to remember when planning a "care-to-patient" mission in which medical equipment will be transported to a foreign hospital during retrieval of a patient (75).

## Medical Equipment

Before embarking on CCT, the equipment necessary to perform any and all of the tasks enumerated in Table 15.1 must be aboard. This includes a laryngoscope, endotracheal tubes, emergency cricothyroidotomy kits, chest tubes, and intravenous and central venous infusion kits. Other standard equipment includes a bag-valve-mask apparatus, a defibrillator, and a portable, battery-powered suction unit. Other special packs and equipment may be needed for the neonatal, pediatric, obstetric, orthopedic, cardiac, or burned patient. Such equipment might include mechanical ventilators, continuous intravenous infusion pumps, incubators, splints, and sometimes equipment as sophisticated as an intraaortic balloon pump.

## Documentation

It is important that both sending and receiving centers coordinate telephonically before a CCT. All medical records must travel with the patient and be annotated regularly during the transport with respect to observations and therapy (45). Many CCT teams have formulated their own "transport forms" for use during a mission, which also serve as checklists to ensure that nothing is forgotten (76).

# MEDICAL CONDITIONS REQUIRING SPECIAL CONSIDERATION DURING CRITICAL CARE TRANSPORT

Some conditions require special consideration and/or therapeutic schemes before embarking on a CCT. Each of these conditions, which may be found alone or in multiple combinations in the TP, will be discussed briefly in this section. For the most part, issues will be viewed from the standpoint of an extended high-altitude, long-range transport, as this presents the harshest set of conditions. The individual CCT physician can then "downgrade" the situation and weigh the benefits and detriments of transport versus delayed evacuation in each case.

## Hemorrhage/Anemia

TPs with acute or chronic anemia (demonstrated as a low hemoglobin level or hematocrit) are predisposed to the amplified effects of altitude hypoxia. Indeed, there are differences in the effects of altitude in patients with chronic versus acute anemia (Table 15.5). The U.S. Armed Forces (Air Force, Army, Navy) follow the general guideline of delaying transportation until the hemoglobin is elevated to at least 7 g/dl or the hematocrit is greater than 21% (46).

For immediate, short-range evacuation, which is normally conducted with land ambulances or helicopters (which are not usually exposed to extremes of altitude), these considerations are generally waived in favor of rapid transport ("load and go" philosophy) to the TC. Oxygen is supplied by face mask, esophageal obturator airway, or endotracheal tube, and blood volume is augmented with a crystalloid solution. In a military situation, in which the service members are wearing an identification tag ("dog tag"), blood type and Rh group can be transmitted to the dispatching center and appropriate blood can be placed on the helicopter before its departure. Long-range transport TPs with anemia or reduced circulating blood volume have an increased oxygen requirement. Supplementary oxygen, replacement of blood volume, and restoration of oxygen carrying capacity are mandatory as soon as possible.

## Thoracic Trauma/Pneumothorax (43, 49)

All patients with a history of thoracic trauma and, for that matter, with a history of recent intubation and institution of positive-pressure ventilation should have a recent chest roentgenogram examined for the presence of a pneumothorax. As described in Chapter 14, the volume of a pneumothorax will expand as altitude increases (Fig. 15.6). This requires immediate puncture of the thorax with a needle or, more ideally, placement of a chest tube with a Heimlich valve at its extrathoracic end. If the TP previously had an intercostal tube (chest tube) placed and is connected to a water suction system, the tube should be detached from the system and capped with a Heimlich valve. However, if the transport aircraft is dedicated to aeromedical evacuation and has a suction system available, the water seal system may be utilized.

## Sickle Cell Trait/Disease/Crisis (49, 77)

When one considers the elevated number of young black men who are victims of

**Table 15.5.  Patient at Sea Level: Altitude-Equivalent Related to Hemoglobin**[a]

| Hemoglobin | Altitude-Equivalent (feet) | |
|---|---|---|
| | Acute Anemia | Chronic Anemia |
| g/100 ml | | |
| 15 | 0 | 0 |
| 14 | 1,200 | 800 |
| 13 | 2.400 | 1,500 |
| 12 | 3,500 | 2,300 |
| 11 | 4,800 | 3,200 |
| 10 | 6,000 | 4,000 |
| 9 | 7,200 | 4,800 |
| 8 | 8,400 | 5,600 |
| 7 | 9,500 | 6,300 |
| 6 | 11,000 | 7,200 |

[a] Supplementary oxygen is required at sea level when a patient has only 10 g of hemoglobin per 100 ml reached acutely or 7.5 g/100 ml when chronically anemic if no other reason for supplementary oxygen is present.
From McNeil EL. Hemoglobin levels and altitude: aeromedical care. In McNeil EL (ed): Airborne Care of the Ill and Injured. New York, Springer-Verlag, 1983, pp. 169–171.

**Table 15.6.  Medical Equipment That Contains Gas and Requires Special Attention in Critical Care Transport**[a]

Orthopaedic air splints
Pneumatic antishock suits (MAST)
Intravenous fluid reservoirs containing air
Blood pressure cuffs
Ballon cuffs (endotracheal tubes, esophageal obturator airways, Foley catheters)
Medication, fluid, and suction bottles

[a] From Grande CM. Critical care transport: a trauma perspective. Crit Care Clin 1990;6:165–183.

interpersonal violence compared with young white men, as well as the entire constellation of a traumatic incident (e.g., cold, stress, hypoxia), it is not unusual to be faced with a TP with sickle cell trait, disease, or frank crisis. CCT physicians must weigh the risks and benefits of transporting versus stabilizing the patient. The points discussed in regard to the physical environment of the aircraft may also affect the situation (e.g., hypoxia, low temperature of the cabin, psychologic stress), more so in the case of long-range, high-altitude flight. Based upon the amount of time available and the urgency of the situation, the following steps should be taken: (a) use maximal supplementary oxygen, (b) maintain an adequate level of hydration, and (c) transfuse blood products as necessary. (If time and facilities permit, the CCT physician can attempt to determine the relative percentages of normal and pathologic hemoglobins [e.g., S, SC]). One may attempt to exchange transfuse the patient to lower the relative percentage of abnormal hemoglobin. Maintenance of body temperature, especially in the distal extremities (i.e., fingers and toes) is important. To reduce the level of emotional stress, sedation may be in order.

## Fever/Infection/Sepsis

The manifestations of fever, infection, and sepsis most commonly occur in a TP being maintained in an intensive care unit 7 to 10 days postinjury. Review of the natural history of traumatic disease will show that infection and sepsis, as well as adult respiratory distress syndrome and renal failure, are "late-phase" manifestations of either the severity of the initial injury or the inadequacy of initial resuscitation efforts.

Elevated body temperature signals an increase in basal metabolic rate, which in turn raises oxygen requirements. Generally, for each degree centigrade the body temperature is increased, the oxygen requirements increase proportionately. Meeting these increased requirements may involve obtaining an aircraft capable of full pressur-

ization (1 atm) or electively intubating the patient and instituting positive-pressure ventilation with 100% oxygen.

The febrile TP will also most likely be receiving a regularly scheduled antibiotic, and this schedule must be continued during the CCT.

## Eye Injuries (49, 77)

The retina is one of the most oxygen-sensitive organs in the body, as demonstrated by the acute decrease in night vision at altitude. This becomes significant in patients with retinal detachment. In cases of open eye injury, global contents can be extruded by cabin pressure changes (see Chapter 8).

## Maxillofacial Injuries (49, 77)

Patients with maxillofacial injuries often experience "surgical emphysema" in the soft tissues of the face and neck or partial obstruction of the sinuses by blood and mucus. As altitude diminishes, these pockets of air begin to swell, causing pain and ischemia.

It is not unusual for the airway to be involved; thus, as a minimum, supplemental oxygen must be supplied. It would also be wise to have definitive airway control if even the smallest possibility of compromise exists.

Surgical repair of these injuries frequently involves the placement of fixation devices that require the teeth to be wired closed. During flight, aspiration becomes a possibility. Thus, the CCT physician should ensure that wire cutters are readily available.

Epistaxis may occur in flight. The CCT physician can attempt to quell the bleeding by applying bilateral nasal compression for several minutes. If this is insufficient, the nose can be packed. Merocel nasal tampons (Americal Corporation, Mystic, Connecticut) are a convenient alternative. These tampons are easy to use and come in a compressed, dehydrated state. Blood and mucus cause them to swell. A tube within the tampon maintains the nasal airway.

### Orthopaedic Injuries (49, 77, 78)

Most of the concerns regarding the TP with orthopaedic injuries relate to lower extremity fractures, especially those of the femur or requiring a long-leg cast. TPs with recently placed plaster casts may have a significant amount of soft tissue swelling, which can lead to circulatory embarrassment of the limb. All casts should be bivalved if possible. Pneumatic splints are absolutely contraindicated for aerial CCT, as they are greatly affected by altitude and pressure changes (Fig. 15.6).

Any devices that have been applied for traction (e.g., Hoffman external fixation) and have weights attached must be modified or the weights must be removed. This is important not only because the weight may oscillate and cause pain and destabilization of the fracture but also because the weights may become missiles in the case of impact. Whenever possible, Collins (spring-type) traction should be used. The CCT physician should also be aware that vibration may cause pain and discomfort in a TP with fractures.

### Spinal Injuries (49, 77, 79)

It is now common that TPs with spinal cord injuries are either moved to a tertiary care center with a neurotrauma unit or triaged initially to such a center. For the TP in the latter category, all attempts should be made to stabilize the injury. This can be done by using devices such as the Kendricks extrication device or a backboard (in the case of cervical injury, in combination with a cervical collar and sand bags on either side, reinforced by adhesive tape). All attempts should be made to stabilize the TP in the first category before CCT. Generally this requires the expertise of a neurosurgeon, who can evaluate the x-ray series and who is capable of placing a device such as Gardner-Wells tongs or a halo vest. Moving a TP in a halo vest presents no special problems other

than ensuring gentle handling. A traction system using Gardner-Wells tongs, hanging weights, and a Stryker frame must be modified. One alternative is to use a Rambaud cervical traction frame, which substitutes a spring system for the application of traction and is attached directly to the stretcher. If the available aircraft cannot accommodate a Stryker frame, use of a "scoop" stretcher or a vacuum stretcher can be attempted.

When a neurosurgeon is not available to stabilize the cervical injury of a TP, risks and benefits must be weighed. If the decision is made to transport, such a patient can be stabilized temporarily in the manner described above.

One other pertinent consideration for the TP with a spinal injury concerns the possibility of a paralytic ileus. Gastric distension of the bowel may cause secondary respiratory embarrassment due to interference with diaphragmatic mechanics. In some cases of spinal cord injury, vagal paralysis is also involved. Respiratory embarrassment may already be present for this reason and/or from paralysis of the intercostal muscles. Thus, a nasogastric tube (NGT) should always be placed in these patients and either be maintained on intermittent suction or left open to air. A Foley catheter should also be used and its cuff filled with water (see "Medical Equipment in the Critical Care Transport Environment").

### Abdominal Trauma (49, 77)

The patient with abdominal trauma can be either in an acute condition or already stabilized. In any patient with abdominal trauma, a NGT should be placed. If the patient's condition is acute, internal or external blood loss as well as tissue edema may be occurring, which may result in anemia and/or hypovolemia. Evaluation should progress as the situation permits (i.e., obtain a hemoglobin or hematocrit level in a hospital situation), and blood products and crystalloid should be infused.

The patient with abdominal trauma who

has undergone surgical intervention should be maintained with a NGT. This is important, as expanding gas within the intestinal tract can place stress upon healing suture lines. Patients with colostomies may experience an increase in bowel elimination; thus, extra colostomy bags should be available during transport.

## Pelvic Fractures (49)

TPs with pelvic fractures also may be separated into two groups: those with acute, unstable injuries and those in the recuperative phase, who have undergone surgical intervention. Patients in the former group will often have other severe injuries that manifest as hypotension. In the short-term evacuation scenario, pelvic injuries can be stabilized by application of medical anti-shock trousers (MAST), which also raise the mean blood pressure for short periods (see Chapter 4). If hypotension is not a problem, the pelvic portion of the MAST can be inflated to a lower pressure to stabilize the pelvis. Also, vacuum stretchers work well in this situation. The TP in the second category usually will have been stabilized with a Hoffman external fixation device. This presents no special problems for transport other than the need to ensure gentle handling and the removal of the hanging weights.

## Burns (49, 77, 79)

TPs with complicated burns are frequently transported form the primary care facility to a specialty care burn center. The Advanced Trauma Life Support protocol of the American College of Surgeons (80) defines complicated burns as the following: (a) burns involving more than 25% of the body surface area (20% in children under 10 years of age and adults over 40 years), (b) full-thickness or third-degree burns exceeding 10% of the body surface area, (c) partial-thickness or second-degree burns exceeding 20% of the body surface area, (d) all burns involving the face, eyes, ears, hands, feet, and perineum, (e) burns associated with significant fractures or other

major injury, (f) high-voltage electrical burns, (g) inhalation injury, and (h) lesser burns in patients with significant preexisting disease.

Severely burned TPs can be the epitome of the critical care patient, being maintained with a full array of invasive cardiovascular and ventilatory equipment and receiving all forms of continuous infusions from vasoactive solutions to central hyperalimentation.

One of the most frequent problems in a burn patient who has been transferred within 24 hours after the incident is inadequacy of fluid resuscitation. This occurs for various reasons, for example, the inability of the "sending" hospital to place lines or inexperience with fluid resuscitation in the burn patient. On the other hand, some burn patients are the victims of fluid overload and are in frank pulmonary edema. Thus, these patients may arrive in poor fluid balance: either dehydrated and hypotensive or fluid-overloaded.

Subsequent airway problems in those patients with facial and cervical burns must be anticipated. Either airway compromise becomes an in-flight emergency or it is difficult to achieve airway control (e.g., intubation) at the receiving hospital. It is important to achieve early, definitive airway control in burn patients. In many cases this is done prophylactically.

A different problem in burn patients is that of other occult and/or overt non-thermal trauma (81). For example, many burn patients sustain fractures of the lower extremities when they jump from burning buildings (82). Unless one is familiar with the care of burn patients and common presentations of injury constellations, non-thermal injuries may go undetected and then become an in-flight emergency.

Because the burned TP is one of the most "exotic" types of TPs and the care of these patients is frequently limited to specialized health care providers, it is important to send a knowledgeable CCT team with the aircraft to evaluate and stabilize the burned patient at the sending hospital and to maintain the patient during CCT.

## Cardiac Disease (49, 83–85)

Cardiac pathology in the TP can be seen in three scenarios: (a) the patient with a history of arrhythmias and syncope may have an accident as a result of these conditions, (b) the cardiac problem may be secondary to the trauma, as either a manifestation of a chronic problem (e.g., in an elderly TP with coronary artery disease, which can progress to a myocardial infarction secondary to stress) or an acute condition (e.g., a cardiac contusion secondary to blunt thoracic trauma), and (c) there may be a combination of these two situations.

Physical evidence of cardiac dysfunction in the TP will be (a) skin pallor and diaphoresis, (b) hypotension, (c) arrhythmias, or (d) rales and pulmonary edema. During immediate evacuation from an accident scene, temporizing maneuvers such as oxygen and fluid infusion are performed routinely. Congestive heart failure and pulmonary edema are absolute contraindications to the use of MAST.

When a TP with cardiac complications must undergo long-range transportation, it is wise to attend to any items that may exacerbate the already complex presentation. This may involve elective intubation to ensure adequate oxygenation during the trip to prevent further ischemia, as well as placement of invasive lines for monitoring and/or drug infusion. With proper planning, patients with even the most serious conditions, including those being maintained on intraaortic balloon pumps, can be transported.

If a long-range aerial transport of a cardiac patient is scheduled, it is wise to anticipate the problems that may arise because of gravitational forces. Venous blood pooling caused by acceleration and deceleration can cause decreased cardiac return and output, reduce coronary artery perfusion pressure, and thus raise the possibility of ischemia and/or arrest. Precautions can be taken by determining and maintaining adequate ventricular end-diastolic pressure and by briefing the pilot on the given situation. It should also be ensured that any supplies necessary to perform cardiopulmonary resuscitation are aboard (e.g., a defibrillator). Sedation of these patients can minimize emotional stress.

## Chronic Obstructive Pulmonary Disease (COPD) (49)

Patients with COPD require careful titration of levels of oxygenation and ventilation. These patients may be dependent on either hypercarbic or hypoxic drive to maintain ventilation. If too much oxygen is supplied, spontaneous respirations will cease. It may be wise to intubate these patients electively. A portable pulse oximeter and capnograph may also be useful when transporting COPD patients.

## Head Injury (49, 77, 86)

The TP with a head injury is probably one of the most difficult to transport correctly. Each of the physical differences in the aviation transport environment can adversely affect this type of patient (i.e., hypoxic atmosphere, pressure-volume changes, and gravitational and centrifugal forces). Meticulous critical care is necessary to minimize mortality and morbidity.

Care of the head-injured patient during CCT should proceed as it would in the neurotrauma unit of a sophisticated trauma center. This includes the use of all currently accepted techniques to normalize the ICP, such as maintaining the proper osmotic balance and fluid status and acute hyperventilation. Adequate ventilation and oxygenation must be ensured. At a minimum, this means that oxygen should be supplied by face mask. Because of the possibility of incompetent airway reflexes, more aggressive control of the airway should be exercised (e.g., intratracheal intubation). A pressurized aircraft should be used for CCT, and the flight should be maintained at the lowest possible altitude to minimize hypoxic hypoxia.

Special attention must be given to invasive lines (e.g., for central venous pressure monitoring) to ensure that they do not accidentally become dislodged and that air is not inadvertently entrained. The latter could result in consequences such as systemic air embolism. Systemic air embolism, which is affected by pressure-volume changes, would be especially disastrous when superimposed on a head injury.

Prior coordination with the pilot and the transport company may preclude radical maneuvers such as short-field takeoffs, "tight" turns, and other causes of extreme gravitational and centrifugal forces. These may result in intracranial venous blood pooling and subsequent elevation of ICP. The TP's head should be kept raised. If a "cross-cabin" placement of the patient is not feasible, then the head should be placed forward.

ICP itself may be measured directly or indirectly by using one of the many devices on the market today. As is the case with cardiovascular parameters, ICP may also be monitored during a CCT. Changes in ICP during CCT must be evaluated and managed properly. In those instances where the aeromedical physician believes that the aerial transport is directly contributing to the deterioration of the patient's condition, a decrease in altitude or an emergency landing may be necessary. It is imperative that a baseline neurologic examination be made before beginning the CCT and that serial examinations be conducted throughout the transport until the patient is stabilized at the receiving hospital. If ICP monitoring is not an available option, then the neurologic examination will carry greater importance.

Although not used much anymore in the United States since the advent of CT, air encephalograms still may be performed, especially in less-developed countries. Considerations regarding pressure-volume changes would negate an aerial CCT, except in those conditions where an aircraft capable of 1 atm pressurization is available. These same considerations apply to the TP with an aerocele associated with a skull fracture.

The final consideration in this type of TP

is the ability to "clear" the ears (i.e., equalize pressure in the middle ear with the ambient pressure) because measures designed to open the eustachian tube may not function normally in the unconscious patient. This may necessitate either temporary puncture of the tympanic membranes bilaterally or the placement of polyethylene tubes to maintain a more permanent conduit. This point is discussed in greater detail in Chapter 14.

## Dysbarisms (49, 87, 88)

The term *dysbarism* generally refers to two conditions, decompression sickness and systemic air embolism (AGE), which are results of pressure-volume changes (see Chapter 14). These two conditions are most often seen in underwater divers and in patients and personnel in the hyperbaric chamber environment. However, dysbarism may also occur in association with aviation and hypobaric operations, especially secondary to explosive (rapid, sudden) decompression. The pathophysiologic problems with transport of these patients are discussed in great detail in Chapter 14. These conditions can be greatly influenced by the CCT environment. For example, a cabin altitude of 6000 to 8000 feet ASL will increase the volume of an air bubble by approximately 30% (Fig. 15.6). Patients with dysbarism may be unconscious and thus be unable to cooperate in middle ear pressure equalization.

## MEDICAL EQUIPMENT IN THE CRITICAL CARE TRANSPORT ENVIRONMENT

With respect to medical equipment, the CCT physician is generally concerned with equipment directly involved with either maintaining or monitoring the patient. The amount of equipment will usually increase in proportion to the severity of the patient's condition and can include mechanical ventilators, intravenous fluid infusion pumps, and monitoring equipment necessitated by the specific medical condition.

One immediate area of concern when

considering any item for CCT should be electrical power. As discussed previously in this chapter, the physician should evaluate points such as compatibility of electrical outlets and equipment plugs, capabilities of the particular aircraft to supply power during its various phases of operation (e.g., taxiing, parking, cruising), and accessibility of an emergency battery pack for each item.

Another area of concern is the compatibility of a piece of equipment with the transport environment. Size, weight, durability, and the ability to operate for extended periods on battery power are prime considerations. Many medical equipment companies manufacture items that possess these characteristics and include integrated three- and four-channel monitors to display parameters such as blood pressure, ECG, central venous pressure, and ICP. Compact pulse oximeters (which may prove useful as indicators of the adequacy of oxygenation in the hypoxic environment) and capnographs are available for transport missions. Small, lightweight mass spectrometers are also beginning to appear on the market. Some of this equipment has been specifically designed for the CCT environment. The physician should be aware of how a particular piece of equipment will function in the transport sphere and the degree to which the reliability of its data output will be affected.

The effects of pressure-volume changes on equipment performance in the aviation environment are similar to those in hyperbaric operations, although the effects are probably less. The reader should refer to "Critical Care in the Hyperbaric Chamber" (Chapter 14) and to Table 14.14. These effects will generally occur in an opposite manner as those described for hyperbaric operations. For example, a glass intravenous bottle may *im*plode because of an increase in ambient pressure in the hyperbaric chamber. The same glass bottle will *ex*plode during a flight because of a reduction in ambient pressure. Other pieces of equipment that will undergo significant changes as a result of pressure-volume effects are

listed in Table 15.6. Inflatable air bladders may be necessary to supply the driving pressure for intravenous infusion systems. The amount of fluid in the drip chamber may have to be adjusted as its volume of air increases with altitude. Sphygmomanometer cuffs must be left vented, and any air within them should be expelled forcibly. It is also wise to remove these cuffs from the patient's arm when measurements are not being taken. Endotracheal tube cuffs should be filled with water, instead of air, to obviate the need for continual readjustment of volume and "pressure-checks" with an anaeroid manometer. These same considerations apply to the cuff on a Foley catheter.

Another problem that may be encountered with equipment in the aviation environment is the inability to open bottles with screw-on tops at altitude because of increased pressure within them. The solution is to lubricate the tops with petroleum jelly and ensure that the threads are free of grime.

The following concerns apply to oxygenation and ventilation equipment: (*a*) Mechanical ventilators that are pneumatically driven will not function well at altitude unless a compressed gas source is available. (*b*) Thorpe tube flowmeters, which are usually used to measure the flow of oxygen, are inaccurate in the hypobaric atmosphere. Other types of flowmeters on regulator valves may also be inaccurate above 8000 feet ASL. (*c*) A humidification system must be used in conjunction with mechanical ventilators because of the extreme dryness of the aircraft cabin (89).

Specific information about medical equipment for aviation operations can be sought from the Aeromedical Systems Branch of the U.S. Air Force School of Aerospace Medicine at the Brooks Air Force Base, San Antonio, Texas. There are also other excellent sources that list acceptable equipment (41).

All electrical equipment used in an aircraft environment should be evaluated for the level of electromagnetic interference it produces and should be shielded if the level is excessive. When obtaining replacement oxygen tanks in a foreign country, ensure that the tank does, in fact, contain oxygen. Oxygen tanks in the United States are color-coded as green; however, this is not the case throughout the world.

## ANESTHESIA DURING CRITICAL CARE TRANSPORT

Review of the literature reveals scant information on the conduct of anesthesia at altitude. This might be explained by the facts that, until recently, the necessary equipment has been neither available nor acceptable and that anesthesiologists, for the most part, were not well represented in the transport field (90). As discussed above, the equipment necessary to support an anesthetic (e.g., monitoring equipment) is now available, and sophisticated critical care is being performed during transport. Small, compact anesthesia machines and ventilators have been designed, primarily for the military (91–97).

The reader might wonder why one would want to administer an anesthetic during CCT. Anesthesia during CCT, to varying degrees, is already being induced. One example is found in the cardiac patient who is heavily sedated to minimize the sensory input of the aviation environment and to decrease levels of anxiety. Other examples are the TP with a head injury who is transported while still in a "barbiturate coma" and the TP to whom Entonox is administered. A final example is the TP who is intubated and must be transported within the TC to the radiography suite for evaluation, before which a narcotic, benzodiazepine, and a muscle relaxant are administered to ensure both the patient's comfort and the quality of the study.

Induction of anesthesia reduces an individual's metabolic rate and oxygen requirements. This becomes important in a hypoxic environment such as that found in aerial CCT. Consider this point in relation to the seriously ill cardiac patient or the patient with a cerebral air embolism and secondary cerebral ischemia. On fixed-wing, long-range transports, an additional advantage is that using a closed-circuit anesthesia system with a carbon dioxide absorber will allow rebreathing and thus reduce the quantities of oxygen needed to operate both the mechanical ventilator and the cabin oxygen system, in addition to avoiding contamination of the cabin with exhaust gases.

At present, the technology exists to render a "full-scale" anesthetic during CCT. Documented and anecdotal information from persons practicing anesthesia at relatively high altitudes (e.g., Denver) has increased our understanding of this unique environment (98, 99). Further information on the effects of altitude on the various anesthetic agents is needed, with increased input from CCT anesthesiologists. Already, diverse anesthetizing locations are being designed and implemented, for example, aboard the NASA Space Station presently in development.

## SUMMARY

In this chapter, an attempt has been made to expose anesthesiologists to the realm of CCT. Considering the background of skills and knowledge possessed by an anesthesiologist, he or she is a "natural" for the aeromedical subspecialty. There is definitely a need for the expertise of these individuals in this field. It is hoped that this chapter will serve as an introduction and enticement for more anesthesiologists to pursue involvement in CCT.

## References

1. Baxt WG. Prehospital treatment and transport of the trauma patient. In Baxt WG (ed): Trauma: The First Hour. East Norwalk, CT, Appleton-Century-Crofts, 1985, pp 293–303.
2. Boyd DR. Foreword. In McNeil EL (ed): Airborne Care of the Ill and Injured. New York, Springer-Verlag, 1983, pp vii–viii.
3. McCarthy H. Waterborne ambulance covers 150 square miles in L.I. Sound. Emerg Department News, November 1982, p 5.
4. Hackel A. An organizational system for critical

care transport. Int Anesthesiol Clin 1987; 25(2): 11–13.

5. Gilman JI. Carrier and vendor selection. Int Anesthesiol Clin 1987;25(2):117–137.

6. Pearl RG. Critical care transport: specific issues. Presented at the Second Annual Trauma Anesthesia and Critical Care Symposium, Baltimore, Maryland, June 1989.

7. Ehrenworth J, Sorbo S, Hackel A. Transport of critically ill adults. Crit Care Med 1986;14: 543–547.

8. White RD. The role of the anesthesiologist in emergency medical services. Semin Anesth 1988; 4:102–113.

9. McNeil EL. Preface. In McNeil EL (ed): Airborne Care of the Ill and Injured. New York, Springer-Verlag, 1983.

10. Neel S. Army aeromedical evaluation procedures in Vietnam. JAMA 1968;204:99–103.

11. Trunkey DD. Trauma. Sci Am 1983;249:28–35.

12. Burghart H. The use of helicopters as mobile intensive units in disaster context and rescue services in the Federal Republic. Resuscitation 1974;3:143–145.

13. Burghart H. Helicopter rescue for traffic accidents: the West German experience. Emerg Med Serv, June 1986;72–74.

14. Oestern HJ. The German model for rescue of traumatized patients. Can J Surg 1985; 28:486–489.

15. Brismar B, Dahlgren BE, Larsson J. Ambulance utilization in Sweden: analysis of emergency ambulance missions in urban and rural areas. Ann Emerg Med 1984;13:1037–1039.

16. Felix WR. Metropolitan aeromedical service: state of the art. J Trauma 1976;16:873–881.

17. Duke JH, Clarke WP. A university-staffed, private hospital-based air transport service. Arch Surg 1981;116:703–708.

18. Robert S, Baily C, Vandermere JR, Marable SA. Medicopter an airborne intensive care unit. Ann Surg 1970;3:325–333.

19. Fischer RP, Flynn TC, Miller PW. Urban helicopter response to the scene of injury. J Trauma 1984;24:946–951.

20. Smith PJ, Bodai BI, Hill AS, Frey CF. Prehospital stabilization of critically injured patients: a failed concept. J Trauma 1986;25:65–70.

21. Border JR, Lewis FR, Aprahamian C, Haller JA, Jacobs LM, Luterman A. Panel: prehospital trauma care—stabilize or scoop and run? J Trauma 1983;23:708–711.

22. Berry R. Air transport of the trauma patient. Ala J Med Sci 1982;19:315–317.

23. Dreyfus UY, Faktor JH, Charnilas JZ. Aeromedical evacuation in Israel-A study of 884 cases. Aviat Space Environ Med 1979;59:958–960.

24. Copass MK, Oreskovich MR, Bladergroen MR, Carrico CJ. Prehospital cardiopulmonary resusci-

tation of the critically injured patient. Am J Surg 1984;148:20–26.

25. Baxt WG. The impact of a rotorcraft aeromedical emergency service on trauma mortality. JAMA 1983;249:3047–3051.

26. Wright SW, Dronen SC, Combs TJ, Storer D. Aeromedical transport of patients with post-traumatic cardiac arrest. Ann Emerg Med 1989; 18:721–726.

27. Moylan JA. Impact of helicopters on trauma care and clinical results. Ann Surg 1988;208:673–678.

28. Pepe PE, Steward RD. Role of the physician in the prehospital setting. Ann Emerg Med 1986;15: 1480–1483.

29. Baxt WG. Is there a role for flight physicians on EMS rotorcraft? Trauma Q 1985;1:39–42.

30. Pepe PE, Stewart RD. Prehospital management of trauma: a tale of three cities. Ann Emerg Med 1986;15:1484–1490.

31. Gorman DF, Coals J. Evaluation of a hospital-based accident flying squad using an injury scoring system. Injury 1975;14:513–518.

32. Gervin AS, Discher RP. The importance of prompt transport in salvage of patients with penetrating heart wounds. J Trauma 1982;22:443–448.

33. Lamont D. Accident services. Br Med J 1967; 2:374.

34. Slagel SA, Skiendzielewski JJ, Martyak GG, Brotman S. Emergency medicine and surgery resident roles as the trauma team: a difference of opinion. Ann Emerg Med 1986;15:28–32.

35. Trunkey DD. Is ALS necessary for pre-hospital trauma care? J Trauma 1984;24:86–87.

36. McSwain NE. On site trauma management. Surg Gynecol Obstet 1973;187:581–584.

37. McSwain NE, Kerstein MD. Preface. In McSwain NE, Kerstein MD (eds): The Management and Evaluation of Trauma. East Norwalk, CT, Appleton-Century-Crofts, 1987, pp xv–xvi.

38. Stewart RD, Yong JC, Kenney DA, Hirschberg JM. Field surgical intervention: an unusual case. J Trauma 1979;19:780–783.

39. Finch P, Nancelieviell DG. The role of hospital medical teams at a major accident. Anaesthesia 1975;30:666–676.

40. Sredl DM. The aerohemodynamics concept. In Sredl DM (ed): Airborne Patient Care Management. St Louis, Medical Research Associate Publications, 1983, pp 27–33.

41. McNeil EL: Regulations and operations. In McNeil EL (ed): Airborne Care of the Ill and Injured. New York, Springer-Verlag, 1983, pp 19–85.

42. Merlone S, Hackel A: Care of patients during long-distance transport. Anesthesiol Clin 1987; 25(2):105–116.

43. Lachenmyer J. Physiological aspects of transport. Int Anesthesiol Clin 1987;25(2):15–41.

44. McNeil EL. Aeromedical care: modifications of care. In McNeil EL (ed): Airborne Care of the Ill

and Injured. New York, Springer-Verlag, 1983, pp 91–107.

45. Departments of the Air Force, the Army and the Navy. Worldwide Aeromedical Evacuation, AR-40-535. Washington, DC, May 1979.

46. Departments of the Air Force, the Army, the Navy and Transportation. Aeromedical Evacuation: A Guide for Health Care Providers, Air Force Pamphlet 164-4. Washington, DC, September 1972.

47. Heimbach RD, Sheffield PJ. Protection in the pressure environment: cabin pressurization and oxygen equipment. In DeHart RL (ed): Fundamentals of Aerospace Medicine. Philadelphia, Lea & Febiger, 1985, pp 110–131.

48. Sredl DM. Acceleration. In Sredl DM (ed): Airborne Patient Care Management. St Louis, Medical Research Associates Publications, 1983, pp 74–89.

49. McNeil EL. Aeromedical care: care of the trauma patient. In McNeil EL (ed): Airborne Care of the Ill and Injured. New York, Springer-Verlag, 1983, pp 139–151.

50. Oxer HF. Aeromedical evacuation of the seriously-ill. Br Med J 1975;3:692–694.

51. Oxer HF. Carriage by air of the seriously ill. Med J Aust 1977;1:537–540.

52. Ingham PN. Pitfalls of aeromedical evacuation. Aust Fam Physician 1983;12:881–883.

53. Spoor DH. The passenger and the patient in flight. In DeHart RL (ed): Fundamentals of Aerospace Medicine. Philadelphia, Lea & Febiger, 1985, pp 595–610.

54. Von Gierke HE, Nixon CA. Vibration, noise and communication. In DeHart RL (ed): Fundamentals of Aerospace Medicine. Philadelphia, Lea & Febiger, 1985, pp 250–298.

55. Safar P, Esposito G, Benson DM. Ambulance design and equipment for mobile intensive care. Arch Surg 1971;102:163–171.

56. Snook R. Medical aspects of ambulance design. Br Med J 1976;3:574–578.

57. Snook R. Transport of the injured patient, past, present and future. Br J Anesth 1977;49:651–658.

58. Moles TM. Travel light, travel fast: motorcycle paramedics in Hong Kong. In Sixth World Congress on Emergency and Disaster Medicine, Hong Kong, Abstracts I. Amsterdam, Excerpta Medica, 1989, p 46.

59. Waddell G, Scott PDR, Lees NW, Ledingham I. Effects of ambulance transport in critically ill patients. Br Med J 1975;1:386–389.

60. Young AE. Transporting patients with chest injuries. Br Med J 1971;4:364.

61. Glover JR. Mortality of the ambulance ride. Br Med J 1967;3:678.

62. Stewart AB. Mortality of the ambulance ride. Br Med J 1967;3:797.

63. Cullen CH, Douglas WK, Danzigan AM. Mortality of the ambulance ride. Br Med J 1967;3:438.

64. Waddell G, Douglas LHS, Ledingham I. Cardiovascular effects of movement in hemorrhagic shock dogs. Crit Care Med 1974;2:68–72.

65. Snook R, Pacifico R. Ambulance ride: fixed or floating stretcher. Br Med J 1976;2:405–407.

66. Mann TP, Mount LE. Temperatures in ambulances. Lancet 1969;1:1257–1258.

67. Waddell G. Movement of critically ill patients within hospital. Br Med J 1975;2:417–419.

68. Hanning CD, Gilmour DG, Hothersall AP, Aitkenhead AR, Venner RM, Ledingham I. Movement of the critically ill within hospital. Intensive Care Med 1978;2:137–143.

69. Braman SS, Dunn SM, Amico CA, Millman RP. Complications of intrahospital transport in critically ill patients. Ann Intern Med 1983;107:469–473.

70. Waddell SG, Stuart B, Tehrani MA, McGarrity G, Reyes A, Smith HC, Ledingham I. Intra-arterial monitoring of critically ill patient in ambulances. Br Med J 1975;4:206.

71. Low RB, Martin D. Accuracy of blood pressure measurements made aboard helicopters. Ann Emerg Med 1988;17:604–612.

72. Aitkenhead AR, Willis MI, Barnes WH. An economical mobile intensive care unit. Br Med J 1980;1:1219–1221.

73. Ledingham I, Banks JG. Movement of the critically ill patient. Hosp Update, January 1980, pp 43–49.

74. McNeil EL. International missions. In McNeil EL (ed): Airborne Care of the Ill and Injured. New York, Springer-Verlag, 1983, pp 185–198.

75. McNeil EL. The aviation environment. In McNeil EL (ed): Airborne Care of the Ill and Injured. New York, Springer-Verlag, 1983, pp 19–88.

76. Committee on Trauma. Interhospital transfer of patients. Bull Am Coll Surg 1984;69:29–32.

77. Johnson A. Treatise on aeromedical evacuation: II. Some surgical considerations. Aviat Space Environ Med 1977;48:550–554.

78. Moylan JA, Pruitt BA. Aeromedical transportation. JAMA 1973;224:1271–1273.

79. Lee G. Transport of the critically ill trauma patient. Nurs Clin North Am 1986;21:741–749.

80. Committee on Trauma. Advanced Trauma Life Support Course Manual, ed 3. Chicago, American College of Surgeons, 1989.

81. Wong L, Grande CM, Munster AM. Burns and associated nonthermal trauma: an analysis of management, outcome and relation to the Injury Severity Scale. J Burn Care Rehabil 1989;10:512–516.

82. Grande CM, Wong L, Bernhard WN, Furman WR. Mechanisms of injury in the burn patient: thermal, nonthermal and mixed multiple trauma. Crit Care Rep (in press).

83. Pearl RG, Mihm FG, Rosenthal MH. Care of the adult patient during transport. Int Anesthesiol Clin 1987;25(2):43–75.

84. Kaplan L, Walsh D, Burncy RE. Emergency

aeromedical transport of patients with acute myocardial infarction. Ann Emerg Med 1986; 16:55–57.

85. McNeil EL. Aeromedical care: airborne cardiac care. In McNeil EL (ed): Airborne of the Ill and Injured. New York, Springer-Verlag, 1983, pp 151–161.

86. Vermeer M. Air transport of a patient with head injury. J Emerg Nursing 1982;8:60–62.

87. Parsons CJ, Bobechko WP. Aeromedical transport: its hidden problems. Can Med Assoc J 1982;126:237–243.

88. Reddick EJ. Movement by helicopter of patients with decompression sickness. Aviat Space Environ Med 1978;49:1229–1230.

89. McNeil EL. Aeromedical care: oxygenation. In McNeil EL (ed): Airborne Care of the Ill and Injured. New York, Springer-Verlag, 1983, pp 91–107.

90. Poulton TJ, Kisicki PA. Medical directors of critical care air transport services. Crit Care Med 1987; 15:784–785.

91. Donchin Y, Wiener M, Grande CM, Cotev S. Military medicine: trauma anesthesia and critical care on the battlefield. Crit Care Clin 1990; 6:185–202.

92. Redden JF, Little K. Anaesthesia and the accident flying squad: a new anaesthetic machine. Br Med J 1973;1:788–790.

93. Fryer ME, Boulton TB. Apparatus for emergency anesthesia outside of main hospitals. Anaesthesia 1977;32:189–196.

94. Gabriel RW. Medical equipment for an accident team. Anaesthesia 1977;32:179–188.

95. Marsh RHK, Ledingham I. Equipment for mobile intensive care. Br J Hosp Med 1981;4:377–385.

96. Adams AP, Henville JD. A new generation of anesthesia ventilators. Anaesthesia 1977; 32:34–40.

97. Gary AJG. Portable lung ventilators. Br J Hosp Med 1981;2:173–178.

98. James MF, White JF. Anesthetic considerations at moderate attitude. Anesth Analg 1984; 63:1097–1105.

99. Weaver RH, Virtue RW. Blood oxygenation as affected by tidal volume and tension of nitrous oxide and oxygen at one mile altitude. Anesthesiology 1955;16:57–66.

# 16

# Occupational Hazards for Trauma Health Care Workers

*Henry E. Rice and Bruce F. Cullen*

Providing anesthesia and surgical care for the trauma victim presents many hazards for the health care worker. The emergency room and operating theater are workplaces which, much like the car factory or machine plant, have their own set of occupational risks. Specifically, infectious hazards associated with trauma and the psychologic stress of care for these patients affect all members of the anesthesia and surgical team. This chapter addresses these occupational hazards.

## INFECTIOUS HAZARDS

Health care providers for trauma victims are exposed to a wide variety of infectious agents, including viral, bacterial, and fungal organisms. Bacterial and fungal infections, despite their prevalence, are rarely transmitted to otherwise healthy personnel. Two viruses are of great concern to the provider of trauma care, human immunodeficiency virus and hepatitis B virus. Although many other agents have reportedly been transmitted within the operative setting, these two agents are responsible for a great deal of

interest within the current literature and deserve detailed description.

### Human Immunodeficiency Virus

The human immunodeficiency virus (HIV) has been identified as the causative agent of multiple life-threatening diseases, with the acquired immunodeficiency syndrome (AIDS) representing the most lethal manifestation of the virus. Occupational transmission of HIV has been under investigation since AIDS was first recognized in 1981 and is of concern to all operating room personnel (1). It is the purpose of this section to review current studies of occupational transmission of HIV and recommendations to limit possible risk of exposure to the virus.

HIV has three main modes of transmission: sexual contact with an infected person, exposure to blood or blood products, and perinatal transmission from mother to fetus (1). Although HIV has been isolated from saliva (2), breast milk (3), tears (4), urine (5), cerebrospinal fluid (6), vaginal fluid (7), and alveolar fluid (8), only blood and semen have been directly implicated in viral transmission (1). Preliminary studies of viral transmission by saliva to dental workers have shown a low risk of HIV transmission (9). Nevertheless, many health care workers continue to be concerned about the risk of salivary transmission.

## HIV TRANSMISSION IN THE HEALTH CARE SETTING

Since the discovery in 1983 of the HIV (10), occupational transmission of HIV has been a topic of great study. Two approaches have been used to define the risk of transmission: longitudinal studies of workers exposed to HIV-infected blood or body fluids and isolated case reports of workers who have become infected with HIV via occupational exposure.

Currently, six major centers have initiated studies of health care workers exposed to blood or blood product inoculums through the work place (Table 16.1). Only health care workers with both no other known risk factors for HIV and documented seroconversion (antibody conversion from negative to positive between acute and convalescent sera) can properly document occupational viral transmission. Seroprevalence (antibody presence without known conversion after occupational viral exposure) has been used in other studies but does not clearly demonstrate acute HIV transmission.

The largest of the longitudinal studies is the ongoing Center for Disease Control (CDC) investigation of 938 health care workers with documented exposure to HIV … infected blood who otherwise have no known risk factor for HIV (11). Of those

938, 451 were tested for HIV antibody immediately and at intervals after percutaneous HIV exposure. Three persons had documented HIV seroconversion, for a rate of 0.3%. One other worker was seropositive, but no serum was obtained to document that seroconversion resulted from occupational exposure.

Geberding et al. have been following a group of 95 health care workers with documented viral exposure at the University of California in San Francisco. No worker demonstrated seroconversion over a 2-year follow-up (12). Hirsch et al. examined 85 employees with nosocomial exposure to HIV and found no cases of documented seroconversion of antibody (13). Weiss et al. followed 44 workers through the National Cancer Institute. Three health care workers were seropositive, although no one had documented seroconversion (14).

Henderson et al. followed 150 health care workers at the National Institutes of Health who reported percutaneous or mucous membrane exposure to HIV-infected blood or body fluids. No case of documented seroconversion was noted (15). In a British study of health care workers with percutaneous HIV exposure, McEvoy et al. were not able to demonstrate any seroconversion among 150 workers (16).

### Isolated Case Reports

In addition to the large institutional studies of HIV exposure, there have been several isolated case reports of health care workers with HIV seropositivity after percutaneous exposure (17–29). A review of current literature shows at least 24 cases of health care workers who became seropositive for HIV. Additional reports about further viral transmissions appear almost monthly.

These case studies, however, do not offer concrete data concerning the actual risk of viral transmission. Many case reports have poor documentation of other risk factors for HIV. Usually these studies do not detail testing for actual seroconversion. However,

**Table 16.1.  HIV Infection Rate in Health Care Workers with Percutaneous HIV Exposure**

| Study | No. Patients | No. Seropositive | No. with seroconversion |
|---|---|---|---|
| Marcus | 963 | 4 | 3 |
| Geberding | 94 | 0 | 0 |
| Hirsch | 85 | 0 | 0 |
| Weiss | 44 | 3 | 0 |
| Henderson | 150 | 3 | 0 |
| Total | 1336 | 10 (0.7%) | 3 (0.2%) |

these reports do support a need for further investigation of HIV transmission patterns.

## HIV PREVALENCE IN THE TRAUMA VICTIM

In the trauma setting, health care workers are in frequent contact with blood and other body fluids from patients about whom little medical or social history may be known. Subsequent identification of HIV-infected patients is often impossible, and the risk of occupational exposure to HIV may be difficult to quantify. Baker et al. tested blood from 203 critically ill patients when they presented in the emergency room. Six patients (3%) were seropositive for HIV (30). All seropositive patients were trauma patients between 25 and 34 years of age, representing a seropositivity of 16% for trauma patients.

Later follow-up studies with this group of patients have supported a high rate of HIV seroprevalence in trauma victims (31, 32). Kelen et al. noted a 13% risk of seropositivity in all victims of penetrating trauma regardless of known risk factors for HIV (32). Other trauma patients had a HIV seroprevalence rate comparable to that of other emergency room patients. An overall risk of 3.6% was found in all surgical patients, regardless of known risk factors (32). This seroprevalence rate is much higher than that in the general population and suggests that trauma health care workers may be exposed to a higher rate of HIV-infected blood than previously thought.

## SUMMARY

In short, the cumulative results from studies of percutaneous exposure to HIV demonstrate that the risk of seroconversion is relatively low, approximately 0.2%. Limitations may make the actual risk of occupational transmission either higher or lower than expected. In the absence of parenteral contact with HIV-infected blood, the risk of transmission is exceedingly low. No case of HIV transmission from direct contact with patients, exposure during surgery or anesthesia, or routine handling of laboratory specimens has been documented (1). Kuhls

et al. followed 246 health care workers, of whom 102 were classified as having high exposure to HIV-positive patients, with no case of seroconversion noted (33).

On the other hand, studies of percutaneous exposure to *known* HIV-infected patients may largely underestimate the number of health care workers exposed to the virus from *undiagnosed* HIV-infected patients. These reports examine a relatively small number of individuals. No conclusions can be drawn from the current studies as to risk of HIV transmission from undiagnosed patients, a potentially much larger population.

### Hepatitis

There are four common types of viral hepatitis in the United States, hepatitis A (Hep A), hepatitis B (Hep B), δ hepatitis, and non-A non-B (NANB) hepatitis. The viruses responsible for Hep A and Hep B have been clearly identified, but the exact etiology of NANB hepatitis has not been defined. δ Hepatitis occurs concurrently with Hep B or can be superimposed on a hidden Hep B infection.

## HEPATITIS A

Hep A is usually a self-limited illness, with patients having a 2 to 4-week period of malaise, jaundice, and anorexia. There is rarely a prolonged course with Hep A infection. The disease is caused by a picornavirus, with diagnosis confirmed by detection of immunoglobulin M antibody to the Hep A virus in acute and convalescent sera.

Transmission of Hep A is by the fecal-oral route, with most outbreaks due to contamination of food or water products. Hospital personnel do not seem to be at increased risk for Hep A, as patients with Hep A are rarely hospitalized. Staff of hemodialysis centers have no higher incidence of antibody to Hep A than is expected in the general population (34).

## HEPATITIS B

Hepatitis B virus (HBV) is a major cause of acute and chronic hepatitis, cirrhosis, and hepatocellular carcinoma worldwide. The severity of Hep B infection ranges from subclinical abnormalities of liver function tests to fulminating hepatic necrosis. Prolonged HBV antigenemia may be found in up to 10% of infected individuals. The CDC estimates that there are up to 300,000 HBV infections each year in the United States alone (35).

The HBV is a double-stranded DNA virus composed of a nucleocapsid core and a protein surface with a number of distinct subtypes based on surface antigen determinants. The diagnosis of Hep B can be made on the basis of serologic testing. Early in the course of the illness, Hep B surface antigen (HBsAg) is detectable. Later HBsAg disappears from serum and antibody to surface antigen (HBsAb) appears. During the window period in which HBsAg and HBsAb are not detectable, antibody to core protein (HBcAb) may be measured. Chronic Hep B carriers are likely to have HBsAg and HBcAb present in serum.

### Transmission of Hepatitis B to Health Care Workers

The transmission of Hep B to health care workers is an occupational health care issue of much greater magnitude than exposure to HIV. Approximately 12,000 cases of occupational Hep B transmission are documented each year (35). Of these infected patients, 500 to 600 are hospitalized, approximately 1,000 become hepatitis carriers, and 250 die from complications of hepatitis (35).

Occupational transmission of HBV occurs through several methods, including percutaneous transmission with infected blood, blood products, or body fluids (35). The role of the HBV carrier is central in the epidemiology of HBV transmission. Carriers and persons with acute infection have the highest concentration of HBV in blood and serous fluids (35). Unlike HIV, HBV is a relatively hearty virus that has been documented to be infectious for at least 7 days in dried blood on certain environmental surfaces (36).

In contrast to HIV, the risk for acquiring HBV after percutaneous exposure ranges from 10 to 35% (37). Transmission of HBV, without transmission of HIV, after percutaneous exposure to blood from an AIDS patient has been described (38). The higher rate of HBV transmission may be related to the higher titer of HBV in blood, although other hypotheses for this finding have been proposed, including cofactors such as concomitant viral infections or preexisting immunologic abnormalities (12, 39).

Anesthesia personnel seem at high risk for hepatitis exposure despite the use of operating room infection control techniques. Within the United States, the prevalence of HBV seropositivity among anesthesiologists ranges from 4 to 49% (40–43). Berry et al. have demonstrated that HBV seroprevalence among anesthesiologists increases with the length of time of anesthesia practice, suggesting that risk of infection is accumulated over time of exposure to infected blood (44).

### Hepatitis B Transmission in the Trauma Setting

Multiple groups have examined the incidence of hepatitis B in the emergency room setting and transmission to emergency health care workers. Studies from Seattle, Houston, and Boston have estimated the rate of HBV seropositivity in paramedics and emergency medical technicians at 13 to 25% (45–47). Pepe et al. showed that duration of employment as an emergency medical technician or paramedic was associated with increased incidence of Hep B seropositivity (47).

Paramedics are often involved in emergencies with uncontrolled bleeding, poor lighting, and patients covered with broken glass, which is difficult to remove without suffering percutaneous blood exposure. Paramedics also perform invasive procedures that increase exposure to blood, including intravenous line placement, thoracocentesis, and endotracheal intubation (45).

## Hepatitis B Prophylaxis

Hep B vaccine, licensed in 1981, provides active immunization against Hep B infection. Since 1987, the U.S. Government Department of Health and Human Services (DHHS) has mandated that Hep B vaccine should be provided to all health care workers at no cost. The DHHS has also encouraged workers exposed to significant amounts of blood and body fluids to be immunized against Hep B (37).

Effective immunologic response to commercially available Hep B vaccine, whether derived from human plasma donors or produced by recombinant DNA methods, is approximately 85% (37). Recent studies have shown that nonresponse to Hep B vaccine may be due to an absence of a major histocompatibility gene (48). The risk of HIV with Hep B vaccine is essentially nil (1). Prophylaxis with Hep B vaccine should be encouraged for all trauma and emergency health care personnel.

## Prevention and Control Strategies against Viral Transmission

Within the health care setting, general infection control procedures for the prevention of disease transmission have been adapted to the unique status of HIV. In 1983, the CDC published a document entitled "Guidelines for Isolation Precautions in Hospitals" (49). This document, amended in 1987 and referred to as the "Universal Precautions," now states that *all* patients should be considered potentially infectious for HIV, HBV, and other blood-borne pathogens (Table 16.2) (37).

Application of the universal precautions includes the rigid use of protective barriers including gloves, gowns, and eyeware (37). The CDC guidelines address issues of the body fluids to which precautions apply, the use of protective barriers and gloves, and the need for making changes in waste management programs. Rubber gloves will not reduce penetrating injuries due to needle and sharp instrument sticks but will reduce contamination due to blood spillage. When gloves are contaminated, they must be removed before one touches any other patient, anesthetic equipment, syringes, etc.

Several studies have examined the emergency health care practice of infection control techniques (12, 50). Adherence to the universal precautions is far from adequate despite encouragement from employers. It is crucial in the trauma setting to make it strict operating room policy to follow the CDC guidelines. As health care workers develop an increased commitment to universal precautions, worker anxiety may decrease and transmission of infectious agents may be better controlled.

Given the small but real risk of occupational exposure to HIV despite precautionary measures, new strategies of postexposure management are being defined. Studies have demonstrated that the course of some retroviral illnesses in animals can be altered by the prophylactic administration of zidovudine (AZT) (51, 52). These findings have led to interest in the use of AZT as postexposure prophylaxis for health care workers with exposure to HIV (53). However, the relatively low risk of viral transmission and the toxicity of AZT make the use of AZT as a prophylactic agent difficult to assess (53).

### Summary

Despite extensive advocation of control policies and the weight of epidemiologic evidence suggesting that the rate of HIV transmission to health care workers is relatively low, many workers perceive a

**Table 16.2.   CDC Recommendations to Control Transmission of Nosocomial Pathogens**

| Activity | Precautions |
| --- | --- |
| Patient contact | Handwashing before and after |
| Injections or phlebotomy | Gloves available, proper disposal of sharps, no needle recapping |
| Direct exposure to blood or body fluids | Protective barriers worn |
| Environmental contamination | Disinfection with germicide, proper waste management |

much greater risk of infection than actually exists. In part, these fears are based on a lack of knowledge of the mode of transmission of viral agents, but some workers remain fearful of AIDS and Hep B patients even after learning the facts.

In the trauma setting, where patients' medical histories are usually not known at the time of initial care, fear of patient contact could lead to disastrous results. These fears are in part derived from the complex psychologic issues surrounding AIDS patients, including homosexuality, mortality, and the looming mortality of the disease (54). For some health care professionals, it is easier to avoid the AIDS patient than to deal with the emotional conflicts encountered while providing care.

Still, health care workers who care for trauma patients are at a higher risk for occupational infections than are those in other areas of medical care. Trauma victims have an unusually high rate of HIV and HBV seropositivity. Personnel who care for these patients are at a greater risk for accidental percutaneous exposure or mucosal contact with patients' blood.

Physicians and other health care providers must assume the responsibility to educate themselves and the public about the possible occupational transmission of viral agents. Strict adherence to accepted guidelines for the prevention of transmission should be encouraged. At the very least, the need for Hep B immunization should be stressed.

## PSYCHOLOGIC HAZARDS

Of the potential hazards of trauma care, stress is universal among trauma health care providers. In psychologic terms, stress occurs when an individual must deal with a situation in which typical response patterns are inadequate and may negatively affect the outcome of the situation. There are several conditions within the trauma setting that contribute to the stress of patient care, including a need for rapid action and decision making, the treatment of critically

ill patients, fatigue, night duty, and interpersonal tensions (55, 56).

Several studies have focused on personality characteristics that predispose one toward maladaptive responses to stress (57). Vaillant et al. reported that students who demonstrate pessimism, passivity, self-doubt, and feelings of insecurity are more likely than controls to have their subsequent medical careers disrupted by substance abuse, psychiatric illness, and marital disturbances (58). Conservative estimates suggest that approximately 5 to 6% of all physicians are impaired by alcoholism, drug abuse, or mental illness (59). Suicide among medical students is the second most common cause of death (60).

An area of recent concern in the popular press has been the effect of "on-call" schedules on physician performance. Many studies have demonstrated decreased psychomotor performance after a 24-hour shift (61). McDonald and Peterson (62) and Cooper et al. (63) report fatigue as a major source of human error associated with anesthesia-related accidents. As the majority of trauma occurs at night, sleep deprivation may affect clinical care. The effect of physician fatigue and work-related psychologic stress on health care deserves more study.

## SUMMARY

Trauma care is virtually unequaled in the large number of infectious, physical, and psychologic hazards to health care providers. The risk of contracting HIV and hepatitis is an increasing concern among hospital staff, and these diseases are now recognized as potentially catastrophic effects of providing care to trauma victims. Current studies have followed small cohorts of health care workers percutaneously exposed to HIV-infected blood and have found the risk of seroconversion to be approximately 1 in 200. Further studies now in progress will further detail the patterns of HIV transmission in the workplace.

# References

1. Friedland GH, Klein RS. Transmission of the human immunodeficiency virus. N Engl J Med 1987;317:1125–1135.
2. Groodman JE, Salahuddin SZ, Sarngadharan MG, et al. HTLV-III in saliva of people with AIDS-related complex and healthy homosexual men at risk for AIDS. Science 1984;226:447–449.
3. Thiry L, Sprecher-Goldberger S, Jonckheer T, et al. Isolation of AIDS virus from cell-free breast milk of three healthy virus carriers. Lancet 1985;2:891–892.
4. Fujikawa LS, Salahuddin SZ, Palestine AG, et al. Isolation of human T-lymphotropic virus type III from the tears of a patient with the acquired immunodeficiency syndrome. Lancet 1985;2:529–530.
5. Levy JA, Kaminsky LS, Morrow WJW, et al. Infection by the retrovirus associated with the acquired immunodeficiency syndrome. Ann Intern Med 1985;103:694–699.
6. Hoa DD, Roa TR, Schooly RT, et al. Isolation of HTLV-III from cerebrospinal fluid and neural tissue of patients with neurologic syndromes related to the acquired immunodeficiency syndrome. N Engl J Med 1985;313:1493–1497.
7. Vogt MW, Witt DJ, Craven DE, et al. Isolation of HTLV-III/LAV from cervical secretions of women at risk for AIDS. Lancet 1986;1:525–527.
8. Ziza JM, Brun-Vezinet F, Venet A, et al. Lymphadenopathy-associated virus isolated from bronchoalveolar lavage fluid in AIDS-related complex with lymphoid interstitial pneumonitis. N Engl J Med 1985;313:183.
9. Klein RS, Phelan JA, Freeman K, et al. Low occupational risk of human immunodeficiency virus infection among dental professionals. N Engl J Med 1988;318:86–90.
10. Barre-Sinoussi F, Chermann JC, Reg F, et al. Isolation of a T-lymphotropic retrovirus from a patient at risk for the acquired immune deficiency syndrome (AIDS). Science 1983;220:868–871.
11. Marcus R. The CDC cooperative needlestick surveillance group: surveillance of health care workers exposed to blood from patients infected with the human immunodeficiency virus. N Engl J Med 1988;319:1118–1123.
12. Geberding JL, Bryant-LeBlanc CE, Nelson K, et al. Risk of transmitting the human immunodeficiency virus, cytomegalovirus and hepatitis B virus to health care workers exposed to patients with AIDS and AIDS-related conditions. J Infect Dis 1987;156:1–8.
13. Hirsch MS, Wormser GP, Schooly RT, et al. Risk of nosocomial infection with human T-cell lymphotropic virus III (HTLV-III). N Engl J Med 1985;312:1–4.
14. Weiss SM, Saxinger WC, Rectum D, et al. HTLV-III infection among health care workers: association with needlestick injuries. JAMA 1985;254:2089–2093.
15. Henderson DK, Saah AJ, Zak BJ, et al. Risk of nosocomial infection with human T-cell lymphotropic virus type III/lymphadenopathy-associated virus in a large cohort of intensively exposed health care workers. Ann Intern Med 1986;104:644–647.
16. McEvoy M, Porter K, Mortimer P. Prospective study of clinical laboratory and ancillary staff with accidental exposures to blood or body fluids from patients infected with HIV. Br Med J 1987;294:1595–1597.
17. Needlestick transmission of HTLV-III from a patient infected in Africa. Lancet 1984;2:31 (editorial).
18. Stricof RL, Morse DL. HTLV-III/LAV seroconversion following a deep intramuscular needlestick injury. N Engl J Med 1986;314:1115.
19. Neisson-Veinant C, Arfi S, Mathez D, et al. Needlestick HIV seroconversion in a nurse. Lancet 1986;2:814.
20. Oskenhendler E, Harzic M, LeRoux JM. HIV seroconversion after a superficial needlestick injury to the finger. N Engl J Med 1986;315:582.
21. Update: Acquired immunodeficiency syndrome and human immunodeficiency virus infection among health care workers. MMWR 1988;37:229–239.
22. Michelet C, Cartier F, Ruffault A, et al. Needlestick HIV infection in a nurse. Presented at the Fourth International Conference on AIDS, Stockholm, June 1988.
23. Barnes DM. Health workers and AIDS: questions persist. Science 1988;241:161–162.
24. Wallace MR, Harrison WO. HIV seroconversion with progressive disease in a health care worker after needlestick injury. Lancet 1988;1:1454.
25. Update: Human immunodeficiency virus infections in health-care workers exposed to blood of infected patients. MMWR 1987;36:285–289.
26. Apparent transmission of HTLV-III/LAV from a child to a mother providing health care. MMWR 1986;35:76–79.
27. Bygbjerg IC. AIDS in a Danish surgeon. Lancet 1983;1:925.
28. Belani A, Dunning R, Dutta D, et al. AIDS in a hospital worker. Lancet 1984;1:676.
29. Update: Evaluation of HTLV-III associated infection in health care personnel—United States. MMWR 1985;34:575–578.
30. Baker JL, Kelen GD, Sivertson KT, et al. Unsuspected human immunodeficiency virus in critically ill emergency patients. JAMA 1987;257:2609–2611.
31. Kelen GD, Fritz S, Quaquish B, et al. Substantial increase in human immunodeficiency virus (HIV-1) infection in critically ill emergency patients: 1986 and 1987 compared. Ann Emerg Med 1989;18:378–382.

32. Kelen GD, Fritz S, Quaquish B, et al. Unrecognized human immunodeficiency virus infection in emergency department patients. N Engl J Med 1988;318:1645–1650.

33. Kuhls TL, Viker S, Parris N, et al. Occupational risk of HIV, HBV, and HSV-II infections in health care personnel caring for AIDS patients. Am J Public Health 1987;77:1306–1309.

34. Szmuness W, Dienstag JL, Purcell RH, et al. Type A hepatitis and hemodialysis: a seroepidemiologic study in 15 U.S. centers. Ann Intern Med 1977;87:8–11.

35. Update: Recommendations for protection against viral hepatitis. MMWR 1985;34:313–335.

36. Bond WW, Favero MS, Peterson NJ, et al. Survival of hepatitis B virus after drying and storage for one week. Lancet 1981;1:550.

37. Update: Guideline for prevention of transmission of human immunodeficiency virus and hepatitis B virus to health care and public safety workers. MMWR 1989;38:1–36.

38. Geberding JL, Hopewell PC, Kaminsky LS, et al. Transmission of hepatitis B without transmission of AIDS by accidental needlestick. N Engl J Med 1985;312:56.

39. Drew WL, Mills J, Levy J, et al. Cytomegalovirus infection and abnormal T-lymphocyte subset ratios in homosexual men. Ann Intern Med 1985;103:61–63.

40. Siebke JC, Degre M. Prevalence of viral hepatitis in the staff in Norwegian anaesthesiology units. Anaesthesiol Scand 1984;28:549–554.

41. Berry AJ, Isaacson IJ, Kane MA, et al. A multicenter study of the epidemiology of hepatitis B in anesthesia residents. Anesth Analg 1985; 64:672–677.

42. Janzen J, Tripatzis F, Wagner V, et al. Epidemiology of hepatitis B surface antigen (HBsAg) and antibody to HBsAg in hospital personnel. J Infect Dis 1978;137:261–266.

43. Fryman PN, Hartung J, Weinberg S, et al. Prevalence of hepatitis B markers in the anesthesia staff in a large inner-city hospital. Anesth Analg 1984;63:433–437.

44. Berry AJ, Isaacson IJ, Hunt D, et al. The prevalence of hepatitis B viral markers in anesthesia personnel. Anesthesiology 1984;60:6–11.

45. Valenzuela TD, Hook EW, Copass MK, et al. Occupational exposure to hepatitis B in paramedics. Arch Intern Med 1985;145:1976–1977.

46. Kunches LM, Craven DE, Weiner BG, et al. Hepatitis B exposure in emergency medical personnel. Am J Med 1983;75:269–272.

47. Pepe PE, Hollinger FB, Troisi CL, et al. Viral hepatitis risk in urban emergency medical service personnel. Ann Emerg Med 1986;15:454–457.

48. Alper CA, Kruskall MS, Marcus-Bagley D, et al. Genetic prediction of nonresponse to hepatitis B vaccine. N Engl J Med 1989;321:708–712.

49. Garner JS, Simmons BP. Guideline for isolation precautions in hospitals. Infect Control 1983; 4:245–325.

50. Gerberding JL, Henderson DK. Design of rational infection control policies for human immunodeficiency virus infection. J Infect Dis 1987;156: 861–864.

51. Ruprecht RM, O'Brien LG, Rossoni LD, et al. Suppression of mouse viraemia and retroviral disease by $3^1$-azido-$3^1$-deoxythymidine. Nature 1986;323:467–469.

52. Tavares L, Roneka C, Johnston K, et al. $3^1$-Azido-$3^1$-deoxythymidine in feline leukemia virus-infected cats: a model for therapy and prophylaxis of AIDS. Cancer Res 1987; 47:3190–3194.

53. Henderson DK, Gerberding JL. Prophylactic zidovudine after occupational exposure to the human immunodeficiency virus: an interim analysis. J Infect Dis 1989;160:321–327.

54. Gerberding JL. Occupational health issues for providers of care to patients with HIV infections. Infect Dis Clin North Am 1988;2:321–328.

55. Clarke TZ, Maniscalco WM, Taylor-Brown S, et al. Job satisfaction and stress among neonatologists. Pediatrics 1984;74:52–56.

56. Mawardi BH. Satisfactions, dissatisfactions, and causes of stress in medical practice. JAMA 1979;241:1483–1487.

57. Vaillant GE, Sobowale NC, McArthur C. Some psychological vulnerabilities of physicians. N Engl J Med 1972;257:372–375.

58. Vaillant GE, Brighton JR, McArthur C. Physicians use of mood-altering drugs. N Engl J Med 1970;282:365–369.

59. American Medical Association: The impaired physician: an interpretive summary, Department of Mental Health. Presented at the AMA Conference on Impaired Physicians, San Francisco, April 1975.

60. Bittker TE. Reaching out to the depressed physician. JAMA 1976;236:1713–1718.

61. Denisco RA, Drummond JN, Granvenstein JS. Effect of fatigue on performance of a simulated anesthetic task. Anesthesiology 1984;61:A467–A470.

62. McDonald JS, Peterson S. Lethal errors in anesthesiology. Anesthesiology 1985;63:A497–A504.

63. Cooper JB, Newbower RS, Long CD, et al. Preventable anesthetic mishaps: a study of human factors. Anesthesiology 1978;49:399–404.

# 17

# Clinical Information Systems and Computers

*Barry Burns*

As the delivery of medical care becomes more complex and technically sophisticated, there is a parallel need to develop comprehensive clinical information systems to integrate information, streamline human operations, and control medical equipment and subsystems. A major goal is efficient data entry and sharing of data without *duplication of data entry* at different points within a system, which is costly and results in inconsistencies. A few secondary goals are listed in Table 17.1, demonstrating the wide range of features that must be considered when designing a medical information system (MIS). A key performance objective is the ability to support diverse activities while being able to accommodate future technologies and interact with other centralized information systems.

The typical problems faced by physicians, nurses, and administrators arise from unfamiliarity with computer technology and a resultant lack of insight into just what computers *could* or *should* do for them. Users are extremely capable of criticizing an existing system but are not too good at articulating or anticipating their needs. This is compounded by a lack of knowledgeable computer specialists with experience in more advanced operating systems and by the fact that both computer technology and medicine are evolving rapidly. The desktop computer of today was the supercomputer of yesterday, and obsolescence is occurring

**Table 17.1.  Secondary Goals**

| Capability | Components |
|---|---|
| Support of diverse applications | Clinical charting<br>Medical records<br>Physicians' notes/nurses' notes<br>Pharmacy/medication history<br>Patient billing/admitting<br>Inventory control/purchasing<br>Field services<br>X-ray, MRI, CT image storage/retrieval<br>OR schedule/utilization<br>Office automation<br>Continuous, real-time patient data collection<br>Computerized diagnoses<br>Electrocardiogram analysis |
| Communication with different types of computer systems | Support for all standard communication proto-<br>cols<br>Intelligent network control and administration<br>Least-cost automatic routing<br>International communication capability<br>Image, voice, video, and data over the network |
| User-friendly features | Menu-driven<br>Windowing software<br>19-inch color displays<br>Optical mouse/trackball for cursor control<br>Transparent communication/networking |

within roughly a 2-year time frame. It is the purpose of this chapter not to make a technical guru of the reader, but rather to explore some of the issues and answers relating to the more efficient use of computer technology in the medical environment.

## CURRENT TRENDS

The evolutionary trends today reflect movement away from the centralized computer mainframe connected to hundreds of terminals toward a more heterogeneous array of hardware in which intelligence is distributed throughout the network. In the distributed model, access to shared data bases (patient data, CT image files, etc.) or communication with systems inside and outside the network is provided by servers—special computers with very large disks that store large amounts of data, act as gateways for network communication protocols, maintain lookup tables for network user I.D.'s, etc. This is referred to as a client-server relationship (Fig. 17.1) and permits network communications that are *transparent* to the user (client) regardless of the type of system the individual user may have—PC, workstation, MRI image station, etc.

## STRATEGY

Let us approach this chapter from two perspectives. (*a*) *The first perspective* is that of an individual user who does not have adequate computer support for patient data analysis, research, word processing, teaching, slide presentations for meetings, special courses of instruction given by computer (cardiac arrest, anesthetic reactions), etc., but yet does not quite know where to begin and would like some good advice in the face of a bewildering array of hardware and software currently available. The process for the individual is similar to that of configuring a MIS for an institution, albeit on a smaller scale. As will be evident in the second perspective, a logical problem solv-

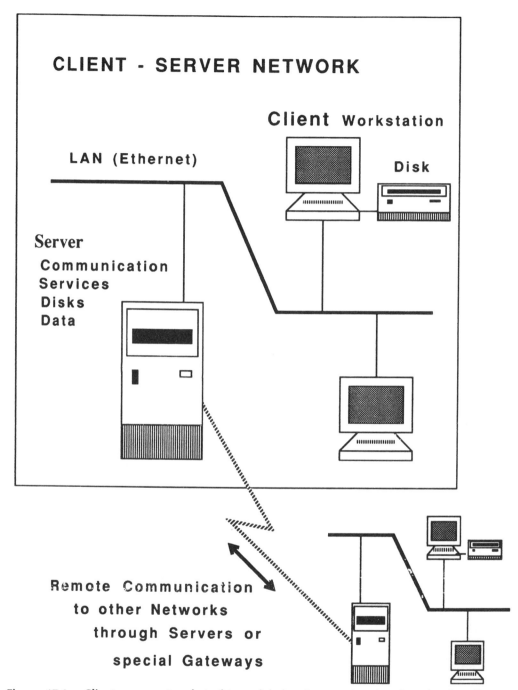

**Figure 17.1.    Client-server network.** In this model, the client workstations have local intelligence and are able to function independently of the status of the server or other clients. The purpose of the network is to allow increased communication among clients on the network and through the server to clients and resources on other networks. The benefits include file sharing; disk storage savings (large disks are present in the server and available to all clients); automatic crash recovery; the ability to mix and match PCs, workstations, mainframes, servers, etc.; simplified network administration; and cost reduction.

ing approach will clarify the objectives and highlight the types of obstacles that must be overcome. (*b*) *The second perspective* is that of an individual faced with the responsibility of computerizing an entire hospital or department starting from scratch. This is instructive because many departments are as large as some small hospitals. In addition, this exercise will provide insight for the individual computer user.

After completing the second perspective, we will explore implementation specifics relating to computers and networks (LAN selection, cabling and communication, electrical power, and application software considerations).

## THE INDIVIDUAL COMPUTER USER

The single user should make one of the three purchase decisions listed under "Specific Recommendations," based upon the application and funds available. Rapid advances in technology will make any system obsolete within 24 months; however, it is still possible to make intelligent choices that will have present benefit yet provide upward compatibility with new technology in the near future. These recommendations are based upon the author's experience in acquiring computers for research applications, installing systems, advising users, and providing computing resources for a variety of applications ranging from publication graphics to real-time data acquisition and networked systems.

More computer power for the personal computer (PC) user is not the ultimate goal. The objective is rather to get greater productivity from PCs at lower cost, i.e., to create more powerful users and not more powerful systems. The choke point is knowing how *low* a cost is too low and how *high* a cost is too high for an entry-level single-user system. As a business investment, companies that purchase large numbers of PCs find that 70% of the effective real cost goes for training and support and only 30% is applied to hardware and software. Furthermore, most individuals with PCs tend to use only one or two software packages routinely.

The following system recommendations incorporate IBM's MS-DOS operating system at the entry and intermediate levels (A, B), with graduation to the current industry standard UNIX operating system at the intermediate or low-end workstation level (C). MS-DOS is a better choice at the entry level for several reasons: (*a*) There are literally thousands of software programs available under MS-DOS. (*b*) MS-DOS itself is relatively well developed with few bugs. (*c*) Application software will execute faster and with fewer problems on an MS-DOS computer than on a different operating system that attempts to emulate MS-DOS. (*d*) Custom application software will be easier to obtain because more programmers are familiar with MS-DOS. (*e*) Finally, costs for both software and hardware will be lower because of the larger installed base of systems and associated volume discounts.

### Specific Recommendations

A. For system A, the user may elect to purchase an IBM-compatible PC and run MS-DOS programs in the single-user mode. Minimal system features should include:
- processor consisting of Intel 80386 32-bit chip, or better
- processor clock speed of 16 MHz minimum
- 1 Mb of memory
- 2-serial and 1-parallel port
- 14-inch autosynch VGA color monitor; 640 × 480 resolution
- autoswitch VGA card
- 40-megabyte hard disk
- 1.2-megabyte 5.25-inch and 1.44-megabyte 3.5-inch floppy drives
- Hayes-compatible autodial internal modem (2400 baud)
- impact printer (132-column) with 24-pin print head; tractor feed; optional dual sheet feeder
- 101 enhanced keyboard
- line conditioner or uninterruptible power system (UPS) with lightning arrestor

B. For package B, additional features may be added to upgrade package A for the intermediate to advanced user: features such as larger memory and hard disk, optical and tape drive backup and storage systems, a high-resolution color display (1280 × 1024 screen resolution), laser printer and publication graphics software, FAX boards, networking capability (Etherned board), image processing hardware and software, computer-aided design (CAD) packages and plotters, etc. For optimal performance, the intermediate-level user may wish to configure a PC to act as server with a large disk and networking software that would support additional diskless terminals for multiple simultaneous users. With a system of this type, the user could install and run the UNIX operating system under which MS-DOS could execute as a subprogram. Using this strategy, which consists of building a technical workstation from scratch, one must purchase application software and hardware from independent third-party vendors and install it oneself. If the system does not work because the software or hardware components are incompatible, the users become "system integrators" in essence and will have to learn more than they ever cared to know about computers to make the system work. A technical consultant is always the best option for system integration. Following is a list of items that would be added to the basic system in A to create the functional capability in system B of a file server or desktop workstation for the advanced user, a department, or a small business:

- 8 megabytes of main memory, minimal
- 140 megabytes of disk storage space, minimal
- math coprocessor chip (80387)
- laser printer for graphics applications; shared resource
- line printer; impact printer for word processing
- optical drive system backup (WORM— write once read only memory) of 1-gigabyte capacity
- power distribution unit and line conditioner/regulator with lightning arrestor
- Ethernet communications board
- UNIX Operating System (System V or BSD4.3) or, alternatively, MS-DOS with third-party network software

C. In the final package option the more advanced user may elect to purchase a desktop workstation or *bundled system* that uses the UNIX operating system and is shipped complete with graphics, networking, and commu-

nication software (Sun, Hewlett Packard, Sony, etc.). There is a common misconception that the technical workstation is too costly for the individual user. This may have been true in the past; however, the rapid evolution of workstations and PCs has closed the gap in both price and performance between the high-end PC and the low-end workstation. The typical user preference for the PC has been likened by some systems planners to a trap, preventing computer users from realizing the benefits of the truly integrated software and hardware available at the workstation level. In fact, when all of the equivalent hardware and software are assembled and added to the PC, it will still only approximate the capability of the workstation but will actually cost more. Furthermore, no single vendor can service or support the integrated PC system (caveat emptor), and small problems with a complicated PC network may assume large proportions. One of the biggest complaints about networking under MS-DOS is that the network software uses up so much memory that there is very little left over for the users in today's 640k DOS environment.

One of the advantages in using a workstation as a network server is that individuals who need a PC are able to communicate with the workstation for file storage, database access, etc., allowing a mix of high- and low-cost stations (clients) on the network and thereby optimizing its cost-effectiveness. Other advantages to the use of UNIX workstations relate to ease of system administration; enhanced security and user access control (virtually nonexistent with PCs); perfected networking and communication software; trouble-free access to shared peripherals such as printers, modems, etc.; the standard incorporation of high-resolution color graphics; windowing; and operating system utilities such as mail, text processing, software debuggers, and others.

The preceding general recommendations will guide the user in acquiring core pieces of computer equipment that are upward-compatible and thereby offer some protection against technical obsolescence. Exact component specifications will change with time.

In selecting a workstation vendor, Sun

Microsystems may be one of the current best selections, partly because their operating system is based on a converged version of AT&T's UNIX System-V and Berkeley UNIX 4.3; furthermore, Sun will not be a here-today-gone-tomorrow vendor. Sun has forged strong working relationships with AT&T, the originator of UNIX, and the Sun file system is considerably faster than many other UNIX file systems. Sun's virtual memory management accommodates programs that may be too large for other UNIX versions and, more importantly, programs written for other UNIX versions work on Sun systems because Sun has not altered the Unix file system and memory management interface—only the implementation. As with the PC, a large amount of third-party software is now available for the UNIX workstation.

Now that we have touched on the individual computer user, let us advance to the *second perspective* for a more comprehensive view of the planning and implementation process for medical information systems. At the system level, UNIX (Fig. 17.2) remains the operating system of choice for several reasons: it is not tied to any particular vendor, software is easy to develop for specific applications, it is superior in its file handling and shared resource capabilities, it contains the necessary building blocks (networking and communications) for an open distributed processing environment, and it is the industry standard internal operating system for high-performance workstations and PCs. Alternatives to UNIX are generally machine-dependent, proprietary systems and do not support the "open systems architecture" needed in the clinical environment, where a heterogeneous array of hardware is encountered.

## CONFIGURING A MEDICAL INFORMATION SYSTEM IN 10 EASY STEPS

### 1. Statement of the Problem

A general description of what is needed is

enlightening. For example, is it important to enhance patient care, reduce the workload for declining numbers of doctors and nurses, evaluate and improve therapies, support research, streamline operations and administration (billing, materials management, purchasing), provide for automatically entered patient data, maintain lab values and census information in the computer database, automate physician orders and nurses' notes, schedule the operating rooms or individual departments, provide patient demographic data, maintain a drug data base and computerized pharmacy, provide automated report writers and dictation services, restrict access to narcotic medications, schedule preventive maintenance for medical monitors and equipment, inventory controls, etc.? Obviously the more things the MIS has to do, the more sophisticated and expensive it will be to install and maintain. It is important to define the problem because its proper resolution will determine such things as type of hardware, network topology, physical site requirements, transmission media (coaxial cable, fiberoptic, twisted pair copper wire), etc.

### 2. Present Environment

Describe the environment where the problems exist. This is helpful because it may reveal certain obstacles to implementing simple solutions. Obstacles such as physical separation of buildings, which would require laying cables in utility tunnels requiring city government approvals or the use of microwave links or special satellite earth uplinks, are an expensive alternative. The environment description will assist vendors in accurately bidding the work to be performed and suggesting problem solutions. It is also possible that the problem exists primarily in a single department within an institution, and it may be cost-effective to restrict the scope of the MIS if the objectives can be narrowed.

### 3. Approach

This section would consist of a condensed

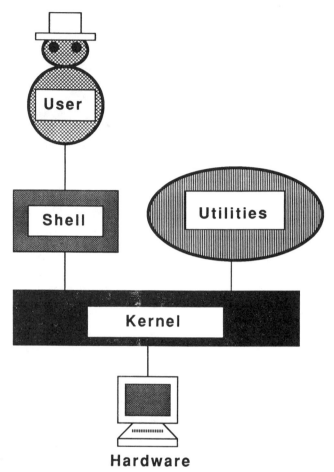

**Hardware**

**Figure 17.2.   Structure of UNIX.** UNIX is an operating system and not a language like C, FORTRAN, BASIC, etc. In this simple model, the UNIX system consists of various software programs written in the C language (*Shell, Utilities*, and *Kernel*) interposed between the user and the hardware (workstation). The Kernel manages the hardware and provides special services (filing, etc.) not enabled by the hardware. The shell is the immediate software interface between the Kernel and the User and acts both as a programming language and as a command interpreter. Utilities are special programs that make life easy for the user and include compilers, editors, debuggers, mail, typesetting software, spelling checker, dictionary, etc., numbering in excess of 200 individual routines. UNIX comes in several versions that are largely but not completely compatible. The name "UNIX" is not an acronym but was derived as a conceptual version of "castrated MULTIX," the operating system that was the basis for much of the UNIX development at Bell Laboratories. Enhancements have been added by the University of California at Berkeley, AT&T, Sun Microsystems, and others to fit different environments better—both commercial and academic. UNIX is the current industry-standard computer operating system.

review and argument in support of the rationale. The approach to the problem should be outlined, the schedule of implementation of the plan tentatively and briefly specified, and the rationale supported by logical arguments, cost-effectiveness, etc. General performance specifications should be included in the approach. This will help to target specific vendors and subcontractors who will contribute to the "Detailed Analysis."

## 4. Detailed Analysis

This part of the exercise requires the most work because it is a description of exactly what the computer system is supposed to do. It is necessary to define the type of network, performance standards, hardware (such as workstations, printers, magnetic or optical disk drives, mainframes, network servers, communication gateways, etc.), operating system and network control software, management personnel, system performance benchmarks, user interface, and cabling requirements. The detailed analysis should include the pro's and con's, with cost-effectiveness of any alternatives that might fulfill the primary objective of the system. Detailed specifications will determine the type of database management software required, the operating system needed, etc.

A variety of secondary considerations would be important to include in the detailed analysis. For example, is it necessary to consider communications system integration? What provision is needed for connection to the international disaster system network? How will chemical hazard and environmental emergencies be handled? Is communication with the center for infectious diseases control important? Should access be provided for poison center communication? Is it necessary to maintain radio links with emergency field personnel? Consideration might also be given to sharing patient databases with other hospitals and the federal government or accessing the National Library of Medicine database.

Specify any office automation aspects in this section; i.e., should the system provide for text processing, personal mail, telephone control (call restrictions for long distance dialing) and least-cost routing for long distance calls, publication graphics support, etc. A serious failing of most computer systems is that they fail to include support for the everyday activities that could be integrated very easily into a properly configured computer network. The simple ability to send electronic mail to an office secretary from a home or office computer terminal in the form of voice or text files would vastly increase office efficiency, help to eliminate transcription errors, and free up

considerable time for patient care that is wasted in trivial and relatively backward daily office activities that everyone must perform. Special consideration must be given to the selection of the operating system, telephone modem hardware, and even special security precautions necessary to protect such systems from unauthorized access. Security considerations are reviewed in more specific detail in later sections of this chapter.

## 5. Potholes

Configuring a MIS is much like planning a military campaign, with an overall strategy, battle plans, the use of new technology, preliminary skirmishes, and contingency plans for "worst-case" scenarios. The intelligent MIS planner will recognize and plan escapes from the following types of problems: hardware faults, operating system defects (is there an automatic and graceful recovery from failure without data loss?), application software faults (maintain dual patient database, provide for file and record locking, etc.), failed implementation plans due to personnel problems, acts of God, "institutional politics," or simply the pervasive and unstated administrative desire for tradition unhampered by progress.

## 6. Political Reality

Often during the planning process, technical issues seem to predominate for those most immediately involved in the system specifications. The likelihood of implementation of any particular plan is every bit as important as the selection of the operating system, workstation vendor, etc. To maximize planning efficiency, one must incorporate financial constraints and cost-benefit strategies into the system specifications. For example, will the system cost be too high, how many terminals can actually be purchased, are there institutional or departmental constraints to access to shared databases or equipment compatibility, among others.

Cost savings and revenue enhancements can be enormous with a properly configured

MIS that would serve anesthesia, nursing, radiology, surgery, administration, OR, ICU, general medical wards, pathology, clinical labs, pharmacy, blood bank, materials management, respiratory and physical therapy, biomedical engineering, purchasing, payroll, etc. How much time is spent each day charting patient data? These data could be entered automatically from monitoring equipment *without* transcription errors—not to mention the reduction in workload and higher levels of job satisfaction (and employee retention) such an automated computer system would allow. Consider even simple things such as medication errors: why not improve health care delivery by having specialized programs that will replace hand calculations with more accurate information in a form that is effortless to access and will include checks and balances for obvious magnitude errors or drug incompatibilities? How often is medication continued unnecessarily because the physician forgot to countermand the medication order at a later date? This situation is easily remedied by having standardized menus for physician's orders with an absolute requirement for duration of medication specified before the system will accept an order.

Issues of confidentiality and liability can be used to advantage in justification arguments. As an example, it is clear that more careful documentation of patient care and computerized reports of intraoperative records could be used as a valuable defense in malpractice cases, e.g., continuously sampled and stored blood pressure, pulse oximetry, and mass spectrometry data might reveal that at no time during surgery did the patient suffer a hypertensive, hypotensive, or hypoxic episode or an overdose or insufficiency of the anesthetic agent. However, for such information to qualify as a "legal document" it must reside in the computer database with specific access restrictions and there must be an audit trail of all transactions affecting this database, including dates, times, person accessing information, old information deleted, and

new information added. Malpractice insurance costs may also be reduced if retrospective stratified sampling of patient data substantiate lower incidence rates, i.e., if the documentation is positive. If a computer system is to be of much clinical value, a relatively sophisticated operating system and equivalent user application software are essential. "Wait," you say, "this is getting too complicated for me and I'm afraid that I couldn't use such a sophisticated system." Quite the opposite is actually true. Just remember that the more sophisticated the system, the more user-friendly it can be made and the less you will have to know about computers to use it.

## 7. Implementation

There is an optimal logical sequence for installing a MIS. It is important to schedule various phases such as ordering equipment, preparing the site, cabling and introducing physical elements, training personnel and establishing user groups with departmental representatives actively involved in these processes, testing at the various installation stages, and developing application software. The "old system" (if any) should be kept running until the new system is in place and debugged—this will help to avoid catastrophic outages that can generate immense user dissatisfaction.

A typical implementation program may have the following phases:
- system configuration and detailed specifications
- vendor selections
  —hardware
  —software
  —benchmark and performance tests
- network and support services installation
  —HVAC
  —electrical power distribution and conditioning
  —communication links and network backbones
- hardware installation
  —physical security
  —systems integration
- software development
  —team organization

—specification development
—writing, testing, and debugging of software and special device drivers
—preliminary user evaluations
—final modifications
—user inservice and final testing

## 8. Maintenance

What types of maintenance will be required? Clearly there will be both hardware and software maintenance. It should be possible to perform routine system maintenance while the system is running *without* interfering with its normal operation. The frequency of hardware maintenance should be scheduled (on the computer, of course), and predicted life should be used as a guide in the upgrading or acquisition of replacement hardware. Upgrades and expansion are included under maintenance and include such items as network expansion, the addition of new performance features to the operating system or hardware, database changes and improvements, the introduction of remote communication links (satellite, radio, or ground), and the interfacing of intelligent devices to the system.

## 9. Application Software Development

Hardware costs have fallen with the advent of new technologies, and wages for personnel have risen. The result is that only

about 20% of the total cost of a MIS will be spent on hardware and 80% will be spent on software, maintenance, and salaries over a typical 5-year operating period. It is extremely helpful if key members of the MIS management and software development staff can be identified and brought on-board before the detailed system configuration is established. Because they are going to be responsible for making the system work, they generally would know more about what to specify and how to hook it up than would a hospital administrator. One or two of these key people should actually be hired before the planning is begun. When asked, many clinicians and administrators profess to know a lot about computers and are quite willing to develop specifications themselves. Beware of this trap. A surgeon would not ask the janitor to recommend a surgical approach that he was about to attempt, nor would an anesthesiologist feel comfortable letting the surgeon attempt to give anesthesia.

Individual users will constantly want new programs, and the development of application software with proper system integration is a full-time job for several persons. Installing a computer network is just the first step. Staff will take the responsibility for writing new application software, solving network-related problems, and providing real-time system management (Table 17.2).

**Table 17.2.   Data Processing Manpower Costs for Software Development (Sample Project Development Costs)**

| Typical Project | Cost | Effort | Duration |
|---|---|---|---|
| | ×1000 | man-months | mo |
| Admission registration | $10 | 3 | 3 |
| Telephone directory | 70 | 11 | 6 |
| Personnel system | 50 | 7 | 9 |
| Calendar of events | 7 | 2 | 2 |
| OR schedule[a] | 560 | 64 | 24 |
| Personnel recruitment | 85 | 12 | 3 |
| Billing and accounting | 216 | 30 | 13 |

[a] OR schedule to include operative data record, sponge counts; OR sheet (turnover, transport, etc.); nursing notes/physician notes; anesthesia notes; unit dose/drug compatibility; emergency procedures; equipment availability; materials & supply lists/utilization; housekeeping/transport coordination; patient fluid administration/balance; bloodbank coordination; audit trail/corrections; transcription/dictation; medical/pharmaceutical dictionary; procedure lists/instrument lists; billing report; OR utilization review/staffing needs.

## 10. Staffing

There are certain key personnel for any reasonably sophisticated MIS. These personnel will be responsible for maintaining system security, 24-hour operation, hardware and software maintenance, data storage and retrieval, the interfacing of new devices to the system, and the development of new application software. As stated previously, it is desirable to hire one or two key persons before the planning phase is started.

## NETWORKS AND DISTRIBUTED PROCESSING

This section deals with specifics relating to networks, communication, security, electrical power requirements of computers, and important user application software issues such as selection of database management and statistical packages. The trend toward distributed intelligence in computer networks creates special problems in maintaining network security and providing clean electrical power with proper isolated grounds. Some aspects of the centralized computer systems of the past (such as site preparation and security) must be carried forward into the new distributed environment for user and database protection.

## Basic Topology of Local Area Networks (LANs)

A LAN could be defined as a user community working in the same general vicinity or environment, e.g., a department, a building, or several buildings linked by a communication cable (copper or glass fiber), laser, or radio link. It is desirable for LANs to communicate with each other either across town or around the world using a common language and standard communication protocols. There are several communication protocols that are used worldwide, including Ethernet, X.25, IEEE 802.3, 802.4 Token Bus, and 802.5 Token Ring.

Ethernet is the most popular hardware technology for local area networking and was invented by Xerox in 1973 to connect large computers with printers. The IEEE specification for Ethernet defines both signal characteristics and type of wire that is acceptable (50-ohm-thick coaxial cable, thin coaxial cable, and optical fiber). Ethernet uses a bus topology, with each station broadcasting to all other stations on the network. Terminating resistors are placed at each end of the Ethernet cable to keep signals from reflecting back onto the bus and causing unwanted collisions. A collision is the result of two devices or stations attempting to access the Ethernet bus at the same time, in which case a time-out is called and then successive attempts are permitted. The more users on an Ethernet, the more collisions and timeouts will occur and the longer user response times will be. Ethernet can be configured with standard telephone wire networks that function acceptably—although they do not meet the IEEE specification.

Two other network configurations are encountered frequently: these are the *ring* and *star* topologies (Figs. 17.3 and 17.4). These two alternate topologies accomplish essentially the same goals. Depending upon the application, however, one may be preferred over the other. The primary distinction between Ethernet and ring versus star topologies is that the ring and star configurations require special hardware and software for the network to function. The unique network control point permits ring or star network services to be handled in a manner that is transparent to the individual user, but there is a higher cost for both hardware and personnel to maintain the network as compared to Ethernet (Fig. 17.5). The advantages of ring and star over Ethernet include speed, better security, rapid fault location, and the potential for rerouting traffic around broken links. The fail-safe aspects of a ring or star network take on greater significance in a busy clinical environment.

Other desirable features of networks allow users access to distributed databases, provide transparent communication with

# LOCAL FIBER RING

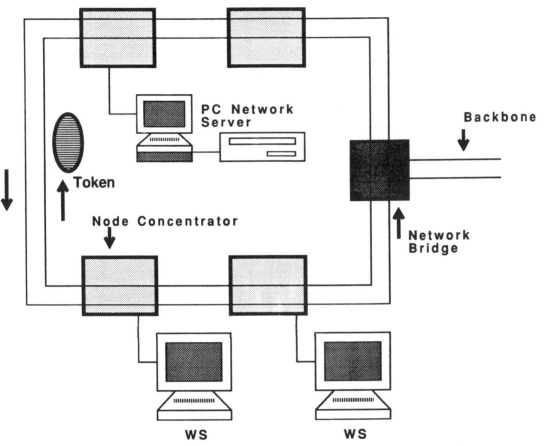

**Figure 17.3.   Token ring network topology.** The dual ring configuration provides a certain measure of redundancy. Should the link between any two node concentrators be broken, the local network server will reroute the token in the opposite direction on the second fiber in the two nodes adjacent to the break in the communication cable and all of the network nodes will remain in constant communication. A fiber token ring configuration would operate in excess of 100 Mb/sec, and communication over the backbone with other local fiber rings would be in excess of 200 Mb/sec. Unless the token is somehow encoded, a drawback of this configuration is that every node has access to all information in the token packet, resulting in poor system security. Additional problems arise should the token get "lost," in which case the entire local fiber ring is nonfunctional until the system adminstrator can resolve the problem. Workstations are represented (WS). The network server would consist of a microcomputer running special network software and dedicated to the local fiber ring. This type of network requires continuous human oversight and intervention in the form of a network manager.

the outside world through gateways or servers, and provide more efficient communication with each other over the same LAN. In addition, special services such as publication graphics support, large statistical packages, etc., can be provided to many users simultaneously with a properly configured network and operating system.

## Making LAN Decisions

The dilemma over which LAN technology to implement is heightened by the slow

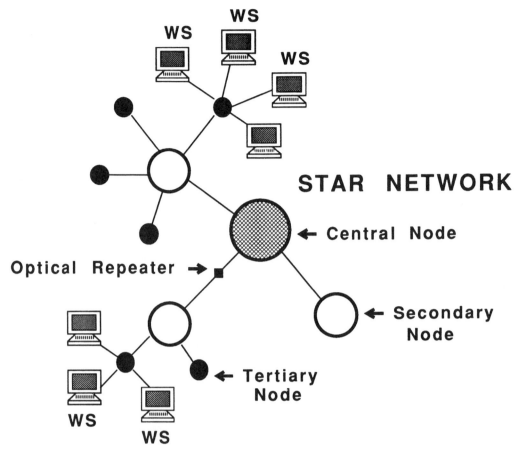

**Figure 17.4.   Star network topology.** Each node in the star topology has the capability of transmitting into the central node and of having its transmitted data received by all other nodes in the network. Likewise, each node has the capability to receive all of the data that are transmitted by all other nodes on the network. Star networks can have either active or passive nodes, the latter giving higher reliability by eliminating the single point of failure in active star networks. Ethernet transceivers conforming to IEEE standard 802.3 can be used throughout if the network is implemented with a fiberoptic Ethernet physical layer. Because fiber has a virtually infinite bandwidth, such a network should serve for many years as data rates are increased from the future FDDI standard (100 Mbits/sec) through 1,000,000 Mbits/sec. Any fiber network has the capability to carry voice, video, and data simultaneously. If a cable in a fiberoptic star-configured network is damaged or severed, only the node on that cable is affected. If any part of a standard Ethernet coaxial cable system is damaged or severed, the resulting reflections will cause continuous data collisions, making the entire network useless until the damaged cable is located and repaired. Optical repeaters may be used for long lengths of fiber between nodes in a star network. Also, for data speeds in excess of the 10-Mbit/sec Ethernet rate, the star network requires additional network server hardware in a manner equivalent to the token ring in Figure 17.3. The requirement for additional network software increases the total cost and also requires the physical presence of staff dedicated to network administration and maintenance. *WS*, workstation.

and erratic movement toward standards that incorporate higher-level protocols for LAN users. There are both de facto standards and those that are legally sanctioned. The user is advised not to wait for final resolution of "standards wars" because some of the most widely used de facto standards, such as TCP/IP (Transmission Control Protocol/Internet Protocol: specifications for a subset of the capabilities needed to

# Multiple Ethernet Network

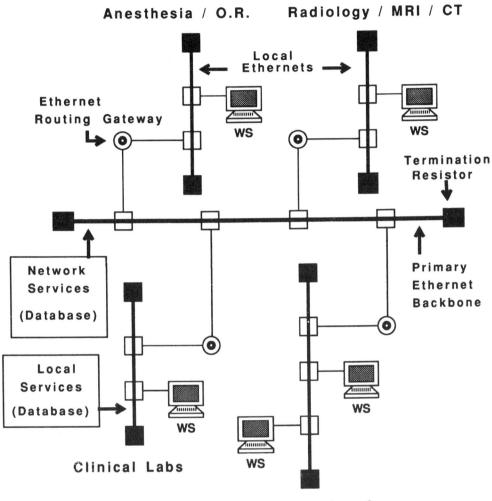

communicate on a network), often perform adequately. TCP/IP became accepted as a de facto standard in 1982 when it was incorporated into the UNIX 4.2 BSD operating system kernel and embodied a protocol mapping Ethernet to Internet addresses—permanently connecting TCP/IP to Ethernet. The Sun Microsystems Network File System (NFS) uses TCP/IP as a conduit through which intermachine communication is achieved. It is only a matter of time before one standard is replaced by another. OSI protocols (Open Systems Interconnection), which will specify all of the capabilities for communication on a network, will someday replace TCP/IP.

The problems involved in standardizing networks are formidable because for years customers have been buying the latest in computer equipment, which runs different operating systems, represents files in different ways, has different performance capabilities, and cannot communicate between vendors. Approximately half of all LANs are PC LANs with diverse third-party networking software.

It is unlikely that any single LAN technology will prevail in the future, and users often tend to select LANs supported by their hardware and software system vendors. For example, IBM users often choose the token ring topology, whereas Ethernet dominates most technical and workstation environments. Installation of a particular wiring technology may preclude certain LAN technologies. If a user selects "DEC-connect," the site cannot then support either Star LAN or Token Ring. It is wise to make vendor decisions first and then select the LAN second.

Speed is not usually a primary LAN consideration except in image storage and analysis or large database applications. For example, a PC typically has an Ethernet throughput of 400 kbps (400,000 bits per second)—or less if limited by hard disk speed. This represents only 4% of the 10-megabit per second Ethernet bandwidth (Fig. 17.6). The PC can only use a fraction of the existing Ethernet bandwidth, primarily because of limitations created by its internal bus (wiring) structure. Even newer and faster processor chips such as the Intel 80386 and 80486 will not provide much

**Figure 17.5.    Ethernet topology.** It is often said that "one of the nice things about standards is there are so many to choose from," and Ethernet is no exception, with three different transceiver standards: version 1, version 2, and the IEEE standard 802.3. Unfortunately, these three versions cannot talk freely to one another. For example, version 1 does not provide for 802.3's 0-volt idle state, and some of the commercial network software interface packages are sensitive to anomalies such as this. The lesson to be learned here is that Ethernet versions must be matched when systems are being fashioned. As can be seen from this figure, Ethernet is a relatively simple configuration with no requirement for an intelligent network control computer (and associated administrative staff, diagnostic equipment, etc.). By logical arrangement of local activities, local Ethernets can function without the need to send information over the "primary backbone" to remote locations. This will reduce the frequency of collisions (because only one station can talk at once following Ethernet protocols) and help to maintain short response latencies for individual users. Using this concept, distributed data can be autonomously maintained by departments, yet still be available for remote access through specialized software such as the network file system (NFS), which runs under the UNIX operating system and was developed by Sun Microsystems. The NFS allows transparent file access, which means that users on the network with different types of computers can share files without having to know anything about the other machines—and need not even be aware that they are using a remote file on another machine. Even though Ethernet is widely accepted, users over the next few years should be prepared for movement away from the 10-Mbit/sec Ethernet to the 100-Mbit/sec fiber distributed interface (FDDI) networks; 1-Gbit/sec networks will follow. *WS*, workstation.

# Ethernet Bandwidth

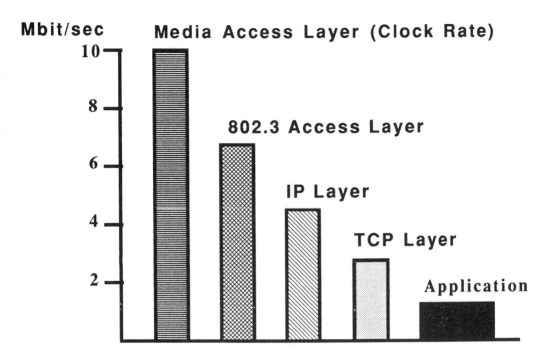

**Figure 17.6.    Ethernet bandwidth.** This figure reveals that only 6.7 Mbit/sec of the stated 10-Mbit/sec Ethernet bandwidth is available to a host at the 802.3 access layer, as would be represented by an Ethernet interface chip in a workstation or PC. Successive functional layers between this chip necessary for communication with the network and the user program reduce the final bandwidth to only 1.2 Mbit/sec for the end -user application, which means that very little of the original bandwidth is actually available and users occasionally find Ethernet to be intolerably slow in such things as downloading image files across the network (CT scans, CXRs, etc.), transferring large data files, etc.—preventing other users from having speedy access to the network and reducing overall system efficiency. Otherwise, Ethernet is an acceptable compromise, and there is vendor hardware and software available to accelerate markedly the communication rate over Ethernet. *IP* = Internet protocol; *TCP* = transmission control protocol; *Application* = user program.

relief until there is a 32-bit communication bus standard for the PC and high-speed intelligent disks with larger memory buffers utilizing caching techniques become available. Caching refers to retrieval from disk and placement into a special memory buffer of information most likely to be needed next as a means of speeding up program execution.

The PC is rapidly being replaced by the intelligent workstation with its 32-bit or 64-bit bus, high-speed disk with caching controller, and high-resolution graphics dis-

play. Users selecting LAN technology should look ahead to those technical performance specifications that are acceptable in a workstation environment where >100-megabit per second LAN speed may be needed.

### Transmission Media

Communications links within a network include microwave, radio frequency, infrared, laser, fiberoptic, coaxial copper cable, and twisted-pair copper wire. One of the newest advances in digital communication technology is called Integrated Services Digital Network (ISDN); it will merge digital image, voice, and data transmissions on the same line using unshielded twisted-pair or standard telephone wiring.

Use of copper cable has the advantage of low cost but is associated with several disadvantages: (a) distance limitations on bandwidth, (b) electrical interference, (c) bulk and weight, (d) difficulty in reconfiguration (cost of installing new copper cable dwarfs all other network costs), (e) poor security, and (f) limitations on numbers of users. Fiberoptic voice/data transmission, on the other hand, is noise-free and secure. Glass fibers have the strength of steel cable, and ruggedized field versions are virtually unbreakable. The fundamental problem with copper wires is that the attenuation over distance rises with the transmitted frequency. This relationship makes telephone trunk lines unsatisfactory for 10-megabit Ethernet, which is optimized with coaxial cables—and even these have a distance limitation of 200 meters between nodes (thinwire). There is no distance limitation for bandwidth on glass fibers, but there is a need for repeaters to boost signal strength every few kilometers. Fiberoptic cables excel at carrying high bandwidth (>100 megabits per second) over long distances. It is well accepted now that the next generation of LAN will be 62.5-μm glass fiber using the Fiber Distributed Data Interface (FDDI) standard. Fiber is probably the only viable choice for the FDDI networks and can easily accommodate up to 1000 nodes with a 2-km internode spacing or a 200-km token ring size.

Fiber networking of entire buildings and complexes of buildings is both cheap and efficient. Compared to copper cable, glass fiber is always cheaper to install when the distance exceeds 200 feet and a single small strand can replace a 6-inch-thick conduit of copper cables. In addition, the bandwidth of glass fiber is wide enough to eliminate the need for special cables for very-high-speed terminals and permits a central processor and high-resolution graphics display to be located more than 50 feet apart. The nonconductive glass fiber can be routed adjacent to power cables, relays, etc., with absolutely zero electrical interference. Fibers are difficult to tap without cutting into the cable or otherwise interfering in a manner that causes a detectable reduction in signal strength. Because the fibers are nonconductive, they can also be used in explosive or hazardous environments with complete safety (OR, hyperbaric chamber, etc.). Other medical applications of glass fibers will continue to evolve. They are being used in diverse areas such as the manufacture of disposable catheter-tip blood pressure sensors.

## Principles of Fiberoptics

In contrast to electrical current in copper cables, fiberoptics uses pulses of light for digital communication at a wavelength around 1.0 μm. The light pulses are typically transmitted through a "multimode" glass fiber 50 to 100 μm in diameter. The fiber cladding is selected to give either a step-change in refractive index (step-index fibers) or a graded change in refractive index (graded-index fibers). These are technical distinctions but are important considerations depending on the light source (LEDs or semiconductor lasers). Graded-index fibers are designed to minimize modal dispersion by minimizing travel time differences for different modes (wavelengths) of light. Chromatic dispersion increases with the range of wavelengths produced by the light source and results from wavelength-dependent variations in refractive index. Because LEDs produce a wider range of wavelengths than do semiconductor lasers, they are more susceptible to chromatic dispersion.

Common graded-index multimode fibers have core diameters of 50, 62.5, 85, or 100 μm and, with the cladding, add up to 140 μm to the minimal overall diameter. Certain applications with ultra-high-bandwidth requirements (such as 4000 × 4000-pixel high-resolution medical images—MRI or x-ray films) or transmission over extremely long distances may require special fibers referred to as "single mode." These fibers have a core that is about 3 μm in diameter and utilize a single wavelength of light between 1.3 and 1.5 μm. Single-mode fibers have very little attenuation and are used mainly in point-to-point communications. Their expense usually precludes their use in a typical fiber LAN.

### Fiber Termination Devices

At the ends of each fiber, there must be devices to convert the photons to electrons (reception) or electrons into photons (transmission). Some termination devices also function as multiplexers, combining signals to get higher throughput. The most costly termination devices are token-ring multiplexers, followed by Star LAN multiplexers and simple Ethernet transceivers. As intelligent workstations become the standard delivery platform, they will incorporate the fiber termination device internally and connect directly to the network via glass fiber.

### Image Transmission and Data Compression

A logical application of fiberoptic systems is in medical image transmission, storage, and data compression. X-ray films, MRI and CT scans, ultrasound films, and other medical diagnostic images will be incorporated into digital image management systems (DIMSs) and picture archiving and communication systems (PACSs) in the filmless imaging department of the 1990s. DIMSs and PACSs will confer many advantages over current methods: digitized images are easily stored and retrieved; poor image quality can be improved through the use of special computer routines referred to as image enhancement; images can be made available from remote locations; substantial cost savings will be realized (silver in archived x-ray films, cost and maintenance for developing systems, personnel expenses, etc.).

Image quality is the major concern in DIMSs. The standard CT scan is composed of a matrix of 512 × 512 pixels with 12 bits ($2^{12}$ or 4096 shades) of grey-scale data per pixel. At a data transmission rate of 9600 bits per second (baud), it would take more than 5 minutes to transmit this simple image over narrowband transmission media such as ordinary telephone lines. Furthermore, for diagnostic x-ray purposes an image of at least 2048 × 2048 pixels may be necessary. Image quality is affected primarily by matrix size and pixel depth, and even fiberoptic systems of the future may not be fast enough without incorporating data compression techniques.

Image compression is an electronic technique that identifies redundancies in the digitized image and encodes and compresses pixel data in ratios ranging from 4:1 to 30:1. The limits of data compression depend on the specific mathematical algorithms used and the diagnostic value of reconstructed images compared with the originals. Compression will also reduce data storage costs substantially. Often the compressed image is adequate for routine referral while the patient is under treatment. Fiberoptic systems with their much higher potential data transfer rates in conjunction with data compression and computerized diagnostic techniques will constitute the next revolution in medical imaging procedures.

## NETWORK AND SYSTEM SECURITY

### The Computer Room

Movement to the client-server network with distributed intelligence does not eliminate the requirement for a "computer room"—the definition is just changed slightly. There is always a need for physical security and environmental controls for servers and shared network resources such as large magnetic or optical disk storage systems, magnetic tape drives, tape libraries, operating system software, and proprietary application software. For larger multiuser systems there should be an organized group of rooms and work areas that are strategically located to restrict access and provide administrative, networking, and electrical power control nodes. Do not use a basement if flooding may occur; likewise, check elevator size and load capacities for rooms above the ground floor unless you plan to rent a crane and make deliveries through a window.

For future expansion, it is a good rule of thumb to acquire electrical and air conditioning systems with at least 50% more capacity than you currently require. Likewise, provide 50% more floor space in these rooms than necessary to save "down-time" for future expansion/renovations—not only will this space be used quickly, but you will have more flexibility in relocating systems as you add new technologies to the system. Insist on a 9- to 12-inch raised floor in areas housing servers, tape drives, disk drives, and tape and media storage, and avoid water-cooled air conditioning systems at all cost. Remember, media, paper, and peripheral equipment should be kept in the same environmental conditions (temperature, humidity, and filtered air) as your important system components. Some manufacturers claim that their servers will not require special air conditioning—don't believe it. There can be a 30°F gradient between the inside and the outside of a file server cabinet, and wide fluctuations of room temperature or shutdown of the physical plant will cause electronics that must be left turned on 24 hours a day to overheat, become unreliable, or fail altogether.

### External Access and Communication Controls

#### SECURITY AND FILE LOCKING

Once a network has been established, it then becomes important to establish security and protective measures to prevent access or tampering by unauthorized users. Unfortunately, the system with distributed intelligence is rather exposed and even more prone to problems of this sort. The recently sensationalized computer virus problems and unauthorized system logins promise to be the leading causes for headaches in modern information systems. Envision the scenario in which decisions relating to patient care in life-or-death situations are based upon stored patient data from a database that has been modified by an unauthorized user or deleted altogether. Determination of liability could be a very complicated task indeed.

Three layers of security must be present to ensure complete protection for the data and programs within a system: (a) physical security with restricted physical access to important system or network components, (b) operating system security to limit both authorized and unauthorized user access to the system, and (c) routine daily security checks and audit reports with some intelligent system administration software to take action for repeated failed login attempts, identify users who fail to log out properly, etc. A secure operating system should be heirarchical (Fig. 17.7), with complete access to all configured hardware and software resources given only to the security administrator. The next level in the hierarchy would include associate administrators given access privileges to maintain the system on a day-to-day basis, followed by principal users, data entry personnel, and others.

Most operating systems have file protection schemes to limit access to sensitive user data files. In a secure system, file protection must be expanded to include peripheral devices such as removable disks and tape drives that can copy information. Only the security administrator and associate administrators should be allowed to write to tapes or removable media. Principal users and all others below that level should be permitted only to read tapes or disks, whereas data entry personnel and "guest users" should be denied access to all removable media. A complete image of all data, user files, and the operating system should be maintained as a backup on read-only optical disks in the event that the entire system is disabled or

# Hierarchical Security

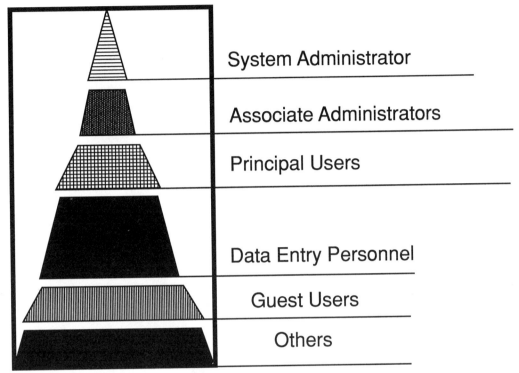

System Administrator

Associate Administrators

Principal Users

Data Entry Personnel

Guest Users

Others

**Figure 17.7.    Hierarchical security pyramid.** All users should receive security-level ratings. Access to the system and data bases may be controlled by terminal location, building, day of the week, time of day, field or data type within a data base, etc. Different levels of access to shared data make the system more efficient and avoid unnecessary duplication of information entry. Simple tasks such as logging users out automatically at unattended terminals after a finite time interval help to maintain system security. In future networks, security will be enhanced by voice recognition, individual user typing patterns at the keyboard, signature recognition, etc.

corrupted by a virus, vandalism, or electronic component failure.

In a secure system there should also be mechanisms to prevent users from reading an executable module, making changes to it, and then saving it under a new name. These protections are embodied in resource accountability features, which can generate audit trail reports to indicate when security violations occur. The accountability features also alert users that there will be a record made if they attempt to go beyond their approved limits. In a secure system, only the security or associate administrators should be able to initiate system boot processes by password control. These same persons should be the only ones authorized to initiate a system (server) shutdown, which should be executed only from the system console and which will alert users of the impending shutdown of the system or network in a timed and graceful manner.

It is extremely rare nowadays that a system would have to be physically shut down because backups, routine maintenance, and software modifications can be accomplished simultaneously with system operation—assuming that the proper selection of operating system and computer hardware has been made. Furthermore, with intelligent stations the users may continue to function even with failure of the network server (until shared data or resources must be accessed).

## CALLBACK

A variety of measures have been tested for limiting access to the LAN by external users through telephone modems. Perhaps one of the simplest and most secure is the "callback" feature. Both digital and analog callback security systems are in existence. Their basic function is to allow callers to identify themselves by typing in their authorized telephone numbers; then the host computer (server) or modem will automatically disconnect the line, consult memory to check the number's validity, and return the call to the authorized location. A unique advantage of this system is its inherent audit trail capability to monitor both authorized and unauthorized users. An audit trail provides summary information that helps to deter intruders even if they have knowledge of a valid identification number and its associated location. Another advantage of the callback system is that remote-user access can be controlled simply by deleting access number and location information without changing the host system user password.

## ANALOG MODEMS

Analog telephone modem systems are not widely used. The analog systems provide a higher degree of telephone line control than do digital systems because they have the ability to reject unauthorized users at the modem handshake request stage. The unauthorized users are not given a handshake recognition tone so they (or their computers) are totally unaware that they have reached a computer system.

## ELECTRICAL POWER REQUIREMENTS

The first thing that must be realized when analyzing power problems is that clean and consistent utility power does not exist. Dirty power constantly surges through the lines and is also created locally by relays, equipment, etc. If not dealt with properly, this army of electrical mutations will enter your computer system or network, where it will not be well received. "Dirty power" is a rather vague term and includes such things as electrical noise, transients, frequency deviations, voltage fluctuations (surges and sags), brownouts, and periodic blackouts. Electrical noise is the main cause of chip and device failure, and the more sophisticated the chip, the more sensitive it is to electrical noise, partly because newer chip components are closer together (1 to 4 µm) and it takes less voltage to "bridge the gap."

Electrical noise occurs in normal and common mode forms. Normal mode noise appears from line to line, and common mode noise occurs from common to ground. Both versions are equally destructive. Common mode noise poses a special threat to medical equipment and computers because the safety ground is often used as the computer logic reference point for communication purposes.

Transients represent another special type of problem. The most devastating transient for electrical equipment is lightning, which will easily destroy sensitive equipment. Smaller switching transients occur when power is turned on or off for various utility systems, creating high voltage and high current pulses that travel down the line acting as small bolts of lightning on their way to your computer. Small transients will corrupt programs, cause permanent memory loss, and destroy discrete components on circuit boards. Longer-lasting transients (surges) can damage disk drive motors and memory devices.

### Clean Power

The solution to all of the above problems, excluding blackouts, is the installation of power distribution units (PDUs) with tab switching technology that will isolate, filter, and regulate utility power. With a PDU, dirty power comes in and clean power goes out to your computer system. Not only does the isolation transformer provide spike suppression, it also eliminates common- and normal-mode noise while regulating the output voltage to your computer within precise limits (prevention of brownouts or sustained overvoltage).

### Battery Backup

A solution for blackout electrical problems is to provide an uninterruptible power supply (UPS); these are battery-based systems, however, which will provide power only for short periods (15 minutes to 2 hours). An UPS usually requires more space and maintenance than it may be worth except for the most critical applications or the individual user with a small PC-based system. If the power fails for a long period at night, even an UPS will not keep your computer from going down unattended.

### Motor Generator

The ultimate solution for power problems is your own private motor generator, which allows you to become a power company. Very few installations can afford, much less justify this approach. Even a motor generator is not without problems; there must be a backup unit that is either periodically brought on line or alternated with the primary unit, creating momentary outages and switching transients akin to the electrical noise discussed previously.

### The Best Solution

The cheapest solution is just to condition your power properly and disregard temporary loss of electrical power. In a practical sense, any good operating system should be able to handle power outages gracefully and *automatically* restore the user to the same point in the task under way when the power returns. This recovery ability should be one of the selection criteria for the operating system and computer hardware during the acquisition and planning stages. This solution applies to both the single-user PC system and the distributed network. A single-user UPS is a good investment for the stand-alone system. In a client-server environment, at least the server should be protected with an UPS of adequate capacity.

### DATABASE MANAGEMENT SYSTEM

### Desirable Features

A database management system (DBMS) is an aid to managing and interpreting increasingly large quantities of clinical data. Many of the existing systems are either so limited or difficult to use that they present barriers to convenient use. Clinicians rarely have the technical expertise (or the time or desire to acquire it) to master these aids. Some of the newer versions, however, promise to end much of the frustration users have experienced. A properly configured DMBS is an invaluable tool for clinical research.

In recent years, relational DBMS systems have gained acceptance with their easy handling of ad hoc queries and application prototyping. The goal of the user is to find a relational system that can also perform real-time, on-line applications for the single or multiple user. In such situations, network access may be required. From the user's perspective, desirable features would include a window-based set of tools for building and running decision support and on-line applications. The DBMS software should support a range of hardware (computer and terminal) types, distributed data management, and the client/server systems approach. The DBMS data server should have a backup utility that will enable the data server to stay on-line during backup operations. Most DBMSs do not permit use of the database while it is being backed up, and routine backup could be performed several times a day in a busy clinical environment. In addition, a fast recovery time (interval defining the length of time it will take to recover the database) is essential to minimize disruption of operations.

### SUMMARY AND CONCLUSIONS

The individual computer user must decide to use either a PC or personal workstation (PW). PCs are easier to set up and run;

however, networking, systems integration, software selection, and support limit their desirability. The PC is best applied as a simple tool for a relatively simple task, and it has a definite utility for the low-end single user or as a low-cost node on a client-server network providing access to shared data (as in data entry applications). Considerably higher productivity and lower support costs can be achieved with a PW that combines the following features: speed and power to run more user-friendly software; high-resolution display for greater information density and better utility; flexible and transparent networking that encourages shared information; enhanced security; and the ability to run programs that incorporate aspects of artificial intelligence. The problem with more powerful PCs is that they are evolving into workstations with brains but no education—and a limited capacity to obtain one. The use of these powerful PCs is developing into a software and systems integration nightmare. The user is trapped because the apparent low cost of a PC masks the crushing burden of expense related to training, support, and systems integration (add a frustration factor for all of the third-party software and hardware that are incompatible in one way or another).

New technologies for networking are appearing yearly, and each has its strengths and weaknesses. For the forseeable future, the computer user is advised to utilize Ethernet in the form of either a simple "Ethernet backbone" or "star LAN" configuration. In the multi-user environment the client-server approach is preferred, as long as the server can support a respectable operating system and is not just a "souped-up" PC with little software support and a lot of loose ends.

Site preparation remains important for the PC and the PW. Adequate cooling is important, and systems will generally perform better if kept on continuously. Electrical power fluctuations and outages can be handled easily with the provision of an inexpensive mini-UPS for key components (servers, network controllers, etc.) or single PC or PW users.

## References

1. Booker E. Fiber optics shed light on university communications. Communications Age October 1986; pp 32–35.
2. Courington B. The Unix System: A SUN Technical Report. SUN Microsystems, Inc, 1985.
3. Garrett RD. Hospital Computer Systems and Procedures, Volume II, Medical Systems. Mason/Charter, Publs, 1976.
4. Hime JA. Development and direction of network services. IEEE Circuits Devices 1986;2(4):17–21.
5. Schneider M, Tolchin SG, Kahane SN, Goldberg HS, Barta P. A workstation-based inpatient clinical system in the Johns Hopkins Hospital. In Proceedings of the 9th Annual Symposium on Computer Applications in Medical Care, November 10–13, 1985, pp 388–393.

# Medical, Legal, and Ethical Issues: General Principles of Medical Jurisprudence and Special Modifications When Applied to Trauma Anesthesia

*Christopher M. Grande, Jonathan Greenberg, and William N. Bernhard*

It is well established that cases of an emergency nature are more likely to lead to legal action than are elective situations, and trauma management is often emergent (1). The reasons are multifactorial but include the type of patient population usually involved (e.g., drug abusers); the circumstances of the relationship formed with the physician (i.e., the patient does not choose the physician and vice versa); the level of emotional anxiety, which is high (for both the patient and relatives); and the fact that the outcome is often poor, unexpected, and/or unappreciated. Approximately 85% of cases that involve bodily injury and involve two or more cars terminate in litigation (2).

It is also well established that the practice of anesthesiology carries a high risk of litigious outcome. The reasons for this have been summarized (3):[a]

1. Anesthesia is practiced in a high-risk environment (e.g., emergency room, operating room).
2. Anesthesia involves working with other high-risk medical professions (e.g., surgery, obstetrics).
3. Anesthesia uses some of the most "dangerous" pharmacologic agents in medicine (e.g., narcotics, muscle relaxants).
4. Personal error is prominent.

For physicians, what is legal may not be ethical; what is ethical may not conform to what the law allows or demands of physi-

---

[a] Due to variations in state law, a competent local attorney and/or the department of risk management at the involved hospital should be consulted before basing significant actions upon statements in this chapter.

cians. There is inevitable friction whenever the respective value systems of law and medicine interfere. All physician-patient interactions, however, including those in the context of emergency medical care, are defined and regulated not only by medical ethics but also by precepts of law.

After reviewing the medicolegal literature, it becomes apparent that several different categories of existing laws and guidelines are relevant to caring for the trauma patient (4–11). These codes are not all contained within the written law. Frequently, other standards are used in conjunction with the law to establish criteria to govern the activities of the medical community and to decide the fate of suits in the courts. Included are publications such as the *Accreditation Manual for Hospitals* compiled by the Joint Commission on Accreditation of Health Organizations (JCAHO) and the written policies (bylaws) of a given hospital, as well as textbooks and the testimony of recognized experts in a particular field. Further, the law allows for variations of a given situation, such as emergencies.

Common issues that arise in the course of rendering treatment include (*a*) whether there exists an obligation to treat; (*b*) what constitutes emergency lifesaving therapy; (*c*) whether it is necessary to obtain a consent (and, if so, what constitutes an informed consent); (*d*) how to deal with refusals of lifesaving therapy; and (*e*) specific problems, for example, those arising from administration of blood transfusions and treatment of the pregnant patient and fetus.

First, let us look at the basic principles that exist and thus must be addressed in every case, whether an emergency or not (12). These principles are referred to as *tort laws*. The word "tort" signifies a "wrongful act" or "injury" and represents the liability to which every citizen is subject for committing a "wrong" against another person, as opposed to a "wrong" committed against society (criminal laws). These torts may be divided into intentional or unintentional. An act that leads to an unintentional tort is termed *negligence*. Negligence can occur in

situations where something was done that should not have been done or, vice versa, when something that should have been done was not done. It is implied that the standard for comparison is what a "reasonable person" would have done in a given situation. What is considered "reasonable" may vary. The acts of an intern who manages a multitrauma victim alone in an emergency situation during his first month of training cannot fairly be compared with the acts of a board-certified trauma surgeon.

It is thought by some that more stringent requirements for proving negligence are demanded in medical cases (13). The following reasons are given: (*a*) society wishes to nurture the health care professions; (*b*) it is generally recognized that adequate judgment and appreciation of the acts of a highly trained medical professional are beyond the ability of lay jurors and judges; (*c*) the element of unpredictability associated with the human organism is such that a poor result does not necessarily indicate malpractice. One author reported that, despite popular opinion within the medical community, the volume of medical malpractice suits has not increased (although settlements have), only 1 of 10 cases of negligence ever become the focus of a suit, and the defendants (physicians) usually prevail (13).

In a recent study conducted by the Committee on Professional Liability of the American Society of Anesthesiologists, the most frequent critical incidents leading to patient injury and death were related to (mis)management of the respiratory system. These included inadequate ventilation, esophageal intubation, air embolism, and respiratory obstruction. Esophageal intubation was the most common of the specific respiratory problems that caused injury (14).

Other common plaintiff complaints in suits against anesthesiologists include "too much anesthesia"; death from anesthesia; injury to the eyes, teeth, or skin; injury due to mask, airways, or improper positioning on the operating table or from struggling, fires, or explosions; pneumonia; complications of spinal anesthesia; injury in the recovery room; failure to document proceedings or follow-up; failure to obtain proper consent; problems related to the choice, proper maintenance, or use of equipment; and problems related to airway maintenance and ventilation (e.g., unrecognized esophageal intubation) (15, 16). Review of the claims made involving anesthesia entered in the Closed Claims Study of the American Society of Anesthesiologists reveals no significant differences in the types of problems that produce claims when trauma patients are compared with others (17).

The key to a defendant's success in lawsuits is *documentation*. Hospital and physicians' records are routinely subpoenaed in medicolegal cases. The basic tenet that, "if it is not written, it wasn't done" should always be kept in mind.

Basically, four major areas of tort law apply to medicine (16, 18): consent and informed consent, standard of care, creating the duty, and respondeat superior. In most instances, the plaintiff must sequentially prove wrongful action: (*a*) that a particular obligation (duty) of the physician existed, (*b*) that this obligation was unfulfilled, (*c*) that a close causal relationship exists between what the physician did or failed to do and the results, and (*d*) that the results of such actions or inaction resulted in actual "damages" (4–16).

In situations in which a breach of one of these conditions cannot be demonstrated, for example, because of the unavailability of an expert witness, the plaintiff may plea *res ipsa loquitur*, which translates to "the act speaks for itself" (19). In this case, proof of transgression of one of the four conditions is unnecessary and negligence is inferred. With regard to this concept, it must be shown that the wrongful act would not have occurred in the absence of malpractice, that such results were under the exclusive control of the defendants, and that the patient's actions did not contribute to the result. In anesthesia-related cases, because patients are not in control of their facilities, they

often cannot be held responsible. The *res ipsa loquitur* doctrine may be invoked more often in these types of cases (12).

This chapter reviews some of the salient legal principles governing the physician-patient relationship, how it is modified in the emergency/trauma situation, and potential areas of ethical conflicts. To focus the discussion, a hypothetical patient problem is presented.

## HYPOTHETICAL CASE PRESENTATION

A 16-year-old, pregnant Jehovah's Witness is struck by an automobile while crossing a street. She sustains bilateral tibia-fibula open fractures, several left-sided rib fractures, a cerebral concussion, and possible pelvic or intraabdominal injuries. She arrives in the triage area mildly hypotensive, with tachycardia, confused, and screaming, "Save me!" She is noted to have poor dentition, is approximately 6 months pregnant, and has a small amount of blood in her vagina. A diagnosis of possible traumatic placenta previa is made. Her parents, arriving with her, state that they are Jehovah's Witnesses and demand that no blood products be given to their daughter; they request that everything possible be done to save the fetus. Both paracentesis and thoracentesis demonstrate hemorrhage; the patient may require an exploratory laparotomy for possible splenic injury or liver lacerations.

Numerous questions arise: Should the patient be given a blood transfusion if medically indicated? What if the patient herself refused a blood transfusion? Should she undergo surgery? Fetal monitoring? If there is fetal distress, should she have a cesarean section? Should she have dilation and curettage at the expense of the fetus' survival? What if the parents did not know she was pregnant? Does it make a difference whether she is 5 months pregnant or 6 months pregnant? Should the physician team decline to treat the patient altogether, or should they temporize while arrangements are made to transfer the patient to a trauma center 1 hour's travel away? To answer these questions, we will review the basis of each of the four areas of tort law and their special application to the emergent trauma patient.

## CONSENT AND INFORMED CONSENT

Whenever a physician touches a patient, this is legally done by *implied consent*. Without this form of consent, the doctor would be committing an intentional tort: assault and battery (unconsented bodily contact). Under certain circumstances, this may involve *criminal* laws. In the case of more invasive procedures such as surgery, *express written informed* consent should be obtained (13). Oral consent may be valid, but it is difficult to prove in court; thus, hospital policies usually require written consent.

The concept of informed consent is based on a classic case from 1914, when these words were spoken by Judge Cardozo (20): "Every human being of sound mind has a right to determine what shall be done with his own body; and a surgeon who performs an operation without this patient's consent commits an assault for which he is *liable damage . . ."

To fulfill the requirements for a legally valid informed consent: (*a*) the patient must be competent; (*b*) the physician must disclose to the patient the facts, outcomes, and risks about what is intended to be done; and (*c*) there must be no pressuring or coercion of the patient.

An adult is assumed to be competent to consent to or refuse treatment (*informed refusal*) unless the person is *formally* declared incompetent. However, a determination of competency involves the circumstantial analysis of a person's ability to make a responsible decision. The presence or lack of competence may vary depending on the particular issue (e.g., a person who is not competent to handle personal business affairs may nonetheless have sufficient understanding to give or withhold consent competently regarding medical treatment) (21, 22).

Constitutional considerations of personal privacy and autonomy, particularly in light of *Roe* v. *Wade* (23) and its progeny (21), affect issues of legal capacity and competence. They are indicative of the great value attached to allowing individuals to give or withhold consent freely in our system of law. The rights of minors to terminate pregnancies without parental consent (legal capacity) under certain circumstances underscore this point (21).

Not all parties are interested in medical recovery at all costs in every instance. A patient with legal capacity and competence to consent to treatment may also legally refuse emergency lifesaving medical treatment, with certain exceptions (24). The physician must respect the patient's personal autonomy (23) and, on occasion, accept the derivative right to refuse treatment, however much this contravenes a physician's instincts for preserving life.

Currently there are two procedures that allow decision making on the behalf of an incompetent person with respect to therapy: durable power of attorney and committee of the person (13).

Whenever the issue of competence arises, as in this hypothetical case, the hospital administrator should be apprised immediately and should be prepared to obtain a court order allowing emergency medical therapy and, if necessary, to make the hospital the guardian for the patient. The physician should be prepared to document the circumstances of the refusal and whether, in his or her professional opinion, the patient is medically competent to make a considered judgment regarding emergency lifesaving therapy. Obvious brain injury, whether direct (concussions, contusions, hemorrhages) or secondary to systemic pathology (shock, multiple organ failure) or drug intoxication, physically impairs the patient's cognition. A psychiatrist may have to assess a patient's nonorganic (functional) cognitive deficits. Lifesaving medical care should not be delayed pending judicial resolution of the issue.

In the hypothetical case, the administrator may obtain a court order to proceed with lifesaving therapy for the patient, including blood transfusions (in spite of her parents' refusal), to protect the life of a minor. Blood transfusion can be further justified in terms of preserving the fetus, especially during the second and third trimesters. Even if the patient refused blood transfusions, an argument could be made that this would jeopardize the fetus. If the fetus were nonviable (by virtue of gestational age or intrauterine damage) and emergency dilation and curettage were necessary to stop a life-threatening vaginal hemorrhage, the physicians would be justified in taking the actions necessary to preserve the patient's life.

A minor normally must have consent given by his or her legal guardian. Exceptions include most emergencies (25); medical care for pregnancy, venereal disease, and drug dependency; and physical examination for rape (rules regarding all of which vary from one location to another). Although not a hard and fast rule, minors who live independently and earn most of their income without parental support may be considered emancipated.

In some states, a minor may be considered emancipated by virtue of marriage, pregnancy, parenthood, or judicial declaration; the patient may be able to give a valid consent although he or she may not yet have attained the state's age of majority. However, a court may decide that a particular minor is not sufficiently mature (competent) to make such decisions (22). This point should be reviewed, if possible, with the administrators and legal counsel of a given hospital.

A consent must be informed to be valid. Unless an exception to the requirement of consent applies, treatment of a patient without informed consent is both a battery (a tort) (26, 27) and a violation of the standards of medical treatment (professional negligence) (28). It may also be a basis for liability for invasion of privacy.

A lucid formulation of this precept was enunciated in *Cantebury* v. *Spence* (25):

[T]he patient's right to self decision shapes the boundaries of the duty to reveal. That right can be effectively exercised only if the patient possesses enough information to enable an intelligent choice. The scope of the physician's communication to the patient, then, must be measured by the patient's need ... And to safeguard the patient's interest in achieving his own determination on treatment, the law must itself set the standard for adequate disclosure.

This is an objective, patient-oriented approach to obtaining informed consent (25, 29–31). Some courts have gone beyond that standard, requiring that a physician reveal all information needed by a particular patient to ensure a fully informed consent (32); this is a subjective standard of consent. Still other courts have adopted a materiality test, holding that a physician's duty to disclose includes the disclosure of all information that would be material to a patient's decision to accept or to reject medical treatment (33). This has led, more recently, to the development of a doctrine of "informed refusal" (34) by which a physician may be liable for not disclosing risks inherent in refusing medical therapy.

What is adequate disclosure for obtaining an informed consent? Based on a synthesis of various judicial rulings, an adequate disclosure should include the following elements:

1. An explanation of the procedure
2. The indications for the procedure
3. The material risks of the procedure (Materiality is determined by the severity of the complication in relation to the chance of that complication occurring. For example, even though the risk of death for a given procedure may be only 0.5%, the catastrophic nature of the complication makes it material. Similarly, even though a chipped or broken tooth may be only a minor annoyance, if there is a 25% chance that it will happen because of poor dentition or other predisposing factors, the patient must be informed.)
4. The putative benefits to be obtained (Patients

should never be offered either express or implied guaranteed results. Failure to deliver guaranteed results is a breach of contract (35, 36), not professional negligence, which is covered by liability insurance.)

5. Any reasonable alternatives to the procedure (Salient considerations in choosing one alternative over another should be made known to the patient. If there are no alternatives, that should be disclosed to the patient.)
6. Potential risks inherent in refusing a specific medical treatment (including missed diagnosis, delayed treatment increasing the risks, or associate morbidity or mortality of a disease process)
7. An opportunity for the patient or guardian/representative to ask questions

Still, it is not entirely clear what constitutes an adequate disclosure of information to the patient. Many physicians hold to a "paternalistic" view and thus feel that they know what is best and which risks should be undertaken by the patient. This view is not condoned legally. Presently, there is a debate between the "reasonable physician" standard (information is disclosed to the extent that other competent physicians would disclose) and the "reasonable patient" standard (the amount of disclosure that the average person would need to make a rational decision). In general, full and frank disclosures reduce the risk of a lawsuit. Conversely, how many patients who have a great need for a medical procedure refuse that procedure on the basis of highly unlikely, but fully disclosed, complications? How many patients in similar situations refuse recommended treatments because of an unfounded fear of a procedure, such as spinal anesthesia? This dilemma remains unsolved. However, under circumstances in which the physician thinks that disclosure of information would "pose an immediate threat to a patient's well-being," the physician is granted a "therapeutic privilege" to withhold the information (37). The physician should scrupulously document in the medical record the basis for finding that any exception exists, particularly when the "therapeutic privilege" exception is invoked.

## Special Situations

### JEHOVAH'S WITNESSES

A controversial medicolegal topic that comes under the general heading of informed consent is transfusion of exogenous blood to a Jehovah's Witness. These persons believe, through their interpretation of the Bible, that they will lose their chance of salvation if they receive "one drop of blood which has left the body" (38). Refusal of treatment, particularly blood transfusions (by Jehovah's Witnesses) or therapeutic intervention (by Christian Scientists), may be based on First Amendment considerations of freedom of religion (24). In reality, some Jehovah's Witnesses will accept blood that is sequestered by an autotransfusion device if it is explained that this is a "closed circuit." In elective situations, the law permits the Jehovah's Witness to refuse transfusion; in turn, the surgeon and/or anesthesiologist may elect to refuse to care for the person (39, 40). Of course, the situation becomes more difficult when an emergency arises or when the child of a Jehovah's Witness is involved. Usually, the right of refusal is a personal right only: refusal of emergency lifesaving therapy for dependents conflicts with the state's interest in preservation of life. Both federal and state courts have been of one voice in denying a parent's right of refusal of lifesaving therapy for their child; the state's interest in protecting the life of an innocent minor has been invoked to override parental rights based on the First Amendment (41, 42). Parents and guardians are held to an affirmative obligation to provide essential medical care for their children or dependents, and they may be held criminally liable for failure to do so, notwithstanding religious beliefs to the contrary. Also, the state's interest in protecting the welfare of minor children has been sufficient to mollify a parent's refusal of lifesaving blood transfusions when he or she has been the sole provider for minors. In such cases, hospitals usually have a mechanism in place by which an emergency writ may be obtained.

## TRAUMA AND EMERGENCIES

The general principles of informed consent are somewhat modified during emergency situations. An unconscious or disoriented trauma patient in direct need of medical intervention is presumed to give the *implied* consent of a "reasonable person" in the same situation (1). This implied consent applies only to those problems that must be addressed immediately to preserve life and limb. Such provisions no longer apply once the patient becomes conscious or is otherwise able to give informed consent. Under these conditions, the law provides for a short-term involuntary protection services order (STIPSO). Such a STIPSO is usually limited to 72 hours, with one renewal for 72 hours (43). However, if the opportunity presents itself, attempts should be made to obtain consent from the spouse (*espousal consent*), the next of kin (*familial consent*), or someone legally authorized to act on the patient's behalf. Additionally, if the trauma patient regains consciousness or becomes lucid, an effort to obtain at least verbal consent should be made. Further, if the person has expressly refused therapy before becoming unconscious, the situation is changed. The same is true if it becomes known that the trauma patient made prior arrangements to avoid resuscitation for some reason (see below).

There is also some controversy over the use of implied consent for procedures involving "loss of life" versus "loss of limb." If the procedure to be undertaken will produce a degree of "physical mutilation" (e.g., amputation of an extremity), it may be wise to delay as long as possible while trying to obtain consent (while simultaneously bearing in mind the "loss of chance" concept [see below]). These types of cases may be tried under the principle of technical assault and battery, based on loss without proper informed consent, and do not require the use of witnesses. Thus, they are easier for lawyers to try and win.

Nonemergency treatment initiated in good faith, on the grounds that it might reduce the risk of later complications that would interfere with the patient's recovery, is technically a battery, but it may be validated retroactively by a court if adequate documentation exists and the risks to the patient were adjudged reasonable in light of the outcome. Whether such a benign outlook would hold true if a complication ensued might become a question of fact for later adjudication (11).

Another facet of the informed consent doctrines that applies to emergencies and trauma concerns documentation of blood alcohol levels (BALs). In most states, merely having a valid driver's license *implies* consent for a blood sample for a BAL determination to be taken *at the direction of a police officer*. If the patient does not have a valid driver's license and does not give consent, the physician may be liable for malpractice if he or she draws such a sample. An interesting point here is that, if the police officer removes the vacutainer vial from the needle while it is still in the patient's vein, he or she is legally considered to have drawn the sample. In this way, the physician is spared legal involvement in these cases. Of course, appropriate consent must be verified.

Lack of informed consent in and of itself is rarely a cause for a lawsuit. It is usually an issue in conjunction with a claim based upon another premise of malpractice.

## CREATING THE DUTY

When a physician begins discussion of a medical problem with a person, it can be said that a physician-patient relationship has been created. This can occur even when a case is being discussed over the telephone (13). Once this relationship has begun, the physician is obligated to meet certain standards of health care and is subject to all of the provisions of the tort laws described herein.

By merely "advertising" in the form of road signs and directions, certain hospitals (and physicians, as their agents) have, in effect, "created the duty" to provide emergency care to those who seek such care. Traditionally, a physician was under no obligation to treat a person, even in an emergency situation, if a physician-patient contractual relation had not been entered (44). This rule is changing, however, as courts have become more willing to find agreements through third-party contracts, which infer patient reliance on the availability of medical services (45, 46). Thus, a physician who has agreed to provide emergency medical services as a condition of appointment to the medical staff of a hospital may be held liable for failure to do so (47). In addition, courts have searched for some "minimal contact" with a patient (48) as a basis for finding the existence of a physician-patient relationship sufficient (e.g., telephone consultation) to invoke an obligation and subsequent hospital liability for "negligent termination" of services (45, 46). A hospital that holds itself forth to the community as being a provider of emergency medical services may be liable for the failure of physician staff to provide adequate medical services (45). Statutory or regulatory requirements for treating patients (e.g., Hill-Burton Act) may provide additional obligations to provide medical care and may impose liability for failure to do so.

This evolution in the legal analysis of the physician-patient relationship effectively extends the contractual obligations of the physician to provide emergency medical care to the community at large as third-party beneficiaries of practice agreements between community hospitals and physicians. Quasi-contractual concepts of equity and tort law, based on the reliance of patients in presenting themselves to a particular medical facility for emergency medical care and foregoing alternative services, foreclose invocation of the defense of the absence of an agreement to treat.

More recent court decisions have focused on the "loss of a chance" concept in determining the proximity of causality of injury. Whether a patient might have lost an opportunity for potential recovery or might have increased the risk of certain complications or death, based on a failure of or delay in medical treatment, is analyzed retrospec-

tively. The development of the "loss of chance" legal doctrine may significantly affect the physician's options for accepting or declining to treat a patient in an emergency. Failure to act decisively early may lead to ultimate liability for lessening the patient's chances for survival, even if those chances were initially poor or if the patient ultimately received adequate treatment. Some jurisdictions have adopted the "all or nothing" approach (49), whereas others have used a "more likely than not" balancing test (50, 51). Still others have found physician liability stemming from deprivation of a "substantial or appreciable chance" for recovery or survival (52–54). Several recent decisions have extended this to the loss of any chance for recovery as being potentially compensable (55, 56).

In the context of the above hypothetical case, one may safely assume that the admitting physicians would be liable for any delay in initiating emergency lifesaving therapy at least sufficient to enable the patient's transfer to an accepting facility. The onus therefore falls on the physician to determine what should and must be done.

Additionally, when a physician has intervened as a "Good Samaritan," for example, by helping the victim of a "heart attack" in a restaurant ("cafe coronary"), he or she has "created the duty" to treat the patient. Subsequent action will be judged on the basis of the standards of care that are described below.

Once the physician-patient relationship has begun, the physician must treat the patient to the best of his or her ability, as his or her training dictates, and as the medical community expects (see "Standards of Care"). The physician *may not* terminate the relationship intentionally by unilaterally withdrawing from the case without (*a*) proper and timely notification of the patient, (*b*) discussion of the difficulties with the patient, and (*c*) appropriate planning to ensure the medical welfare of the patient (e.g., follow-up care, physician referral or substitution). A physician who fails to take these steps would be liable for breach of duty and abandonment (1, 11). For example, an anesthesiologist who has performed a rapid sequence intubation on a head-injured trauma patient who is then taken to the CT suite must ensure that proper monitoring, observation, and therapy of that patient continue. It is not enough simply to "lube, tube, and leave." On the other hand, a patient *may* unilaterally end the relationship by dismissing the physician and/or by leaving the hospital "against medical advice."

## STANDARDS OF CARE

In today's mobile society, the traditional standards of due care, which legally prescribe guidelines for physician behavior, are changing quickly. Originally, doctors' actions were compared with those of their peers within a regional medical community. However, because medical education is becoming increasingly similar throughout the country (due to conferences, journals, etc.), a "national" standard of care is now commonplace. Standards of care include Advanced Cardiac Life Support (ACLS) and Advanced Trauma Life Support protocols, adopted hospital and departmental policy and procedure manuals, and, most recently, those that have been developed by legislation and by administrative agencies (as in New Jersey and New York) to promote standards for intraanesthetic monitoring (17, 57). Once a practitioner deviates from these various types of written standards and patient injury occurs, the burden of proof transfers to the defendant, and the case is very difficult to win. Expert testimony provided by authorities imported into the jurisdiction from outside the locality is preferred by plaintiff counsel because of the unwillingness of professionals to testify against someone with whom they would have subsequent contact. Those who regularly serve as expert witnesses prefer this arrangement also. Expert witnesses base their opinions upon established guidelines (57).

Deviation from standards of care usually will involve lack of an indication for therapy, the presence of a contraindication to the therapy provided, incompetence in the performance of a procedure, failure to diagnose, misdiagnosis, and/or failure to obtain appropriate consultation (7). Generally, if it can be shown that the physician's conduct was within the bounds of current medical practice (even within that of a certain "unpopular" faction), the defendant will probably be acquitted (7). A physician is expected to demonstrate a level of knowledge and skill commensurate with other similarly trained physicians. A specialist is expected to meet the standards of other specialists. When a nonspecialist undertakes a nonemergency service that is usually provided by a specialist, his or her actions may be compared against the standard expected of a specialist.

Physicians working in a specialized emergency facility such as a level I trauma center, who have received advanced training in the management of the critically ill or who have been at that job for some time, are expected to be capable of providing a higher level of care than someone without such a background. Thus, the way in which a trauma patient is handled at a trauma center and the actions of the doctors involved will be compared against the standards of care rendered at other such facilities by similarly experienced physicians.

After the duty has been created, which necessitates a given standard of care, *outcome* itself is not warranteed. The standard of care applies only to the training and level of expertise of the physician and stipulates that appropriate methods and techniques be applied in a standard fashion. However, a physician who binds himself or herself to a given result (i.e., by verbal promises to the patient or family) may be liable for *breach of warranty* (2).

### Special Situations

#### GOOD SAMARITAN LAWS

The concept of the Good Samaritan law, which involves elements of both "creating the duty" and "standards of care," was first developed in California in 1959. The Good Samaritan laws were created partly to induce professionals and nonprofessionals to render necessary emergency assistance without the hesitancy brought about by fear of legal liability. In fact, certain states (Vermont and Minnesota) have gone so far as to *require* citizens (physicians and lay public) to become involved when an emergency presents itself (13). Good Samaritan laws are influenced by the principles of standards of care and consider the expertise of the person rendering the care. Thus, if a gynecologist cares for a multitrauma patient on a deserted highway and then becomes involved in a lawsuit, the doctor's actions possibly could be judged against a "standard of care" that would describe the actions expected of a similarly trained person under similar circumstances. On one hand, the fact is that the person is a physician and should be current at least on techniques of basic life support. On the other hand, the fact is that the management of this type of patient is not truly within this physician's area of expertise; the fact that the situation occurred under adverse conditions and away from a hospital would probably also be considered. Further, if a doctor who is board-certified in emergency medicine were to be involved in this same situation, different considerations would apply. It may be recognized that circumstances such as lack of equipment, support personnel, and an optimal environment contribute to the outcome of the situation. Therefore, the Good Samaritan laws hold different interpretations for different persons. They are not a license for total immunity from the consequences of one's actions, except perhaps for someone completely inexperienced in matters of health care. Furthermore, protection may be related only to treatment rendered for certain types of accidents (e.g., motor vehicle accidents). Also, most state statutes require that aid be rendered without consideration of professional fee.

## DO NOT RESUSCITATE (DNR) ORDERS

The concept of withdrawing or withholding life-sustaining measures touches all three of the medicolegal principles discussed thus far: informed consent, creating the duty, and standards of care. A competent person can make the decision ahead of time, either in consultation with his or her primary physician (in which case *orders* to not resuscitate should be *written in advance*) or in the form of a legal document (will). The law recognizes that compliance with the patient's prior arrangements is mandatory. Usually, such patients have been suffering from a chronic terminal disease (46). If, for some reason, resuscitation has begun on a patient who has made such prior arrangements, the attending physician who initiated the DNR orders should probably come to the scene and personally discontinue such efforts because of the emotional reluctance of a "code team" to abruptly stop resuscitation in such cases (1). Further, if the patient is conscious when the decision is being made whether to institute resuscitative measures and refuses such therapy, this request must be honored. Frequently (perhaps too frequently) such a refusal serves as a stimulus to raise questions about the patient's competence to make decisions. In emergencies, this creates a difficult situation. If circumstances permit, psychiatric consultation should be sought and the competence of the patient should be examined. If a guardian or surrogate is available, one may attempt to obtain consent from such a person. Generally, guardians are expected to decide in a manner that a "reasonable" person acting to achieve his or her own best interests would act. Decisions to discontinue life-sustaining treatment made by such persons are less well accepted than decisions to continue therapy. One author recommends that, in an emergency situation where doubt exists as to whether to discontinue life support, it is more appropriate legally, ethically, and morally to continue "full-blown" efforts until either the patient dies or the situation stabilizes. At that time, decisions concerning the plan of action may undergo more careful deliberation (1).

Some patients are brought to the trauma center or emergency department in conditions that raise questions regarding the *futility* of treatment, for instance, a trauma patient who has been without vital signs for an undetermined time or for an allegedly prolonged time. For these "dead on arrival" patients, one must exercise caution when evaluating reports of bystanders as to such details and must also be wary of complicating secondary factors such as drug overdose, hypothermia, or lightning strikes, in which cases prolonged resuscitation is indicated until these conditions have been reversed adequately. In all cases, the American Heart Association's doctrines concerning ACLS state that the decision to discontinue resuscitation may be made on the basis of medical futility *only after* the institution of full basic and advanced cardiac life support fails to be successful (58).

Another scenario is that in which a "limited, slow, partial, or chemical" code is performed. Purists would condemn such practices on medical and ethical grounds. However, these types of resuscitative efforts can be appropriate if the patient has agreed to them ahead of time. For example, a patient with terminal emphysema may not want to be intubated but is willing to undergo other lifesaving measures, such as cardiopulmonary resuscitation or the administration of emergency intravenous drugs (although such actions may be contradictory to the integrated care concepts of ACLS). Additionally, these "limited" codes may reassure the family that "everything was done" (59).

## RESPONDEAT SUPERIOR

The term *respondeat superior* translates to "the superior one will answer." Under this doctrine, an attending physician is held responsible for the actions of subordinate interns, residents, and fellows. This also involves the concept of *caput respondeat* ("the captain of the ship is responsible"). Likewise, an attending anesthesiologist will be responsible for the actions of a nurse anesthetist (CRNA), who may or may not be immune to legal action for malpractice (although CRNAs usually carry their own malpractice insurance). In the absence of a supervising anesthesiologist or surgeon, the hospital becomes responsible for the nurse anesthetist's actions. Similarly, physicians who are involved in emergency medical services and manage field teams may be held responsible for the actions of emergency medical technicians and paramedics (60).

## SPECIFIC POINTS FOR TRAUMATOLOGISTS

In today's climate of heightened litigious awareness, it would be highly unlikely for the practicing physician involved on a routine basis with the management of trauma patients to "escape" interaction with the medicolegal system. The physician may be called to give a deposition, appear as a witness in court, or serve as an expert witness. These interactions can often be emotionally stressful and can extend over several years before they are resolved (61). In this section, we briefly touch upon points that apply directly to the daily functioning of the traumatologist. Other excellent sources may be consulted for more detailed information (2, 12, 62–67).

### Communications with the Family

It will usually be the surgeon who first has contact with relatives of the patient, although the anesthesiologist will have contact with them postoperatively, preoperatively for secondary procedures, while serving as a critical care physician, or when billing for renumeration.

While maintaining a polite, professional demeanor, it is usually best to focus on the family member who seems to be the most collected and then take that person aside to act as a family representative. Anxious family members approached as a group will often "read into" what the physician is saying or "put words in his mouth." Statements may thus be distorted, become difficult to track, and later appear as issues in court.

Further, while giving comfort to the family it is unwise to "paint a rosy picture." It is much easier to update an initial guarded prognosis if and when the patient's situation improves. To do otherwise may invoke a condition of "breach of warranty" and make the patient eligible to collect charges for an undelivered but promised result. "How" something is said is as important as "what" is said.

## Operating Room Conduct

If the patient is undergoing a general anesthetic, it is difficult to predict the level of consciousness at a given moment. Thus, a patient may actually hear and remember parts or all of the events during the perioperative period. This is obviously even more important if the patient is receiving a regional or local anesthetic with or without sedation. Thus, all personnel should behave accordingly. Innocent statements, jokes, and petty arguments may be remembered and misinterpreted by the patient and may cause future damage.

All equipment should be tested thoroughly and certified by the bioengineering department of the hospital. Under "respondeat superior," the physician-in-charge may be held liable for malfunction of a piece of equipment, for example, if "Bovee burns" are caused by improper placement of a grounding pad. Safety guidelines for anesthesia must be followed (e.g., preparation and check-out of the anesthesia machine).

## Documentation

Medical records will be scrutinized by the legal team and will be used, and often misinterpreted, to their best advantage. Although documentation and procedures for preservation of important patient rights may seem needlessly ritualistic and extraneous when all medical attention is being directed at preservation of a patient's life and limb, it is essential to keep accurate notes (2). This applies not only to the physician's notes but also to nurses' notes, operating records, orders, and laboratory results. One should be compulsive about the way "verbal orders" are handled. In tenuous situations (e.g., proceeding with a controversial "lifesaving" procedure such as an amputation without informed consent), a detailed written explanation should be entered in the chart, which includes details of attempts to obtain consent. Further, the written agreement of a consultant is invaluable.

Dictations should be performed within 24 hours. If a defense attorney can prove that a dictation was made much later than this, its validity will be contested in court (2).

## Interaction with the Legal System

If an untoward event does occur, be it as simple as an altercation with the family, it is probably wise to notify the legal counsel or risk management services of the hospital.

Even if a physician has no direct culpability with respect to a given case, it is still possible to become involved involuntarily as a subpoenaed "witness of fact" to describe one's involvement and interpretation of the case. This will usually consist of giving a deposition at the attorney's office. The physician should bear in mind the seriousness of this function and the fact that anything said can be introduced later in court during the actual trial.

The behavior, attitude, and appearance of the physician in court will undoubtedly influence the jury. It is very easy to alienate the jury through a haughty demeanor or the use of technical jargon. Commonly, the opposing attorney will attempt to discredit the physician by confusing him, causing him to lose his composure, or questioning his credentials. It is important to remain level-headed. Specific questions require specific answers, and one should not elaborate, discuss irrelevant points, or volunteer unsolicited information. However, some answers do require more than a simple "yes" or "no." If the opposing attorney is trying to pressure one of these answers, an appeal may be made to the judge by the witness.

If the expert witness for the opposing legal team presents contradictory testimony, interpersonal attacks are to be discouraged, as the opposition will try to capitalize on this. It should simply be pointed out that a number of valid opinions may be available for a given case, that they do not necessarily all agree, and that more than one may be correct.

## SUMMARY

The physician faced with life and death situations increasingly is held to a societal duty to treat the patient expertly, expeditiously, and effectively. Complex legal analysis of the patient's capacity or competence to consent to or refuse treatment is an inappropriate consideration for the physician in the emergency setting. The rule of thumb for provision of emergency medical care, opting in favor of preservation of life and limb whenever there is a question, is sound. The physician who becomes involved in a physician-patient relationship involuntarily should be circumspect and (*a*) initiate administrative review of therapy as soon as possible, particularly whenever there is a question of patient refusal of care; (*b*) evaluate which therapies are truly justified by the emergency situation and which are less urgent or elective; (*c*) initiate therapy in accordance with his or her best medical judgment; and (*d*) document findings and actions in light of the patient's wants and needs.

## References

1. Sanders AB. Unique aspects of ethics in emergency medicine. In Iserson KV, Saunders MD, Buchaman AE (eds): Ethics in Emergency Medicine. Baltimore, Williams & Wilkins, 1986, pp 9–12.
2. Gorney M. Medicolegal aspects of automobile injuries. Clin Plast Surg 1975;2:167–171.
3. Brunner EA. The National Association of Insurance Commissioners: closed claims study. Int Anesthesiol Clin 1984;22:17–30.
4. Rinaman JC. The tort liability system: overview for the anesthesiologist. In Gravenstein JS, Holzer JF (eds): Safety and Cost Containment in Anesthesia. Boston, Butterworth, 1988, pp 55–69.
5. Scarzella v. Saxon, 436 A.2d 358 (DC 1981).
6. Weigel CJ. Medicolegal aspects of trauma. In Mattox KL, Moore EE, Feliciano DV (eds): Trauma. Norwalk, CT, Appleton & Lange, 1988, pp 53–60.
7. Burroughs JT. Medico-legal aspects of trauma. In Maull KI (ed): Advances in Trauma. Chicago, Year Book, 1988, pp 15–36.
8. Averbach A. The patient sues the anesthesiologist—or, malpractice cases don't belong in court. Int Anesthesiol Clin 1973;11:141–158.
9. Schwachman B. Legal issues. In Vanstrum GS (ed): Anesthesia in Emergency Medicine. Boston, Little, Brown & Co, 1989, pp 378–397.
10. Peters JD, Fineberg KS, Kroll DA, Collins V. The law of malpractice. In Peters JD, Fineberg KS, Kroll DA, Collins V (eds): Anesthesiology and the Law. Ann Arbor, MI, Health Administrative Press, 1983, pp 3–60.
11. Kolber JL. Malpractice law and emergency department medicine. Emerg Med Clin North Am 1988;3:625.
12. Kroll DA. Professional Liability and the Anesthesiologist. Park Ridge, IL, American Society of Anesthesiologists, 1987.
13. Capron AM. Legal setting of emergency medicine. In Iserson KV, Saunders MD, Buchaman AE (eds): Ethics in Emergency Medicine. Baltimore, Williams & Wilkins, 1986, pp 13–28.
14. Cheney FW, Posner K, Caplan RA, Ward RJ. Standards of care and anesthesia liability. JAMA 1989;261:1599–1633.
15. Snow JC. Medicolegal aspects of anesthesia. In Snow JC (ed): Anesthesia in Otolaryngology and Ophthalmology. Springfield, IL, Charles C Thomas, 1972, pp 193–198.
16. Ochsner AJ. Medicolegal aspects of anesthesiology. South Med J 1988;52:958–960.
17. Heckel CG. Medicolegal aspects of trauma care. Presented at the Second Annual Trauma Anesthesia and Critical Care Symposium, Baltimore, June 1989.
18. American College of Legal Medicine: Legal Medicine: Legal Dynamics of Medical Encounters. St Louis, CV Mosby, 1988.
19. Rosenberg AR, Goldsmith LS. What is res ipsa loquitur? In Rosenberg AR, Goldsmith LS (eds): Malpractice Made Easy. New York, Books for Industry, 1976, pp 52–57.
20. Shloendorf v. Society of New York Hosp, 211 NY 125.105 NE 92 (1914).
21. Planned Parenthood v. Danforth, 428 US 52 (1976). But see Cage v. Wood, 428 So.2d 850 (La 1986).
22. In the Matter of T.H., 484 NE.2d 568 (Ind Sep Ct 1985).
23. Roe v. Wade, 410 US 113 (1973).
24. In re Brown, 478 So.2d 1033 (Miss Sup Ct 1985).

25. Cantebury v. Spence, 464 F.2d 772, 780 (DC Cir 1972), cert den 409 US 1064 (1972).

26. Abril v. Syntex Laboratories, Inc, 364 NYS.2d 281, 283 (Sup Ct 1975).

27. Karl J Pizzalotto, MD, Ltd v. Wilson, 437 So.2d 859 (La 1983).

28. Harnish v. Childrens Hospital Medical Center, 387 Mass 152, 439 NE.2d 240 (1982).

29. Nathanson v. Kline, 186 Kan 393, 350 P.2d 1093, reh-g den 187 Kan 186, 354 P.2d 670 (1960).

30. Petersen v. Shields, 654 SW.2d 929 (Tex 1983).

31. Karp v. Cooley, 493 F.2d 408, 422 (5th Cir), cert den 419 US 845 (1974).

32. Scott v. Branford, 606 P.2d 554 (Okla 1979).

33. Cobbs v. Grant, 8 Cal.3d 229, 502 P.2d 1, 104 Cal Rptr 505 (1972).

34. Truman v. Thomas, 27 Cal.3d 285, 611 P.2d 902, 165 Cap Rptr 308 (1980).

35. Sciacca v. Polizzi, 403 So.2d 728 (La 1981).

36. Scarzella v Saxon, 436 A.2d 358 (DC 1981).

37. Salgo v. Stanford University Board of Trustees, 154Cal App2d 560, 578, 317 P.2d 170, 181 (1957).

38. Ford JC. The refusal of blood transfusions by Jehovah's Witnesses. Linacre Q, February 1955 pp 3–10.

39. Jonsen AR. Blood transfusions and Jehovah's Witnesses: the impact of the patient's unusual beliefs in critical care. Crit Care Clin 1986; 2:91–100.

40. Dornette WHL. Jehovah's Witnesses and blood transfusion: the horns of a dilemma. Anesth Analg 1973;52:272–278.

41. Jefferson v. Griffin Spaudling County Hospital Authority, 247 Ga 86, 274 SE.2d 457 (1981).

42. Raleigh Fitkin-Paul Morgan Memorial Hospital v. Anderson, 42 NJ 421, 201 A.2d 537, cert den 377 US 985 (1964).

43. Ciccone JR. The elderly and medicolegal trends in consent. NY State J Med, December 1986, pp 635–638.

44. Findlay v. Board of Supervisors, 72 Ariz 58, 65, 230 P.2d 526, 531 (1951).

45. Wilmington General Hospital v. Manlove, 54 Del 15, 174 A.2d 135 (1961).

46. Brownsville Medical Center v. Gracia, 704 SW.2d 68 (Tex Ct App 1985), reh'g den 1985.

47. Hiser v. Randolph, 126 Ariz 608, 617 P.2d 774 (Ct App 1980).

48. O'Neill v. Montefiore Hospital, 11 App Div.2d 132, 202 NYS.2d 426 (1960).

49. Cooper v. Sisters of Charity, Inc. 272 NE.2d 97 (Ohio 1971).

50. Gooding v. University Hospital Building, Inc., 445 So.2d 1015 (Fla 1984).

51. Curry v. Summers, 483 NE.2d (Ill App Ct 1985).

52. Hicks v. United States, 368 F.2d 626 (4th Cir 1966) (Virginia law).

53. Jeanes v. Milner, 428 F.2d 379 (8th Cir 1970).

54. Thomas v. Corso, 288 A.2d 379 (Md 1972).

55. Herskovitz v. Group Health Cooperative, 664 P.2d 474 (Wash 1983).

56. Aasheim v. Humberger, 695 P.2d 824 (Mont 1985).

57. Hirsh HL. The legal impact of professional standards of anesthesiology care. Practice Management Anesthesiol 1987;3:1–9.

58. American Heart Association. Medicolegal aspects of cardiopulmonary resuscitation (CPR) and emergency cardiac care (ECC). In Textbook Advanced Cardiac Life Support. Dallas, TX, American Heart Association, 1987, pp 271–285.

59. Katz LE. Bioethical issues in anesthesia: termination of life support. Semin Anesthesia 1986; 5:277–285.

60. Page TO. Medical legal considerations in prehospital care. Top Emerg Med II 1979;1:55.

61. Charles SC, Wilbert JR, Franke KJ. Sued and nonsued physician's self-reported reactions to malpractice litigation. Am J Psychiatry 1985; 142:437–440.

62. Gore G. Factors that influence who wins a malpractice suit. In Gravenstein JS, Holzer JF (eds): Safety and Cost Containment in Anesthesia. Boston, Butterworth, 1988, pp 129–137.

63. Taraska JM. The physician as a witness. In Taraska JM (ed): Legal Guide for Physicians. New York, Matthew Bunder & Co, 1988, pp 9-1-9-56.

64. Fish RM, Ehrhardt ME. Malpractice Depositions: Avoiding the Traps. Oradell, NJ, Medical Economics, 1987.

65. Horsley JE, Carlova J. Testifying in Court: A Guide for Physicians, ed 3. Oradell, NJ, Medical Economics, 1988.

66. Belli MM, Carlova J. Belli for Your Malpractice Defense, ed 2. Oradell, NJ, Medical Economics, 1989.

67. Fish RM, Ehrhardt ME, Fish B. Malpractice: Managing Your Defense, ed 2. Oradell, NJ, Medical Economics, 1989.

# Index

whole blood, 134
Blood donation, 160-165
    autologous, 123-124, 124-125, 164. See also
        Autotransfusion
    directed, 164-165
        arguments against, 164
        compared with volunteer donations, 164
        definition of, 164
        policies regarding, 164-165
    infectious disease screening and, 160-163
        AIDS, 161-163
        cytomegalovirus, 163
        hepatitis, 160-161
        HTLV-I, 163
Blood pressure
    in children, 318, 318t
    effect of hemorrhage on, 103-104
    effect of inhalational anesthetics on, 198
    effect of nalbuphine on, 200
    intraocular pressure and, 281
    invasive monitoring of, 191
    noninvasive monitoring of, 189
Blood substitutes, 122-123, 165
Blunt trauma, 50-58, 184-185
    compartment syndrome due to, 56
    degloving injuries, 56
    due to falls, 56-58
    due to motor vehicle accidents, 51-56
    due to motorcycle accidents, 56
    forces in, 50-51
    indications of, 51t
Body temperature. See also Hypothermia;
    Malignant hyperthermia
    in burn victim
        intraoperative loss of heat, 294
        monitoring techniques, 292
    correlation with severity of injury, 187, 188
    equipment for monitoring of, 190
    in injured children, 318-319
    intraoperative factors affecting, 342
    monitoring methods for, 343-344
    normal regulation of, 340-343
    operating room temperature and, 342
Bone marrow fluid infusion, 114
Bowel, wound ballistics in, 49
Boyle's law, 377, 377t
Brachial plexus block, 334-335
    axillary approach for, 334
    interscalene approach for, 334
    supraclavicular approaches for, 334
Brain
    edema of, 254
    oxygen requirements of, 251
    swelling of, 254
    wound ballistics in, 49

"Breath-hold" rule, 73
Brooke formula, 287, 288t
Bullets. See Missiles
Bupivacaine, 335
Burns, 286-298
    of airway, 89
    airway management for, 88-90, 288-290,
        289
        carbon monoxide poisoning, 288
        causes of respiratory dysfunction, 288
        chest wall restriction, 289-290, 290
        intraoperative, 294-295
        subglottic thermal injury, 289
        upper airway edema, 288-289
    anesthesia outside of operating room for,
        291
    anesthetic agents for, 295-296
        chlordiazepoxide, 296
        depolarizing muscle relaxants, 295
        diazepam, 296
        inhalational anesthetics, 296
        ketamine, 291
        narcotics, 296
        nondepolarizing muscle relaxants, 296
        succinylcholine, 199, 290-291, 295
        vecuronium, 199
    critical care transport for, 432
    debridement phase of care for, 291-298
        blood loss vs. excision size, 293, 293-294
        monitoring techniques, 291-292
        thermal conservation, 294
        vascular access, 293
    degrees of, 286
    edema due to, 89
    fluid replacement for, 287-288
        determining adequacy of, 287
        resuscitation formulas for, 287, 288t
        venous access for, 287
    hyperbaric therapy for, 392-393, 393t
    immediate resuscitation for, 287-291
    inhalation injury and, 89, 286, 286t-287t
    injuries associated with, 290
    intubation in patient with, 294-295, 295
    mechanical ventilation for, 298
    mortality from, 286, 286t-287t
    myoglobinemia/myoglobinuria and, 297
    in patient with cardiac disease, 297-298
    in pregnancy, 309-310
    reconstructive phase of care for, 298
    renal failure and, 297
    septic complications of, 296-297
    use of burn case book, 291, 292

Caffeine-halothane contracture test, 357
Caffeine skinned fiber tension test, 357-358